Food for Today

Seventh Edition

Helen Kowtaluk

Alice Orphanos Kopan, M.Ed., M.A., CFCS

Glencoe
McGraw-Hill

New York, New York   Columbus, Ohio   Woodland Hills, California   Peoria, Illinois

Front Cover Photo
FPG International/Denis Scott

Back Cover Photo
Corbis/Westlight
    Japack

Title Page Photo
Food Pix

Interior Design
MKR Design, Inc.

Brand Name Disclaimer:
Publisher does not necessarily recommend or endorse any particular
company or brand name product that may be discussed or pictured
in this text. Brand name products are used because they are readily
available, likely to be known to the reader, and their use may aid
in the understanding of the text. Publisher recognizes other brand
name or generic products may be substituted and work as well
or better than those featured in the text.

Glencoe/McGraw-Hill

A Division of The **McGraw·Hill** *Companies*

Copyright © 2000, 1997, 1994, 1990, 1986, 1982, 1977 by Helen
Kowtaluk and Alice Orphanos Kopan. All rights reserved. Except as
permitted under the United States Copyright Act, no part of this
publication may be reproduced or distributed in any form or by any
means, or stored in a database or retrieval system, without prior
written permission of the publisher.

Send all inquiries to:
Glencoe/McGraw-Hill
3008 W. Willow Knolls Drive
Peoria, Illinois 61614-1083

ISBN 0-02-643048-7 (Student Text)
ISBN 0-02-643049-5 (Teacher's Wraparound Edition)

Printed in the United States of America

3 4 5 6 7 8 9   071/043   04 03 02 01 00

Nutrition Consultant
Elizabeth Shipley Moses, M.S., R.D.

Contributors

Gwen Bagaas
Jamestown, New York

Gayle Gardner Erskine, M.S., CFCS
Home Economics Department Chair
Cherry Creek Schools
Aurora, Colorado

Brenda Barrington Mendiola, M.S.
Home Economics Teacher
Irion County Schools
Mertzon, Texas

Elise Zwicky
Pekin, Illinois

Technical Reviewers

Sherri Hoyt, R.D.
Outpatient Nutrition Counselor
Missouri Baptist Medical Center
St. Louis, Missouri

Virginia Messina, M.P.H., R.D.
Nutrition Consultant
Nutrition Matters Inc.
Port Townsend, Washington

Tamara Vitale, M.S., R.D.
Clinical Assistant Professor
Utah State University
Logan, Utah

Teacher Reviewers

Linda Brown
Foods and Nutrition Teacher
Sanderson High School
Raleigh, North Carolina

Regina Chaney
Family and Consumer Sciences Teacher
Hazen High School
Hazen, Arkansas

Gayle Dickinson, M.S.
Family and Consumer Sciences
    Department Chairperson
Edison Junior Senior High School
Lake Station, Indiana

Lanell Early, M.S.
Food Management, Production &
    Service Instructor
West Point Vocational Center
West Point, Mississippi

Mary Koch
Family and Consumer Sciences Teacher
Kewaskum High School
Kewaskum, Wisconsin

Sheila Bartley Kratzer, M.Ed.
Counselor/Teacher
Sulphur High School
Sulphur, Louisiana

Joyce P. Littlejohn
Teacher
Wolfson Senior High School
Jacksonville, Florida

Ann Marin
Food Production, Management &
    Services Coordinator
Garland High School
Garland, Texas

LaVoy Myers, M.Ed.
Family and Consumer Sciences Teacher
Pocatello High School
Pocatello, Idaho

Diann Pilgrim, M.A.T.
Teacher-Coordinator
Birmingham Public Schools
Birmingham, Alabama

Kadee Przysiecki
Family and Consumer Sciences Teacher
Rossford High School
Rossford, Ohio

Connie D. Toole
Family and Consumer Sciences Teacher
Jeff Davis High School
Hazlehurst, Georgia

3

CONTENTS IN BRIEF

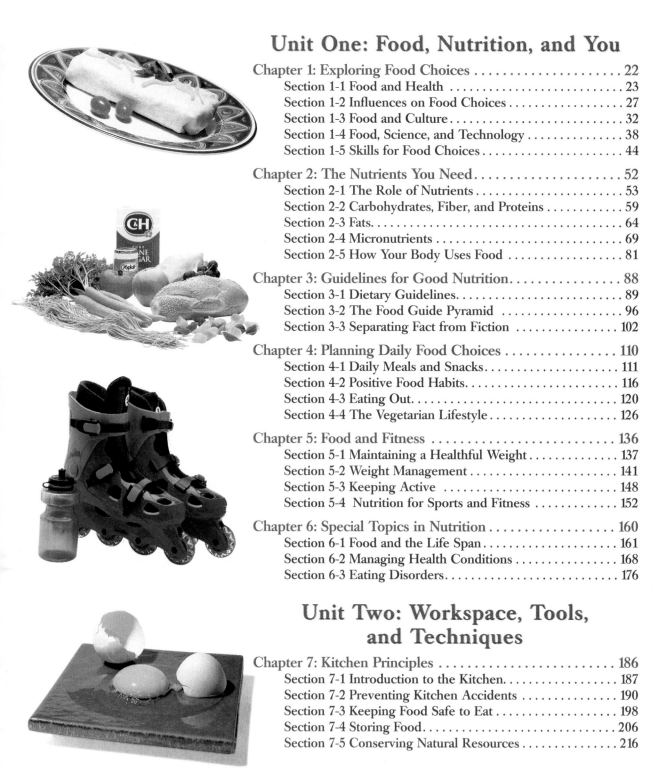

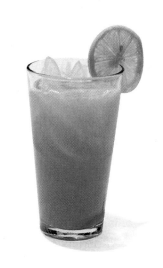

Unit Three: Consumer Decisions

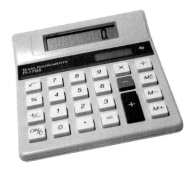

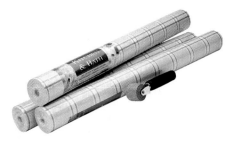

Unit Four: Foods for Meals and Snacks

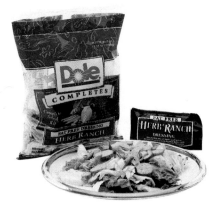

Unit Five: Expanding Your Horizons

TABLE OF CONTENTS

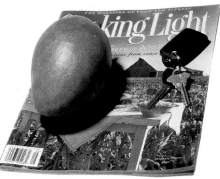

Unit One: Food, Nutrition, and You

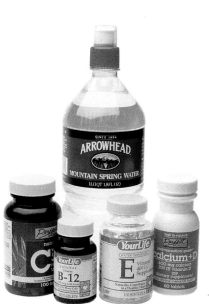

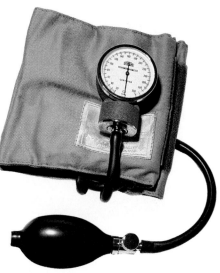

Unit Two: Workspace, Tools, and Techniques

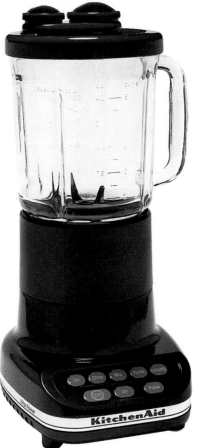

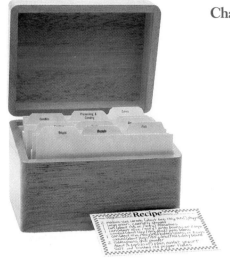

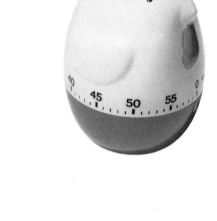
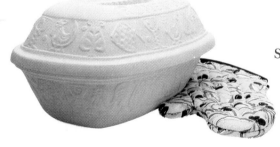

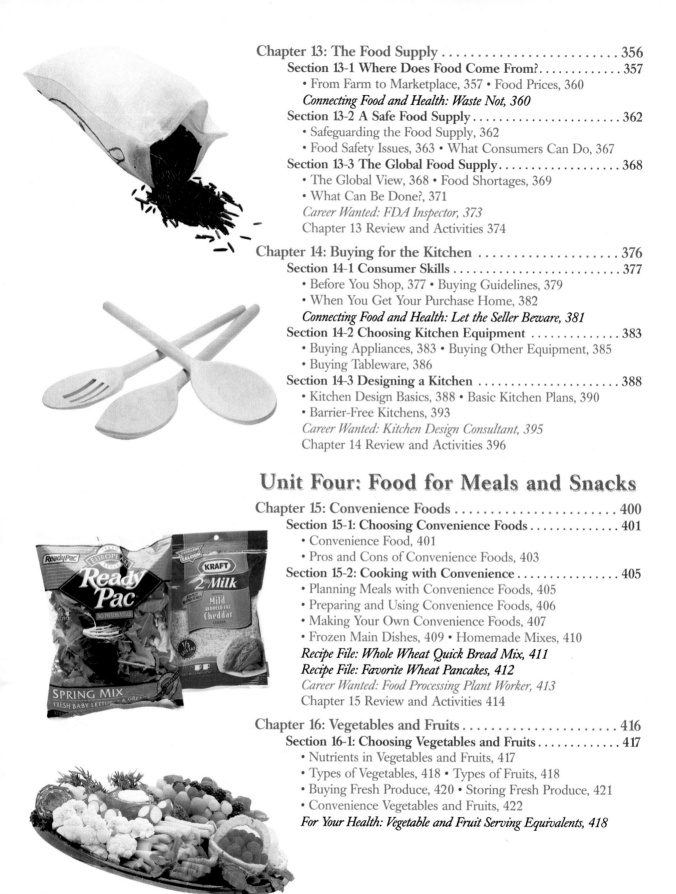

Unit Four: Food for Meals and Snacks

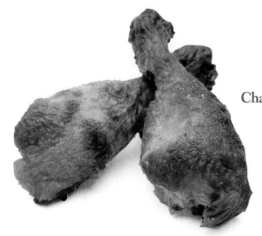

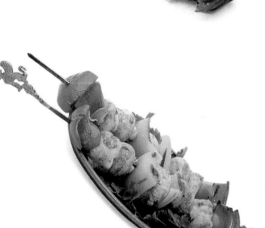

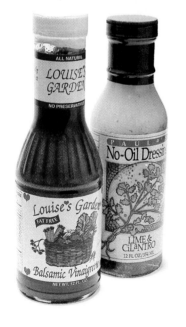

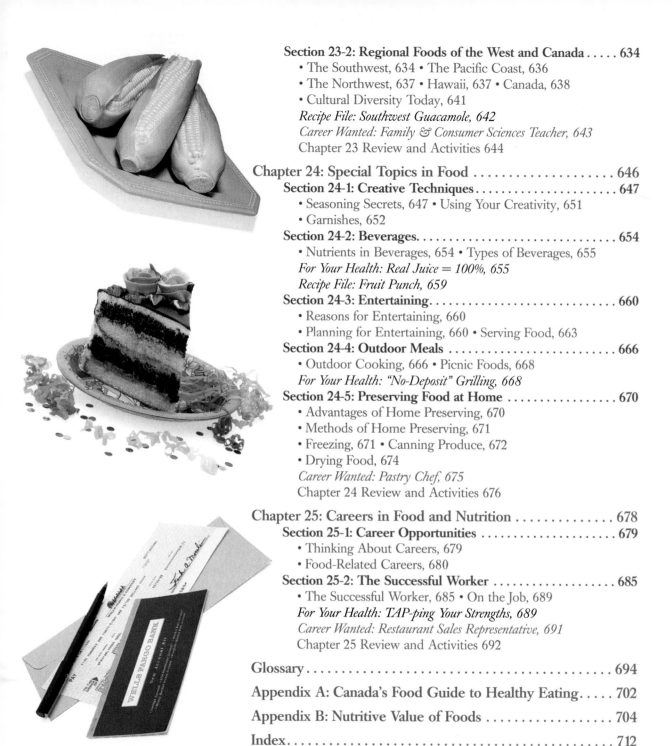

SPECIAL TEXT FEATURES

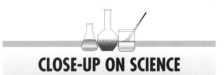
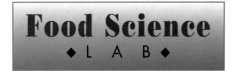

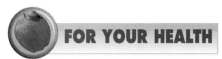

FOR YOUR HEALTH

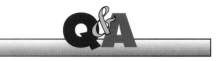

Safety Check

Food safety, accident prevention, and health precautions are highlighted in these features throughout the text.

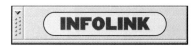

Helpful suggestions on a variety of topics are highlighted throughout the text.

INFOLINK

Special cross-references to information presented in specific sections of the text.

PHOTO CREDITS

Unit Openers
Paul Rico Photography

Chapter Openers
Tim Fuller Photographers

Section Openers, Contents
Joe Mallon Photography

Career Features
Roger B. Bean 181
Corbis
    Nathan Benn 107
    Ed Eckstein 257
    Richard T. Nowitz 85, 487
    Bob Rowan/Progressive
        Images 643
Corbis/Westlight
    Brent Bear 435
    Ril Premium 413
    Paul A. Souders 525
Joe Mallon Photography 49, 157,
    221, 293, 307, 330, 353, 395,
    459, 555, 587, 623, 675, 691
Stock Market/Ariel Skelley 133
Tony Stone Images/
    Don Smetzer 373

Text Credits
Comstock 24, 30, 359, 636R
Corbis/Bettmann 42, 106, 156,
    431B
Corbis/Westlight
    Adamsmith Productions 164
    Australian Picture Library/
        John Carnemolla 153T,
        456R
    Cradoc Bagshaw 630
    D. Baswick 469
    Brent Bear 607
    Steve Chenn 57
    Jay Dickman 639L
    Randy Faris 638T
    Fotografia 165
    Lois Frank 573B, 670B
    Owen Franken 578B
    Philip Gould 635L
    J. Habel 628T
    Richard Hamilton Smith 498T
    D. & J Heaton 611R
    R. W. Jones 33
    Catherine Karnow 628B
    Robert Landau 336

Warren Morgan 150
Chuck O'Rear 37, 217, 613R,
    638B, 682
Douglas Peebles 638M
Jim Richardson 358
Bill Ross 41
Kevin Schafer 611L
Steve Smith 167, 595
Nik Wheeler 599B
Mike Yamashita 617T

David Frazier 594B

Tim Fuller Photographers 25, 34L,
    34R, 43, 45, 54L, 78, 90, 94,
    104, 117L, 117R, 118, 132,
    139, 145, 149, 163, 173, 174,
    177, 179, 186, 188, 191T, 194,
    204, 207, 209, 218L, 218R,
    233T, 264, 265, 268, 269, 270,
    277, 283, 287, 288, 303, 304,
    312, 314, 316, 323, 324, 328,
    340, 343L, 343R, 351, 359,
    367, 383B, 385, 389, 391, 400,
    404L, 404, 408, 409, 420L,
    421, 428B, 430, 440T, 440B,
    441, 447B, 452T, 465, 470,
    473, 483B, 500, 505, 514, 521,
    522, 531, 532, 545, 549, 552,
    563, 568T, 571, 581R, 585,
    593B, 594T, 608T, 608B, 609,
    611RT, 611LT, 617B, 620B,
    649, 661, 674, 680, 686,

Ann Garvin 581L

Health Connection 127

Joe Mallon Photography 40, 60,
    61T, 61B, 65, 70, 74, 102,
    112B, 113L, 113R, 121B, 123,
    124, 142, 153B, 155, 191B,
    192L, 192R, 195, 201, 212,
    213, 220, 229, 230, 231, 233B,
    237, 243R, 246, 248, 249,
    262L, 262R, 281, 298L, 298R,
    305, 329T, 329B, 339, 342L,
    342R, 342B, 345, 346, 348,
    35OL, 350R, 364B, 379, 380T,
    423, 425T, 426, 431T, 442,
    445, 452B, 456L, 471B, 483T,
    486, 543, 544, 550, 553, 559B,
    561, 562, 569, 576, 596, 610R,
    612, 619B, 635R, 648, 655,
    656, 657, 664, 688T

Joe Mallon Photography/
    Universal Studios Hollywood 55

mkw Creative 226, 252, 253T,
    253B, 378, 662, 687

Morgan-Cain & Associates 29,
    243T, 243B, 272, 327, 362,
    364T, 380B, 407, 499T, 499B,
    501, 511, 681

Morgan-Cain & Associates/
    David Ashby 504, 665

Morgan-Cain & Associates/
    Carol Barber 58, 67, 144, 203,
    263, 273, 280, 285, 365, 384,
    390, 392, 493, 495, 498B, 667,
    672, 673,

Mary Moye-Rowley 82, 234, 235,
    244, 245, 247, 317, 352, 425B,
    439B, 475B, 492T, 507B, 517,
    538, 564, 568B, 570L, 570R,
    574, 579, 583, 653,

National Pork Council 546

Paul Rico Photography 39R, 46,
    83, 91, 100, 112T, 114, 121T,
    128, 130, 138, 162, 169, 170,
    200, 202, 238, 255, 271, 275,
    278, 279, 289, 300, 315L,
    315R, 322, 338, 386, 394,
    402L, 402R, 403R, 406, 418,
    420R, 432, 446, 449, 454, 455,
    463B, 464, 472, 477, 479T,
    479B, 485, 492B, 502, 506,
    509, 515, 519, 520, 530, 536,
    539, 540, 548B, 560, 565, 566,
    580, 601, 602, 604, 613L, 629,
    631L, 631M, 631R, 636L, 651,
    669, 679B, 683, 688B, 690

Tony Stone Images 600
    Neil Gunderson 370
    David Joel 39L
    Bob Krist 610L
    Mark Lewis 620T
    Yves Marcoux 639R
    Frank Oberle 361
    Richard Passmore 35R
    Jim Pickerell 363
    Alan Sacks 366
    Rene Sheret 103
    Hugh Sitton 369
    James Strachan 618
    Erik Svenson 35L
    J.M. Truchet 619T
    Robert Torrez 54R

UNIT
1

Food,

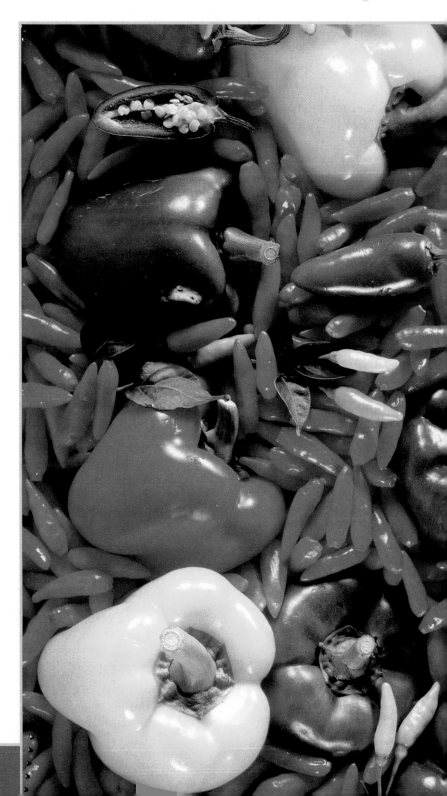

Nutrition, and You

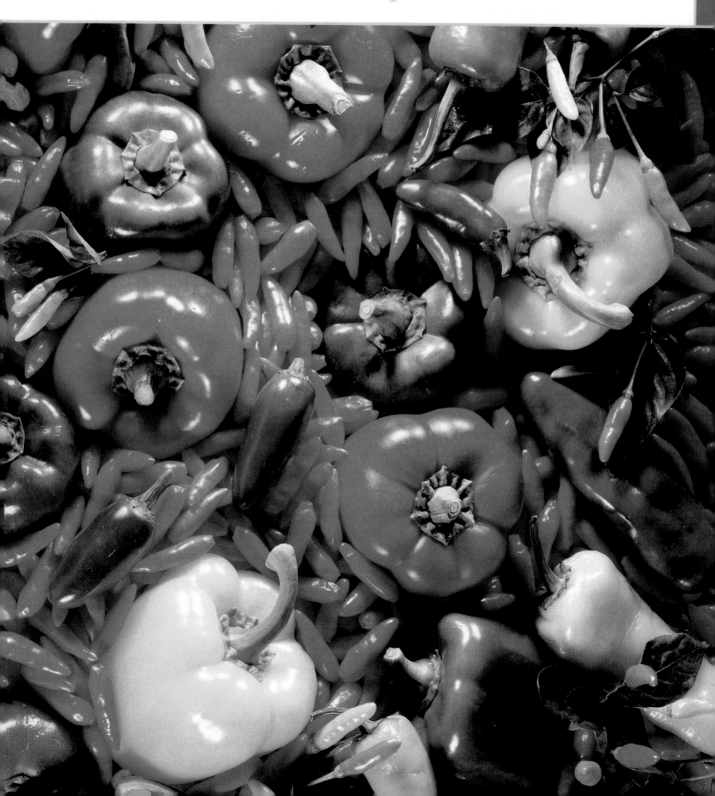

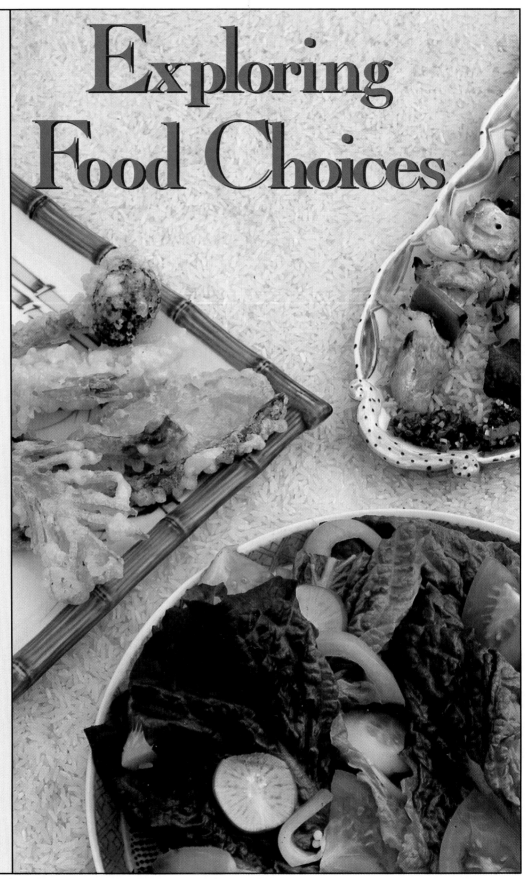

Exploring Food Choices

Have you ever noticed what an important role food plays in people's lives? In this chapter, you will find out.

Food and Health

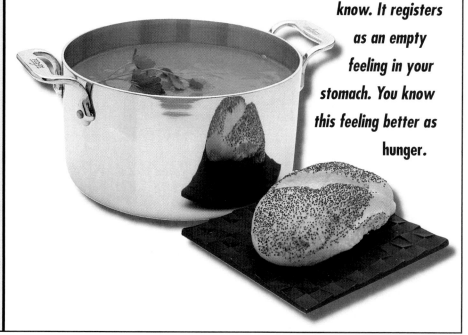

If you were asked to identify the three things you need most to survive, how would you respond? Probably, one of your answers would be "food." Food is basic to life. When your body needs food, it lets you know. It registers as an empty feeling in your stomach. You know this feeling better as hunger.

Objectives

After studying this section, you should be able to:

- Describe the importance of nutrition and wellness.

- Explain how food helps meet physical and psychological needs.

Look for These Terms

nutrients

nutrition

wellness

psychological

Physical Needs

Food does more than stop hunger pangs. It supplies you with **nutrients**, chemicals from food that your body uses to carry out its functions. These chemicals are so important that they have given rise to a branch of science. That science, called **nutrition**, is the study of nutrients and how they are used by the body.

You have probably also seen or heard the term *nutrition* used in a more popular sense to refer to the effects of a person's food choices on his or her health. If your food choices provide all the nutrients you need in the right amounts, you are said to be practicing good nutrition.

Good nutrition has many benefits. It helps you not only feel and look your best but also grow and become strong. In addition, it helps you stay energetic and healthy, both now and later in life. In this program, you will learn all about good nutrition and how to make wise food choices.

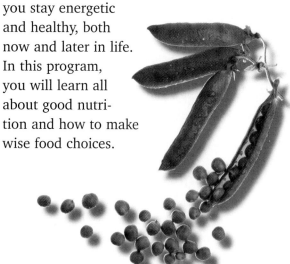

FOR YOUR HEALTH

All's Well That Starts Well

Wellness is affected by many decisions you make. Do your decisions promote wellness? To find out, privately answer the following statements "true" or "false" on a separate sheet of paper. Be honest with yourself.

- I eat at least three regular meals each day, beginning with breakfast.
- I have a varied eating plan that includes plenty of fruits, vegetables, and whole grains.
- I drink at least six to eight cups of water every day.
- I get between seven and eight hours of sleep each night.
- I exercise at least 20 to 30 minutes three to four times a week.
- I take safety precautions such as wearing a seat belt and using protective sporting gear.
- I avoid harmful substances such as tobacco, alcohol, and other drugs.
- I ask for help when I need it.
- I know where to turn for current and reliable health and nutrition information.
- I can manage stress.
- I get along well with others.
- If I have a problem, I try to work it out.

If you answered "true" to eight or more statements, your health and wellness levels are high. Seven or fewer "true" answers means you should take a close look at your wellness plan. Learning about nutrition and wellness is a good place to start.

Following Up

- In your Wellness Journal, list the items above to which you answered "false." In the weeks ahead, look for ways of changing the responses for those statements to "true."

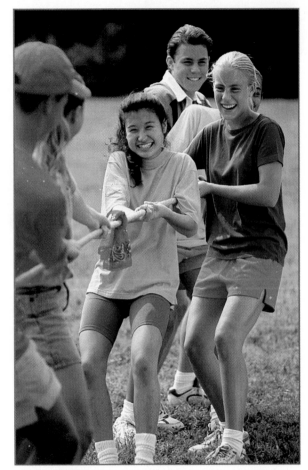

◆ Getting the most out of life depends on feeling your best. Name two daily routines or habits you take part in that promote wellness.

Wellness

Good nutrition is part of a bigger health picture known as wellness. **Wellness** is a philosophy that encourages people to take responsibility for their own health. Wellness is reflected in both your attitudes and your behaviors. Wellness decisions that influence your health include:

◆ The food choices you make.

◆ The amount of physical activity you get.

◆ How you manage your feelings and emotions.

◆ How you handle certain social situations.

By developing habits that promote wellness, you have a better chance of staying healthy and happy throughout your life.

Practicing wellness doesn't guarantee you will never get sick or feel upset. It will, however, help you achieve the highest level of health you possibly can.

Psychological Needs

Although you may not know it, food also helps you meet psychological needs. **Psychological** (sye-kuh-LODGE-ih-kuhl) means having to do with the mind and emotions. The psychological needs that food helps meet include security, a sense of belonging, and enjoyment.

Security

Security is feeling free from harm and want. The love of family and friends is an important source of security. Another type of security comes from knowing you have the basic necessities of life. Having an ample supply of food helps you feel secure.

Security can also be related to emotional needs and desires. During stressful periods, some people turn to foods that they believe will make them feel better. They may crave "comfort" foods from childhood, which they associate with feelings of being cared for or rewarded. Later in this chapter, you will learn more about how emotions influence food choices.

A Sense of Belonging

People are social beings. They need to feel that they are accepted by others—that they belong. Food can help create a bond between people, giving them a sense of belonging.

Food is associated with social events such as parties and weddings. Even when a friend comes over to your house, you probably offer something to eat or drink. Food makes people feel welcome and at ease.

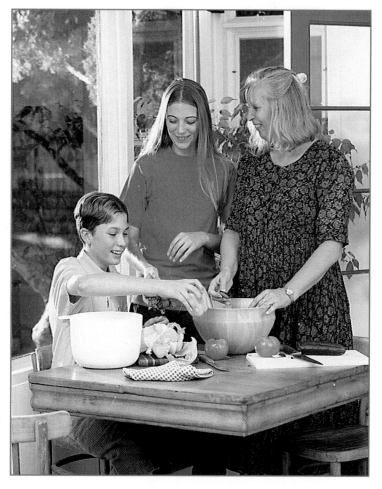

◆ Involving the whole family in food preparation is not only fun but provides opportunities for passing on family traditions. Write a short paragraph about one family food tradition practiced in your home or in the home of a relative.

Food can also help strengthen family relationships. Do you help with the preparation of family meals or the shopping? Tasks like these make a positive contribution to the family's health. They also can create feelings of self-pride. When families are able to share meals together, they have a chance to talk and laugh together.

Food can also help you feel a part of a larger group—all the people with whom you share customs and traditions. In Section 1-3, you will learn more about the relationship between food and culture.

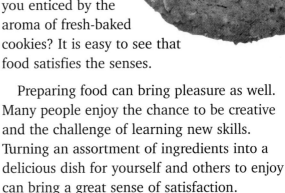

Enjoyment

What are your favorite foods? Do you most enjoy sinking your teeth into a slice of pizza oozing with cheese and zesty tomato sauce? Are you enticed by the aroma of fresh-baked cookies? It is easy to see that food satisfies the senses.

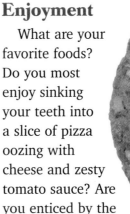

Preparing food can bring pleasure as well. Many people enjoy the chance to be creative and the challenge of learning new skills. Turning an assortment of ingredients into a delicious dish for yourself and others to enjoy can bring a great sense of satisfaction.

Section 1-1 Review & Activities

1. What is nutrition? Identify two health benefits of good nutrition.

2. What are three psychological needs that food can help meet?

3. What psychological need is being met when family members share a meal together?

4. **Synthesizing.** How might a flood or other natural disaster threaten food supplies? How would this affect people's sense of security? How might the people react?

5. **Analyzing.** Do you think physical and psychological needs for food could ever conflict? Explain.

6. **Applying.** List foods you might serve at each of the following events: a school team victory party, a surprise birthday party for a friend, a wedding anniversary celebration for an adult couple with whom you are close. Identify how these foods could help meet the physical and psychological needs of the people present.

Influences on Food Choices

Tom loves parmesan cheese, but his sister Abby can't stand the smell. Which foods do you like or dislike? More important, where do these preferences come from? Even though you may not be aware of them, many influences are at work when you make food choices.

Objectives

After studying this section, you should be able to:

- Identify social influences on food choices.
- Describe how food choices are influenced by available resources and technology.
- Identify personal influences on food choices.

Look for These Terms

culture

media

resources

technology

lifestyle

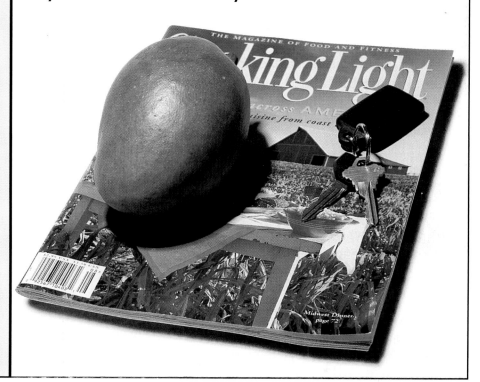

Social Influences

Although you are an individual, you are also a member of various social groups. Many of your preferences begin with the influence of culture, family, friends, and the media.

Culture

Culture refers to the shared customs, traditions, and beliefs of a large group of people, such as a nation, race, or religious group. These customs are part of what defines a group's unique identity.

Food customs are one aspect of culture. Every culture has its own traditional ways of preparing, serving, and eating foods. Some of these customs are one of a kind. The Mexican dish pollo con mole poblano, for instance, combines chicken with chocolate. Other customs are dictated by geography. The hot climate throughout much of southeastern Asia is ideal for growing rice, which is why rice is a staple starch in most southeast Asian cuisine.

Modern trends that have "shrunk" the world —high-speed transportation and communication, for instance—have made it possible for people to share and experience the foods of many cultures. Most cities in this country have Chinese and Italian restaurants. What foods from other cultures have you tried?

Family

Your family probably has had the single greatest influence on your food choices. When you were very young, family members made most of your food choices for you. As you grew, you learned food habits by following your family's example. You saw them enjoying certain foods at certain times of the day, for instance.

A family's food customs often reflect cultural background. For instance, the Masinelli family always has two main dishes at Thanksgiving—turkey and lasagna.

Families sometimes develop their own food rituals. In one family, pancakes might be a traditional Saturday night meal. Another family might never think of serving pork chops without applesauce.

People tend to feel comfortable with foods that are familiar. If certain foods were never served in your home, you may think you dislike them. Part of the adventure of eating, however, is trying new foods and finding ones that you enjoy.

Friends

As you grow older, friends play an increasingly greater role in your food choices. Because eating is a social experience, part of the time you spend with friends involves food. When you are out together, your friends influence where and what you eat, and vice versa.

If your friends are from cultural backgrounds different from your own, you might

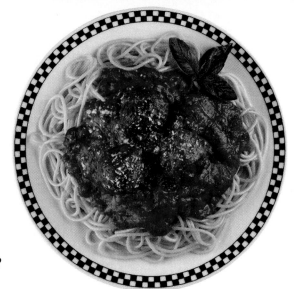

learn to enjoy the foods they commonly eat. Can you think of foods you have learned to enjoy as a result of a friendship?

The Media

We live in an information age. Each day, we are bombarded with messages from a multitude of communication sources, including television, radio, movies, newspapers, magazines, advertisements, and the Internet. These sources, known collectively as the **media**, are a major influence in the food choices you make. News reports may shape your decision to eat—or not eat—a certain food. Magazines may make you aware of new food trends.

One medium that has an especially powerful influence in your food choices is advertising. Have you ever bought a particular cereal or snack food because a TV commercial made it sound so good?

In order to make wise food choices, you need to be aware of media influences. You need to analyze the messages you see and hear.

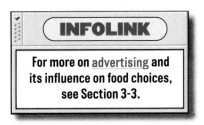

INFOLINK

For more on advertising and its influence on food choices, see Section 3-3.

Connecting Food and Math

Food Advertising and Your Health

Each year, advertisers spend millions of dollars to sell food products. What types of foods are advertised the most? Study the pie chart below. Use the data in the chart to answer the questions that follow.

Think About It

1. Which food category gets the least advertising? Why do you think this is so?

2. Approximately how much more is spent on desserts, snacks, and soft drinks than on all the other categories combined?

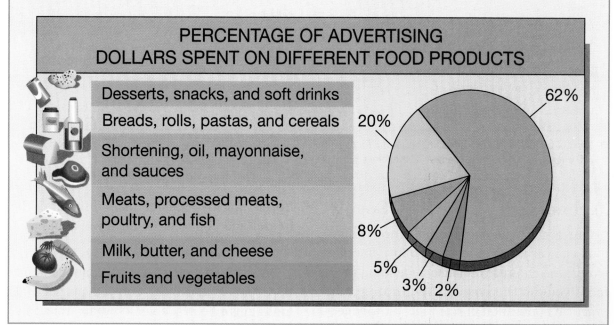

PERCENTAGE OF ADVERTISING
DOLLARS SPENT ON DIFFERENT FOOD PRODUCTS

Desserts, snacks, and soft drinks — 62%

Breads, rolls, pastas, and cereals — 20%

Shortening, oil, mayonnaise, and sauces — 8%

Meats, processed meats, poultry, and fish — 5%

Milk, butter, and cheese — 3%

Fruits and vegetables — 2%

Available Resources

Your choice of foods depends a great deal on the resources that are available to you. **Resources** are objects and qualities that can help you reach a goal. For example, this textbook is a resource that helps you learn about food and nutrition.

Many resources are involved in obtaining the food you need. Money is an obvious one. Time, knowledge, abilities, equipment, and a place to buy food are also important.

People's food choices differ because their resources differ. No one has an endless supply of all the resources, but everyone has some.

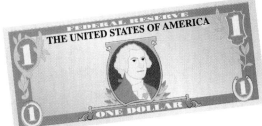

You can often substitute one resource for another that is in short supply. For instance, if you have time and skills, you can save money by cooking at home instead of eating out.

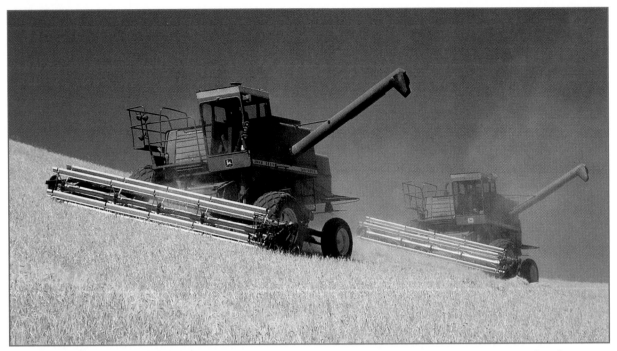

◆ **Technology has had an enormous impact on the foods available to us.** Look up the term *agriculture* in an encyclopedia or other resource. Explain how changes in technology have increased the availability of foods to enjoy.

Technology and the Food Supply

One of the resources that influences your food choices is the basic food supply. In other words, the choices you make depend on the foods you can choose from. **Technology**, the practical application of scientific knowledge, influences the food supply and, therefore, your choices.

Suppose you could step into a time machine that could whisk you 300 years into the past. What would your food choices be like? In this world of long ago, almost everything you ate would be grown by your family or your neighbors. In warm weather, food would be plentiful, but spoilage would be a problem. In cold weather, the challenge would be to make food last until the next harvest.

Today, modern technology has greatly increased the options available to you. Planes and trucks bring food from around the world to your local market. You can also take a frozen, already-prepared main dish out of the freezer and pop it in the microwave. In just minutes it's hot and ready to eat.

Advances in technology will continue to add to people's food choices. Can you imagine what foods might be available 300 years from now?

Personal Influences

Your lifestyle, values, priorities, and emotions also influence your choice of foods. They are part of the reason that your food choices are uniquely your own.

Your Lifestyle

Lifestyle refers to a person's typical way of life. Your lifestyle includes how you spend your time and what is most important to you. Lifestyle has a strong influence on what and where you eat, how and where you shop, and how you prepare food.

A teen's lifestyle commonly revolves around school, family, friends, leisure activities, and possibly, a part-time job. A busy lifestyle can affect your food choices. For instance, you may buy a snack from a vending machine just because the food is available, easy to carry, and easy to eat quickly.

Values and Priorities

Not everyone spends time or money in the same way. People make choices based on their personal values and priorities.

Food choices also depend on personal values and priorities. Some people enjoy the time they spend preparing meals. Others would rather spend the time on another activity, such as a hobby or a sport.

It's not always easy to juggle your priorities. Time, money, health, enjoyment—all are important to most people. As you continue to study food, you will learn ways to meet the challenge of a busy lifestyle.

Your Emotions

Emotions and mood can influence food choices. Some people rely on certain foods to make them feel better when they are sad or depressed. They may choose different foods if they are happy or when they are celebrating an event.

Food often carries strong associations—both pleasant and unpleasant. For instance, Jarod can still remember being forced to eat spinach as a child. He does not like spinach to this day. On the other hand, Tonya loves spinach. It reminds her of meals at her grandmother's house and the associated feelings of comfort and security.

As you can see, even a decision as seemingly simple as what to have for lunch is influenced by many factors. Your background, your lifestyle today, and the world around you all play a part in your food choices.

Section 1-2 Review & Activities

1. What is culture? How does it relate to food choices?

2. What is a resource? Name five resources that are involved in obtaining food.

3. What is a lifestyle? Give an example of how a particular lifestyle can influence a person's choice of foods.

4. Analyzing. Think about ways in which your family has influenced your personal food choices. Identify one or two of your family's food traditions, and explain where they came from and why your family observes them.

5. Extending. Imagine that you are an inventor in the next century. Describe a new food product or kitchen appliance you would like to invent. Tell how it would affect people's food choices.

6. Applying. Find three food advertisements in magazines. Tell whether each makes you want to buy the product. Explain your reactions.

Food and Culture

SECTION
1-3

Food and Culture

Eric, Cyrise, and Amber were having lunch in the food court at the mall. Each went to a different food stand. Eric returned with wonton soup and stir-fried chicken. Cyrise chose a burrito, while Amber decided on shish kebab and pita bread.

Objectives

After studying this section, you should be able to:

- Identify three aspects of culture.
- Give examples of cultural food customs.
- Explain how food customs have evolved throughout history.

Look for This Term

ethnic group

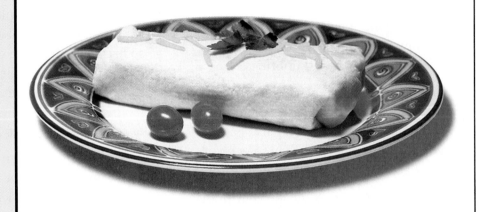

Understanding Culture

The foods Eric, Cyrise, and Amber chose were all made from basic ingredients, such as grains, vegetables, and meat or poultry. However, each dish was distinctly different. Each represented the food customs of a different culture.

As noted in the previous section, *culture* refers to the shared customs, traditions, and beliefs of a group of people. What, however, constitutes "a group of people"? This question has several possible answers:

- **Geography.** People who live in a particular region or part of the world may be said to make up a cultural group.

- **Heritage.** A common heritage, or past, is another defining feature of a cultural group. Native Americans, descendants of the first people to live in the Americas, are

one such group. Some people now living in the United States were born or have ancestral roots in other cultures. A cultural group based on common heritage is often called an **ethnic group**.

- **Religion.** Religion is another basis for defining cultural groups. Members of a particular faith usually have a common set of beliefs and follow specific practices.

Blending Cultures

If you were to take a survey of students in your school, you would probably find many cultures represented. Some students might trace their cultural roots to Ireland, others to Korea, still others to Venezuela. As such a mix reveals, the United States is a society of many cultures. Many people view this cultural richness as a great strength. People within the society are free to share and explore the customs of all the different cultures.

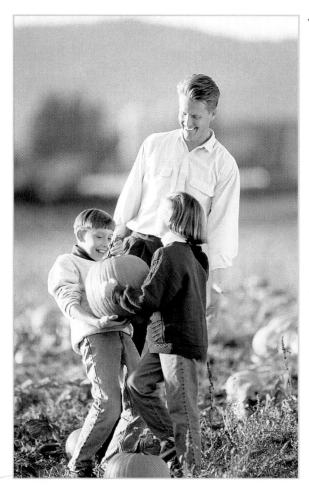

◆ Food-related celebrations are common in this country. One town's annual pumpkin festival offers everything from pumpkin ice cream to pumpkin chili. **Name a food custom associated with each of the four seasons.**

Understanding Cultural Food Customs

Food is essential in the everyday life of individuals and families. It can also play an important role in celebrations and ceremonies. It is not surprising that food customs are often a focal point in cultural traditions.

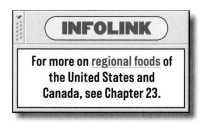

INFOLINK

For more on regional foods of the United States and Canada, see Chapter 23.

Examples of Food Customs

Food customs usually involve certain kinds of food, but that's just the beginning. They also include how food is prepared, how it is served, and how it is eaten.

Unique Foods

The foods chosen by Eric, Cyrise, and Amber have their roots in different parts of the world. For instance, wonton soup is a dish that originated in China. Wontons are dumplings filled with minced vegetables and meat. Shish kebab, chunks of meat threaded on a skewer, originated in the Middle East. So did pita bread, a distinctive flat bread that forms a pocket.

Within a nation, there may also be distinct regional food traditions. In the United States, well-known regional foods include cornbread and grits from the South, chili and barbecue from Texas, sourdough bread from San Francisco, and clam chowder from New England. Although these foods are now available all over the United States, each was developed in a particular section of the country.

Dietary Laws

Religious beliefs often include dietary laws, or rules about what foods may be eaten. For example, Jews who follow a kosher diet do not eat meat and dairy products in the same meal. Hindus do not eat beef because they consider cattle sacred animals. Muslims eat no pork.

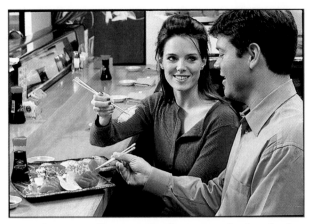

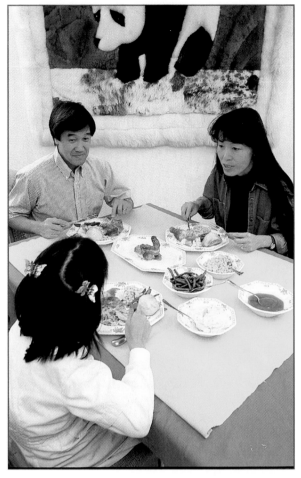

◆ **Food customs affect not only what is eaten, but how foods are served.** With what cultures do you associate the eating utensils in these two pictures? In what ways have lines between the customs of these cultures been blurred?

Cultural Etiquette

Social customs for serving and eating food also vary depending on the culture. Not all cultures use forks, knives, and spoons for eating. In China, Japan, and Korea, chopsticks are the traditional eating utensils. In some countries, such as India, Afghanistan, Algeria, and Morocco, it is considered proper to eat many foods using the fingers. In some nations of Africa, food is scooped up with a flat bread called *injera*.

Special Occasions

Some food customs relate to holidays, festivals, and religious observances. To celebrate the Chinese New Year, Judy Chen helps her mother make New Year's dumplings. The small, smooth, round dumplings are made of rice powder and water and are filled with a sweet soybean paste. Their shape symbolizes good fortune. For Easter, Poles and Ukrainians color eggs in complex designs. In Italy, a popular Easter food is a ring-shaped coffee cake with colored eggs tucked into the top.

Sometimes food itself is the theme for a festival. Harvest festivals have been common since ancient times. In the United States, Thanksgiving is the official harvest festival. Many communities also have their own festivals to celebrate the harvest of locally grown foods.

Not all holiday customs involve special foods. On Yom Kippur, the Jewish faith observes the Day of Atonement by fasting. Catholics refrain from eating meat on certain church holy days. During Ramadan, a month-long religious observance, Muslims do not eat or drink during the daylight hours.

How Food Customs Evolve

The many cultural groups dispersed throughout the world have many varied ways of preparing, serving, and eating food. None of these food customs can be considered better than any other. Different customs arise naturally as a result of different circumstances. For instance, you may be used to eating leftovers for lunch or dinner. In Japan, this would be considered unusual, even strange. This cultural difference can be understood if you realize that most Japanese do not have large refrigerators for food storage. Food is purchased fresh to be eaten that day. Dining on leftovers would be viewed as eating "old" food.

Food Customs Throughout History

A journey through history can help you understand food customs. In the distant past, cultural groups were limited in their food choices to items they could raise or gather locally. How these foods were cooked often depended on the types and amount of fuel available. For example, in many Asian countries, cooking fuel was scarce. To conserve fuel, food was cut into small pieces that would cook quickly.

Economic conditions in some cultures led to food distinctions along social class lines. The rich, who could afford the finest foods, dined on elegant fare prepared by top chefs. The rest of the people ate simple meals—typically, soup made from whatever food was available, accompanied by coarse, dark bread made from ground whole grains.

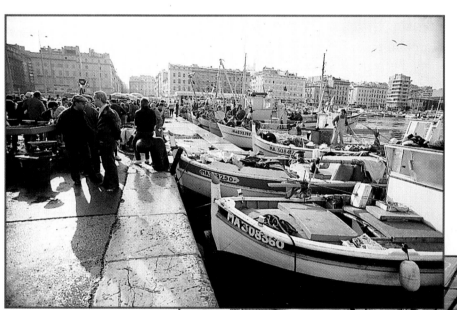

◆ The status of regional dishes sometimes changes. Bouillabaisse, an elegant fish stew served in the south of France, began as a "peasant" dish consisting of leftover fish sold at day's end to local housewives. Investigate the origins of a dish from another culture that you have sampled.

These and other food traditions were passed down from one generation to the next. Additionally, changes occurred along the way. Explorers took some of their own foods with them on their journeys and brought back strange foods from distant lands. Invading armies often brought new food customs with them.

European explorers who reached the Western Hemisphere found an abundance of foods eaten by the Native Americans. The explorers brought back samples and seeds of foods that were not found in Europe, such as dry beans, corn, tomatoes, potatoes, sweet potatoes, and cassava, a type of root. Over the centuries, some of these foods became popular in the Eastern Hemisphere.

As food customs traveled around the world, they were often changed because of a lack of availability of certain ingredients or as a result of personal tastes. Sometimes an entirely new dish resulted. For example, chop suey is not an authentic Chinese food, but an American invention based on the Chinese style of cooking.

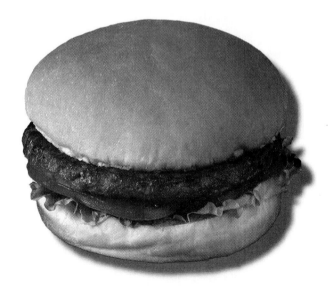

A World of Food Choices

Today, the world is becoming "smaller." People and foods can be flown thousands of miles in a few hours. Satellite links and the Internet allow instant communication between people in remote corners of the globe. As a result, food customs are shared the world over. Foods grown halfway around the world are sold in your local supermarket. Television programs and Internet sites can show you the sights of another country or tell you how to prepare dishes from foreign lands.

It is no surprise, therefore, that ethnic and international foods are now an everyday part of American life. Supermarkets routinely stock a wide variety of ethnic foods, and many restaurants include an assortment on their menus. You probably enjoy many such foods, from tacos to pasta, without thinking of them as being unusual. They have become as familiar to Americans as steak and potatoes.

This variety is one of the benefits of living in a society of many cultures. Consider the mingling of international flavors in this meal, which Katie's family ate recently: chicken vindaloo and rice (India), steamed snow peas and water chestnuts (China), and a dessert of guava shells and cream cheese (Mexico).

Flavors from around the world are being combined in recipes. Rachel makes pizza with chili-seasoned ground meat and tops it with grated sharp cheese and salsa—a spicy Mexican fresh tomato sauce. American fast-food chains featuring fried chicken and hamburgers have sprung up around the globe. Such global diversity enriches everyone's life. No matter where people go, they can find foods they enjoy and can experience the adventure of new flavors.

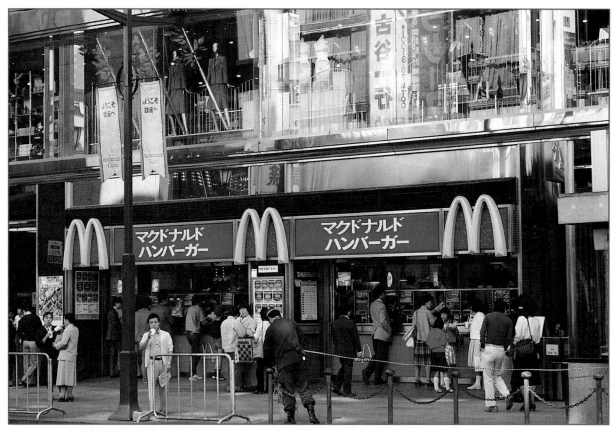

◆ **Evidence that the world is "shrinking" may be seen in the American fast food restaurant chains cropping up in other cultures.** Identify two foods from Japan, China, or another Asian culture that you have sampled or are familiar with.

Section 1-3 Review & Activities

1. What are three aspects of culture?

2. Name four categories of cultural food customs. Give an example of each.

3. What often happens when food customs are introduced into new areas? Why?

4. Evaluating. Do you think it is important for members of a particular culture to retain some distinct food customs? Why or why not?

5. Synthesizing. Do you think differences in food customs will continue to exist? Why or why not?

6. Applying. List some of your own or your family's favorite foods. Indicate the cultures that are represented.

Food, Science, and Technology

Objectives

After studying this section, you should be able to:

- Explain how science is related to nutrition and food preparation.
- Discuss the impact of food-related technology in the food industry and in the home.

Look for These Terms

food science

ergonomics

Stacey wandered down the supermarket aisles trying to decide on food for her party Saturday night. Finally, she chose a few old favorites as well as several new items that looked good, including fat-free cookies, mini-pizzas made for the microwave, and red, tomato-flavored tortilla chips.

It never occurred to Stacey that science and technology were responsible for the wide variety of foods that made her choices so difficult. Science and technology have had a tremendous impact on food, from the kinds of food available to the ways in which food is prepared.

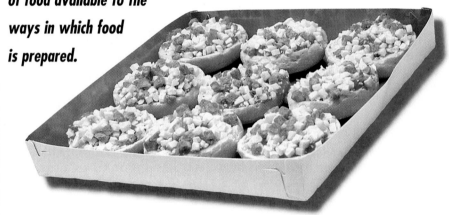

Scientific Aspects of Food

The science of nutrition has links to a number of other basic sciences, including chemistry, biology, physics, and a recently developed science known as *ergonomics* (err-guh-NAHM-iks). Here is a brief look at these relationships.

Nutritional Research

The foundation of any scientific inquiry is research. The science of nutrition is no exception. So far, nutritional research has uncovered about 40 nutrients. No one knows how many other nutrients remain to be discovered. Once nutrients are discovered, scientists continue to investigate the role they play in health.

One promising direction of nutritional research in recent years has been into the realm of nutrient chemicals that occur naturally in plants. Research so far has offered hope that this class of nutrients may reduce the risk of certain forms of cancer and other potentially life-threatening diseases.

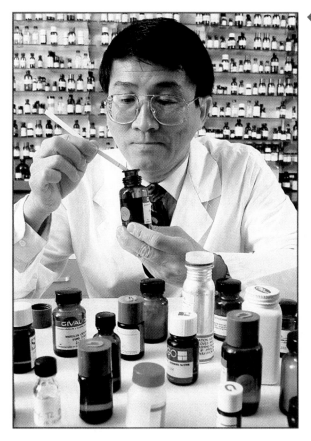

◆ Food technologists help develop new foods and improve existing ones by relying on knowledge of food, nutrition, science, and technology. This technologist is testing flavors in a food research laboratory. Investigate olestra, a synthetic form of fat being used in some fried-food products. What information is available regarding the healthfulness of this product?

and a hard, flat one? The answer isn't found in magic but in science.

Food preparation is governed by natural laws. When certain foods are heated, chilled, mixed, or manipulated in other ways, they undergo chemical and physical changes. In fact, a recipe might legitimately be compared to a chemistry experiment. If you change the conditions of the experiment, the results are likely to change. In the same way, even a slight change in a recipe can cause the final product to turn out differently.

A knowledge of **food science**—the scientific study of food and its preparation—can help you understand why certain instructions in a recipe are important. If something doesn't turn out right, food science can help you understand why so that you'll be able to keep the problem from happening again.

The Science of Food Preparation

Moira's friend Keisha is a whiz in the kitchen. Inspired by Keisha's example, Moira tried making a cheese soufflé, an airy blend of eggs and cheese. She followed Keisha's recipe exactly—well, almost exactly—but the soufflé didn't turn out right. "I guess I just don't have Keisha's magic touch," Moira decided.

What makes the difference between a light, fluffy soufflé

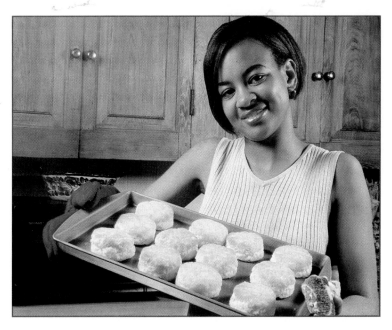

◆ Creating delicious tempting foods is not the result of kitchen "secrets" but hard science. In your Wellness Journal, keep a running list of science tips you learn from your reading. Refer back to these from time to time.

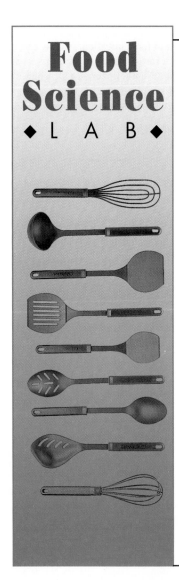

Food Science ◆ L A B ◆

How Does Temperature Affect Egg Whites?

Throughout this program, you will perform experiments in food science. You will learn how different factors affect different foods. In this experiment you will discover what effect, if any, temperature has on beaten egg whites.

Procedure

1. Place three refrigerated egg whites in a quart-size glass mixing bowl that is clean and free of grease. With a rotary beater or electric mixer, beat the whites until they form peaks that bend over slightly when the beaters are lifted out of the whites.

2. Scoop the contents into a clean measuring cup and record the results.

3. Repeat the procedure with three egg whites that have been at room temperature for 30 minutes.

Conclusions

◆ Which egg whites produced the greatest volume?

◆ How might this information help you if you were preparing meringue for a pie or a cake that called for beaten egg whites?

Ergonomics

Have you ever experienced a headache or eye strain after staring at a computer screen for a long period? If so, you understand the need for ergonomics. **Ergonomics** is the study of ways to make tools and equipment easier and more comfortable to use. In addition to computer hardware, ergonomicists have developed types of seating that cause less wear and tear on the muscles, bones, and joints than conventional chairs.

Ergonomics has played a key role in the design of kitchens, appliances, and food preparation equipment. Cookware and kitchen tools are ergonomically designed to make food preparation easier and faster.

Work simplification, an important part of ergonomics, means looking for the fastest and easiest method for getting a job done. Using work simplification in the kitchen or foods lab can save time and energy, as you will discover.

Technology and Food

Through technology, new or improved products and processes are developed. Examples can be found in the food industry and in the home.

The Food Industry

Technology plays a major role in how foods are produced, processed, packaged, and shipped. For instance:

◆ Food processing plants are using computers and robots to help control the quality of their products.

◆ New forms of packaging have been developed to keep food safe longer. In some cases, special packaging methods allow foods that traditionally require refrigeration to be stored at room temperature.

◆ Food scientists continue to develop new fat and sugar substitutes and new ways to use them in foods.

◆ Scientists are using a technique called genetic engineering to improve and refine foods.

In later chapters, you will learn more about the food industry and the products that have been developed as a result of technology.

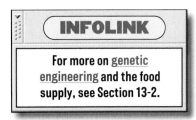

INFOLINK

For more on genetic engineering and the food supply, see Section 13-2.

◆ Hydroponic farming—the growing of crops without soil—is still a relatively new industry. Learn more about other cutting-edge areas of technology. Share your findings with classmates in a brief report.

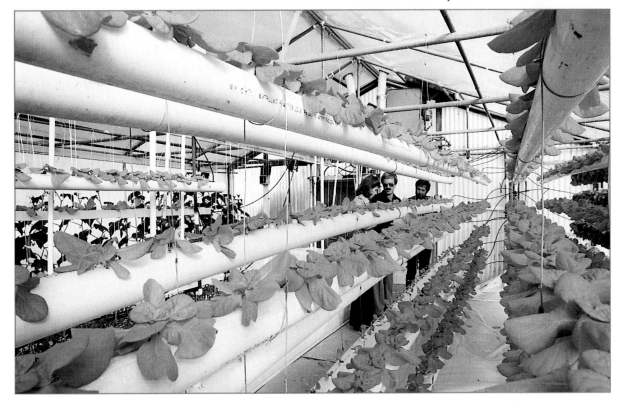

Learning to use new technology can be exciting, but don't forget about safety. Always read the instructions before using an appliance or other device for the first time.

The Home

Do you have a microwave oven in your home? Today, 90 percent of U.S. households do. These devices, which cook many foods in a fraction of the time required by conventional ovens, are one of many examples of how technology has benefited the home. Another standard fixture in many home kitchens nowadays is the food processor, which has made chopping, dicing, and similar preparation tasks easier than ever.

Technology has led not only to the development of new kitchen tools but also to the updating of older ones. Both major appliances—such as ranges, refrigerators, and dishwashers—and small appliances have become increasingly more reliable and easier to use while using less energy. Many of today's appliances contain a "brain" in the form of a computer chip. Some even alert the user when repair is needed.

New technology does have its drawbacks. Appliances with advanced features are more costly than basic models. In some cases, the advanced features may add to the difficulty and cost of repairs. Learning to use new features and controls can be time-consuming.

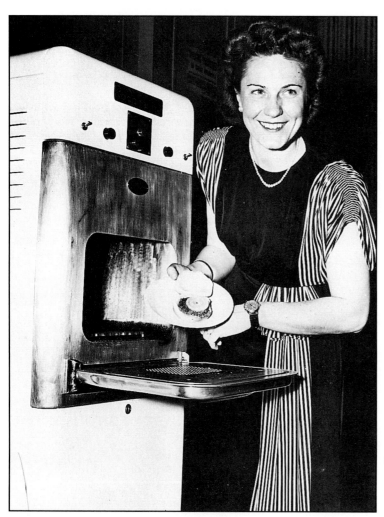

◆ **This picture shows what the earliest microwave ovens looked like.** In addition to changes in size, what other differences can you see between this and microwaves now?

Personal Computers

Personal computers are proving helpful in the planning of meals. Some people use computers to store recipes, plan menus, and prepare shopping lists. A computer can also help you keep track of food spending and supplies. Software and Internet sites are available to evaluate both individual foods and entire meals for their nutritional content.

Food for Tomorrow

What you have read is just a sample of the ways in which science and technology influence the foods you prepare and eat. Discoveries are being made every day. Staying informed about the latest developments in science and technology is one way of keeping up on changes that can have an impact on your life. In the next section, you will learn about ways of sharpening this and other key life skills.

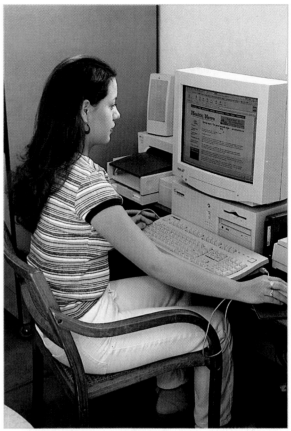

◆ **There is quite a bit of information available on the Internet about food choices and their nutritional value.** Identify at least two other types of information that might be found by using a computer to help you manage food selection and preparation.

Section 1-4 Review & Activities

1. How is a recipe like a chemistry experiment?

2. What does *ergonomically sound* mean when applied to a kitchen tool?

3. Give an example of two recent technological advances in the food industry.

4. Evaluating. Analyze this statement: "The benefits of technology outweigh the drawbacks."

5. Comparing and Contrasting. Name one advantage and one disadvantage of using a personal computer to help with meal planning.

6. Applying. Using ads from the newspaper or a home-shopper catalogue, compare the price and features of a basic model and a high-tech model of a common kitchen appliance, such as a toaster. Present your conclusions in a brief report.

Skills for Food Choices

Life is filled with choices, many of which involve food. No matter what the decision is, every food choice becomes easier when you have a grasp of four related skills. These are thinking, communication, leadership, and management.

Objectives

After studying this section, you should be able to:

- Identify skills related to the food choices you make.
- Give examples of how management techniques relate to the study of food and nutrition.
- Explain the steps in the decision-making process.

Look for These Terms

critical thinking

management

Thinking

Most of the thinking you do each day is an automatic process that begins the instant you wake up. It is this type of thought that enables you to carry out routine tasks, such as finding your way to school. Yet, there is another type of thought, unique to humans, known as directed thinking. Directed thinking is using higher-level reasoning skills in a deliberate and purposeful way to arrive at a desired outcome.

One especially important aspect of directed thinking is **critical thinking**, which involves examination of printed and spoken language in order to gain insights into meanings and interpretations. When you read between the lines of a health claim for a food product that sounds too good to be true, you are using critical thinking.

In a society in which you are confronted with many food choices, critical thinking can be a valuable skill. It can help you, for example, recognize and resist negative influences on your overall pattern of food choices.

Communication

Critical thinking is tied closely to a second skill that can guide healthful food decisions— communication. Communication is the sending and receiving of thoughts, feelings, opinions, and information. Communication is made up of a number of subskills, including speaking, listening, writing, and reading. An effective communicator is able to process and evaluate advertisements and other media messages concerning foods. He or she is then able to react to the information in an appropriate fashion.

Leadership

Do you think of yourself as a leader or as a follower? As a food-related skill, leadership may be defined as helping those around you develop positive food goals and attitudes. Leadership skills may be targeted at groups as small as a family and as large as a community, a nation, or the world. On its most immediate level, leadership might mean setting a good example for younger brothers

or sisters by making healthful food choices at home. On a broader level, a leader might be a concerned citizen who alerts government officials about pollution or other practices that pose a risk to the food supply.

INFOLINK

For more on the global food supply and factors that have a negative impact on it, see Section 13-3.
For more on comparison shopping as it relates to food purchases, see Section 12-3.

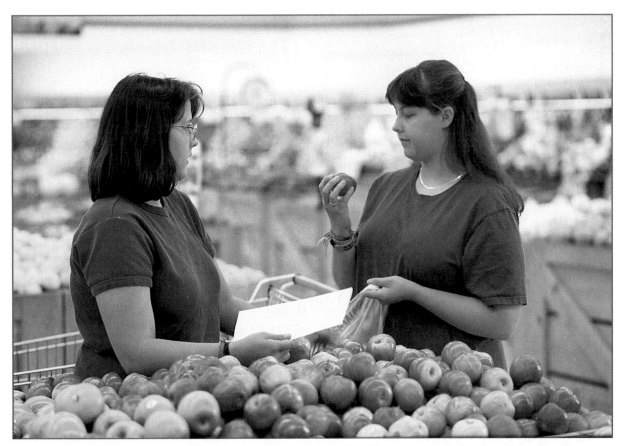

◆ **With good management you can use whatever resources you have most effectively. For example, price information is essential when shopping for food.** Name two other kinds of information that play a role in good management skills when shopping.

Management

Management refers to specific techniques that help you use resources wisely. Among the many ways in which management techniques play a role in sound food choices are the following:

♦ **Managing your time.** Helps you accomplish what you really need and want to do within given time constraints. An effective manager is able to find time in even the busiest of schedules to ensure getting the nutrients his or her body needs.

♦ **Managing your money.** Enables you to meet financial goals and get the most value for your dollar. An example of money management is comparison shopping— examining the cost of similar food items to see which offers the best value.

♦ **Record-keeping.** Helps you make plans and evaluate how well you use your resources. For instance, keeping a record of the foods you eat for a few days can help you make better food choices.

♦ **Organizing.** Arranging items in an orderly and logical way. For example, organizing a shopping list by grouping similar items together cuts down on shopping time.

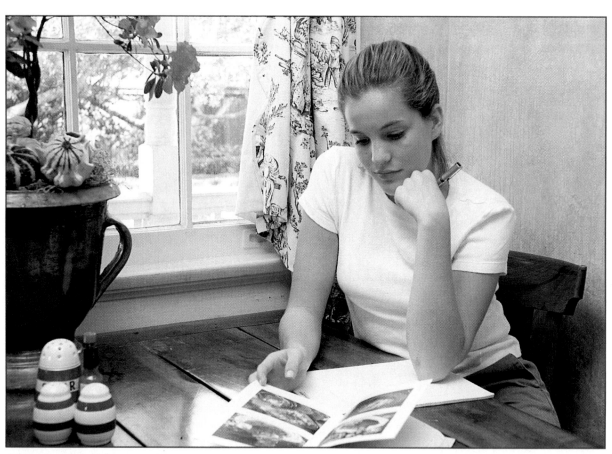

♦ With practice, the decision-making process will become automatic. Think about a difficult decision you have made or might be faced with in the future. Use the steps in the decision-making model to help you make your decision.

Making Decisions

A common link among the four food-related skills is that each involves decisions of one kind or another. Think about the decisions you make in a typical day or week. Some, such as what clothes to wear, are minor. Others—for example, whether to study for a final exam or attend a rock concert with friends—are not.

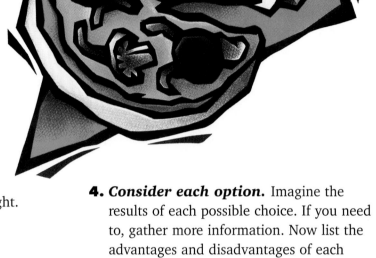

In spite of their importance, some people make big decisions without thinking them through. They may simply pick an option at random. Sometimes they put off making a decision until they no longer have any choices. However, important decisions deserve more careful thought.

Steps in Decision Making

With practice, making decisions becomes easier. Try using this simple seven-step process on a problem or decision you have faced or are facing:

1. ***Identify the decision to be made and your goals.*** What do you want the result to be? Suppose you are cooking for a party. Your goal might be finding something easy to fix and easy to keep hot or cold, and something most people will like.

2. ***Consider your resources.*** What do you have available that could help you in this situation? A resource for finding recipes might be a cookbook. A resource for keeping food hot at the party might be an electric slow cooker.

3. ***Identify your options.*** Be creative and open to new ideas. As you think of solutions that might work, make a list.

4. ***Consider each option.*** Imagine the results of each possible choice. If you need to, gather more information. Now list the advantages and disadvantages of each option. How well would each meet the goals you originally set?

5. ***Choose the best option.*** Often there is no perfect solution. Weigh and compare options; then choose the one that seems best. What if none of the choices is acceptable? Try going back to step 3 to see if there's a solution you overlooked.

6. ***Carry out your decision.*** Make a plan based on your choice. If you decide to make mini-pizzas for the party, plan when and how you will make them. Then put your plan in action.

7. ***Evaluate the result.*** How did your decision turn out? If it worked well, take pride in what you accomplished. If it didn't, don't be discouraged. Accept that you did your best; then try to learn from the experience.

Decision Making and Food Choices

Some decisions that seem small can turn out to have major consequences. Think about the food choices you make each day. Deciding what to choose from the lunch menu or what to snack on can seem minor until you realize that a lifetime of good or poor health depends, in part, on small decisions like these. Often, poor food choices are made out of habit. Yet good choices can also become a habit.

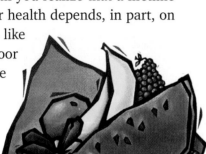

Career Decisions

One of the most important decisions you will ever make is how you will earn your living as an adult. Too often, people decide on a line of work without really knowing much about it. They are unaware of many other possible careers, any one of which might prove even more satisfying to them.

You might be surprised at the wide range of careers that relate to food and nutrition. This textbook will help you explore many of the possibilities. At the end of each chapter, you will find a career feature that focuses on a particular worker and his or her job. The final chapter will provide more in-depth information to help you think about and prepare for a career.

Section 1-5 Review & Activities

1. What four skills are associated with food choices?

2. Name three management techniques. Tell how each relates to food and nutrition.

3. Identify the seven steps in the decision-making process.

4. **Analyzing.** Which food-related skills would be involved in organizing a letter-writing campaign addressing unfair prices at a local food store?

5. **Evaluating.** Jorge has band practice at 3:30 and a basketball game at 5:30. What management skill could help him determine the kind of snack he should eat?

6. **Applying.** Imagine that your class has been asked to cook a meal for a local senior citizen's group. Identify at least three decisions that would have to be made. Choose one and explain how you would use the decision-making process in this situation.

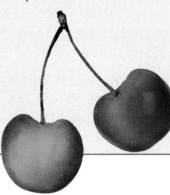
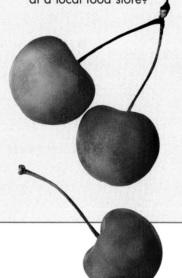

CAREER WANTED

Individuals who enjoy working with others, use deductive reasoning, and are creative problem solvers.

REQUIRES:

- some postsecondary training in food production or dietetics
- on-the-job training in laboratory procedures

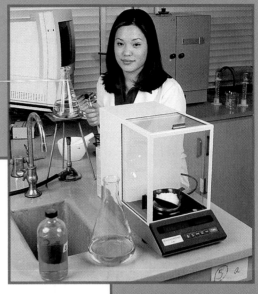

"The proof really *is* in the pudding,"
says Test Kitchen Worker Mei Chin

Q: Mei, how did you get started as a test kitchen worker?

A: During high school, I had a great part-time job as a short-order cook. And, I've always enjoyed science. So, after graduation, I wanted a job that combined both interests. My counselor helped me find this job as a test kitchen worker for a major food manufacturer.

Q: Is your job only to test new products?

A: No. For example, the manufacturer is always looking for ways of getting products out faster. As new technology is brought in to help accomplish that, we are there to make sure that quality is still inside every package. Test kitchen workers also help food scientists create "lite" versions of a product that taste exactly the same, but have only a fraction of the fat.

Q: Then you work as part of a team?

A: Sometimes. Often the same challenge is given to individual technicians to see who comes up with the best recipe. Or, one of us might also be asked to do the preparation and cooking tasks, while the others run nutritional analyses.

Career Research Activity

1. Research two of the careers listed on the right. Make a chart comparing and contrasting the training, educational background, salary range, and other aspects of the work involved.

2. Imagine you have the education and experience to be a Cuisine Specialty Cook. What type of cuisine would be your specialty? Write a one-page essay explaining why.

Related Career Opportunities

Entry Level
- Short-Order Cook
- Kitchen Helper
- School Cafeteria Cook

Technical Level
- Cafeteria Manager
- Test Kitchen Worker
- Specialty Cook

Professional Level
- Cuisine Specialty Cook
- Executive Chef

Chapter 1 Review & Activities

Summary

Section 1-1: Food and Health

- Good nutrition is an important part of physical health and wellness.

- Food can contribute to psychological health by providing security, a sense of belonging, and enjoyment.

Section 1-4: Food, Science, and Technology

- The science of nutrition is linked to other sciences, including chemistry and ergonomics.

- Food science is the scientific study of food and its preparation.

- New technology is changing the way food is produced and processed, as well as the way people plan and prepare meals.

Section 1-2: Influences on Food Choices

- Social influences on food choices include culture, family, friends, and the media.

- Food choices also depend on available resources.

- Technology has increased the options available.

- Factors affecting personal food choices include lifestyle, values and priorities, and emotions.

Section 1-5: Skills for Food Choices

- Four skills related to food choices are thinking, communication, leadership, and management.

- The decision-making process can help in many situations.

Section 1-3: Food and Culture

- Different cultures have distinct food customs.

- Many food customs that originated in the distant past have changed and mingled with others along the way.

- With technology, the world has shrunk, increasing the sharing of cultural customs relating to food.

Working IN THE Lab

1. **Taste Test.** Wearing a blindfold, taste food samples prepared by your teacher. Describe the aroma, texture, and flavor. Try to identify the food. Discuss how the senses contribute to the enjoyment of food. What role do they play in making food choices?

2. **Food Preparation.** Prepare popcorn in the microwave oven, on the range, and in a popcorn popper. Compare the methods for time, cost, and taste. What are the advantages and disadvantages of each method? Which would you be more likely to choose in the future?

Checking Your Knowledge

1. Give two meanings of the word *nutrition*.

2. How can food provide a sense of belonging?

3. Define *media*. How does the media affect food choices?

4. Identify three resources that might affect food choices.

5. How does living in a society relate to food customs?

6. How did geography affect food customs in the past? Why does it have less influence today?

7. What do natural laws of science have to do with food preparation?

8. Name two results of technology that have streamlined food preparation and cooking in the home.

9. How is critical thinking different from the thought processes used in daydreaming?

10. What should you do if a decision doesn't turn out as you expected?

Thinking Critically

1. Recognizing Values. Mark and Ina's family and consumer sciences class is holding its annual international dinner. As in years past, each person is asked to bring a homemade dish. Mark plans to make a delicious Spanish soup of white beans, collard greens, fresh garlic, and sausage. Ina has decided to look through the cookbooks and computer files in the classroom library and see which dish would take the least time and effort to make. What values and priorities are reflected by each approach to the task of preparing food?

2. Recognizing Fallacies in Logic. Angelina is thumbing through a magazine and comes upon an article proclaiming that the microwave oven has changed daily life. Without reading even the opening paragraph, Angelina flips ahead to the next feature in the magazine, mumbling under her breath that this is just another underhanded effort to sell appliances and, in so doing, cater to the magazine's advertisers. Explain what, if anything, is wrong with the position Angelina has taken.

Reinforcing Key Skills

1. Directed Thinking. Rory is watching TV when a commercial comes on for a candy bar that claims to provide all the nutrients your body needs in a given day. State whether or not you would advise Rory to buy the product. Explain your advice.

2. Communication. Ella and Sean have volunteered to bake cakes for a charity bake sale. As they work, Ella notices that Sean is spending a lot of time on the phone with friends. She is beginning to fear that the two will miss their deadline, which is in two days. What would you advise Ella to do?

Making Decisions and Solving Problems

You are helping your family shop for a new microwave oven. A basic model, which is in your price range, looks easy to use. However, you think your family would like some of the special features found in higher-priced models. How would you help your family decide which oven to buy?

Making Connections

1. Social Studies. Using cookbooks, food magazines, or online sources, learn about three foods eaten in the United States that originated in other cultures. Prepare a map that shows the place of origin of each food and the route it took to reach this country. Use a different colored line for each food. Be sure to include a legend indicating what the colors represent.

2. Economics. Interview a local supermarket manager or other community merchant to investigate the role management skills play in his or her job. Prepare by drafting questions regarding each of the management techniques detailed in the chapter. Learn what other management skills are used in business. Share your findings in the form of a tape-recorded interview or a brief oral report.

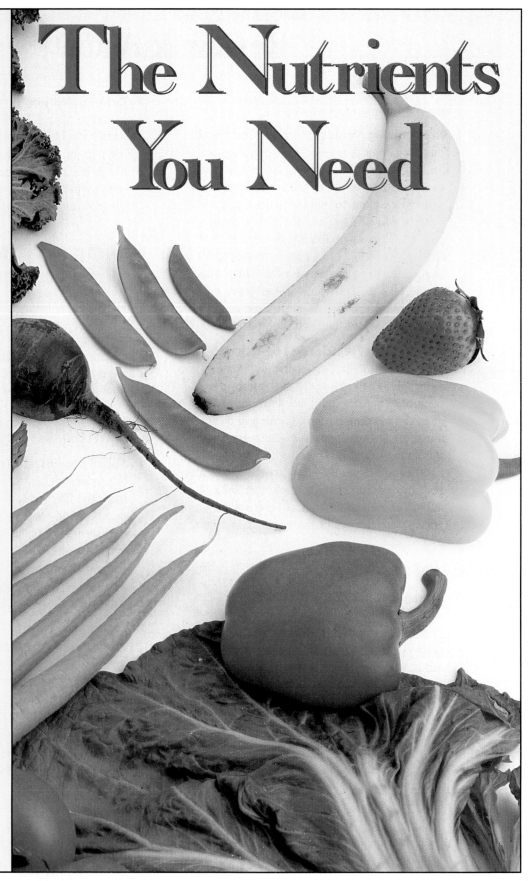

The Nutrients You Need

You may know the saying "You are what you eat." As you'll soon find out, there is much truth in those words. In this chapter, you'll learn about the many nutrients your body needs.

The Role of Nutrients

If you have ever looked under the hood of a car, you know that its engine is made up of many interconnected parts and systems. The human body is organized in much the same way. Just as a car needs gasoline to run, so the body needs its own type of fuel. Like a car, the body requires periodic maintenance if it is to work efficiently.

Objectives

After studying this section, you should be able to:

- Name the six major types of nutrients.
- Explain the purposes of DRIs, RDAs, and AIs.
- Give guidelines regarding calorie needs and calorie sources.

Look for These Terms

carbohydrates

dietary fiber

fats

proteins

vitamins

minerals

nutrient deficiency

malnutrition

DRIs

RDAs

AIs

calorie

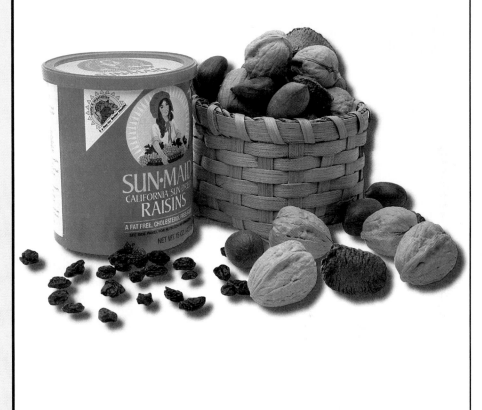

The Six Main Nutrients

The nutrients your body uses are divided into six major types. All these types work together as a team, each one playing its own special role in your health and well-being.

- **Carbohydrates** (kar-boh-HY-drayts) are the body's main source of energy. One unique and important form of this major nutrient is **dietary fiber**, a mixture of plant materials that is not broken down in the digestive system. All forms of carbohydrates, except fiber, provide energy.

- **Fats** are a concentrated source of energy. You need fats in moderate amounts to perform important functions in your body, including transporting nutrients.

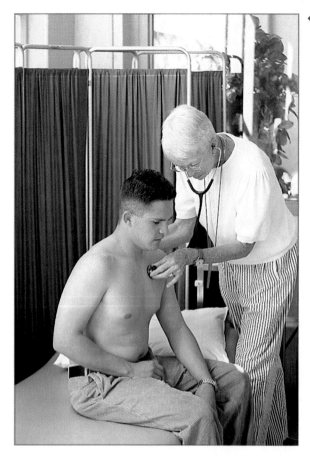

◆ Good nutrition is essential for good health. Name two other benefits associated with good nutrition.

Nutrient Teamwork

What would happen if a school's football team went out onto the field for a game without one or two of the players? To play well, a team must have all its members. Each has a specific job to do and needs to be present to do it.

The same is true of the key nutrients in your eating plan. No one nutrient can be substituted for any other. If any of the six main nutrients is absent, your entire body—and your health—suffers.

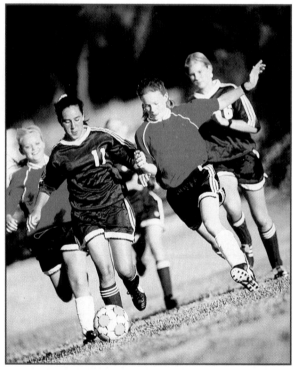

◆ Just as a team relies on the contributions of each member, so the food you eat must include all vital nutrients for your body to function smoothly. Use the table "Nutritive Value of Foods" in Appendix B at the back of this book to analyze a food you regularly eat. Identify the amount of each nutrient it contains.

◆ **Proteins** are nutrients that help build, repair, and maintain body tissues. Proteins are also a source of energy.

◆ **Vitamins** are chemicals that help regulate many vital body processes and aid other nutrients in doing their jobs. Your body requires only small amounts of vitamins.

◆ **Minerals** are nonliving substances that help the body work properly and, in some cases, become part of body tissues, such as bone. Like vitamins, minerals are needed in only small amounts.

◆ Water is a nutrient because it is essential to life. It makes up most of your body weight too.

You will learn more about these nutrients in the next two sections of this chapter.

Effects of Poor Nutrition

When people make poor food choices or do not have enough to eat, serious health conditions can result. One such condition is a **nutrient deficiency**, a severe nutrient shortage. A nutrient deficiency can have far-reaching consequences. A lack of vitamin D, for instance, can keep children's bones from growing properly. Their bones become weak, and the children develop bowed legs. In adults, a lack of vitamin D results in brittle bones, which break easily. It may also cause muscle weakness and spasms.

Malnutrition refers to serious health problems caused by poor nutrition over a prolonged period. Generally, malnutrition occurs when people don't get enough to eat. Bad weather, inadequate transportation, political problems, or other factors can cause food shortages. Malnutrition can also result from poverty. In the United States alone, it is estimated that 20 percent of all children live below the poverty line.

Poor nutrition can also occur among people who have an abundant food supply and can afford to buy enough food to eat. Nutrition problems occur when people consistently choose foods that do not supply enough of the nutrients needed for good health. They may also get too much of some nutrients, such as fat.

The food choices you make have long-term effects on your health. An unbalanced eating plan can increase the risk of diseases that can shorten life or reduce the quality of life. Although there are no "bad" foods, too much

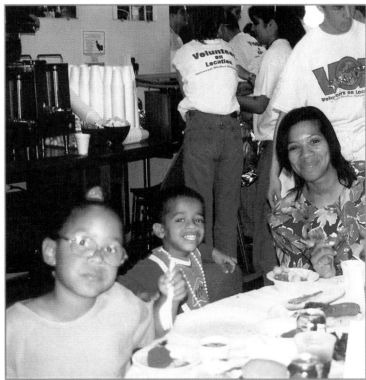

◆ **These children and their mother are enjoying a nutritious meal served to them by a group of teen volunteers.** Visit the Web site of the World Health Organization (WHO) and learn about the important work WHO does.

or too little of one food can create an unhealthful eating plan. Making balanced choices increases your chances of staying healthy, strong, and active throughout your life.

How Much Do You Need?

Everybody needs the same nutrients, although not necessarily in the same amounts. Females require more iron than males. Athletes and others who are physically active need more of most nutrients than inactive people. Older adults require less of many nutrients.

Scientists have developed a series of standards for assessing nutrient needs among people of different age and gender groups. These standards have different names but are known under the general label "Dietary Reference Intakes," or **DRIs**.

Two examples of DRIs are Recommended Dietary Allowances (RDAs) and Adequate Intake (AI). **RDAs** are the amounts of a nutrient needed by 98 percent of the people in a given age and gender group. When a lack of scientific information makes it impossible to establish the RDA for a particular nutrient, approximate nutrient measures, or **AIs**, are set instead. Both RDAs and the AI are used to determine average individual needs.

The DRIs, including RDAs and AIs, are updated periodically as new information becomes available. They are used by dietitians, nutritionists, and other health professionals. DRIs are an important tool in shaping U.S. nutrition policy and for developing educational programs. They are also used by the food industry for product development.

The U.S. Food and Drug Administration (FDA) has used the DRIs as the basis for another set of guidelines. These are known as Daily Values (DVs) and are used in nutrition labeling.

> **INFOLINK**
>
> For more information on Daily Values (DVs) and how to use them when shopping for food products, see Section 12-2.

How Nutrients Are Measured

Most nutrients are needed in relatively small amounts. It's easier to measure them using the metric system, the system of measurement used by scientists. The metric system includes small units of measure, such as the milligram (mg). For example, female teens need 15 milligrams (mg) of iron each day. That's equivalent to about 0.0005 ounce—about the size of a single dry bean.

Energy from Nutrients

Running, walking, sitting, and even reading this sentence all require energy. Your body gets this energy from carbohydrates, as well as protein and fats. The energy is measured in units called *kilocalories* (KIL-oh-KAL-uh-reez). A kilocalorie—or **calorie**—is the amount of energy needed to raise the temperature of 1 kilogram (a little more than 4 cups) of water 1 degree Celsius. In the metric system, energy is measured in kilojoules (KJ).

Your Energy Needs

The number of calories your body needs for energy in a given day depends on a number of factors. These include your activity level, age, weight, and gender. If you are still growing, the number is affected by increased energy demands for building muscles and bones.

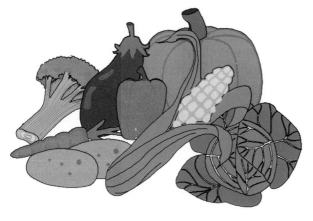

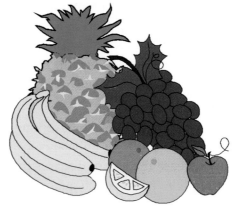

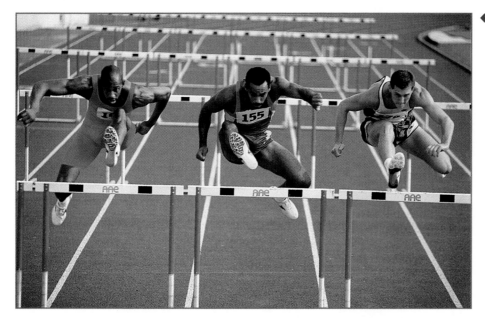

◆ Vigorous activity, such as running or swimming, uses large amounts of energy. Speak with a physical education teacher or athletic trainer in your school about the calorie requirements of athletes. Share your findings with the class.

The U.S. Department of Agriculture recommends the following calorie intakes:

◆ 2,800 calories for teen males, many active men, and some very active women.

◆ 2,200 calories for most children, teen females, active women, and many inactive men. Women who are pregnant or breast-feeding may need more.

◆ 1,600 calories for many inactive women and most older adults.

Keep in mind that these calorie levels vary with the amount of physical activity in your life. For instance, teens who spend most of their leisure time in front of the computer or TV will need to adjust their caloric intake if they take up hockey or soccer.

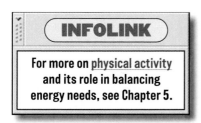

INFOLINK

For more on <u>physical activity</u> and its role in balancing energy needs, see Chapter 5.

Recommended Sources of Calories

Scientists have determined that carbohydrates and proteins in their purest forms each provide 4 calories per gram, whereas fat provides 9 calories per gram. Notice that fat has more than twice the number of calories per gram as either of the other energy-producing nutrients.

Health experts recommend that you get less than 30 percent of the calories you take in from fat, approximately 60 percent from carbohydrates, and at least 10 percent from protein. This ratio provides the healthiest balance of the three nutrients.

For instance, Julie, who needs about 2,200 calories a day, should get less than 660 of those calories from fat ($2,200 \times 0.3 = 660$). How many grams of fat will supply 660 calories? Since there are 9 calories in 1 gram of fat, divide 660 by 9. The answer is about 73 grams. If Julie eats a fast-food double cheeseburger and fries for lunch (about 47 grams of fat), she will need to eat lower-fat choices the rest of the day to stay under 73 grams of fat.

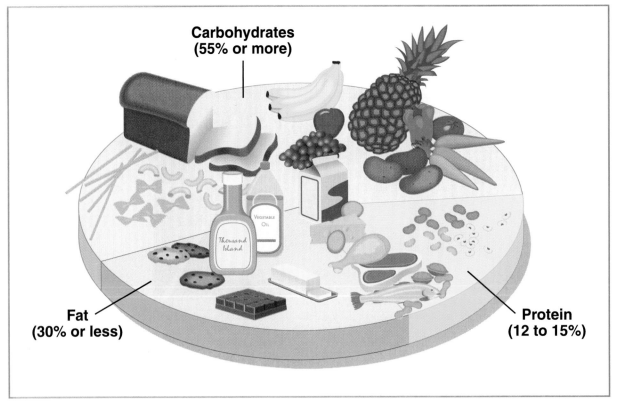

**Carbohydrates
(55% or more)**

**Fat
(30% or less)**

**Protein
(12 to 15%)**

◆ It is not just the number of calories you take in that is important but the sources of those calories. This drawing shows the recommended percentages for the healthiest balance of carbohydrates, protein, and fat. What percentage of your daily food intake should include fruits, vegetables, and grains?

Section 2-1 Review & Activities

1. What are the six major types of nutrients? What are the main functions of each?

2. What are DRIs? How are they used by professionals or industry?

3. Which nutrients supply your body with energy? How is food energy measured?

4. Comparing and Contrasting. Juan is a moderately active 15-year-old male. His mother, Inez, is a very active 40-year-old. What calorie levels are suggested for each? How are they the same? How are they different?

5. Analyzing. Some fad diets recommend levels of fewer than 1,000 calories per day. Why is such an approach unhealthful for reaching a healthy weight?

6. Applying. Use the information in this section to determine your approximate calorie needs. Make a list of the days of the week you exercise or play sports. Which day(s) of the week will you need the most calories? Which day(s) will you need the fewest calories? Why?

SECTION 2-2

Carbohydrates, Fiber, and Proteins

Objectives

After studying this section, you should be able to:

- Name sources of simple and complex carbohydrates.
- Explain why soluble and insoluble fibers are important.
- Distinguish between complete and incomplete proteins.

Look for These Terms

insoluble fiber

soluble fiber

refined sugars

amino acids

complete proteins

incomplete proteins

As you read in Section 2-1, for good health you need six basic nutrients, plus fiber. Read on to learn more about these, beginning with carbohydrates, fiber, and proteins.

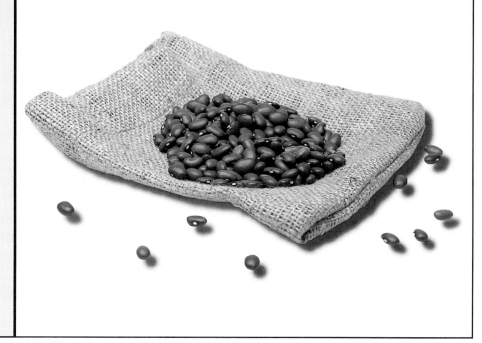

Carbohydrates

The body's main source of energy is carbohydrates. You may know them as starches and sugars. They are found mainly in foods from plant sources, such as fruits, vegetables, grain products, and dry beans and peas. For good health, eat a variety of these foods every day. Generally, they are the least expensive form of energy you can buy.

If you don't eat enough carbohydrates, your body will use the other energy-producing nutrients for energy. When it does this, however,

it keeps those nutrients from doing their specialized jobs.

Depending on their source, carbohydrates fall into one of two categories—complex and simple carbohydrates.

Complex Carbohydrates

Complex carbohydrates are broken down into two subcategories: starches and dietary fiber. Both are found in dry beans, peas, and lentils; vegetables, such as potatoes and corn; and grain products, such as rice, pasta, and breads. Foods high in starch are usually good

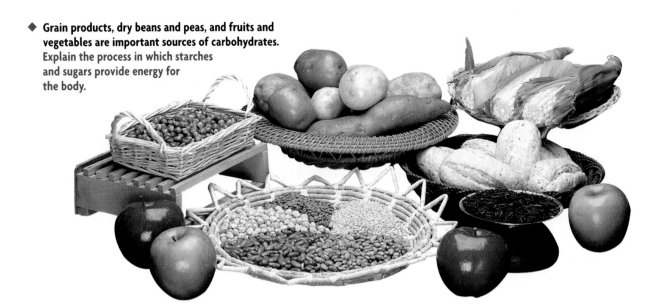

◆ Grain products, dry beans and peas, and fruits and vegetables are important sources of carbohydrates. Explain the process in which starches and sugars provide energy for the body.

sources of proteins, vitamins, minerals, and dietary fiber.

Dietary Fiber

As noted in Section 2-1, dietary fiber is the only form of carbohydrate that does not provide energy. It consists of nondigestible plant materials. This complex carbohydrate is found only in foods from plant sources, such as fruits, vegetables, grain products, and dry beans and peas.

There are two kinds of fiber, insoluble and soluble. Most fiber-containing foods provide both.

Insoluble Fiber

Insoluble fiber is fiber that will not dissolve in water. Insoluble fiber absorbs water, much like a sponge does, and contributes bulk. It helps food move through the large intestine at a normal rate. It promotes regular bowel movements and helps prevent constipation. This type of fiber appears to lower the risk of colon cancer. You can find it mainly in fruit and vegetable skins and in whole wheat or wheat bran products.

Soluble Fiber

Soluble fiber is fiber that dissolves in water. Soluble fiber increases the thickness of the stomach contents. Studies show that it may reduce blood cholesterol levels. You can find soluble fiber in fruits, vegetables, dry beans, peas, lentils, and oat products.

How Much Fiber?

How much fiber do you consume? If you are like most other Americans, you get only about half the recommended fiber intake. The American Dietetic Association recommends 20 to 35 grams of dietary fiber a day for adults. To compute your daily fiber needs during the growth years, which include adolescence, add 5 to your age. For instance, a 14-year-old needs 19 grams of fiber daily (14 + 5).

To get enough fiber, eat a wide variety of plant foods every day. Bean burritos, chili with beans, vegetable stir-fry dishes, and vegetable pizza are all excellent choices. Increase fiber gradually, and be sure to drink plenty of fluids to avoid digestive upset.

Simple Carbohydrates

Simple carbohydrates, or sugars, are a natural part of many foods. These sugars include *fructose* (FROOK-tohs), found in fruits; *maltose* (MALL-tohs), found in grain products; and *lactose* (LACK-tohs), found in dairy products. Most foods that contain these sugars also provide other nutrients, such as proteins, vitamins, and minerals.

Refined sugars are sugars that are extracted from plants and used as a sweetener. The most widely used refined sugar is *sucrose* (SOOK-rohs), or table sugar. Sucrose comes from plants such as sugar cane or sugar beets. Other refined sugars include corn syrup, honey, maple syrup, molasses, and brown sugar. Refined sugars do not supply nutrients other than simple carbohydrates. Eating large amounts of sweetened foods can lead to excess weight, which can contribute to health problems.

Proteins

When it comes to the energy they provide, complex and simple carbohydrates and proteins are all created equal. However, unlike their sweet and starchy counterparts, proteins have unique building roles in the body. They are used mainly to help the body grow and repair worn-out or damaged parts. About one-fifth of your body's total weight is protein. Your hair, eyes, skin, muscles, and bones are made of proteins. The proteins you eat help maintain them in good condition.

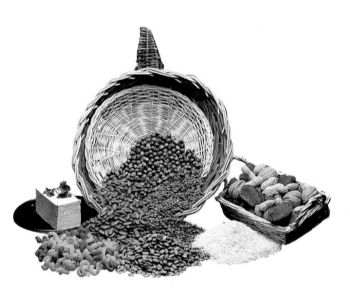

◆ Good sources of protein include animal foods, which are called complete proteins, and plant foods, such as the ones pictured. Describe a meatless meal that would provide the protein your body needs.

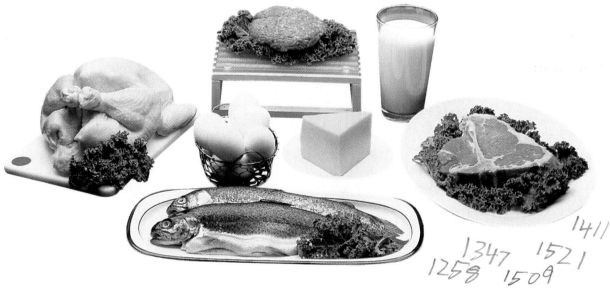

How Much Protein Should You Eat?

To meet the demands of a more active lifestyle and the growth spurt associated with the teen years, your body needs more protein now than it may later in life. How much protein do you need? This formula will help you find out:

1. **Multiply your body weight in pounds by one of the following numbers.** If you are between the ages of 11 and 14 and do light activity, use the number 0.45. If you are between the ages of 15 and 18, use the number 0.40. If you are between the ages of 11 and 18 and are very active—for example, if you participate in a sport—use the number 0.55.

2. **Write the number you arrive at in your Wellness Journal.** This is your recommended daily allowance of protein expressed in grams.

Note: Nutritionists recommend that no more than a third of your protein come from animal sources, which are higher in fat than vegetable sources of protein.

Proteins also regulate important body processes. For instance, they play a major role in fighting disease because parts of the immune system are proteins.

Proteins can do their job only if you consume enough carbohydrates and fats for your energy needs. If not, the body uses proteins for energy instead of for building and repairing.

Proteins are found in all foods from animal sources, including meat, poultry, fish, eggs, and dairy products. They are also found in foods from plant sources, especially dry beans and peas, peanuts, vegetables, and grain products. Most Americans eat more protein than they need. Excess amounts are broken down and stored by the body as fat.

Complete and Incomplete Proteins

Proteins are made of chains of chemical building blocks called **amino** (uh-MEE-noh) **acids**. Just as letters of the alphabet are arranged to make countless different words, so these chemical substances that make up body proteins can be arranged in numerous ways. Your body can make all but 9 of the 22 known amino acids. These nine are called *essential amino acids* because they must come from foods you eat.

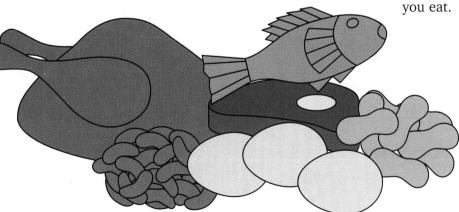

Complete proteins—proteins that supply all nine essential amino acids—include meat, poultry, fish, eggs, dairy products, and soy products. Except for soybeans, all foods from plant sources supply **incomplete proteins**, proteins lacking one or more essential amino acids. Although such foods by themselves fail to deliver all the essential amino acids, it is possible to obtain them all by eating a variety of foods and enough calories throughout the day. This is especially important for people who follow a vegetarian eating plan.

Most Americans get the largest amount of their protein from animal sources. Health experts, however, recommend that people get more of their protein from plant sources. Why? Plant sources generally have less fat, and low-fat choices are recommended. You will learn more about fats in the next section.

INFOLINK

For more information on specific nutrient needs in a vegetarian eating plan, see Section 4-4.

Section 2-2 Review & Activities

1. List three foods that supply simple carbohydrates and six foods that supply complex carbohydrates.

2. Why is it important to obtain both soluble and insoluble fiber?

3. What is the difference between complete and incomplete proteins?

4. Synthesizing. Studies show that most Americans eat less fiber than is needed for good health. Identify some possible reasons this would be true.

5. Analyzing. Years ago it was suggested that sugar was the biggest culprit in weight gain. Is this belief still true? Why or why not?

6. Applying. Think back to the last meal you ate. Which foods supplied carbohydrates? Fiber? Proteins? What types of carbohydrates, fiber, and proteins were they?

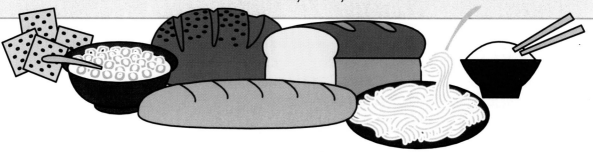

Fats

Objectives

After studying this section, you should be able to:

- Describe the functions and sources of fats.
- Discuss the effects of cholesterol and fatty acids on health.
- Identify three basic types of fatty acids.

Look for These Terms

cholesterol

LDL

HDL

saturated fatty acids

polyunsaturated fatty acids

monounsaturated fatty acids

hydrogenation

"Eat Less Fat!" "New Study Links Disease with Excess Saturated Fat!" Headlines like these seem to be everywhere these days. So, it seems, are fat-free and low-fat foods.

Although reducing fat in your eating plan is sound advice for most people, fat is not always the villain you may have been led to believe. In fact, as you will see, you can't live without some fat.

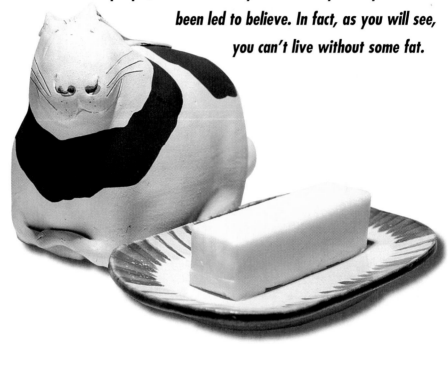

Functions and Sources of Fats

Fats—or, more specifically, substances called *essential fatty acids,* found mainly in vegetable oils—are an essential nutrient with several important functions. Fats promote healthy skin and normal cell growth, and carry vitamins A, D, E, and K to wherever they are needed. In addition, fats stored in the body provide a reserve supply of energy and act as a cushion to protect your heart, liver, and other vital organs.

From a sensory standpoint, fats add flavor to food. Because they move through the digestive system slowly, they help you feel full longer.

What, then, is the problem with fat? Studies show that most Americans eat too much fat—and the wrong kinds. Doing so can increase the risk of illness such as heart disease and cancer. It can also create a health risk by contributing to overweight or obesity. Remember, fats have twice as many calories per gram as carbohydrates or proteins.

◆ **Some of the foods shown here are obvious sources of fat.** Which of the foods pictured do you regularly eat? List other foods that you eat that may contain hidden fat.

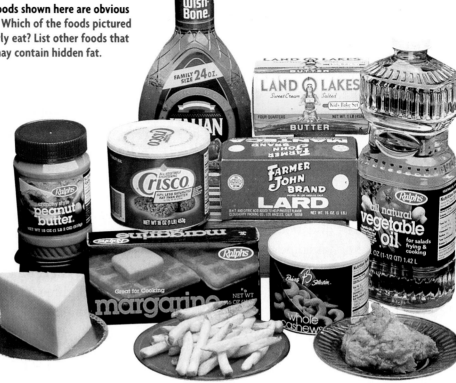

Although fats cannot, nor should not, be eliminated from one's eating plan completely, it is important to limit their use. One way of accomplishing this is to eat more complex carbohydrates. Another is to choose low-fat foods. Foods high in fat include butter, margarine, oils, cream, sour cream, salad dressing, fried foods, some baked goods, and chocolate. Moderate to large amounts of fat are also found in some cuts of meat, nuts and seeds, peanut butter, egg yolks, whole milk, and some cheeses.

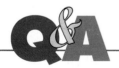

Q Is avoiding fat completely the best approach for healthful eating?

A No. Your body has an essential need for some fat. A good guideline is to follow a low-fat eating plan (less than 30 percent of total calories from fat).

Cholesterol, Fats, and Health

"Is cholesterol the very same thing as fat?" "Do I need any cholesterol, or can I eliminate it from my eating plan?" Questions like these about cholesterol are common. You may have asked some yourself.

What Is Cholesterol?

Cholesterol (kuh-LES-tuhr-ol) is not fat. Rather, it is a fatlike substance present in all body cells that is needed for many essential body processes. It contributes to the digestion of fat and the skin's production of vitamin D. Adults manufacture all the cholesterol they need, mostly in the liver. Infants' and children's bodies, on the other hand, don't produce enough cholesterol. So they need it in their eating plans.

A certain amount of cholesterol circulates in the blood. It does not float through the bloodstream on its own, but in chemical "packages" called lipoproteins (LIH-poh-PROH-teenz). There are two major kinds of lipoproteins, LDL and HDL.

- **LDL**, which stands for "low-density lipoprotein," is a chemical that takes cholesterol from the liver to wherever it is needed in the body. However, if too much LDL cholesterol is circulating, the excess amounts of cholesterol can build up in artery walls. This buildup increases the risk of heart disease or stroke. Thus, LDL cholesterol has come to be called "bad" cholesterol.

- **HDL** stands for "high-density lipoprotein" and refers to a chemical that picks up excess cholesterol and takes it back to the liver, keeping it from causing harm. For this reason, HDL cholesterol has come to be known as "good" cholesterol.

Medical tests can determine the amounts of total cholesterol, LDL cholesterol, and HDL cholesterol in the bloodstream. The risk of heart disease may increase if LDL and total cholesterol levels are too high and if the HDL level is too low.

Making wise food choices can help reduce the amount of harmful cholesterol in the bloodstream. As you will see, both cholesterol and fat in foods may affect blood cholesterol levels. The good news is that cholesterol can't make you fat since it doesn't provide energy.

Cholesterol in Foods

Did you also know that all animals have the ability to manufacture cholesterol? This means that if you eat any animal product, including meat, poultry, and fish, you will likely be consuming some cholesterol. Other foods high in cholesterol are egg yolks, liver and other organ meats, and some shellfish. Eating less of these foods may help reduce blood levels of LDL cholesterol.

Saturated and Unsaturated Fats

For most people, the amounts and types of fats eaten have a greater effect on blood cholesterol levels than does the amount of cholesterol eaten.

The fats found in food, such as butter, chicken fat, or corn oil, are made up of different combinations of *fatty acids*. There are three basic kinds of fatty acids. Each has a different effect on cholesterol levels. All fats include all three kinds of fatty acids, but in varying amounts.

- **Saturated** (SAT-chur-ay-ted) **fatty acids** are fats that appear to raise the level of LDL ("bad") cholesterol in the bloodstream. Foods relatively high in saturated fatty acids include meat, poultry skin, whole-milk dairy products, and the tropical oils— coconut oil, palm oil, and palm kernel oil.

- **Polyunsaturated** (PAH-lee-un-SAT-chur-ay-ted) **fatty acids** are fats that seem to help lower cholesterol levels. Many vegetable oils, such as corn oil, soybean oil, and safflower oil, are high in polyunsaturated fatty acids.

- **Monounsaturated** (MAH-no-un-SAT-chur-ay-ted) **fatty acids** are fats that appear to lower LDL ("bad") cholesterol levels and may help raise levels of HDL. Foods relatively high in monounsaturated fatty acids include olives, olive oil, avocados, peanuts, peanut oil, and canola oil.

A simple rule of thumb is that fats that are solid at room temperature, such as butter, are made up mainly of saturated fatty acids.

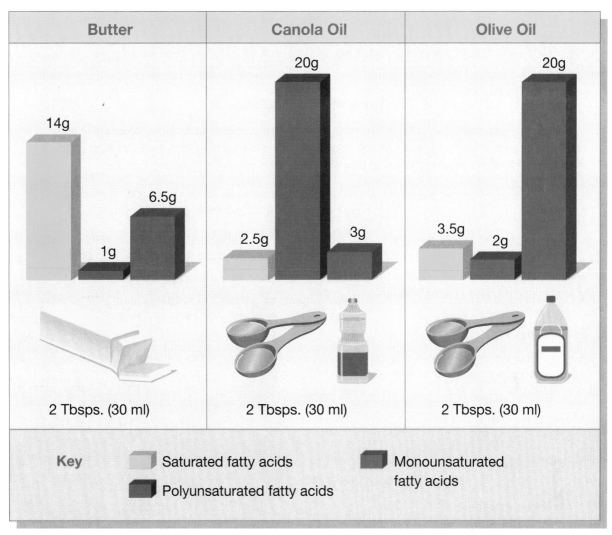

Butter	Canola Oil	Olive Oil

Butter: 14g, 1g, 6.5g — 2 Tbsps. (30 ml)

Canola Oil: 2.5g, 20g, 3g — 2 Tbsps. (30 ml)

Olive Oil: 3.5g, 2g, 20g — 2 Tbsps. (30 ml)

Key
Saturated fatty acids
Polyunsaturated fatty acids
Monounsaturated fatty acids

◆ Butter, canola oil, and olive oil each contain all three types of fatty acids. Identify the type of fat that is highest in each of the following: polyunsaturated fatty acids, saturated fatty acids, and monounsaturated fatty acids.

Fats that are liquid at room temperature, such as corn oil or olive oil, are composed primarily of mainly unsaturated fatty acids.

Hydrogenation

If corn oil is high in polyunsaturated fats, then it would seem logical that margarine made from corn oil is likewise high in poly-unsaturated fats. Unfortunately, this reasoning is flawed. Margarine and vegetable shortening are both examples of hydrogenated fats.

Hydrogenation (hy-DRAH-juh-NAY-shun) is a process in which missing hydrogen atoms are added to an unsaturated fat to make it firmer in texture. Hydrogenation results in a type of fatty acid called *trans fatty acid*. Trans fatty acids have many of the properties of saturated fats.

For better health, many people are making a switch from saturated fats to unsaturated ones. You need to remember too that it's important to limit the total amount of fat eaten.

FOR YOUR HEALTH

Reducing Saturated Fat

For years, consumers cut back on cholesterol, hoping to lower their blood cholesterol levels. However, research now suggests that saturated fat—not cholesterol—is the cause of high blood cholesterol. Here are some ways to cut down on saturated fat, without cutting the flavor.

Instead of . . .

- Butter

- Whole milk
- Ground chuck

Try . . .

- Fruit spread or tub margarine (for spreading)
- Olive oil or canola oil (for frying and stir-frying)
- Applesauce or mashed bananas or prunes (for baking)
- Buttermilk, fat-free milk, or flavored fat-free milk
- Ground round or ground turkey breast meat

Following Up

- Speak with the school nurse, a local physician, or other health professional on other strategies for reducing saturated fat in your eating plan. Share your findings with the class.

Section 2-3 Review & Activities

1. Name two functions of fat. List six foods high in fat.

2. What is cholesterol? Why is LDL cholesterol called "bad" cholesterol?

3. Name three types of fatty acids. Which is considered least healthy? Why? Where is it mainly found?

4. Evaluating. Suppose you are shopping for peanut butter. One brand claims "No Cholesterol" in large letters on the label. The kind you usually buy makes no such claim. Would you switch brands? Why or why not?

5. Comparing and Contrasting. Is switching from butter to olive oil a good approach for weight loss? Why or why not?

6. Applying. Design a magazine ad encouraging people to cut down on fat and cholesterol. Include at least five facts from this section, and point out one common misconception.

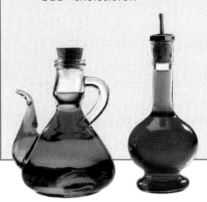

Objectives

After studying this section, you should be able to:

- Identify the types of vitamins and minerals, their functions, and their food sources.

- Tell the potential role phytochemicals play in health.

- Explain the importance of water in the eating plan.

Look for These Terms

antioxidants

water-soluble vitamins

fat-soluble vitamins

major minerals

electrolytes

trace minerals

osteoporosis

phytochemicals

You have probably heard the expression "Good things come in small packages." This expression certainly applies to vitamins and minerals. Although they are among the six key nutrients and are essential for good health, your body requires only the tiniest amounts of them. These micronutrients, along with water and a class of substances called phytochemicals (fy-toh-KEM-ih-kuhls), complete your body's nutrient team.

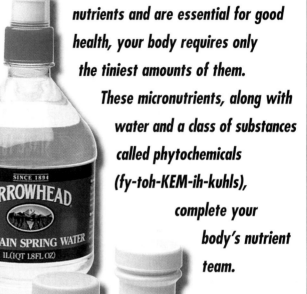

Vitamins

Vitamins help keep your body's tissues healthy and its many systems working properly. They also help carbohydrates, fats, and proteins do their work.

Scientists are still learning about the functions of vitamins. One relatively recent discovery is that some vitamins have antioxidant (an-tee-OKS-ih-dunt) properties.

Antioxidants are substances that protect body cells and the immune system from harmful chemicals in the air, certain foods, and tobacco smoke. Other recent studies suggest that some vitamins may protect against illnesses such as heart disease and cancer. More research is needed, however, before scientists can say for certain what specific roles all the vitamins have in the body.

Types of Vitamins

So far, scientists have identified 13 different vitamins, only one of which—vitamin D—is manufactured by the body. The rest must be derived from food.

Vitamins are classified into two groups:

◆ **Water-soluble vitamins** are vitamins that dissolve in water and thus pass easily into the bloodstream in the process of digestion. Water-soluble vitamins include vitamin C and the eight B vitamins.

◆ **Fat-soluble vitamins** are vitamins that are absorbed and transported by fat. They include vitamins A, D, E, and K.

The charts on pages 71-73 list the functions and food sources of these nutrients.

If you eat more fat-soluble vitamins than you need, they will be stored in the body's fat and in the liver. Your body can draw on these stores when needed. In contrast, water-soluble vitamins remain in your body for only a short time. Therefore, you need them on a daily basis.

Vitamin Sources

Some vitamins can be found in a wide range of foods. Others are limited to just a few food sources. To be sure you are getting the vitamins your body needs, remember the following tips:

◆ Eat plenty of fruits and vegetables every day. These plants are the only naturally occurring source of vitamin C. In particular, eat plenty of dark green vegetables (such as broccoli and spinach) and deep yellow-orange fruits and vegetables (such as carrots, sweet potatoes, and cantaloupe). These foods can help meet your need for vitamin A.

◆ Drink milk. Fortified milk is one of the best sources of vitamin D. The body can also make some vitamin D through the action of sunlight on the skin. That's why it's also called the "sunshine vitamin." If you don't drink fortified milk, be sure to get enough vitamin D from other sources.

◆ When you eat bread or pasta, choose enriched, whole-grain products. These are excellent sources of folate, an important vitamin that builds red blood cells. Other sources include green leafy vegetables, dry beans, and some fruits.

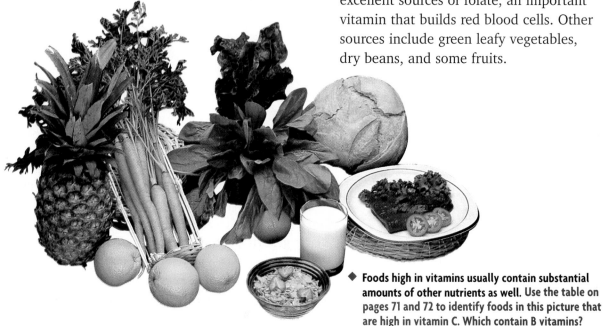

◆ Foods high in vitamins usually contain substantial amounts of other nutrients as well. Use the table on pages 71 and 72 to identify foods in this picture that are high in vitamin C. Which contain B vitamins?

Water-Soluble Vitamins

Vitamin/Functions	Food Sources
Thiamin (Vitamin B$_1$) • Helps turn carbohydrates into energy • Needed for muscle coordination and a healthy nervous system	• Enriched and whole-grain breads and cereals • Dry beans and peas • Lean pork • Liver
Riboflavin (Vitamin B$_2$) • Helps your body release energy from carbohydrates, fats, and proteins	• Enriched breads and cereals • Milk and other dairy products • Green leafy vegetables • Eggs • Meat, poultry, fish
Niacin (Vitamin B$_3$) • Helps your body release energy from carbohydrates, fats, and proteins • Needed for a healthy nervous system and mucous membranes	• Meat, poultry, fish • Enriched and whole-grain breads and cereals • Dry beans and peas • Peanuts, peanut butter
Vitamin B$_6$ • Helps your body use carbohydrates and proteins • Needed for a healthy nervous system • Helps your body make nonessential amino acids, which then make body cells	• Poultry, fish, pork • Dry beans and peas • Nuts • Whole grains • Some fruits and vegetables • Liver and kidneys
Folate (Folacin, Folic acid) • Teams with vitamin B$_{12}$ to help build red blood cells and form genetic material • Helps prevent birth defects • Helps your body use proteins • May help protect against heart disease	• Green leafy vegetables • Dry beans and peas • Fruits • Enriched and whole-grain breads
Vitamin B$_{12}$ • Helps your body use carbohydrates, fats, and proteins • Teams with folate to help build red blood cells and form genetic material • Needed for a healthy nervous system	• Found naturally in animal foods, such as meat, poultry, fish, shellfish, eggs, and dairy products • Some fortified food • Some nutritional yeasts

Water-Soluble Vitamins (cont'd)

Vitamin/Functions	Food Sources
Pantothenic acid • Helps the body release energy from carbohydrates, fats, and proteins • Helps the body produce cholesterol • Needed for a healthy nervous system • Promotes normal growth and development	• Meat, poultry, fish • Eggs • Dry beans and peas • Whole-grain breads and cereals • Milk • Some fruits and vegetables
Biotin • Helps your body use carbohydrates, fats, and proteins	• Green leafy vegetables • Whole-grain breads and cereals • Liver • Egg yolks
Vitamin C (Ascorbic Acid) • Helps maintain healthy capillaries, bones, skin, and teeth • Helps your body heal wounds and resist infections • Aids in absorption of iron • Helps form collagen, which gives structure to bones, cartilage, muscle, and blood vessels • Works as an antioxidant	• Fruits—citrus fruits (orange, grapefruit, tangerine), cantaloupe, guava, kiwi, mango, papaya, strawberries • Vegetables—bell peppers, broccoli, cabbage, kale, plantains, potatoes, tomatoes

Minerals

Like vitamins, minerals are vital for good health. Most minerals become a part of your body, such as your teeth and bones. Others are used to make substances that your body needs.

Types of Minerals

Minerals can be divided into three groups:

◆ **Major minerals** are minerals needed in relatively large amounts. These include calcium, phosphorus, and magnesium.

◆ **Electrolytes** (ee-LEK-troh-lyts) are specific major minerals that work together to maintain the body's fluid balance. These include potassium, sodium, and chloride.

◆ **Trace minerals** are minerals needed in very small amounts, but they are just as important as other nutrients. They include iron, copper, zinc, iodine, and selenium. Scientists continue to research trace minerals and their functions.

Since fat-soluble vitamins are stored in the body's tissues, an excess buildup of them is possible, leading to toxic or other damaging effects. An overdose of vitamin A, for example, can cause nerve and liver damage, bone and joint pain, vomiting, and abnormal bone growth. People who take vitamin supplements are advised to use caution.

Meeting Your Mineral Needs

Though your need for some minerals is small, getting the right amount is important to your health. For example, getting too much or too little iodine can cause thyroid problems. The thyroid gland, located in the neck, produces substances needed for growth and development. For certain individuals, getting too much sodium, or too little potassium, may be linked to high blood pressure.

Fat-Soluble Vitamins

Vitamin/Functions	Food Sources
Vitamin A • Helps protect you from infections • Helps form and maintain healthy skin, hair, mucous membranes, bones, and teeth • Helps you see normally at night • Works as an antioxidant	• Dairy products • Liver • Egg yolks • Foods high in beta carotene (see phytochemicals, p. 78)
Vitamin D • Helps your body use calcium and phosphorus • Helps your body build strong and healthy bones and teeth	• Fortified dairy products • Egg yolks • Higher-fat fish—salmon and mackerel • Fortified breakfast cereals and margarine
Vitamin E • Works as an antioxidant	• Nuts and seeds • Green leafy vegetables • Wheat germ • Vegetable oils
Vitamin K • Necessary for blood to clot normally	• Green leafy vegetables • Fruits and other vegetables • Dairy products • Egg yolks • Wheat bran and wheat germ

Getting the right balance of minerals is not difficult. The key is to eat a wide variety of foods. However, you may need to pay special attention to whether you are getting enough calcium and iron—two major minerals especially important for teens.

Calcium and Strong Bones

As noted in the chart on page 75, calcium has several important functions. One of these is to maintain bone strength. Lack of calcium throughout life is one of the factors that can lead to **osteoporosis** (AH-stee-oh-puh-ROH-sis). This is a condition in which the bones become porous, making them weak and fragile. As a result, posture may become stooped and bones can break easily. Osteoporosis affects over 25 million Americans, both men and women. The condition is most common in women. It is estimated that up to 50 percent of women over age 45 and 90 percent of women over age 75 have osteoporosis.

You can lessen your risk of osteoporosis, but you need to start now. Bone mass builds up during childhood, the teen years, and young adulthood. The more you do to build strong, healthy bones now, the less likely you will be to develop osteoporosis when you are older.

Here are some "bone-building" tips you can follow:

◆ Eat plenty of calcium-rich foods. These include dairy products, dry beans and peas, and dark green, leafy vegetables.

◆ Follow other basic guidelines for healthy eating. Remember, nutrients work in teams. Like best friends on a team, vitamin D and many other nutrients work together with calcium.

◆ Play a sport, take part in some other vigorous activity, or exercise regularly. Weight-bearing exercise, such as walking or jogging, and weight training help build and maintain strong bones.

◆ Avoid tobacco products, alcohol, and excess caffeine (found in coffee, tea, and soft drinks). All may contribute to osteoporosis.

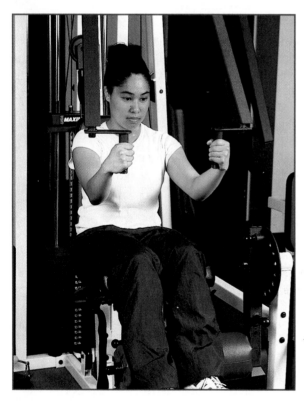

◆ **Weight-resistance training, which includes the activity shown here, helps build and maintain strong bones.** Name two foods you can eat that aid in this process. Identify the nutrient contained in these foods.

Iron and Red Blood Cells

Iron is essential for making hemoglobin (HEE-muh-gloh-buhn), a substance in your red blood cells that carries oxygen to all the cells in your body. If you don't get enough iron, your blood may not be able to carry enough oxygen to your cells. The resulting condition is called *iron-deficiency anemia* (uh-NEE-mee-uh). People with anemia are often tired, weak, short of breath, and pale.

Where can you find iron? Some sources are lean red meat, dry beans and peas, dried fruits, grain products, and dark green, leafy vegetables. Eating foods rich in vitamin C at the same time as foods rich in iron helps the body absorb more of the iron from plant foods. Interestingly, the iron content of foods cooked in an iron skillet gets a boost. Researchers disagree, however, on how much iron can be absorbed from this source.

Major Minerals

Mineral/Functions	Food Sources
Calcium • Helps build bone and maintain bone strength • Helps prevent osteoporosis • Helps regulate blood clotting, nerve activity, and other body processes • Needed for muscle contraction, including the heart	• Dairy products • Canned fish with edible bones • Dry beans, peas, and lentils • Dark green, leafy vegetables—broccoli, spinach, and turnip greens • Tofu made with calcium sulfate • Calcium-fortified orange juice and soy milk
Phosphorus • Works with calcium to build strong bones and teeth • Helps release energy from carbohydrates, fats, and proteins • Helps build body cells and tissues	• Meat, poultry, fish • Eggs • Nuts • Dry beans and peas • Dairy products • Grain products
Magnesium • Helps build bones and make proteins • Helps nerves and muscles work normally	• Whole-grain products • Green vegetables • Dry beans and peas • Nuts and seeds

Electrolytes

Mineral/Functions	Food Sources
Sodium • Helps maintain the fluid balance in your body • Helps with muscle and nerve action • Helps regulate blood pressure	• Table salt • Processed foods
Chloride • Helps maintain the fluid balance in your body • Helps transmit nerve signals	• Table salt
Potassium • Helps maintain the fluid balance in your body • Helps maintain the heartbeat • Helps with muscle and nerve action • Helps maintain normal blood pressure	• Fruits—bananas and oranges • Vegetables • Meat, poultry, fish • Dry beans and peas • Dairy products

Trace Minerals

Mineral/Functions	Food Sources
Iron • Helps carry oxygen in the blood • Helps your cells use oxygen	• Meat, fish, shellfish • Egg yolks • Dark green, leafy vegetables • Dry beans and peas • Enriched or whole-grain products • Dried fruits
Iodine • Responsible for your body's use of energy	• Saltwater fish • Iodized salt
Copper • Helps iron make red blood cells • Helps keep your bones, blood vessels, and nerves healthy • Helps your heart work properly	• Whole-grain products • Seafood • Organ meats • Dry beans and peas • Nuts and seeds

Trace Minerals (cont'd)

Mineral/Functions	Food Sources
Zinc • Helps your body make proteins, heal wounds, and form blood • Helps in growth and maintenance of all tissues • Helps your body use carbohydrates, fats, and proteins • Affects the senses of taste and smell • Helps your body use vitamin A	• Meat, liver, poultry, fish, shellfish • Dairy products • Dry beans and peas, peanuts • Whole-grain breads and cereals • Eggs • Miso (fermented soybean paste)
Selenium • Helps your heart work properly • Works as an antioxidant	• Whole-grain breads and cereals • Vegetables (amount varies with content in soil) • Meat, organ meats, fish, shellfish
Fluoride • Helps strengthen teeth and prevent cavities	• In many communities, small amounts are added to the water supply to help improve dental health.

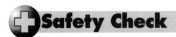

Safety Check

Rich in many vitamins and minerals, eggs can be a valuable contribution to a healthful eating plan. However, if eggs aren't handled properly, a food-borne organism called salmonella can grow. Don't keep eggs and egg-rich foods between 40 and 140° F (4 and 60° C) ("the temperature danger zone") for more than two hours.

Phytochemicals

If you look up *phytochemical* in a dictionary, you will find that this word (from the Greek *phyton*, or "plant") was coined over 150 years ago. It was only in the last decade that an important scientific discovery—the presence of disease-fighting nutrients in plant foods—gave a new meaning to the term **phytochemical**.

Current estimates suggest that every plant has at least 50 to 100 different phytochemicals. So far, most of the research has concentrated on identifying and classifying these substances, though early studies hint that many may play important roles in reducing the risks of cancer and other diseases. Some phytochemicals, like vitamins, are antioxidants.

One of the best-known phytochemicals is beta carotene (bay-tuh KAR-uh-teen), a substance that gives fruits and vegetables their bright yellow-orange and dark green colors. Beta carotene is an antioxidant believed to prevent certain kinds of cancer. The body uses beta carotene to produce vitamin A.

The following table lists just a few of the phytochemicals being studied.

Phytochemicals

Phytochemical	Food Source	Potential Health Benefits
Beta carotene	• Yellow and orange fruits and vegetables • Dark green vegetables	• May play role in slowing the progression of cancer
Allyl sulfides	• Onions, garlic, leeks, chives, shallots	• May play role in cancer prevention • May play role in lowering blood pressure and cholesterol
Indoles	• Cabbage, broccoli, kale, cauliflower	• May play role in cancer prevention
Saponins	• Soybeans, dry beans, peas • Most vegetables	• May prevent cancer cells from multiplying
Lutein	• Kale, spinach, collards, mustard greens, romaine lettuce	• May protect against blindness
Phytosterol	• Soybeans and some soy products • Nuts • Whole-grain products • Many vegetable oils	• May play role in cancer prevention • May lower cholesterol

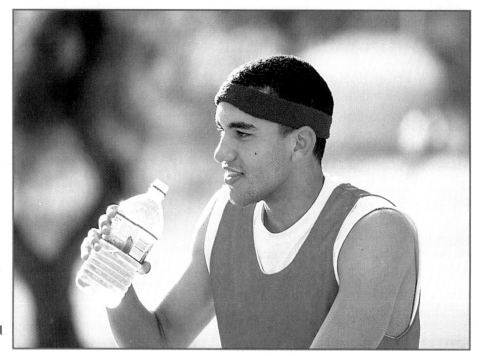

◆ Health experts highly recommend drinking at least 8 glasses of water each day. Name two foods that are good sources of this essential nutrient.

Water

Often called the "forgotten nutrient," water is actually the one most critical to our survival. You may be able to live for weeks without food, but you can live only a few days without water.

About 50 to 60 percent of your body is water. Your blood is 80 percent water.

Water plays a role in many chemical reactions that constantly go on in the body. It also helps keep the body temperature normal. Think of what happens when you get too warm. You begin to perspire. As the perspiration evaporates into the air, it cools your body. Water also helps your body get rid of waste products.

On average, the body uses about 2 to 3 quarts (2 to 3 L) of water a day. To help replace this lost fluid, be sure to drink at least 8 cups (2 L) of water daily. During strenuous physical activity or in hot weather, when you perspire heavily, you usually need even more. A good rule of thumb is to drink 1 cup (250 mL) of water for every ½ pound (250 g) of weight lost through perspiration.

Eight cups of water daily may seem like a large amount. To make it easier to get the amount of water you need, keep bottles of water on hand. Carrying a sipper bottle filled with water is one convenient way to help

meet your daily need. If you like, flavor it with a little fresh lemon juice.

Other liquids, such as milk, fruit juice, and soup, can also help supply your body with water. So can fresh fruits and vegetables, most of which contain large amounts of water. Did you know that watermelon is over 90 percent water?

FOR YOUR HEALTH

Water, Water Everywhere

Don't wait until you are thirsty to drink water. By the time you feel thirsty, you may have already lost a quart (liter) of water or more. To stay well hydrated when water or other beverages are not handy, eat foods with a high water content. Here are a few:

Food	Percent Water by Weight
Lettuce	95
Watermelon	92
Grapefruit	91
Yogurt	75

Following Up

1. Find out about other foods that may have at least 75 percent water.

2. Keep a food and beverage log in your Wellness Journal for one day. Total the approximate amount of water you get, including water, beverages, and foods with high water content.

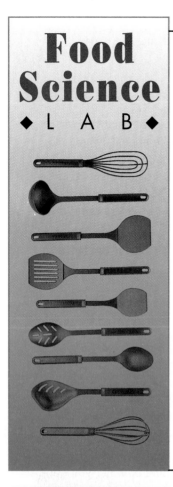

How Much Water Is in Food?

Meeting daily fluid needs can seem challenging to many people. However, many foods contain a lot of water. Which foods have the most? You are about to find out.

Procedure

1. Weigh a raw potato, apple, and carrot, and record the weight of each.

2. Place one of the foods in a food processor, and process until it is a liquidy mash. Pour and scrape the food into a strainer, forcing out as much liquid as possible. Weigh the liquid, and measure it.

3. Calculate the percentage of water by comparing the liquid weight with the original weight.

4. Repeat with each of the remaining foods.

Conclusions

◆ Which food had the highest water content? Which had the lowest?

◆ Do you think it is possible to meet at least half (4 cups; 4 L) of your water needs through solid food? Explain.

◆ Repeat the experiment using a slice of bread. Predict the percentage that is water. Was your prediction right?

Section 2-4 Review & Activities

1. Which vitamins are fat-soluble? Water-soluble? Why is this distinction important?

2. Why do you need calcium? Iron? What foods provide these nutrients?

3. How much water do you need to drink each day to replenish your body's water supply?

4. Define *phytochemical*. Explain the potential role of phytochemicals in good health.

5. Evaluating. Why are trace minerals just as important as other minerals, even though they are needed in such small amounts?

6. Comparing and Contrasting. Cereal A is high in fiber (7 grams per serving) with 75 percent of seven vitamins and minerals. Cereal B is low in fiber (1 gram per serving) with 100 percent of the same seven vitamins and minerals. Which would you choose? Why?

7. Applying. Use the information from this section to create a vitamin and mineral checklist. Armed with your checklist, determine which vitamin and mineral needs can be met by the foods available in your home. Discuss your findings with an adult in your home.

How Your Body Uses Food

While you are reading this page, your body is busily working—inhaling oxygen from the air and exhaling waste products. Your heart is busy, too. In the time it takes to read this paragraph, about 100 million of your body cells will die and new ones will take their place. If you ate in the last several hours, your digestive system is breaking down the food into nutrients.

Objectives

After studying this section, you should be able to:

- Outline the process of digestion.
- Explain how nutrients are absorbed, transported, and stored.
- Tell how the body uses food to produce energy.

Look for These Terms

digestion

esophagus

peristalsis

glucose

glycogen

oxidation

basal metabolism

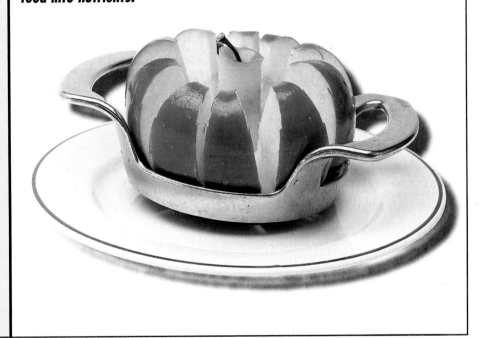

Digestion

The process of breaking down food into usable nutrients is known as **digestion**. It takes place in the digestive system, a long, hollow tube that extends from the mouth through the entire body. Here is what happens to food on its journey through the digestive system.

The Mouth

The digestive process starts before you even begin to eat the food. Just smelling and seeing food, or even thinking about it, can start saliva flowing in your mouth. Saliva is the first of many digestive juices that act on food to break it down chemically.

Food is also broken down physically as your teeth grind it into tiny pieces. Chewing food well is important. It mixes the food with saliva and makes it easier to swallow and digest. Solid food should be chewed until it is the consistency of applesauce.

◆ **Each part of the digestive tract has a specific role in breaking food down into nutrients.** In what body organ does digestion begin?

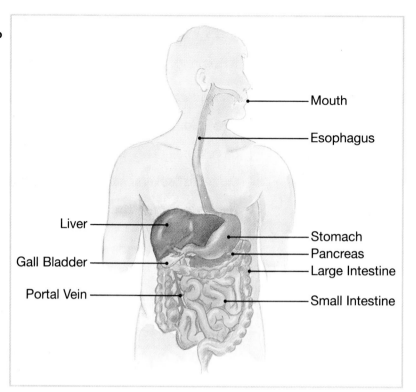

Mouth
Esophagus
Liver
Gall Bladder
Portal Vein
Stomach
Pancreas
Large Intestine
Small Intestine

The Esophagus

Once the food is swallowed, it passes into the **esophagus** (ih-SOFF-uh-gus), a long tube connecting the mouth to the stomach. The muscles of the esophagus contract and relax, creating a series of wavelike movements that force the food into the stomach. This muscular action is called **peristalsis** (PEHR-uh-STAHL-suhs).

The Stomach

The stomach, the next stop on the digestive journey, is the widest part of the digestive system. It is a muscular pouch located on the left side of your body inside the rib cage. On the average, your stomach can hold about 4 cups (1 L) of food.

The walls of the stomach manufacture gastric juices—a combination of acid and enzymes that helps in the chemical breakdown of the food. In addition, the stomach breaks food down physically through peristalsis. The food is churned until it turns into a thick liquid called chyme (KIME).

Different kinds of food take different amounts of time to break down and leave the stomach. Think of your stomach as a holding tank. Carbohydrates take the shortest amount of time, usually one to two hours. Proteins take longer, about three to five hours. Fats take the longest time to digest, up to seven hours. That is why a food with fat will keep you from feeling hungry for a longer time.

The Small Intestine

From the stomach, chyme is released into the small intestine a little at a time. The small intestine is a long, winding tube between the stomach and the large intestine. Here, the chyme is acted on by three types of digestive juices:

◆ Bile, a substance that helps your body digest and absorb fats. Bile is produced in the liver and stored in the gall bladder until needed.

◆ Pancreatic (pan-kree-AT-ik) juice, which contains enzymes that help break down carbohydrates, proteins, and fats. It is produced by the pancreas (PAN-kree-us), a gland connected to the small intestine.

◆ Intestinal juice, produced in the small intestine. This digestive fluid works with the others to break down food.

When fully broken down, carbohydrates are turned into a simple sugar called glucose (GLOO-kohs). **Glucose** is the body's basic fuel supply. Fats are changed into fatty acids. Proteins are broken down into amino acids. Vitamins, minerals, and water do not need to be broken down—they're ready for action just as they are. They can be used by your body in the same form in which they occur in food.

Using the Nutrients

Once food has been broken down into nutrients, digestion is complete. However, your body still has work to do. It must absorb the nutrients and take them to where they can be used or stored.

Absorption

After digestion, the nutrients are absorbed into the bloodstream. Most absorption takes place in your small intestine. The lining of the small intestine is arranged in folds. It is lined with billions of tiny fingerlike projections, called villi (VIL-eye). The villi increase the surface area of the intestine so that more nutrients can be absorbed.

After absorption, some waste mineral, including fiber, is left in the small intestine. This waste material is moved into the large intestine, also called the colon. The colon removes water, potassium, and sodium from the waste. The remainder is stored as a semi-solid in the rectum (REK-tum), or lower part of the intestine, until it is eliminated.

Processing and Storing Nutrients

After the nutrients are absorbed by the villi of the small intestine, they are carried through a blood vessel, called the portal vein, to the liver. One of the liver's many jobs is to turn nutrients into forms the body can use. For instance, it converts amino acids into different kinds of proteins. Then the proteins are carried by the blood to wherever they are needed.

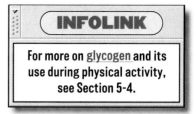

INFOLINK

For more on glycogen and its use during physical activity, see Section 5-4.

Some nutrients, if not needed immediately, can be stored for future use. Extra glucose, for example, is converted by the liver into **glycogen** (GLY-kuh-juhn), a storage form of glucose. Glycogen is stored in the liver and the muscles. If there is more glucose than can be stored as glycogen, the rest is converted to body fat. Fats are then deposited throughout the body as an energy reserve. Excess fatty acids and amino acids are also converted to body fat.

Minerals are stored in various ways. For instance, iron is stored in the liver and in bone marrow. Fat-soluble vitamins are stored mainly in the liver and in body fat.

Some nutrients, including most water-soluble vitamins, are not stored for long periods. If not needed, they are removed from the body with wastes.

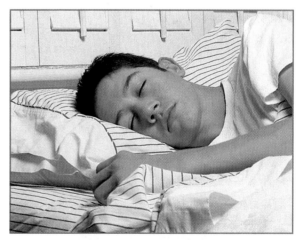

◆ **Even when you are asleep your body continues to work and renew itself.** Name the type of energy your body uses during periods of rest.

How Nutrients Are Used

Nutrients and oxygen are carried through-out the bloodstream to individual cells, where they are used for specialized purposes. As you may recall, one of these is to provide energy. This is done by combining glucose with water. Such a process in which fuel is combined with oxygen to produce energy is known as **oxidation** (AHKS-ih-day-shuhn). Another example of oxidation is a log burning in a fireplace. The fuel in that case is wood. To keep burning, the wood must have oxygen from the air. Energy is produced as light and heat.

In your body, the fuel is glucose. When glucose reaches the cells, it is combined with oxygen. The result is energy as heat and power for the cells.

Your body uses energy for two basic purposes:

◆ *Automatic processes,* such as breathing, digesting food, and creating new cells. Even when you are resting or sleeping,

your body is using minimal amounts of energy. This minimum amount of energy required to maintain the life processes in a living organism is called **basal metabolism** (BAY-zuhl muh-TAB-uh-lih-zuhm).

◆ *Physical activities,* such as work and exercise. The more active you are, the more energy you use. For instance, you would use more energy walking up a flight of stairs than riding in an elevator.

Generally, about two-thirds of the calories used by the body are for basal metabolism. However, this varies from person to person. It depends on factors such as age, body size, and body composition—the ratio of lean tissue to fat. The amount of energy used for basal metabolism is sometimes called the *basal metabolic rate,* or BMR.

As you can see, the human body is an amazing organism. Without even thinking about it, your body carries on thousands of complex processes every moment of your life.

Section 2-5 Review & Activities

1. How do nutrients get from the digestive system to the bloodstream?

2. Name two ways in which excess glucose can be stored.

3. What two substances combine to produce energy in the cells? What is the process called?

4. Analyzing. If someone had a portion of the small intestine removed because of a disease, what nutritional problems could result?

5. Comparing and Contrasting. On Monday, Ben's lunch provided 500 calories and was 90 percent fat, 10 percent protein. On Tuesday, lunch provided 600 calories and was 30 percent fat, 10 percent protein, 60 percent carbohydrate. Which meal do you think stayed in Ben's stomach longer? Why?

6. Applying. Sketch a design for a poster or bulletin board showing how food is broken down into nutrients and how nutrients travel through the body.

CAREER WANTED

Individuals who love science, can reason mathematically, and work well independently.

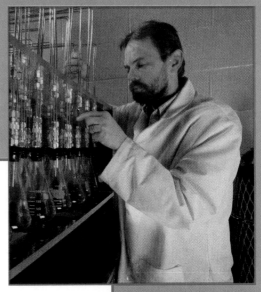

REQUIRES:

- advanced degree in food science or related field
- research and development skills

"An inquisitive mind is a plus!"

says Food Scientist Raynaud Kelly

Q: Raynaud, what you do as a food scientist?

A: I help develop a wide range of vitamins, carotenoids, and polyunsaturated fatty acids supplied to leading companies in the pharmaceutical and food industries. I also customize vitamin mixes for newly manufactured food products.

Q: Do you need to be a whiz at science to become a food scientist?

A: I didn't get all "A's" in science, but a strong science background is required to be a successful food scientist.

Q: What's the most difficult part of your job?

A: My job can be frustrating at times. Research is very time-consuming and much of my day is spent working alone. My lab experiments have to meet exact specifications and high quality standards.

Q: What's the most satisfying aspect of your job?

A: I enjoy combining my results with others to create successful products. My inquisitive mind is a definite plus. The most satisfying part of my job is knowing that my research ultimately leads to nutritious products that may help improve people's health.

Career Research Activity

1. Conduct a web search for "food scientist." Based on the information you find, design a brochure about the career opportunities in food science.

2. Write a "career path" story that explains how being a caterer's helper and then a laboratory test technician helps prepare you for careers in food science, pharmacy, and/or nutrition.

Related Career Opportunities

Entry Level
- Data Clerk
- Cashier
- Caterer's Helper

Technical Level
- Quality Assurance Analyst
- Dietetic Assistant
- Laboratory Test Technician

Professional Level
- Food Scientist
- Nutritionist
- Pharmacist

Chapter 2 Review & Activities

Summary

Section 2-1: The Role of Nutrients

- The six major types of nutrients work as a team.
- Lack of or excess of certain nutrients can result in poor health.
- Recommended amounts have been set for some nutrients.
- The energy supplied by nutrients is measured in calories.

Section 2-4: Micronutrients

- Each vitamin and mineral has specific functions and food sources.
- Some minerals are needed in large amounts and others in small amounts.
- Phytochemicals may prevent diseases.
- Every day you must replace the water lost by the body.

Section 2-2: Carbohydrates, Fiber, and Proteins

- Carbohydrates include complex and simple carbohydrates.
- Both soluble and insoluble fiber are important for good health.
- Complete protein can be obtained by eating animal foods or a wide variety of plant foods.

Section 2-5: How Your Body Uses Food

- Digestion is the process of breaking down food into usable nutrients.
- After digestion, nutrients are absorbed and put to use.
- Some nutrients can be stored if not needed right away.
- The bloodstream carries nutrients to all the cells in the body.
- Glucose and oxygen combine to produce energy for physical activities and basal metabolism.

Section 2-3: Fats

- Fats perform several important jobs.
- Eating too much fat is linked with several health problems.
- The three types of fatty acids—saturated, polyunsaturated, and monounsaturated—appear to have different effects on blood cholesterol levels.
- Experts recommend that people limit their intake of total fat, saturated fat, and cholesterol.

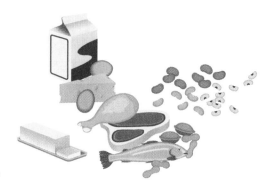

Checking Your Knowledge

1. Name two examples of DRIs and explain how they differ.

2. What percentage of daily calories should come from carbohydrates? From proteins? From fats?

3. What are two types of dietary fiber? List two food sources for each type.

4. What are proteins made of? Why are plant proteins considered incomplete?

5. What is the difference between HDL and LDL cholesterol?

6. Which type of fatty acid is corn oil highest in? Olive oil? Coconut oil?

7. How does your body use beta carotene? In what foods is it found?

8. Which minerals are electrolytes? What do electrolytes do?

9. Name four digestive juices. In what part of the digestive system does each do its work?

10. What is basal metabolism?

Thinking Critically

1. Determining Accuracy. An advertisement claims that a special nutrient supplement will "meet all your daily nutrient needs." What is wrong with this claim?

2. Comparing and Contrasting. One frozen dinner boasts "only 300 calories per serving." The nutrition information shows that the dinner contains 20 grams of fat. A similar product lists 400 calories and contains 10 grams of fat. How do these foods differ? How do they reflect recommendations from nutritionists?

Working IN THE Lab

1. *Taste Test.* Taste samples of ripe fresh fruits provided by your teacher. Which do you think are highest in natural sugar?

2. *Food Science.* Rub a sample of butter or margarine on a piece of white paper. Label the spot left by the butter. Do the same with samples of ten different foods, such as cheese, a potato, an apple, and a cookie. Let the paper dry for 15 minutes. Which foods left a translucent spot that did not disappear? How do those spots compare with the spot left by the butter? What do you conclude?

Reinforcing Key Skills

1. Communication. Reanne, who has iron-deficiency anemia, has been instructed by her physician to cut back on red meat because of her high cholesterol. What solutions can you propose to Reanne?

2. Management. Veejay is overweight. He lives with his father in a tiny apartment without a kitchen. In the main room they have a microwave and a small refrigerator/freezer. They eat only microwaved frozen pizzas and "fast food." Within the constraints posed by his environment, what steps can Veejay take to improve his and his father's food choices?

Making Decisions and Solving Problems

Your uncle tells you he has decided to increase the fiber in his eating plan. Since he hasn't eaten much fiber before, he plans to eat twice the recommended amount for several days. He asks your opinion.

Making Connections

1. Math. Collect and bring to class three food labels that include nutrition information. Multiply the number of grams of saturated fat by 9 to find the number of saturated fat calories per serving. Divide that number by the total calories from fat. Then multiply by 100 to get the percentage of saturated fat compared with total fat. What does this percentage mean for heart health? Compare results with classmates. Hint: An easier way to calculate this percentage is by using grams instead of calories.

2. Social Studies and Health. In regions of the world where food is scarce, certain nutrient deficiencies are common. Using library resources, find information about three specific deficiency diseases. What are the symptoms? How can each disease be prevented? How can each be treated?

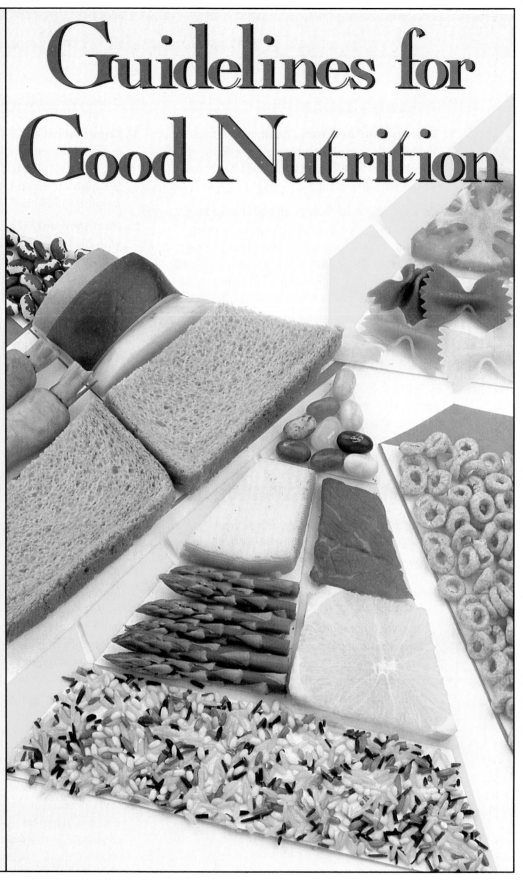

CHAPTER 3

Guidelines for Good Nutrition

Section 3-1
Dietary Guidelines

Section 3-2
The Food Guide Pyramid

Section 3-3
Separating Fact from Fiction

Jenna could scarcely believe her eyes when she first saw the buffet with its endless parade of gleaming dishes and bowls. How would she decide? Go with what she knows or try something new?

Decisions relating to food can be difficult. In this chapter, you will learn what you need to know to make informed, healthful food choices.

Dietary Guidelines

Whether you are deciding what to have for breakfast or packing food supplies for a two-week camping trip, making food choices that promote good health is a difficult challenge. Just think of the thousands of foods and food products lining the shelves in your supermarket. How can you tell which items will give your body the nutrients it needs?

Objectives

After studying this section, you should be able to:

- Discuss what the *Dietary Guidelines for Americans* contributes to good health.
- Explain how each Dietary Guideline contributes to good health.
- Describe ways of reducing fats and sodium in your eating plan.

Look for These Terms

moderation

lifestyle diseases

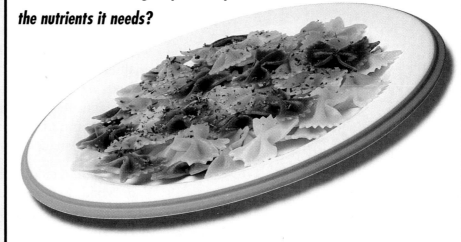

Dietary Guidelines for Americans

To help you make this decision, the U.S. Department of Agriculture (USDA) and U.S. Department of Health and Human Services have published a helpful set of guidelines called the *Dietary Guidelines for Americans*.

The Dietary Guidelines offer six main recommendations, each of which will be explored in this section. These recommendations are

- Eat a variety of foods.

- Balance the food you eat with physical activity—to maintain or improve your weight.

- Choose a diet with plenty of grain products, vegetables, and fruits.

- Choose a diet low in fat, saturated fat, and cholesterol.

- Choose a diet moderate in sugars.

- Choose a diet moderate in salt and sodium.

Following these guidelines will help decrease your risk of eating-related illness now and in the future.

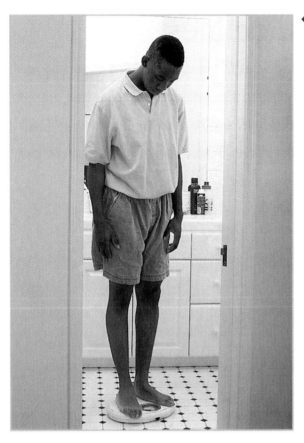

◆ Maintaining a healthful weight can help reduce the risk of lifestyle-related health problems such as high blood pressure. Analyze the statement "A person's eating patterns alone are not enough to ensure total health, even if the person is at an appropriate weight."

A concept that goes hand in hand with variety is **moderation**—avoiding extremes. Do you know someone who eats just a few favorite foods regularly and avoids other foods altogether? People who limit the variety of foods they eat are missing out on essential nutrients. By eating moderately sized servings of many different kinds of foods, you get a wider variety of nutrients for good health.

Keep in mind that there are no "bad" or "good" foods. Any food that supplies nutrients can be part of a healthful eating plan. The key is to balance your food choices so that, overall, they lead to good health. Variety and moderation can help you do just that.

Balance Food Intake with Physical Activity

Balancing the foods you eat with physical activity can help you stay at or reach a weight that is right for you. One-fifth of all teens in the United States today are overweight.

Generally, a few extra pounds can't do much harm. Being truly overweight, however, poses a serious health risk. It may contribute to one or more **lifestyle diseases**—illnesses that relate to how a person lives and the choices he or she makes. These diseases include high blood pressure, heart disease, stroke, diabetes, and certain kinds of cancer.

Being too thin can also be a problem. It may mean that you are not eating enough to meet your body's energy and nutrient needs.

Eat a Variety of Foods

You may know the expression "Variety is the spice of life." When it comes to choosing the foods that make up your eating plan, variety is a good way of making sure you get all the nutrients your body needs. As you learned in Section 2-1, scientists have identified about 40 different nutrients. By eating a variety of foods, you can be sure you get all the nutrients you need, as well as some that have not yet been identified.

No single food can supply all nutrients in the amounts you need. For instance, sweet potatoes are packed with vitamins A and C and fiber, but have no calcium or phosphorus. Fat-free milk is a good source of calcium and phosphorus, but has no fiber and little vitamin C. As you can see, you need to eat a variety of foods for good health.

Maintaining a healthful weight is a balancing act. As noted earlier, food provides energy, and physical activity uses up energy. The key is to balance the energy supplied by the food you eat with the energy your body uses.

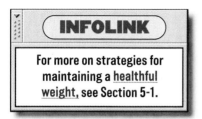

INFOLINK

For more on strategies for maintaining a <u>healthful weight,</u> see Section 5-1.

Choose Plenty of Grain Products, Vegetables, and Fruits

Most of the calories supplied by the food you eat should come from grain products, vegetables, and fruits. They are considered the foundation of a healthful eating plan for several reasons:

◆ Grain products, vegetables, and fruits are key sources of the carbohydrates your body needs for energy. As noted in Chapter 2, carbohydrates should supply about 60 percent of your calories.

◆ Dietary fiber is found only in foods from plant sources. Because these foods contain different types of fiber, choose a variety of grain products, vegetables, and fruits to be sure you get the fiber your body needs.

◆ Grain products, vegetables, and fruits are excellent sources of many vitamins and minerals essential to health. Take another look at the vitamin and mineral charts in Section 2-4. Notice how many of the nutrients listed there are supplied by grain products, vegetables, and fruits. Some nutrients, such as vitamin C and beta carotene, are found only in fruits and vegetables.

◆ Most grain products, vegetables, and fruits are low in fat. Eating more of these foods can help you cut down on the amount of fat in your eating plan—as long as you don't add high-fat toppings, such as butter, sour cream, or rich sauces.

Get in the habit of eating more grain products, vegetables, and fruits. Think of them as central to your food choices rather than as extras to have "on the side." With so many flavorful choices available, you'll find it to be an enjoyable habit as well as a healthful one.

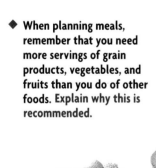

◆ When planning meals, remember that you need more servings of grain products, vegetables, and fruits than you do of other foods. Explain why this is recommended.

Limit Fat and Cholesterol

There are several reasons why the Dietary Guidelines encourage people to eat less fat and cholesterol. A high-fat eating plan is linked with various lifestyle diseases. Regularly choosing foods high in fat can lead to over-weight or other medical problems.

Health experts have suggested the following goals regarding fat in your daily food choices:

◆ **Total fat:** 30 percent or less of the calories you eat. Section 2-1 shows how to calculate the amount of fat that is equal to 30 percent of the day's total calories.

◆ **Saturated fat:** 10 percent or less of your calories. Remember, the highest proportions of saturated fatty acids are found in animal fats and in tropical oils, such as coconut, palm, and palm kernel oil.

◆ **Cholesterol:** Limit the amount of cholesterol eaten. Only foods from animal sources contain cholesterol.

Visible and Invisible Fats

Studies show that on the average, Americans get 34 percent of calories from fat. Many people are unaware of how much fat is in the food they eat.

Some fat is called *visible fat* because it is easily seen. For example, you can see the butter on a baked potato or the layer of fat around a pork chop. People are usually aware of these sources of fats in foods.

Much of the fat people eat, however, is *invisible fat.* It is a part of the chemical composition of the food and cannot be seen. Foods such as whole milk, cheese, egg yolks, nuts, and avocados are loaded with invisible fat. So are fried foods and baked goods.

Suggestions for Lowering Fat

High-Fat Food	Low-Fat Alternative	Fat Savings
Whole milk (1 cup/250 mL)	Fat-free milk	8 grams less fat
Fried chicken (3 oz./84 g)	Baked chicken without skin	8 grams less fat
Regular salad dressing (1 Tbsp./15 mL)	Flavored vinegar, lemon juice, or fat-free dressing	9 grams less fat
Potato chips (1 oz./28 g)	Plain popcorn, air popped (1 cup/250 mL)	10 grams less fat
Premium ice cream (½ cup/125 mL)	Low-fat frozen yogurt	20 grams less fat
Cheddar cheese (1 oz./28 g)	Part-skim mozzarella	4 grams less fat
Sour cream on a baked potato (2 Tbsp./30 mL)	Plain nonfat yogurt Salsa	6 grams less fat

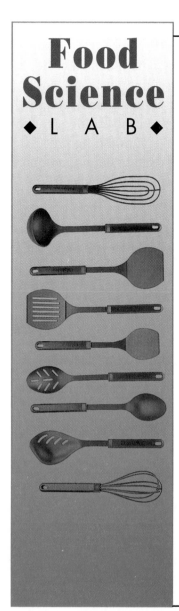

Food Science ◆ L A B ◆

Making Invisible Fats Visible

Have you ever seen a magician make an object seem to suddenly appear? You are about to do something similar. This isn't an illusion. You are about to make the invisible fat in foods visible!

Procedure

1. Start with a clean, dry work surface. Place five or six potato chips on a paper towel, and fold the edges of the towel over the chips. Press lightly to crush the contents.

2. Open the towel. Dump the solid contents into a waste receptacle, and brush away any crumbs that remain. Return the towel to its place on the work surface next to a sticky note or other piece of paper that identifies the food used.

3. Repeat steps 1 and 2 for small amounts of each of the following foods: pretzels, apple, snack crackers, muffin, and air-popped unflavored popcorn.

4. Leave the paper towels undisturbed for 30 minutes. This will allow any water on the towels to evaporate. At the end of the 30 minutes, examine each paper towel by holding it up to a window or other light source. Any grease stains or other light spots show that the product contains some fat.

Conclusions

◆ Which foods produced stains? Which did not?

◆ Are any of the foods you used ones that you regularly eat?

◆ Were you surprised by any of your findings? If so, which?

◆ What changes in your eating habits might you consider making as a result of this experiment?

Lowering Fat

Controlling the amount of total fat in your eating plan can help reduce your risk of lifestyle diseases and other health problems. It also allows you to eat more food without increasing your total calories. Remember, a gram of fat has 9 calories, while a gram of protein or carbohydrate has only 4 calories.

It's easier than you might think to cut down on fat. One way is by substituting low-fat food choices for high-fat ones. As you progress through this program, you will learn other ways of reducing the fat in the eating and cooking you do.

Limit Sugars

You expect to find sugar in foods such as candy, desserts, and baked goods. Did you know, though, that other foods—ketchup, salad dressing, and peanut butter, for example—may also contain refined sugar?

Like natural sugar, the refined sugars that are added to many foods provide energy. However, these sugars are limited in nutrients. The Dietary Guidelines recommend that most healthy people use only moderate amounts of these sugars. Very active people with high energy needs may be able to consume more, as long as their food choices are nutritious ones. People with low energy needs should use refined sugars in very small amounts.

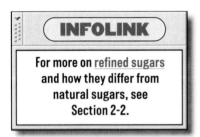

INFOLINK

For more on refined sugars and how they differ from natural sugars, see Section 2-2.

Limit Salt and Sodium

Table salt contains sodium and chloride, both of which are essential nutrients. Most people, however, eat more salt and sodium than they need for good health. Salt is added to most foods and beverages during processing. Many foods also contain natural amounts of sodium. Here are some hints for cutting down on salt and sodium:

◆ Add little, if any, salt to food when cooking and at the table. When you must add salt, shake once—not twice.

◆ Choose salted snacks—chips, crackers, pretzels, and nuts—only occasionally.

◆ Go easy on processed foods. They generally have more sodium than fresh ones.

◆ Check labels for the amount of sodium in foods. Choose those lower in sodium most of the time.

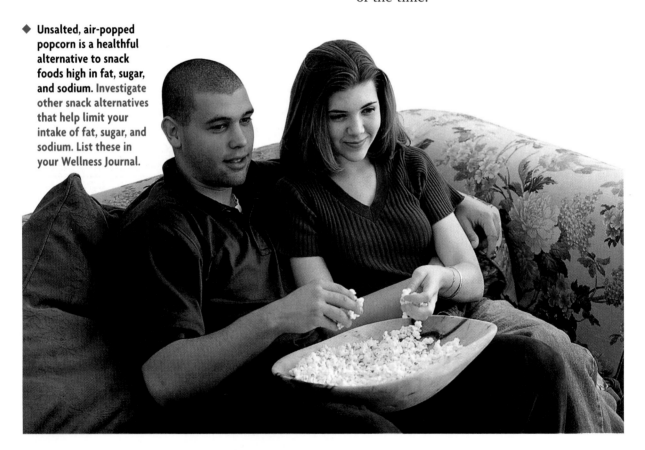

◆ Unsalted, air-popped popcorn is a healthful alternative to snack foods high in fat, sugar, and sodium. Investigate other snack alternatives that help limit your intake of fat, sugar, and sodium. List these in your Wellness Journal.

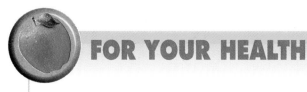

How Sweet It Is!

Because there are many different kinds of sugars, you may not be aware that a product you are buying has been sweetened. Examine the ingredients lists of products you buy. Any of the following terms that appear on the label will tell you that the product contains added sugar:

- Sucrose
- Raw sugar
- Dextrose
- Maltose
- Honey

- Corn sweetener
- High-fructose corn syrup
- Fruit juice concentrate
- Brown sugar
- Glucose

- Fructose
- Lactose
- Syrup
- Molasses

Following Up

1. Check the ingredients labels of three products you regularly eat. Which contain one of the sugars in the list above? Which contain more than one?

2. Three of Theo's favorite foods contain at least one form of sugar. Devise a strategy Theo could use to cut down on the amount of sugar in his eating plan.

Section 3-1 Review & Activities

1. Why is eating a variety of foods important to good health?

2. What is meant by the term *invisible fat?* Name three foods in which it is found.

3. List five examples of different sugars that may appear on food labels.

4. Analyzing. Which of the six recommendations in the Dietary Guidelines do you think is hardest for most people to follow? Why?

5. Evaluating. Research the dietary guidelines of other countries. What are the similarities and differences?

6. Applying. Choose one Dietary Guideline. In your Wellness Journal, list five to ten suggestions for helping yourself and other people to follow it.

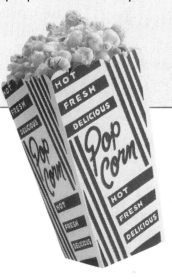

The Food Guide Pyramid

You probably know the expression "A picture is worth a thousand words." The authors of the Dietary Guidelines for Americans *decided to follow the wisdom of these words. They included a graphic tool to help readers better understand the concepts summarized in Section 3-1.*

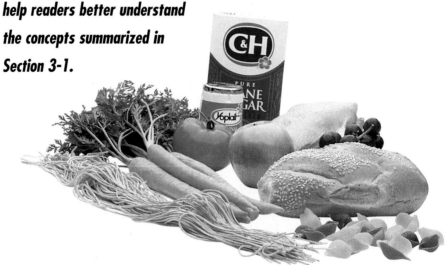

Objectives

After studying this section, you should be able to:

- Describe the food groups in the Food Guide Pyramid.

- Give guidelines for using the Food Guide Pyramid to plan daily food choices.

Look for These Terms

Food Guide Pyramid

nutrient-dense

Understanding the Pyramid

Who hasn't seen the **Food Guide Pyramid** printed on the back of cereal boxes, bread wrappers, and countless other food packages? Subtitled "A Guide to Daily Food Choices," this pyramid-shaped food grouping system is designed to help you choose a variety of foods in moderate amounts, including plenty of grains, vegetables, and fruits.

The Food Guide Pyramid includes five food groups:

- Bread, Cereal, Rice, and Pasta Group.

- Vegetable Group.

- Fruit Group.

- Milk, Yogurt, and Cheese Group.

- Meat, Poultry, Fish, Dry Beans, Eggs, and Nuts Group.

Using the Pyramid

Foods are arranged in the Food Guide Pyramid according to the recommended number of servings. The Bread, Cereal, Rice, and Pasta Group is at the base of the pyramid—and is the largest section—because you need more servings from this group than any of the others. Within each food group is a wide assortment of foods. They differ in nutrients and calories—both naturally occurring and according to preparation methods. Spinach, for example, has more vitamins and minerals than iceberg lettuce. French fries have more fat and calories than a plain baked potato. Peaches canned in syrup have more sugar and calories than fresh peaches.

In addition to the five food groups, the pyramid includes a section labeled "Fats, Oils, and Sweets." Foods in this category include salad dressings and oils, cream, butter, margarine, refined sugars, soft drinks, candies, and sweet desserts. These foods provide calories from fat and sugar, but few or no vitamins and minerals. Fats and sweets are placed at the small tip of the pyramid to show that they should be used sparingly.

On the pyramid diagram, you will notice small circles and triangles. These represent fats and added sugars. Notice that these symbols appear not only at the tip of the pyramid but also within the food groups. This is to show that fats and sugars can occur in some of the foods in each group.

Choosing Nutrient-Dense Foods

In general, the greater the number of servings in a particular group, the larger the space it is given in the pyramid. The most space is given to foods that are **nutrient-dense**, low or moderate in calories yet rich in important nutrients. As a rule, nutrient-dense foods are low in fats and added sugars and high in other nutrients, such as complex carbohydrates, fiber, proteins, vitamins, and minerals. Organizing the pyramid in this fashion is a way of helping you remember to eat more servings of grains, fruits, and vegetables than of any other foods.

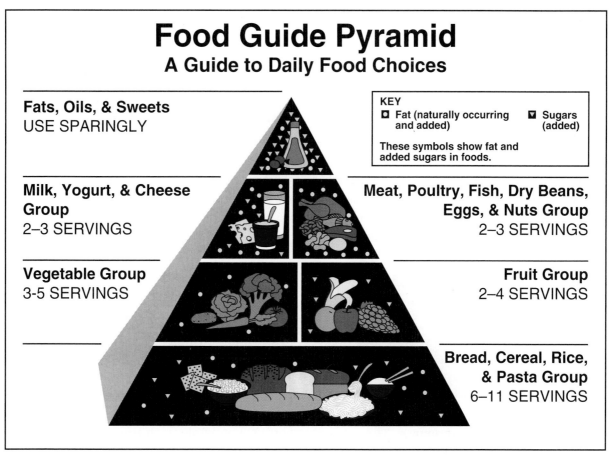

Food Guide Pyramid
A Guide to Daily Food Choices

Fats, Oils, & Sweets
USE SPARINGLY

KEY
▫ Fat (naturally occurring and added)   ☑ Sugars (added)
These symbols show fat and added sugars in foods.

Milk, Yogurt, & Cheese Group
2–3 SERVINGS

Meat, Poultry, Fish, Dry Beans, Eggs, & Nuts Group
2–3 SERVINGS

Vegetable Group
3-5 SERVINGS

Fruit Group
2–4 SERVINGS

Bread, Cereal, Rice, & Pasta Group
6–11 SERVINGS

◆ The Food Guide Pyramid shows the types of foods you need and in which amounts in order to balance your daily food intake. Which three food groups have the highest number of recommended daily servings? Explain why.

The Food Groups

All five food groups are important to health. Each provides some, but not all, of the nutrients you need. One group cannot replace another. You need a variety of foods from the food groups each day.

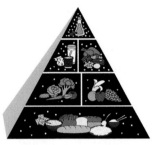

Bread, Cereal, Rice, and Pasta Group

This group includes all kinds of grain products. They supply complex carbohydrates, fiber, vitamins, and minerals.

You need 6 to 11 servings from this group every day. Some examples of a serving are:

- 1 slice bread.
- 1 ounce (28 g) ready-to-eat cereal.
- ½ cup (125 mL) cooked cereal, rice, or pasta.

To get the fiber you need, choose as many whole-grain foods as you can, such as whole wheat bread and whole-grain cereals. This group includes many low-fat choices, but also some higher-fat ones, such as croissants and other baked goods.

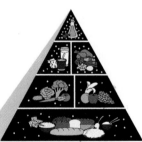

Vegetable Group

Vegetables provide beta carotene, which your body uses to make vitamin A. They also supply vitamin C, folate (a B vitamin), and minerals such as magnesium and iron. They provide fiber and complex carbohydrates and are low in fat.

You should have three to five servings of vegetables daily. Each of the following counts as one serving:

- 1 cup (250 mL) raw leafy vegetables.
- ½ cup (125 mL) other vegetables, cooked or chopped raw.
- ¾ cup (175 mL) vegetable juice.

Different types of vegetables provide different nutrients. For variety, include dark green, leafy vegetables, such as kale; deep yellow-orange vegetables, such as sweet potatoes; starchy vegetables, including corn, peas, and potatoes; dry beans and peas; and others.

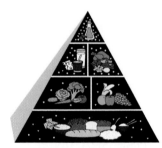

Fruit Group

Fruits provide important amounts of beta carotene, vitamin C, and potassium. Edible skins are good sources of fiber. Like vegetables, most fruits are low in fat and sodium.

You need two to four servings of fruit every day. One serving equals:

- 1 medium fruit, such as an apple, a banana, or an orange.
- ½ cup (125 mL) chopped raw, cooked, or canned fruit.
- ¾ cup (175 mL) fruit juice.

Be sure to have fruits rich in vitamin C regularly, such as citrus fruits, melons, and berries. Eat whole fresh fruits often for the fiber they provide. When choosing canned or frozen fruits, look for products without added sugar. Count only 100 percent fruit juices as a serving of fruit.

Milk, Yogurt, and Cheese Group

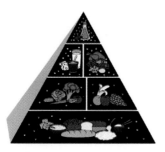

Foods in this group are high in protein, vitamins, and minerals. They are also one of the best sources of calcium.

Most adults need two servings of milk products daily. Three servings are recommended for pregnant or breast-feeding women, teens, and young adults up to age 24. One serving equals:

◆ 1 cup (250 mL) milk or yogurt.

◆ 1½ ounces (42 g) natural cheese.

◆ 2 ounces (56 g) processed cheese.

Low-fat choices from this group include skim milk, nonfat yogurt, and nonfat dry milk. Go easy on high-fat cheese and ice cream. Remember, too, that some milk products, such as flavored yogurt, contain added sugar.

Meat, Poultry, Fish, Dry Beans, Eggs, and Nuts Group

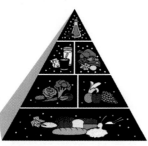

This group is an important source of protein, vitamins, and minerals. Two to three daily servings are recommended.

◆ 2 to 3 ounces (56 to 85 g) of cooked lean meat, poultry, or fish equals one serving. This is about the size of an average hamburger or the amount of meat in half a medium chicken breast.

◆ Each of the following portions is the equivalent of 1 ounce (28 g) of meat: ½ cup (125 mL) cooked dry beans; one egg; or 2 tablespoons (30 mL) peanut butter.

The total of your daily servings should be the equivalent of 5 to 7 ounces (140 to 196 g) of cooked lean meat, poultry, or fish. For instance, you might eat an egg for breakfast, a cup of cooked dry beans in bean soup for lunch, and a lean hamburger for dinner. These foods would give you the equivalent of 6 ounces (168 g) of meat.

To limit the fat in your diet, select lean meats, fish, and poultry without skin. Have dry beans and peas often—they are high in fiber and low in fat. Go easy on eggs, nuts, and seeds. Eggs are high in cholesterol; nuts and seeds are high in fat.

Crossover Foods

Some foods in the Food Guide Pyramid have been identified by the authors of the guide as "crossover" foods. These foods, which include dry beans and other legumes, may be considered as belonging to more than one food group. For example, dry beans may be considered as one serving from either the Meat, Poultry, Fish, Dry Beans, Eggs, and Nuts Group or the Vegetable Group. Note that any crossover food can be used to satisfy a serving requirement from *either* group it is classified in, but not *both*.

How Many Servings for You?

You may have noticed that the Food Guide Pyramid does not give an exact number of servings for each group. Instead, it gives a range, such as three to five servings of vegetables. This is because people have different needs for calories and nutrients, depending on their age, gender, body size, and activity level.

The Food Guide Pyramid

Keeping the Food Guide Pyramid in mind can help you balance your daily food intake.

Look and Learn:

On the Food Guide Pyramid, find each food you have eaten so far today. How many servings from each group have you had? How do these foods stack up in terms of your nutrients needs?

◆ **Fats, Oils, and Sweets**
Use these foods sparingly. They provide calories from fat and sugar, but little or no vitamins and minerals.

◆ **Milk, Yogurt, and Cheese Group**
Foods in the milk group are high in protein, vitamins, and minerals and are one of the best sources of calcium.

◆ **Meat, Poultry, Fish, Dry Beans, Eggs, and Nuts Group**
This group is an important source of protein, vitamins, and minerals.

◆ **Vegetable Group**
Vegetables provide beta carotene, vitamin C, folate (a B vitamin), and minerals such as magnesium and iron. They provide fiber and complex carbohydrates and are low in fat.

◆ **Fruit Group**
Fruits provide important amounts of beta carotene, vitamin C, potassium, and fiber.

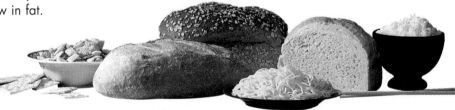

◆ **Bread, Cereal, Rice, and Pasta Group**
This group includes all kinds of grain products. They supply complex carbohydrates, fiber, vitamins, and minerals.

In general, most male teens need the highest number of servings from each food group. Most female teens need the middle number of servings (such as nine servings from the bread group). However, all teens need three servings from the milk group.

You may be used to eating amounts of food that are larger or smaller than what is considered a serving according to the Food Guide Pyramid. For example, if you eat 1 cup (250 mL) of cooked spaghetti, remember to count that as two servings, not one, from the Bread, Cereal, Rice and Pasta Group.

Some foods include ingredients from more than one food group. If you're eating tacos, you would have servings from the bread group (taco shell), meat group (meat or bean filling), milk group (cheese), and vegetable group (lettuce and tomatoes). Depending on the amounts of the different fillings, you might have full or half servings from the different groups.

The Food Guide Pyramid makes it easy to plan for good nutrition. It is a valuable tool for getting all the nutrients you need in the proper balance.

Section 3-2 Review & Activities

1. List the five food groups in the Food Guide Pyramid. Give the range of recommended daily servings for each group.

2. What does the term *nutrient-dense* mean? How does it relate to choosing foods from the pyramid?

3. For each food group, give two examples of serving sizes.

4. **Analyzing.** Do you feel the pyramid design is an effective way to get the desired nutrition message across? Why or why not?

5. **Extending.** Name two combination foods (other than tacos). List the food groups that are represented by the combination food's ingredients.

6. **Applying.** Make up a one-day menu that provides the recommended servings from the Food Guide Pyramid for a female teen.

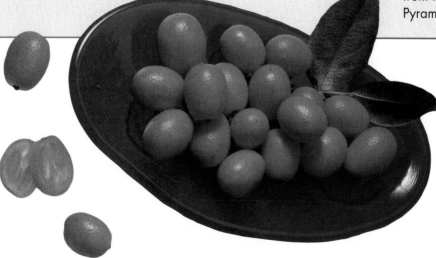

Separating Fact from Fiction

"Now, with less sugar!" a TV ad for a soft drink promises. "Scientists Find That Fried Foods Are Good for You," announces the headline of a tabloid that catches your eye as you stand in the supermarket checkout line.

Each day, dozens of media messages about food and nutrition come your way. With this wealth of information, some of it conflicting, how can you tell what to believe and what to disregard?

Objectives

After studying this section, you should be able to:

- Explain how to evaluate news reports, advertisements, and other information related to foods and nutrition.
- Identify the techniques advertisers use to sell products.
- Discuss how food myths originate.

Look for These Terms

bias

study design

Developing Consumer Skills

Part of the answer to the question above is mastering two of the food-consumer skills you learned about in Chapter 1. Those skills —critical thinking and communication—constitute a first step in learning how to separate fact from fiction. As a critical thinker, you learn to look for the "angle" in a given message. When you see an ad, for example, you are alert to the fact that advertisers have something to sell and, therefore, may not be the most reliable information sources.

As an effective communicator, you learn to consider the source of the information. You become able to discriminate between legitimate sources and popularizers.

◆ **Evaluating competing health claims and information is an important skill to learn.** Make a list of different information sources—for example, scientific journal, newspaper tabloid, television program, etc. Rate each from 1 to 5 in terms of its credibility.

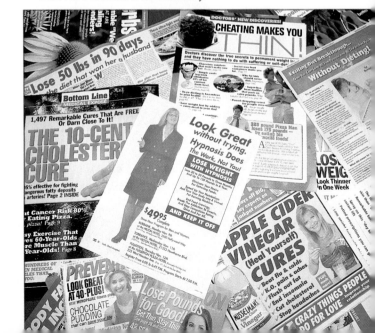

Going to the Source

How often do you read articles or hear news stories about food that contain phrases such as "a recent study shows" or "scientists have found"? On the surface, such reports seem believable enough. How can you tell whether to accept the information at face value? Here are some ways:

◆ Check the original source, when possible. Credible research is carried out by qualified scientists and recognized institutions. The results are then reported in scientific and professional journals. Be wary of the results of research attributed to unnamed sources.

◆ Be alert for bias on the part of the people who performed or reported on the study. A **bias** is a tendency to be swayed toward a particular conclusion. Which would you expect to be more objective, a study of the effectiveness of a food supplement paid for by the supplement's manufacturer or one carried out by an independent research facility?

◆ Read past the headlines. Headlines are designed to get your attention and may be misleading. Don't jump to a conclusion before you have read or heard the whole report.

◆ Consider the body of evidence. Is the report based on preliminary findings? If so, it may be too early to make any changes in your eating habits. Wait until more evidence has been gathered. Remember, too, that different scientists view study results differently and that it takes time to study and adequately test early findings. Be on the lookout for follow-up reports.

◆ Consider the **study design**, that is, the approach used by researchers to investigate a claim. Some studies, known as clinical

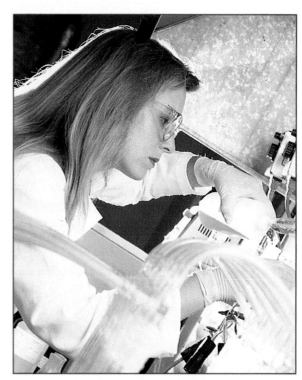

◆ **Valid scientific studies are done by professional researchers under controlled conditions.** Name two sources to which you can turn for reliable results of such studies.

trials, are performed on human subjects. Others are designed around animal subjects. Findings involving animals aren't always reliable.

Evaluating Advertisements

Are there TV commercials you enjoy watching? Advertising can be informative and entertaining. At times, however, advertisements can be misleading. When it comes to food ads, the emphasis is seldom on real nutrition issues. Here are a few of the techniques advertisers use to persuade an unsuspecting public to buy their products:

◆ **Limited information.** Advertisements often give only the facts that will encourage you to buy, without telling the whole story.

What the Terms Mean

Some words and phrases that turn up in reports of scientific studies are often misunderstood. Here are a few of them and what they really mean.

Term	Meaning
• Associated with	• Implies a connection between two things that can't be explained by mere coincidence; does not indicate that a cause-and-effect relationship has been established.
• Double the risk	• If the original risk is 1 in 1 million, double the risk translates to 1 in 500,000.
• Probability	• Refers to the likelihood of an event's taking place; is not the same thing as a certainty.
• Significant	• Also appearing sometimes as "statistically significant"; implies a probability of 95 percent or better.
• Survival	• Indicates the percentage of people with a specific disease or condition who are still alive after a given period; does not mean the same thing as a cure.

◆ **Positive images.** An ad may use images of things that people feel positively about, such as friendship or a good appearance. The advertiser's hope is that the consumer will associate these images and feelings with the product.

◆ **Celebrity endorsement.** Some ads show popular performers or athletes promoting the product. They don't tell you whether the person actually uses the product in real life.

◆ **Appeal to basic needs.** Advertisers may focus on ways the product meets a need for security or self-esteem. They try to convince you that the product will make you look or feel better.

◆ **Scare tactics.** Advertisers may play on people's fears of aging or developing a medical condition by claiming that their product can prevent or relieve the symptoms or provide essential nutrients.

◆ **False claims.** Ads may make claims that are not true, such as fast or guaranteed results. Remember, if a claim sounds too good to be true, it usually is.

◆ **Infomercials.** Infomercials are TV ads made to look like regular consumer programs or televised news reports. Unless you look carefully, you may believe you're watching something you are not!

Besides advertising, companies use other techniques to promote their products. A soft drink company may lend its name to a sports event or arrange to have its product shown in a movie. Coupons and eye-catching store displays encourage consumers to buy. Even product packages are a form of advertising.

Remember that the purpose of advertising is to get people to buy a product. Your goal is to get good nutrition at a fair price. Be sure your buying decisions are based on your own priorities, not the advertiser's.

Food Myths

When Margaret has a cold, her mother gives her a mixture of hot tea and fruit juice flavored with cloves. Margaret's mother learned this remedy from her own mother. In reality, this mixture has no medicinal value. Its use as a cold remedy is nothing more than a food myth.

Where do food myths originate? Some, like Margaret's grandmother's "cure" for the common cold, are handed down through generations of the same family. Others are spread by word of mouth. When a food or nutrition myth becomes so widespread as to be embraced by a fairly large group, it becomes a fad. One weight-loss fad that was popular some years ago was the grapefruit diet. It was grounded in the myth that eating grapefruit at every meal could help a person shed pounds.

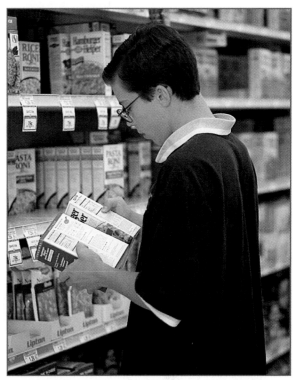

◆ No product can guarantee good health or weight loss. Make your choices based on facts, not false promises. Which aspects of skills for food choices come into play when evaluating product labels?

Connecting Food and Social Studies

Teen Consumerism

The purpose of advertising is to sell, and today's teens are a target market. Think about the kinds of promotions that have inspired you to try a new product. A recent marketing and lifestyle study revealed the following buying habits in response to various promotions:

	AGE		
Promotion	12-15	16-17	18-19
Free sample	48%	47%	38%
Coupon	35%	40%	42%
Contest/sweepstakes	26%	21%	19%
Free gift with purchase	25%	21%	20%
Cash rebate	11%	10%	11%
Frequent-buyer clubs	6%	8%	9%

Think About It

1. Which promotional technique appeals to the greatest percentage of teens? Which appeals to the fewest teens? How do your buying tendencies compare with those of other people in your age group?

2. Which technique would most inspire you to try a new food product? Explain your reasoning.

As with news reports and advertisements, consumer skills can help you avoid becoming the victim of food myths or fads. When you are confronted with a food or nutrition "fact":

◆ Keep a healthy skepticism. Ask the individual who shares the information what his or her source is. Then investigate the source yourself.

◆ Seek a qualified opinion. Consult a registered dietitian, other qualified nutrition expert, or a health care professional.

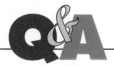

Q What sources can I contact if I am suspicious about any nutrition information I have received or if I just want more facts?

A You might contact any of the following: a local nutritionist or dietitian; your local health department; your food science teacher; a professional organization, such as the American Dietetics Association; or the nutrition department at a nearby university or college.

Remember, your health is your responsibility. Separating nutrition fact from fiction is an important part of exercising that responsibility.

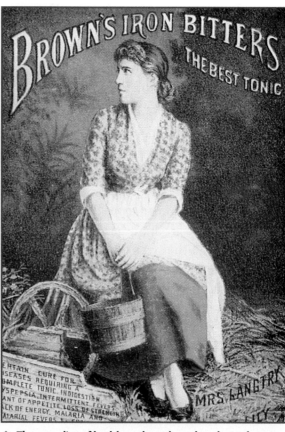

◆ The spreading of health myths and quackery began long ago. Name some products today that make great health claims.

Section 3-3 Review & Activities

1. Why doesn't any one scientific study provide enough evidence from which to draw a conclusion?

2. Name two techniques advertisers use to sell food products.

3. Where do food myths originate?

4. Analyzing. Why do you think some people continue to believe false claims and myths when there is no evidence to support them?

5. Extending. "Scientists Say Miracle Vitamin Stops Aging." You have a friend who wants to start taking large doses of that vitamin. What advice would you give your friend?

6. Applying. Look for ads that you think are false or misleading, and bring them to class. Identify the misleading statements or techniques used in each.

CAREER WANTED

Individuals with good communication skills who can explain nutrition concepts clearly and easily.

REQUIRES:

- associate degree in diet technology
- 1-2 years of work experience

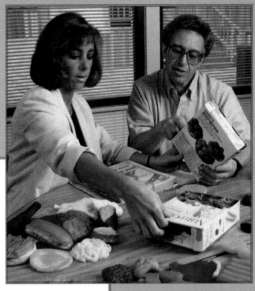

"You really are what you eat,"

says Dietetic Technician Jan Bradshaw

Q: What is the difference between a dietetic technician and a dietitian?

A: It's mostly background. When people think of dietitians, they think of "RDs," or *registered dietitians*. To be an RD, you have to go through a supervised internship program, and, in some places, you need an advanced degree. As a dietetic technician, I have an associate degree in food science from a two-year college and I do counsel people on nutrition.

Q: What exactly are your responsibilities here in the outpatient department of a hospital?

A: I counsel patients with a variety of nutritional needs and medical problems—diabetes, cancer, heart and kidney disease. My supervisor is a clinical dietitian. I discuss my caseload with her and get recommendations. I also teach a healthy cooking class for the community at large.

Q: Where do you see your career in five years?

A: I like my work a lot, but sometimes I think about going back to school and getting an advanced degree. With all the interest nowadays in eating right, I might even become director of a nutrition clinic.

Career Research Activity

1. Working in teams, stage a "news magazine" that focuses on the role of nutrition in the prevention and treatment of disease. Segments of your program should cover the advice of experts in dietetics, pharmaceuticals, and medicine.

2. Create an "ad" that would get students interested in becoming an EMT. Include a list of high school courses that would best prepare someone for this exciting career. Also mention other related career opportunities.

Related Career Opportunities

Entry Level
- Dietary Aide
- Cook
- Kitchen Worker

Technical Level
- Emergency Medical Technician (EMT)
- Dietetic Technician

Professional Level
- Dietitian
- Registered Dietitian
- Clinical Dietitian

Chapter 3   Review & Activities

Summary

Section 3-1: Dietary Guidelines

• The Dietary Guidelines for Americans provide the following recommendations: Eat a variety of foods; maintain or improve your weight; choose an eating plan with plenty of grain products, vegetables and fruits; choose an eating plan low in fat, saturated fat, and cholesterol and moderate in sugars, salt, and sodium.

Section 3-2: The Food Guide Pyramid

• The Food Guide Pyramid, a tool to help you plan daily food choices, shows the approximate number of servings needed each day from each of the five food groups.

• The foods in the Food Guide Pyramid are grouped according to the nutrients they provide.

• Choosing nutrient-dense foods from the food groups will help you get the nutrients you need without excess calories.

Section 3-3: Separating Fact from Fiction

• Food-related skills, including critical thinking and communication, can help you identify information that may be misleading.

• It is important to stay informed about nutrition research, but use food-related skills to evaluate research findings.

• Advertisers use a variety of techniques to persuade you to buy their products.

• Be wary of food myths and fads, and know where to get accurate information about nutrition.

Checking Your Knowledge

1. What are the recommended limits for fat and saturated fat in an eating plan?

2. What are the benefits of choosing an eating plan with plenty of grain products, vegetables, and fruits?

3. Explain how the position of food groups in the Food Guide Pyramid diagram relates to the recommended number of servings of each.

4. Why does the Food Guide Pyramid give the recommended number of servings for each food group as a range instead of an exact number?

5. Briefly describe the main nutrients provided by each food group.

6. What problems are associated with excess sodium? Give three hints for cutting down on salt and sodium.

7. Why is it important to watch for follow-up reports on research findings?

8. Name three techniques used by advertisers to persuade you to buy their products.

9. What makes an infomercial misleading?

10. How can you tell whether the author of a book on nutrition is a reliable source of information on the subject?

Thinking Critically

1. Identifying Evidence. A friend tells you that honey and molasses are better for you than white or brown sugar. How can you decide whether this is true?

2. Recognizing Bias. Suppose that you are reading a magazine or newspaper and happen upon a study on the effectiveness of vitamin C against colds. After reading the article, you discover that the study was financed by a company that makes vitamin C tablets. Why does this suggest a possible bias?

Working IN THE Lab

1. _Taste Test._ Heat three samples of a canned vegetable, such as green beans—one canned with salt and two canned without salt. Season one of the no-salt samples with a salt alternative, such as herbs or lemon juice. Compare the taste of the vegetables. Which do you prefer? Why?

2. _Foods Lab._ Compare the amount of fat in different types of ground beef. Weigh out ¼ pound (125 g) of regular ground beef and the same amount of ground round. Form each portion into a patty. Cook each patty in a separate skillet over medium-low heat until done (about five minutes on each side). After cooking, weigh each patty again. Pour the grease from each pan into a separate measuring cup. Which patty contained more fat? How might you use this information?

Reinforcing Key Skills

1. Leadership. As participants in a schoolwide health fair, your class is planning a presentation on the _Dietary Guidelines for Americans._ List the steps the planning group can take to heighten people's awareness of the guidelines and the Food Guide Pyramid.

2. Management. Eryka is writing a review of a recent nutrition study and has asked for your help in organizing her report. What questions would you suggest that Eryka ask herself about the study in order to evaluate it properly?

Making Decisions and Solving Problems

Your sister has learned that carrots are very nutritious. Therefore, she has stopped eating most other vegetables and eats large amounts of carrots at almost every meal. What would you tell your sister?

Making Connections

1. Language Arts. Find a newspaper or magazine article about a nutrition-related study. Identify the following information in the article: What was the purpose of the study? Who did the study and where? Who paid for it? What type of people or animals did the researchers study? How was the study carried out?

2. Math. Conduct a survey of classmates' eating habits by asking them to write down the number of servings of vegetables eaten the previous day. Calculate the class average. How does this average compare with the servings suggested in the Food Guide Pyramid?

Planning Daily Food Choices

When it comes to eating, different families and individuals follow different patterns. In this chapter, you will learn about some of these patterns as well as reasons for the differences.

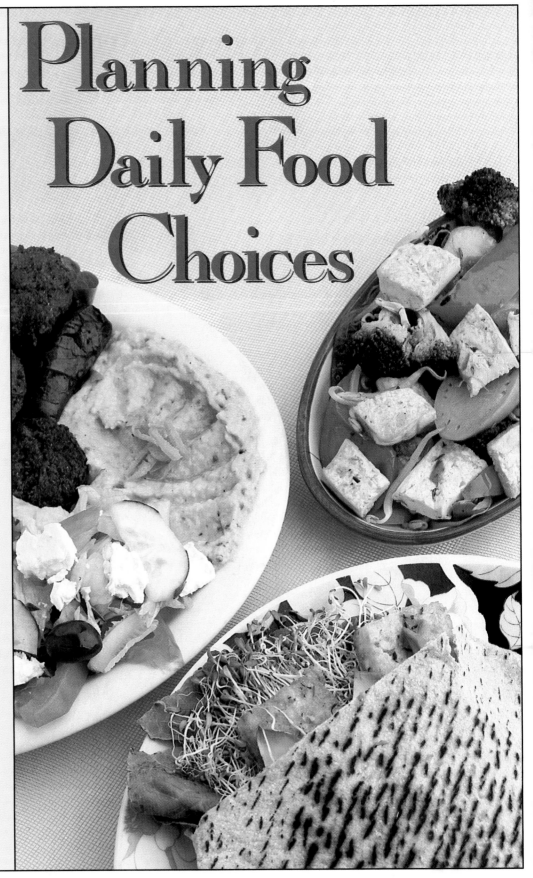

Daily Meals and Snacks

As an exchange student from Italy, Frederica was surprised by some of the "strange" eating customs she encountered on her visit to the United States. For instance, the family she was staying with had their big meal in the evening, instead of at noon, as she was used to doing at home.

Objectives

After studying this section, you should be able to:

- Identify different eating patterns.
- Discuss how nutritional needs can be met through meals and snacks.

Look for These Terms

eating patterns

grazing

Eating Patterns

Have you ever visited or studied the homeland of another culture? If so, you, like Frederica, may have been struck by differences in that culture's eating patterns. **Eating patterns** are food customs and habits, including when, what, and how much people eat. People have different schedules, so people often have different eating patterns. Some people eat the traditional three meals a day, while others prefer to eat five or six "mini-meals." Still others may follow different eating patterns from one day to the next.

Any eating pattern is acceptable as long as the food choices in it reflect sound nutritional practices. It is also important to eat regularly. If you try to go too long without food, your body won't have the fuel it needs. Studies show that people who skip meals make up for it by overeating later. Usually, meal skippers eat more in a day than they would if they chose to eat at regular intervals.

Traditional Meals

Despite the differences noted above, traditional eating patterns in many cultures—including Frederica's—revolve around three main meals. These are breakfast, the midday meal, and the evening meal.

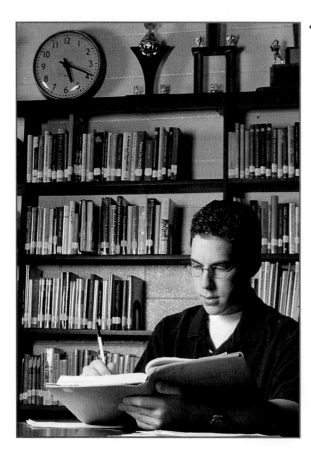

◆ Your daily schedule is one of the factors that influence your eating pattern. Name some others.

time and do better scholastically than those who don't eat breakfast.

Not all breakfasts are equal, however. A breakfast consisting of a complex carbohydrate, protein, and fruit—for example, whole-grain cereal or a muffin, milk, and a banana—gives you more lasting energy than a doughnut and a soft drink. You may feel fine after eating the doughnut and soft drink, but you will probably experience a mid-morning letdown.

Some people skip breakfast because they are bored with standard breakfast fare. Any food, though, can be a breakfast food, as long as it provides some of the nutrients your body needs. Try having pizza, tacos, soup with crackers, or refried beans on toast for breakfast. Round out the menu with a serving of fruit and a glass of low-fat milk.

Breakfast

Breakfast is the most important meal of the day. Why? When you first awaken after seven or eight hours of sleep, your body's fuel gauge reads "empty." Breakfast gives you energy to get your motor running. A good breakfast also helps you feel alert during the morning hours. If you skip breakfast, it's harder to concentrate on your schoolwork. Recent research reveals that students who eat breakfast get to school on

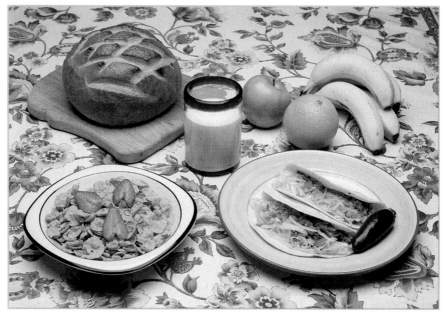

◆ Eating breakfast makes a difference in how you feel all morning. Any of these nutritious choices can give your body fuel for a morning of activity. In your Wellness Journal, list other eye-opening morning meal possibilities you might like to try to add variety.

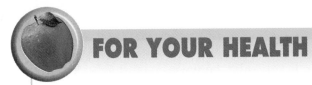

FOR YOUR HEALTH

Beating the Breakfast Blahs

Are you a breakfast skipper? If time is your problem, begin by getting up a few minutes earlier. Make a meal out of foods such as these:

- Low-fat flavored or plain yogurt, whole-grain muffin or bagel, and a banana.
- Peanut butter and jelly sandwich and low-fat milk.
- A breakfast drink made by blending low-fat milk or yogurt, juice, and fruit.

Following Up

1. Using the Food Guide Pyramid in Chapter 3 (page 97), plan a week of breakfasts. Each breakfast must include one or two servings from the grains group, one serving from the dairy group, and one serving from the fruit group.

2. Try the breakfasts. Rate each in terms of variety, originality, ease of preparation, and enjoyment. Keep a list in your Wellness Journal of breakfast ideas that you rate highly. Continually add new ones.

Midday and Evening Meals

Whether you call it lunch, brunch, or some other name, the midday meal gives you energy and nutrients to carry you through the rest of the day's activities. The evening meal is a good time to think about the food you've eaten for the day. It's your chance to fill in any food group servings that are lacking.

Dinner traditionally means the largest meal of the day. It may be eaten at midday or in the evening, depending on your personal preference and your schedule. In some cultures, including Frederica's, people prefer to eat dinner at midday and a lighter meal, sometimes called supper, in the evening. The larger midday meal provides fuel for the day's activities. Some people find they sleep better if the evening meal is light.

The usual custom in American culture is to have a light meal, or lunch, at midday, saving the largest meal for the evening—a time when all or most family members can eat together. On weekends or special occasions, some individuals and families may follow a different pattern.

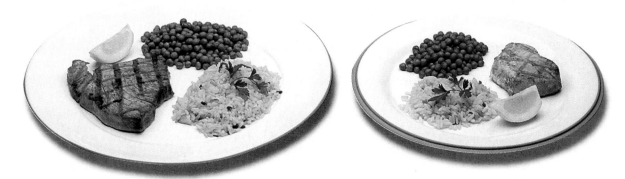

◆ Some health experts are now recommending five or six smaller meals in place of three large ones. Name some possible health benefits of this style of eating.

Dinner

No matter when it is eaten, a dinner usually focuses on a main dish, a grain product, vegetables, a beverage, and sometimes, dessert. With an increasing awareness of nutritional needs, more and more people are preparing main-dish meals that include smaller portions of meat, poultry, or fish, with the grain and vegetables mixed right in. Such a dinner might center on stir-fried chicken with broccoli and water chestnuts, served over rice. Accompanied by a tossed salad, low-fat milk, and a whole wheat roll, and followed by fruit for dessert, such a meal follows the *Dietary Guidelines for Americans*.

Snacks

If you enjoy between-meal snacks, here is good news: Snacking is not necessarily a bad habit. In fact, during the teen years, when your nutritional and caloric needs are at a high point as a result of rapid body growth, snacking can actually help you meet those needs.

Of course, what you choose to snack on can make all the difference. Many snack foods—such as candy, chips, granola, cookies, and other sweets—are high in fat, sugar, and calories.

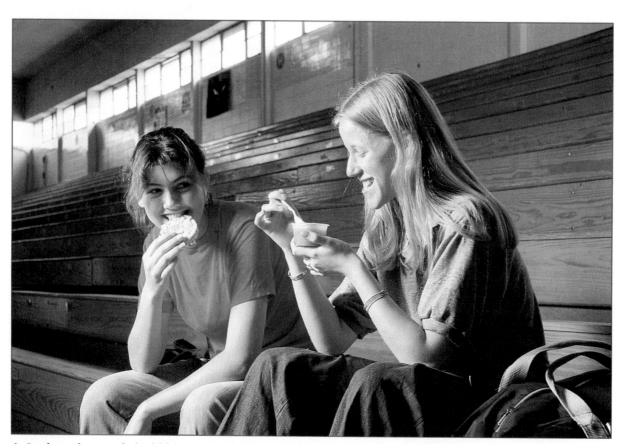

◆ **Snacks can be part of a healthful eating plan when you select wisely.** Using the table "Nutritive Value of Foods" in Appendix B at the back of this book, analyze two or three foods you regularly snack on. Which are low in fat and/or calories? Which are not?

For a nutritious snack, you can choose almost any nutrient-dense food. Try leftovers from the refrigerator, fresh fruits or vegetables, low-fat dairy products, or whole-grain breads and cereals.

Remember, too, to pay attention to the *timing* of your snacks. If you snack too close to mealtime, you may not be able to eat the nutritious foods included in the meal.

Grazing

Some people prefer eating five or more small meals throughout the day instead of three large ones. This eating pattern is sometimes called **grazing**. Some health experts view grazing as a healthful alternative to conventional meal patterns.

If grazing is your eating pattern, think about your food choices toward the end of the day. Are you lacking any servings from any of the food groups? If so, eat those foods so that you'll be sure to meet the daily recommendations. At the same time, check to be sure you are not eating too much. The day's total servings and calories should be the right amount for you, just as if you were eating three traditional meals.

As you have learned, eating patterns vary from person to person and day to day. In the end, *when* you eat is less important than *what* you eat. The eating pattern that helps you get the nutrients you need and the right number of calories is the one that's best for you. Identifying your eating pattern can help you plan for good nutrition.

Section 4-1 Review & Activities

1. Give three examples of different eating patterns.

2. Why is breakfast considered the most important meal of the day?

3. What kinds of snack foods can help you meet your nutrient needs?

4. **Analyzing.** Think about this statement: "Snacking during the teen years has the potential to help as well as the potential to do harm." Write a short paragraph that explains your interpretation of the sentence.

5. **Comparing and Contrasting.** Divide a sheet of paper into two columns. In one column, list as many advantages of grazing as you can. In the second column, list as many disadvantages as you can.

6. **Applying.** In your Wellness Journal, make a list of 15 nutritious snack foods that require little preparation. Put a check mark by those you have already tried. Put a star by those you plan to try.

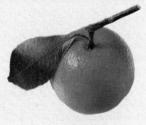
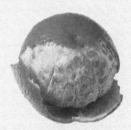
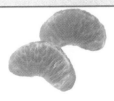

SECTION 4-2

Positive Food Habits

If you are like most people, some of your eating habits are healthful, but others could stand improvement. The first step in improving your eating habits is to recognize the kinds of food choices you make now. Then you can keep your good habits and work on improving the poor ones.

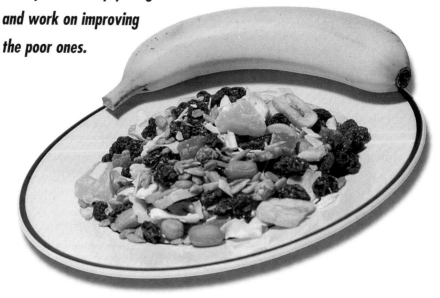

Objectives

After studying this section, you should be able to:

- Analyze your current eating habits.
- Suggest practical ways to improve your eating habits.

Look for This Term

appetite

Analyzing Your Current Habits

People sometimes aren't aware of how often and what they eat. Sometimes, they eat just to be sociable. Maybe you have found yourself making room for dessert at the end of a big meal. In such cases, you are eating not in response to hunger, but to appetite. **Appetite** is a desire, rather than a need, to eat.

Appetite is a learned, rather than an inborn, response. It is shaped by social influences, such as friends, as well as personal ones, such as emotions.

Keeping a Food Record

One way of becoming more aware of your habits is by keeping a food record. This is simply a list of all the foods you eat for a specific period of time—usually three consecutive days, including a weekend. A food record is not a test you have to pass. Rather, it is a way of letting you know the kind of food choices you are making now and how much you are eating.

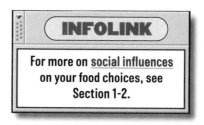

INFOLINK

For more on social influences on your food choices, see Section 1-2.

Whether you keep your food record in a diary, a personal journal, or just a page in your loose-leaf binder, it should include the following:

◆ The time you ate.

◆ The food eaten and the approximate amount.

◆ A brief description of the eating situation, including where you were, what you were doing, your mood, and any other information that could help you understand your food habits.

Reviewing Your Food Record

At the end of the allotted time, take a look at your food choices. For each day, count the number of servings you had from each group in the Food Guide Pyramid (page 97). Compare your totals with the recommended number of servings. Did you eat at least the minimum amount of servings? If not, which foods were you lacking? Were your food choices high or low in fats and added sugars?

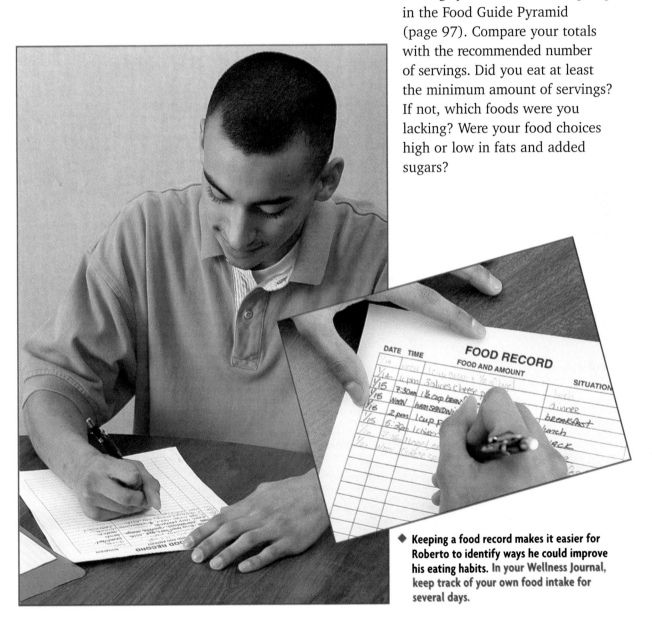

◆ Keeping a food record makes it easier for Roberto to identify ways he could improve his eating habits. In your Wellness Journal, keep track of your own food intake for several days.

Improving Your Eating Habits

Once you have identified any poor eating habits, think about why they occur. Did you tend to make poor food choices in certain situations, such as while watching TV or when you were unhappy? Were you responding to appetite rather than hunger?

Next, think about how you can correct any problems you isolated. Don't just tell yourself, "I'll eat better from now on." That promise is hard to keep because it isn't specific. Instead, decide on specific changes you can make.

Remember, eating is an enjoyable part of life. Don't take the pleasure out of it. You can make changes in your food habits and have fun doing it.

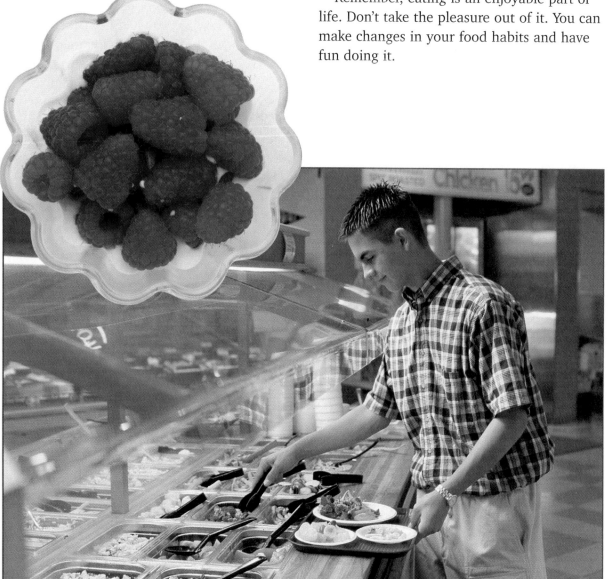

◆ In settings like this one, it is possible to choose foods that are both satisfying and provide needed nutrients. Visit the food court of a mall near you, and make a list of the meal and snack possibilities that help you satisfy your nutrient needs.

FOR YOUR HEALTH

What's a Healthful Portion?

When it comes to eating, a problem for many people is not just *what* they eat. Rather, it's *how much* they eat. Learning to identify healthful portions can be a first step in controlling the tendency to overeat.

To see how much you know about accurate healthful portions, try the following:

1. Consult the Food Guide Pyramid for suggested single servings of each of the following foods: apple, cooked rice, unsalted pretzels, cooked chopped meat (hamburger).

2. Spoon what you imagine to be a single serving of each of these foods onto separate paper plates. Measure out an accurate portion of each food onto a second set of plates.

Record any differences between the two portions of each food.

3. After several days, repeat the entire experiment. Record your results.

Following Up

1. How close were you at estimating correct serving sizes? Did you become more skilled at judging correct amounts when you repeated the experiment?

2. Were the recommended serving sizes less or more of each food than you normally eat?

3. How can learning to estimate accurate healthful servings decrease your risk of having eating-related illnesses now and in the future?

Section 4-2 Review & Activities

1. What is appetite?

2. What is a food record? What is its purpose?

3. When keeping a food record, what information do you need to write down?

4. **Synthesizing.** How could you give encouragement to a friend who is working on new eating habits?

5. **Applying.** Using the instructions in the section, create a food record for yourself in your Wellness Journal. After analyzing your current eating habits, make a list of specific changes you intend to make. Repeat the activity a month from now. Which new behaviors have become habits?

Eating Out

"Let's eat out!" Each year Americans spend about 22 percent of their food dollar on restaurant meals, including meals eaten at fast-food chains. Another 22 percent is spent on take-out foods brought into the home.

Objectives

After studying this section, you should be able to:

- Give guidelines for making nutritious food choices when eating out or ordering ready-to-eat food.

- Explain how home meal replacements fit into overall food choices.

Look for These Terms

home meal replacement

entrée

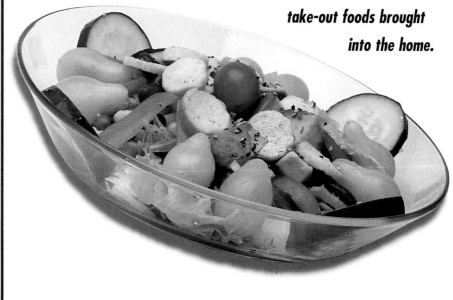

Restaurants

There are three main types of restaurants. Each has its pros and cons with regard to food choices and nutrition.

- **Full-service restaurants.** These are restaurants that offer table service, meaning you sit at a table and a server takes your order. Nutrition varies, depending on the menu. Some restaurants offer a wide variety of choices. Others specialize in certain types of food, such as fish, steaks, or ethnic food.

- **Self-serve restaurants.** Examples are cafeterias and restaurants with buffets or food bars. Some self-serve restaurants, particularly those that advertise "all you

can eat," allow you to return for second and third helpings. Such offers—which appeal to the appetite, not to hunger—are an invitation to overeat.

- **Fast-food restaurants.** These restaurants usually offer a limited range of foods, many of which are high in fat, sugar, and sodium. Some fast-food chains have added more healthful choices to their menus in recent years. You can now find broiled and roasted foods, salads, low-fat milk, and fruit juice.

Many factors enter into your choice of restaurant, such as the price of a meal and how quickly you want to be served. Nutrition should also be a consideration. Try to select a restaurant that you know offers healthful choices.

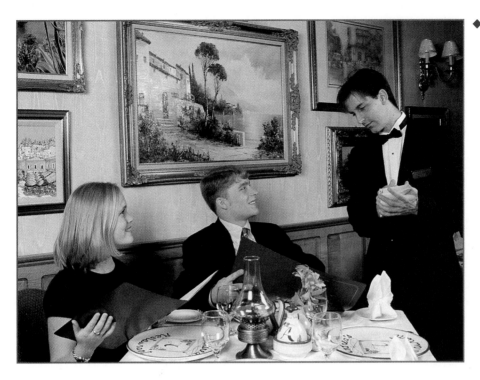

◆ At full-service restaurants, you usually have many food options. How can you use this fact to your advantage to make healthful choices?

Meals to Go

As the pace of daily living speeds up, many people today are choosing to buy ready-to-eat meals to take home. These foods, which you may know better as take-out or carry-out meals, are known in the food service industry as **home meal replacements**.

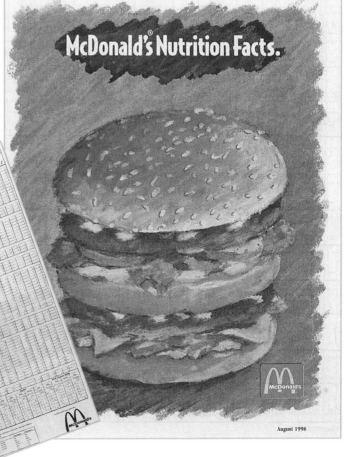

McDonald's Nutrition Facts.

August 1998

◆ Many fast-food restaurants now have information available on the nutritional content of the foods on their menu. Explain why this information is of value to their customers.

According to the National Highway Traffic Safety Administration (NHTSA), nearly 6 percent of all fatal traffic accidents are caused by drivers handling food or beverages while at the wheel. Eating while driving is a major distraction. If you reach for a soft drink or hold food with one hand while you drive, you're asking for an accident to happen. Play it safe. Make your car a "no-food zone."

Home meal replacements may come from delicatessens, fast-food chains, or establishments that specialize in one kind of food, such as pizza. Another popular option is the meal centers found in some supermarkets. Resembling restaurant salad bars and buffets, these centers feature a wide variety of take-out foods, ranging from complete meals to sandwiches. Many meal centers offer fresh cut-up salad ingredients, soups, beverages, and desserts.

Today, many full-service restaurants have take-out menus. Still another recent innovation in some locales is the "meal taxi." Consisting of a fleet of cars operated by an independent food delivery service, the meal taxis will pick up food from any one of a number of participating restaurants and deliver it to your home.

Making Healthful Food Choices

The food choices you make when you eat out or bring food in are important ones. Whether you are dining at a fancy restaurant or having a pizza delivered, you need to count the food as part of your overall eating plan. The following paragraphs explain how.

Eating Out Healthfully

"Am I stuffed," Paul groaned as he and his friends emerged from a restaurant. "I don't think I'll ever eat again!"

Have you ever made a remark like that after eating out? It hints at one of two potential pitfalls associated with eating in restaurants —portion size. The other pitfall is the menu choices you make.

Ordering from the Menu

The meal that made Paul feel so full consisted of fried potato skins followed by batter-dipped chicken with mashed potatoes and gravy. Several words from this description—"fried," "batter-dipped," and "gravy"— are clues that foods are high in fat. Other such terms are

◆ Breaded

◆ Creamy

◆ In a cheese sauce (or *au gratin*)

◆ Scalloped

◆ Rich

◆ Crispy

◆ Parmigiana

◆ Tempura

When ordering from a menu, look for items described as "broiled," "baked," or "steamed." These terms identify foods that are usually relatively low in fat. When in doubt about how a dish is prepared or what ingredients it contains, ask your server. You might also ask whether your food can be prepared differently from how it is described— for example, broiled instead of fried.

Be wary, too, of toppings, such as sauces, mayonnaise, salad dressings, and sour cream. Request either that your food be served without the topping or that the topping be served on the side so that you can use as little as you want. Still another option is to ask for a substitute—for example, a low-fat salad dressing or lemon juice in place of an oily, high-fat dressing, or a simple tomato sauce instead of a cream sauce on pasta.

You can watch your sodium intake by asking the kitchen to eliminate salt and sodium-based seasonings. One such seasoning, monosodium glutamate (mah-no-SO-dee-uhm GLUE-tuh-mate), or MSG, is used as a flavor enhancer, especially in Chinese foods.

Keep in mind that variety is one of the keys to good nutrition. If your choices are limited—as they usually are in a fast-food restaurant—you may come up short on other food groups needed for good health, such as fruits and vegetables. If so, make an extra effort to include those foods in other meals during the day.

How Big Is a Serving?

These are "official" serving sizes from the Food Guide Pyramid.

Look and Learn:
What other strategies can you think of for controlling portion size?

A(n) . . .

is as big as a serving of . . .

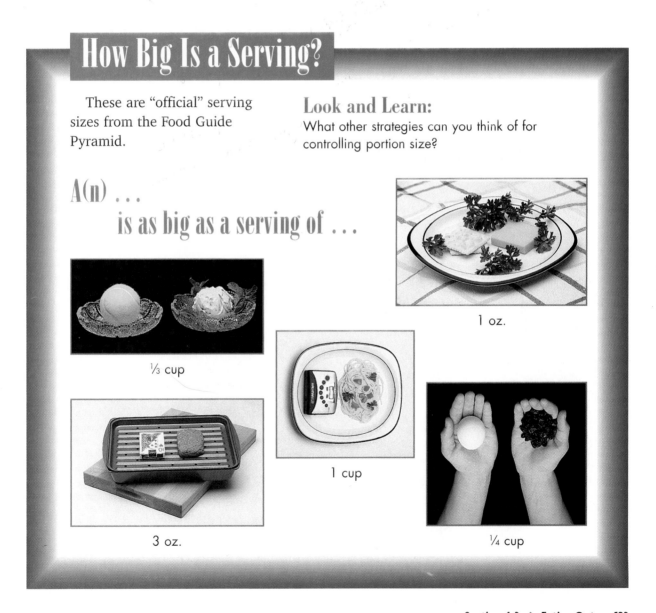

⅓ cup

1 oz.

1 cup

3 oz.

¼ cup

Controlling Portions

Have you ever been served so much food in a restaurant that you were unable to finish? Many restaurants offer very large servings—sometimes two to three times what the Food Guide Pyramid recommends.

When it comes to eating in restaurants, remember that "less is more." There are several ways of accomplishing this:

◆ Build your meal around several appetizers instead of one large main dish, or **entrée** (AHN-tray)—the term used for main dishes on many restaurant menus.

◆ If you do opt for an entrée, do not eat the entire serving. Let your hunger, not your appetite, be your guide. Most restaurants will pack leftover food so that you can take it home.

◆ Make the salad bar your main course. Many full-service restaurants have salad bars, often with soup choices and breads. Choosing from the salad bar is a good way not only of controlling the amount of food you eat but also of getting servings of vegetables and fruits in your meal.

Another practical and healthful solution to controlling portion size and limiting fats, salt, and sugar in your eating plan is to prepare more meals at home. Save eating out for special occasions. This gives you a chance to splurge occasionally on higher-fat and higher-calorie foods without feeling guilty. Just be sure the rest of the time to follow the guidelines in the Food Guide Pyramid.

◆ When preparing a salad, keep in mind that salad dressing isn't the only way to enhance the flavor. Name some other low-fat, low-sodium possibilities for tossed salad.

Food Safety

When you bring food home to eat or have it delivered, is it safe to eat? That question can be answered in one word: *temperature.* To avoid causing foodborne illness, hot food should be served hot and cold food should be cold. If food brought into the home is not going to be eaten right away, refrigerate it to prevent harmful bacteria from starting to grow. Heat it as necessary before serving. Many restaurants that deliver have special equipment that will keep hot food hot and cold food cold until it reaches your door.

Eating at School

Most schools have a cafeteria that serves lunch and sometimes breakfast as well. Usually, the cafeteria offers a complete meal that was planned with good nutrition in mind. Bringing food from home is also an option. You'll learn how to pack a nutritious lunch or snack in Chapter 20.

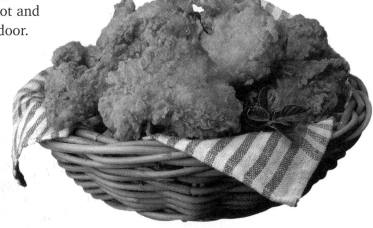

> **INFOLINK**
>
> For more on foodborne illness and keeping food safe to eat, see Section 7-3.

Section 4-3 Review & Activities

1. What does the term *home meal replacement* mean?

2. Give two suggestions for making healthful food choices from a restaurant menu.

3. Identify two ways of controlling portion size when you eat out.

4. Analyzing. Cal was delayed in traffic for nearly an hour on his way back from picking up food for the family's meal. Why should this be a concern?

5. Applying. Develop a lunch menu for a fast-food restaurant that emphasizes foods low in fat, sugar, and sodium. Give names to these food items.

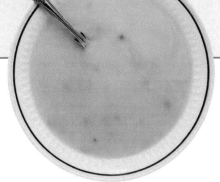

The Vegetarian Lifestyle

Inez and her friends were standing in the lunch line, trying to decide what to eat. After Jennie had made her choices, Inez looked at her tray and said, "What? No hamburger today?"

"No," said Jennie, "I'm thinking of becoming a vegetarian."

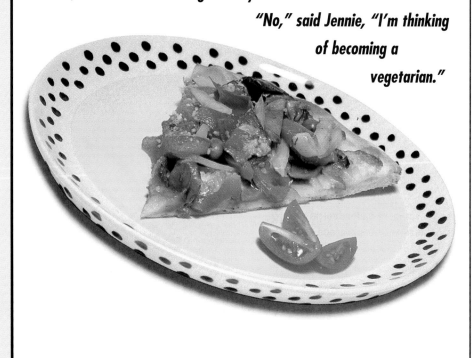

Objectives

After studying this section, you should be able to:

- Identify foods eaten by different types of vegetarians.
- Discuss reasons why people choose to become vegetarians.
- Plan nutritious vegetarian meals.

Look for These Terms

vegetarians

vegans

lacto vegetarians

ovo vegetarians

lacto-ovo vegetarians

Vegetarianism

Vegetarians are people who do not eat meat, poultry, or fish. In addition, some vegetarians do not eat dairy foods or eggs.

A vegetarian eating plan can supply complete nutrition. However, as with any other way of eating, the food choices require some thought and planning. Before Jennie changes her way of eating, she would be wise to learn more about making vegetarian food choices.

Facts About Vegetarians

Some people are confused about what foods vegetarians eat. In fact, there are several kinds of vegetarians, depending on what foods they include in their eating plans:

- ◆ **Vegans** (VEE-guns or VEH-juns), also known as pure vegetarians, are people who eat only foods from plant sources, such as grain products, dry beans and peas, fruits, vegetables, nuts, and seeds.

- ◆ **Lacto vegetarians** are people who eat dairy products in addition to foods from plant sources.

- ◆ **Ovo vegetarians** are people who eat eggs in addition to foods from plant sources.

- ◆ **Lacto-ovo vegetarians** are people who eat foods from plant sources, dairy products, and eggs.

People choose to become vegetarians for many reasons. Some people do so because they feel it is a healthier way of eating. Of course, it's not necessary to become a vegetarian in order to practice healthful eating habits. Still, studies show that well-chosen vegetarian eating plans are healthier than the average American eating pattern. For instance, most Americans eat too much protein and fat, whereas vegetarian eating plans can provide enough protein and be relatively low in fat.

Good Nutrition for Vegetarians

If they make wise food choices, vegetarians can usually get all the nutrients they need. As with any other eating patterns, the key to good vegetarian nutrition is variety. Although vegetarians choose to avoid some foods, they still have plenty of other foods from which to select.

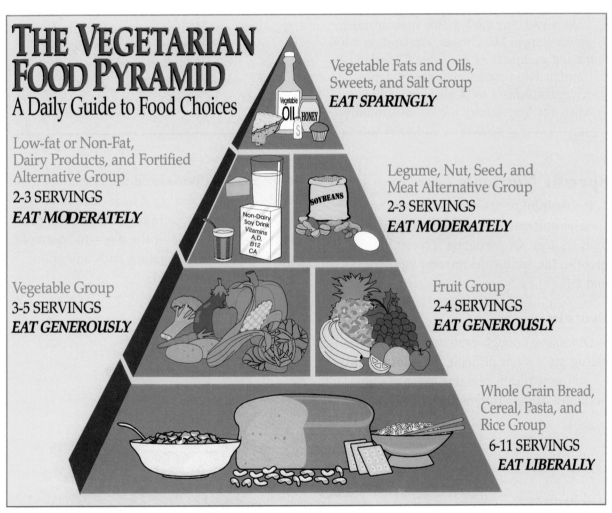

THE VEGETARIAN FOOD PYRAMID
A Daily Guide to Food Choices

Vegetable Fats and Oils, Sweets, and Salt Group
EAT SPARINGLY

Low-fat or Non-Fat, Dairy Products, and Fortified Alternative Group
2-3 SERVINGS
EAT MODERATELY

Legume, Nut, Seed, and Meat Alternative Group
2-3 SERVINGS
EAT MODERATELY

Vegetable Group
3-5 SERVINGS
EAT GENEROUSLY

Fruit Group
2-4 SERVINGS
EAT GENEROUSLY

Whole Grain Bread, Cereal, Pasta, and Rice Group
6-11 SERVINGS
EAT LIBERALLY

◆ **The Vegetarian Food Pyramid gives specifics for people who prefer a meatless eating plan.**
How does it compare to the Food Guide Pyramid?

The Vegetarian View

You may think of vegetarianism as a recent development, but in reality, it dates to antiquity. For over two millennia, vegetarianism has been a religious practice among certain Hindu and Buddhist sects, which consider all animal life to be sacred. Another religious group, the Trappist monks, embraced vegetarianism in 1666. More recently, the practice was adopted by Seventh-Day Adventists.

As a Western movement, vegetarianism got its start in Manchester, England, in 1809, among members of the Bible Christian Church. The first nonreligious practice of vegetarianism took place in 1847, when the Vegetarian Society was founded.

In 1850, the movement spread to the United States, and in 1908, the International Vegetarian Union was founded.

Think About It

1. Some people become vegetarians because they are concerned about the world food supply and believe that eating meat contributes to the problem of world hunger. Learn about this view from outside resources. Summarize your findings in a brief report.

2. Other people become vegetarians for economic reasons. Compare the cost of a typical vegetarian meal with that of a nonvegetarian meal. Show your findings in a graph.

Specific Nutrients

It is helpful to take a look at how some specific nutrients are supplied in vegetarian food choices. Of particular interest are protein, fat, iron, calcium, and vitamins B_{12} and D.

Protein

Obtaining enough protein on a vegetarian eating plan is not difficult, even for vegans. As you may recall, proteins are made up of amino acids. Proteins from plant sources do not provide all the essential amino acids. However, eating a wide variety of foods from plants can provide complete protein over the course of the day—for example, dry beans or peas together with any grain products, nuts, or seeds.

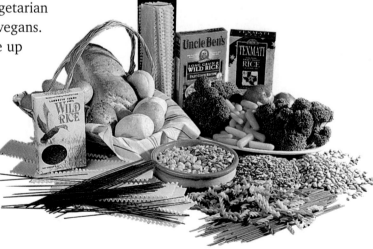

◆ Grain products, dry beans and peas, nuts and seeds, and vegetables are all sources of protein. Identify three other nutrients provided by these products.

Fat

Some people who become vegetarians are surprised to find themselves putting on weight. Often, this is because their eating plans center on whole milk, cheese, or eggs, all of which are high in fat. Nuts and seeds are also high in fat.

The solution to this problem is to choose a meal plan that emphasizes grain products, fruits, and vegetables. These foods provide many important nutrients but are low in fat.

Iron

As noted in Chapter 2, iron is essential in making hemoglobin, a substance in blood that carries oxygen to all body cells. This important mineral is found in many fruits, vegetables, and grain products, especially dry beans and peas and dried fruits. Since the iron in foods from plant sources is not easily absorbed, however, vegetarians run the risk of an iron shortage.

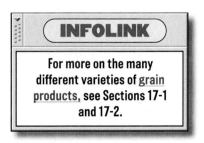

INFOLINK

For more on the many different varieties of grain products, see Sections 17-1 and 17-2.

Because vitamin C aids the body in its absorption of iron, a sensible solution is to eat foods rich in vitamin C together with foods high in iron. If vegetarians eat a wide variety of foods, including rich sources of vitamin C, they will probably meet their iron needs. Another way to get iron is by using cast-iron cookware.

Calcium

Getting enough calcium is of particular concern for vegans as well as others who do not drink milk. As you have learned, a good supply of calcium is essential for healthy bones and teeth.

Calcium needs can probably be met by eating good plant sources of the nutrient. These include dry beans and green, leafy vegetables, such as spinach, kale, and mustard greens.

Even so, it may be difficult for vegans to get enough calcium. They may be advised to drink fortified soy milk. Some health professionals recommend that vegans use calcium supplements.

Vitamins B$_{12}$ and D

Another concern regarding vegan eating plans is vitamins B$_{12}$ and D. Since Vitamin B$_{12}$ is not found in foods from plant sources, the *Dietary Guidelines for Americans* recommends that vegans take supplements. Vegans may also need supplements of vitamin D, which is found mainly in fortified milk.

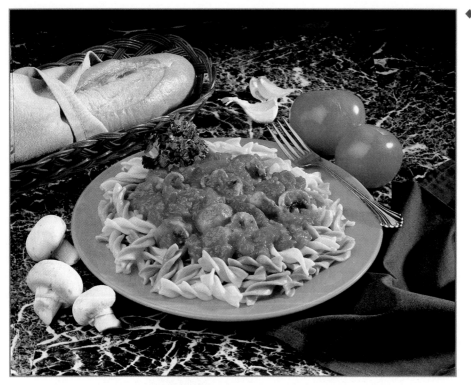

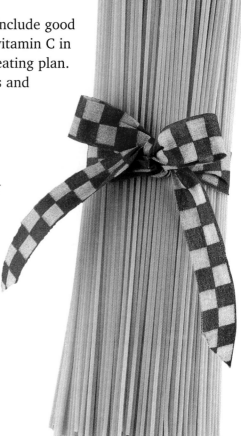

◆ **Even people who aren't vegetarians may want to collect tempting vegetarian recipes like the one pictured.** Locate one vegetarian recipe either online or in a magazine geared toward the vegetarian lifestyle. Discuss trying out the dish with adults at home.

Planning Vegetarian Meals

Planning vegetarian meals can be easy. Just follow the basic guidelines for meal planning covered earlier in this chapter, but with some modifications, as follows:

◆ Substitute products made from soybeans and wheat for foods from animal sources. Many of these items, including soy milk, bean curd (or tofu), and seitan (SAY-tan) —a wheat-based meat substitute—can be found in supermarkets or health food stores.

◆ Get acquainted with the many varieties of grain products and dry beans and peas that are available. For instance, you might want to try grains such as millet, bulgur, and barley.

◆ Be sure to include good sources of vitamin C in your daily eating plan. Citrus fruits and melons are excellent sources.

◆ Use dark green, leafy vegetables, such as kale and mustard greens, liberally.

Vegetarian Recipes

Many vegetarian recipe books are available. They range from basic information on getting started with vegetarian foods to gourmet and ethnic recipes. Since vegetarian recipes are sometimes high in fat, choose them carefully. You can also adapt favorite nonvegetarian recipes, substituting ingredients such as seitan or bulgur for meat.

Many ethnic cuisines, such as Asian and Central and South American, are based on vegetarian foods. They can provide you with a wealth of menu ideas and recipes as well as introduce you to new foods.

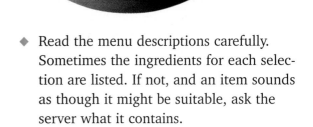

Eating Out Vegetarian-Style

Because of customer demand, many restaurants have begun offering at least one vegetarian meal on their menu. Except for vegans, most vegetarians should have no problems making food choices when eating out. They can usually find meatless meals made with milk, eggs, or cheese. Some food choices might include baked potatoes with cheese toppings, pizza, meatless lasagna, bean soup, and omelets.

Since vegans eat no animal products, their choices are more limited. Many restaurants offer salad bars or a selection of salads on the menu, but for those who eat out frequently, the limited choices can be tiresome.

Here are some suggestions for vegans to consider when eating out:

◆ Read the menu descriptions carefully. Sometimes the ingredients for each selection are listed. If not, and an item sounds as though it might be suitable, ask the server what it contains.

◆ Tell the server that you are a vegetarian, and ask whether the chef would be willing to make up a plate of cooked vegetables.

◆ Ethnic restaurants, such as Chinese, East Indian, Mexican, and Middle Eastern, usually offer some vegan meals.

◆ If a restaurant does not offer any vegan meals except salads, talk to the manager. Restaurants are always looking for ways to attract new customers and may be receptive to your ideas.

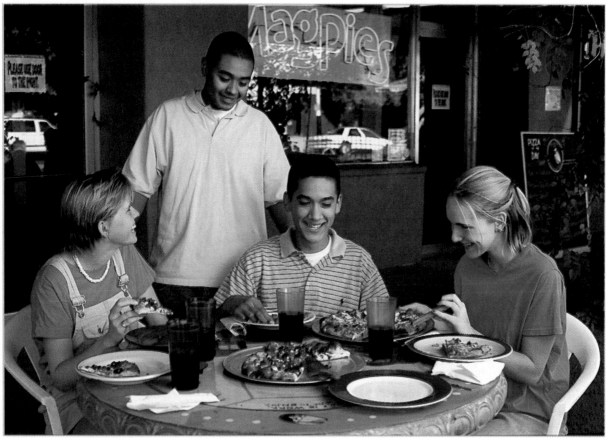

◆ **Today, vegetarians are finding more restaurant choices that suit their way of eating.** Research restaurants in your community, or one nearby, that offer interesting vegetarian options. Create a restaurant guide of such places.

Section 4-4 Review & Activities

1. How are a vegan and a lacto-ovo vegetarian similar? How are they different?

2. What reason do the majority of people give for becoming vegetarians?

3. How can vegetarians be sure to get enough protein? Iron?

4. Give three guidelines for planning vegetarian meals.

5. Evaluating. Do you think restaurants should offer more choices for vegetarian customers? If they did, would nonvegetarian customers also benefit? Why or why not?

6. Applying. Plan one day's meals and snacks for a vegetarian. Be prepared to explain the type of vegetarian the menu is for and why you chose those foods.

CAREER WANTED

Individuals proficient at designing web pages and who stay aware of changing technology.

REQUIRES:
- knowledge of HTML
- long periods of creativity

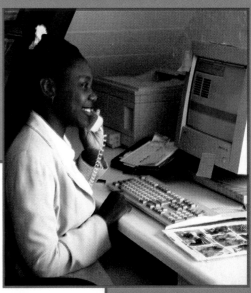

"Food never looked so good in words on a computer screen,"
says Food Web Designer Junilla Dawson

Q: What exactly do you do as a Web designer, Junilla?

A: I have created a web site promoting healthful eating that includes updated recipes and hyperlinks. My responsibilities include making sure this information is intriguing to the public using animations and exciting graphics.

Q: What skills and education are necessary to become a Web designer?

A: You must have a good grasp of HTML, the most common web programming language. To stay competitive, however, a solid background in computers is needed, plus some training or experience in graphic arts.

Q: What is the greatest challenge facing someone who wants to pursue a career in Web design?

A: Without a doubt, the rapidly evolving technology. It's no joke that the computer you bought yesterday was obsolete before you got it home! My greatest challenge is staying current in the latest developments.

Q: What rewards are there for a Web designer?

A: For me, it's knowing that the way my information is presented makes the end-user sit up and take notice. If the public develops more healthful eating habits because of web sites like mine, then I have helped others while doing what I love!

Career Research Activity

1. Investigate advances in cable technology that may impact on the future of the Web. Using this information, write a description of what some people have referred to as the "Next-Net," the Internet of the 21st Century.

2. Visit some food web sites. Identify at least two that match Junilla's description of her web site. Describe why you think these food web sites are exciting. Will they impact people's eating habits? Why?

Related Career Opportunities

Entry Level
- Web Master
- Software Designer

Technical Level
- Web Site Administrator
- Software Technician
- Computer Programmer

Professional Level
- Graphic Artist
- Media Director
- Imaging Specialist

Chapter 4 Review & Activities

Summary

Section 4-1: Daily Meals and Snacks

- People follow different eating patterns, from eating three meals a day to grazing.

- Be sure your daily food choices provide the right amount of calories and nutrients.

- Eat regularly, start the day with a nutritious breakfast, and choose snacks wisely.

Section 4-3: Eating Out

- All types of restaurants have pros and cons with regard to food choices and nutrition.

- Learning to identify the healthful choices on a restaurant menu and controlling portion size are important skills to develop.

- Wise food choices are also important when eating at school or eating on the go.

Section 4-2: Positive Food Habits

- Keep a food record to identify your eating habits. Then you can evaluate your habits and decide whether you want to change them.

- Work at improving your eating habits gradually, and set specific, realistic goals.

Section 4-4: The Vegetarian Lifestyle

- Some vegetarians eat only foods from plants, while others also eat dairy products or eggs.

- People become vegetarians for many reasons.

- The vegetarian way of eating can be healthful as long as sound food choices are made.

- To plan vegetarian meals, modify the basic guidelines for good nutrition.

Working IN THE Lab

1. **Food Preparation.** Using recipe books or magazines, find three ideas for quick and easy foods that would provide needed nutrients. As a group, prepare the foods in class for lunch. Working independently, evaluate the foods on the basis of cost, ease of preparation, and taste. Record your results in your Wellness Journal.

2. **Taste Test.** Taste samples of vegetarian dishes provided by your teacher. Judge them on taste and appearance.

Checking Your Knowledge

1. Describe two different eating patterns.

2. Why is breakfast such an important meal?

3. What is meant by the term *grazing*?

4. Briefly describe how to keep a food record.

5. When you are planning to improve your food habits, why is it important to decide on specific changes?

6. Name three clues that a food on a restaurant menu may be high in fat.

7. How can an awareness of appetite help you eat healthfully when eating out?

8. Name four types of vegetarians and the foods eaten by each.

9. Why do some vegetarians need to be careful about eating too much fat?

10. Why is calcium a concern for some vegetarians? Name two foods that can help meet their calcium needs.

Review & Activities Chapter 4

Thinking Critically

1. Analyzing Behavior. Alyssa was reviewing her food record. She noticed that when she ate alone or with her family, she usually made healthful food choices. However, her choices were less wise when she ate out with friends. Why might this be so?

2. Predicting Consequences. How might consumer complaints or suggestions affect menu items offered by a restaurant? What might happen if restaurant owners ignore consumer complaints and suggestions?

3. Recognizing Stereotypes. Suppose you and a friend are eating out. You hear a person at the next table asking if there are any vegetarian dishes on the menu. Your friend says, "How dumb. People who don't eat meat are weird." Is this a reasonable judgment? What can you say to help your friend better understand vegetarians and their way of eating?

Reinforcing Key Skills

1. Management. Kris has been invited to the home of a friend for the evening meal. Kris knows that her friend's family eats a light meal in the evening because they have their big meal at noon. Because of her hectic schedule, Kris was able to have only a sandwich and piece of fruit at lunchtime. How can she satisfy her nutritional needs and hunger while at her friend's home?

2. Communication. Harris's science club is having a year-end celebration in a local restaurant. Harris, who is very conscious of his nutrient needs, would like to ask how a certain dish is prepared. The server appears to be busy, however, taking orders from other people at the table. How can Harris satisfy his need for information without being a burden to other members of the club?

Making Decisions and Solving Problems

Your dad routinely fixes breakfast for the family. Most mornings he prepares eggs, bacon or sausage, and buttered biscuits, and serves whole milk. You appreciate his willingness to see that you have a hot breakfast each morning. However, you are concerned about the fat and cholesterol in the foods he prepares.

Making Connections

1. Social Studies. Using library resources, research the eating patterns in two other cultures. Present your findings to the class. Discuss why eating patterns vary from one culture to another.

2. Health. Visit two fast-food restaurants or consult a Web site that provides information about the number of calories, grams of fat, milligrams of cholesterol, and milligrams of sodium contained in their foods. Use this information to create a guide to fast-food dining in your area. Include the most healthful options on each of the menus.

CHAPTER

5

Section 5-1
Maintaining a Healthful Weight

Section 5-2
Weight Management

Section 5-3
Keeping Active

Section 5-4
Nutrition for Sports and Fitness

In addition to eating sensibly, one of the most important habits teens should develop is getting regular physical activity. In this chapter, you'll learn about the many benefits.

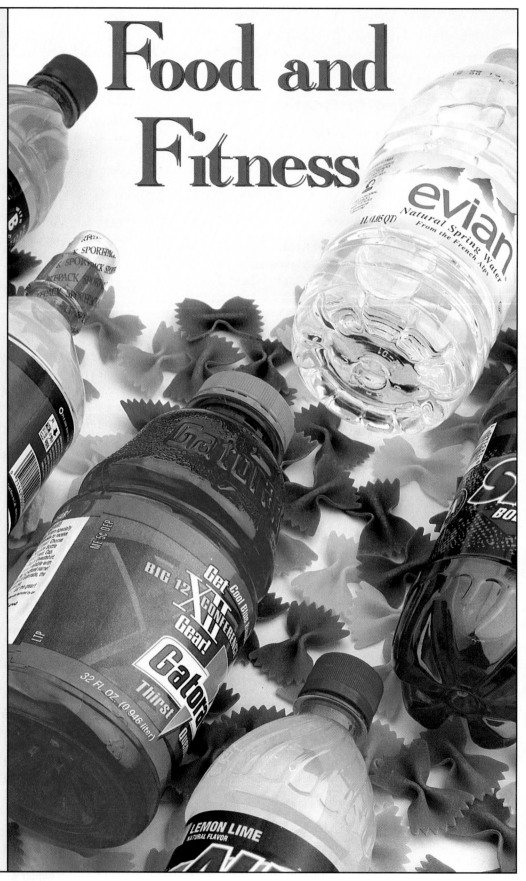

Food and Fitness

Maintaining a Healthful Weight

Objectives

After studying this section, you should be able to:

- Explain why there is no one ideal body shape.
- Describe methods used to determine whether a person's weight is at a healthy level.

Look for These Terms

body mass index (BMI)

skinfold calipers

obese

waist-to-hip ratio

Although Alonza ate sensibly and was physically active, she was still unhappy with her body. Maybe you know someone like Alonza. Some people are dissatisfied with their body shape because they lack realistic goals.

The Myth of the Ideal Body

The human body comes in many different shapes and sizes. These differences have nothing to do with being too fat or too thin. Body shape is one of many traits passed down through heredity. Some people have wide shoulders or hips. Others are tall and thin; still others, short and stocky.

In spite of this, many people carry around in their minds an image of an "ideal" body—and they try desperately to reach that ideal. Usually, it's a losing battle. The tall, slender model you might see on TV inherited her shape, just as you did yours. You can change the amount of fat or muscle you have, but you can't change your body frame.

What Is a Healthy Weight?

Successful weight management starts with accepting the body you were born with. Then you can take steps to achieve a healthy weight within your body limits. You may never look like a model or famous athlete. Few people ever will. However, it's far more important to be fit and healthy, whatever your shape and size.

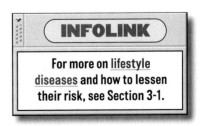

INFOLINK

For more on lifestyle diseases and how to lessen their risk, see Section 3-1.

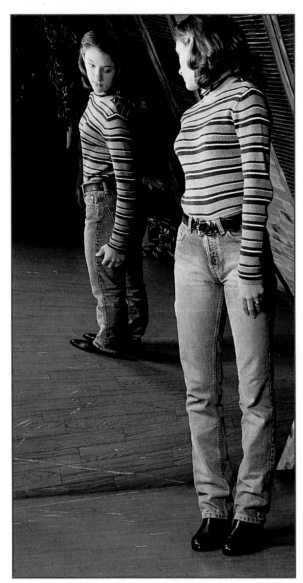

◆ Having a realistic perception of your appearance is a first step toward achieving and maintaining a healthy weight. Find pictures of high-fashion models in magazines and advertisements. Describe what all the models have in common. What message are these ads sending?

Body Mass Index

Body mass index (BMI) uses a ratio of weight to height. You can compute your BMI by doing the following:

1. Record your weight in pounds.

2. Measure your height in inches.

3. Multiply your weight by 703; then divide that number by your height squared (your height times itself).

By locating your BMI in the chart below, you can determine if you are at risk for health problems related to your weight.

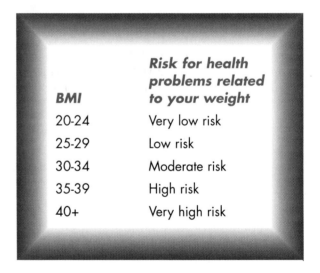

BMI	Risk for health problems related to your weight
20-24	Very low risk
25-29	Low risk
30-34	Moderate risk
35-39	High risk
40+	Very high risk

What is a healthy weight? It is one that will help you stay healthy throughout your life, within the framework of your own inherited shape, and minimizes your risk of lifestyle diseases.

Health professionals use a variety of methods to evaluate whether a person is at a healthy weight, is overweight, or is underweight. Three common methods involve determining body mass index, body fat percentage, and waist-to-hip ratio.

Although it is more accurate than just your weight alone, the BMI is not a foolproof measurement of health or fitness. For example, a bodybuilder may have a BMI of 30 or higher. Athletes and other individuals with large muscle masses are not necessarily at risk even if they have high BMIs. In such cases, body fat measurements may be taken.

Body Fat Percentage

Instead of BMI, some health professionals prefer to check the amount of body fat a person has in relation to muscle. In many instances, this gives a truer picture of healthy weight than the BMI—or just the number on a scale. Measuring body fat percentage can show when extra pounds are from muscle, not fat.

You may have given yourself a "pinch test" to see how much body fat you have, like the teen in the photo. Health professionals do a similar, but more sophisticated, test using **skinfold calipers**, a device that pinches the skin to measure body fat. Healthy body fat percentages for nonathletes are approximately 15 to 19 percent for males, and 20 to 25 percent for females. Individuals with percentages above these ranges are said to be **obese** (oh-BEESE), a term that means having excess body fat. Many athletes have body percentages in the range of 5 to 12 percent for males, and 10 to 20 percent for females. Body fat percentages lower than these ranges may indicate an eating disorder, which you'll read about in Chapter 6.

Waist-to-Hip Ratio

You probably know the saying, "You can't compare apples and oranges." A variation on this saying applies to body types. In this case, the comparison is of apples and pears. Some health professionals divide all individuals into one of two groups depending on their **waist-to-hip ratio**, a measure of how fat is distributed in the body.

Adults with pearlike shapes carry most of their fat on the thighs and hips. Those with applelike shapes carry most of it over the abdomen. Research shows that "apples" may have greater risks of health problems than

"pears." Apples, however, seem to be able to lose excess weight more easily than pears.

Adults can check body shape very easily: Stand relaxed and measure the waist without pulling in the stomach. Then measure the hips where they are largest. Dividing the waist measurement by the hip measurement gives the waist-to-hip ratio.

Adult women should have a ratio no higher than 0.80; adult men should have no higher than 0.95. Ratios above these limits may increase the risk of health problems, even if the BMI shows that weight is at a healthy level.

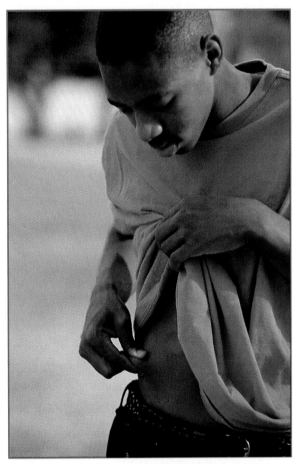

◆ Measuring the ratio of body fat to muscle gives a more reliable picture of a person's weight than the "pinch test" shown here. **What is a desirable body fat-to-muscle ratio for females? For males?**

The Healthy Weight for You

As you can see, there's more to evaluating a person's weight than meets the eye. If you're wondering about your weight, don't compare yourself to your friends or to a picture in a magazine. Instead, talk to a health professional. He or she can use reliable methods to judge whether your weight is healthy for you.

No matter what your shape or size, following a sound weight management program is beneficial. In the next section, you'll learn some basic guidelines to help you maintain a healthy weight throughout your life.

Section 5-1 Review & Activities

1. Why do people have different body shapes and sizes?

2. Name three methods that health professionals may use to evaluate the healthfulness of a person's weight.

3. **Synthesizing.** What "ideal" body shape is shown in the media? Why do you think that images of the ideal body have such a powerful effect on people?

4. **Analyzing.** How does the statement "You can't change your genes" apply to a person's weight goals?

5. **Applying.** In magazines, find pictures of men and women who have "ideal" body shapes. Compare and contrast their body shapes with more typical body shapes.

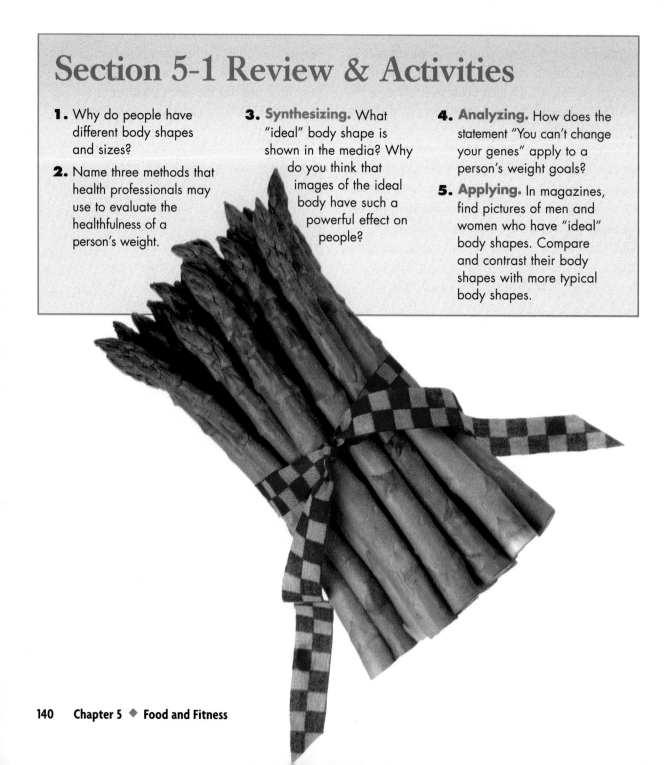

Weight Management

"Lose ten pounds in ten days." "Eat all you want and lose weight." "Gain muscle and lose fat without exercise." If claims like these sound too good to be true, it is because they generally are.

So what is a healthy approach to weight management? Whether you need to lose weight, gain weight, or maintain your current weight, you'll find tips in this section to help you achieve and manage a healthy weight throughout your lifetime.

Objectives

After studying this section, you should be able to:

- Recognize question-able weight-loss methods.
- Describe techniques for successful weight loss and weight gain.
- Give guidelines for maintaining a healthy weight.

Look for These Terms

overweight

fad diets

over-the-counter drugs

behavior modification

underweight

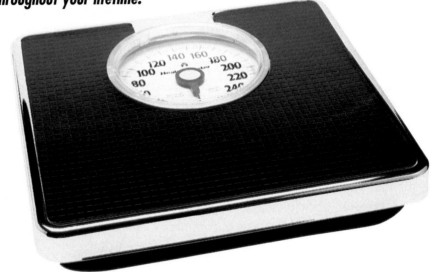

Losing Excess Weight

Excess weight can be a health risk. Studies show that **overweight**—weighing more than 10 percent over the standard weight for one's height—is a risk factor in heart disease, diabetes, cancer, and high blood pressure. For many people, losing weight is a positive step toward better health. If you begin a weight management program now, it can lead to a lifetime of better health.

Evaluating Weight Management Methods

With so much attention focused on health and appearance, weight-loss methods are a big business. Everywhere you turn, you can find books, articles, and advertisements that claim to provide the answers to weight loss.

Some popular types of weight manage-ment methods include:

- ◆ **Weight management diets.** Eating plans that reduce calorie intake for weight loss.

- **Weight management centers.**
  Organizations that provide both an eating plan and psychological support.

- **Weight management products.**
  Pills, shakes, prepared meals, and more, all sold with the promise of helping people lose weight.

Some of the weight management methods that are promoted are based on sound nutrition principles. A counseling session with a dietitian who provides you with an individualized eating plan is an example of a sound weight management method. Many methods, however, are not based on sound nutrition. Some methods can even be dangerous to health.

Fad Diets and Other Dangers

Every now and then, a scheme comes along that promises quick and/or easy weight loss. The best-known of these schemes are **fad diets** —popular weight-loss methods that ignore sound nutrition principles. Fad diets vary considerably but have one trait in common: They are risky.

Here are some other fad approaches to watch out for:

- Very low-calorie diets (800 calories or less per day). These may not provide enough energy or enough of the nutrients needed for good health.

- Eating plans based on a single food, such as grapefruit. As you know, your body needs a variety of foods every day.

- Fasting—going without food. This can be extremely damaging to your health.

- Diet pills. Some drugs can be obtained by prescription only and may play a small role in treating obesity. They're not for people with just a few pounds to lose. Alternatively, some **over-the-counter drugs**—drugs

that can be obtained without a prescription —may contain herbs or other ingredients that could create serious health problems.

- Plans that promise quick weight loss (over 2 pounds, or 1 kg, per week).

Even a weight-loss plan that would be acceptable for adults may pose problems for teens. At this point in your life, you are probably still growing. If you follow a weight-loss plan now, you might not get enough nutrients to grow into a healthy adult. If you are overweight now, see a health professional before you begin a weight-loss plan.

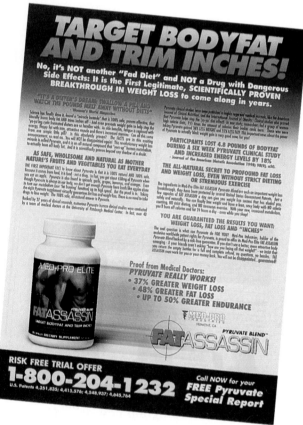

◆ There are no magic ways to lose weight. The advertisements for diet pills, for example, don't tell you that they can cause serious health problems. Write a paragraph about a sensational advertisement for a weight-loss product you have seen. Identify why the promises will most likely prove false.

Ten Red Flags of Junk Science

If you want to follow a weight management program, check it out first. Compare statements or claims made by the program with any combination of these "red flags" to help determine if the program is a healthful plan.

1. Recommendations that promise a quick fix.

2. Warnings of danger from a single product or regimen.

3. Claims that sound too good to be true.

4. Simplistic conclusions drawn from a complex study.

5. Recommendations based on a single study.

6. Dramatic statements that are refuted by reputable scientific organizations.

7. Lists of "good" and "bad" foods.

8. Recommendations made to help sell a product.

9. Recommendations based on studies published without peer review.

10. Recommendations from studies that ignore differences among individuals or groups.

Source: Food and Nutrition Science Alliance (FANSA)

Disadvantages to Consider

Certain weight-loss methods, although not dangerous to health, have other disadvantages.

Some methods simply don't work and are frauds. For instance, some products that claim to suppress appetite may use too little of an ingredient to actually have an effect.

Cost is another consideration. Weight management centers and special diet products can be expensive. Think carefully about what you are getting for your money.

Some weight-loss plans offer very limited food choices. Favorite foods are denied and the diet becomes monotonous. As a result, people find it difficult to stay on the plan long enough to get the results they want. Imagine giving up your favorite food for a year or more. Could you do it?

Of those who do manage to lose weight by dieting, approximately 95 percent gain it back. The most likely reason is that weight-loss diets are seen as temporary ways of eating. Instead of learning to make healthful food choices, dieters often rely on printed menus or prepackaged meals. As soon as they have lost the weight, they tend to go back to their old eating habits.

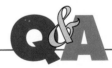

 What can I do to make my low-calorie, low-fat meals look more satisfying?

 Use small plates to help you moderate portion sizes. A full small plate of food will look much more appealing than a sparse large plate of food. In addition, don't forget to get a variety of food shapes, textures, and colors for more lively meals.

Successful Weight Management

If so many weight management methods don't work, what does work? The most successful way to lose and manage weight is through **behavior modification**, making gradual, permanent changes in your eating and activity habits. That is the key to keeping your weight at a healthy level throughout your life.

Set Reasonable Goals

Setting specific goals for weight loss can help motivate you and give you a way to see your progress. However, be sure your goals are reasonable.

First, be realistic about the size and shape of your body. Don't try to reach a weight or clothing size that's not right for you.

If you have a large amount of weight to lose, divide the task into a series of smaller goals. For instance, David needed to lose 40 pounds (18 kg), but his first goal was to lose just 10 pounds (4.5 kg). The smaller goal was easier to reach and gave him the encouragement he needed to stick with his program.

Give yourself plenty of time to reach your goal. Excess weight isn't gained overnight, so it can't be lost overnight. It has taken you a lifetime to develop your eating and exercising habits. Aim for a weight loss of no more than ½ to 1 pound (0.25 to 0.5 kg) a week. The more slowly you lose weight, the better your body can adjust. Your weight loss has a greater chance of coming from body fat—and of being a long-term loss.

Be More Active

Inactivity is one of the basic causes of overweight. Just increasing your physical activity, even without cutting down on food, can often result in a leaner body. This doesn't mean you have to start jogging ten miles a day. If you're not highly active, a good place to start is simply by increasing your lifestyle physical activity. Taking the stairs instead of the elevator or walking the dog instead of simply watching it play outside are two examples. Just like setting reasonable weight-loss goals, setting reasonable activity goals is important.

Calories Burned in Activities	
Degree of activity	Calories per minute
Sitting or standing quietly	1 to 2 calories
Light activity: cleaning house, playing baseball	4 calories
Moderate activity: brisk walking, gardening, cycling, dancing, playing basketball	6 calories
Strenuous activity: jogging, playing football, swimming	9 to 10 calories
Very strenuous activity: running fast, playing racquetball, skiing	12 calories

◆ Vigorous physical activity is a key to successful weight loss. In which of the activities above do you participate?

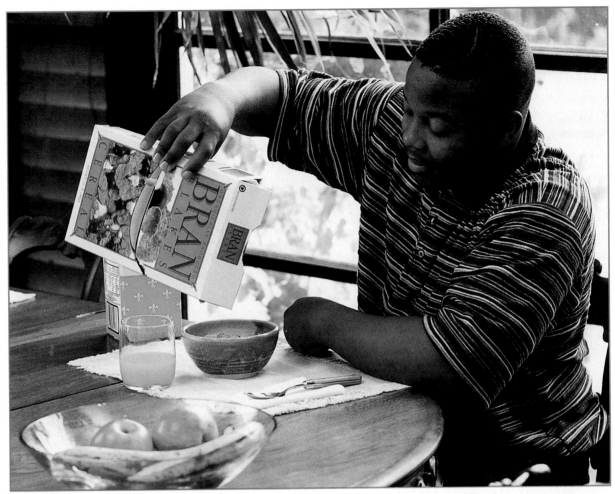

◆ **By eating sensibly, you can maintain a healthy weight.** What other measures can a person take to achieve a healthy weight?

Remember, the balance between energy in food and the energy you use for activities affects your weight. If you use up in activities about the same number of calories you get from food, your weight should stay at about the same level. If the food you eat provides more calories than you need for your activities, your body stores the extra as fat—and you gain weight. If you use up more calories in activities than you take in from food, you should lose weight.

In theory, you could change your energy balance just by eating less. In reality, however, it's better to increase your activity level as well.

Why? Studies show that exercise not only burns calories during the activity, but also increases metabolism for a short time afterward. In other words, it increases the amount of energy used for basic body processes. Regular activity also helps ensure that the weight you lose comes from body fat, not muscle.

Whatever your level of physical activity when you start a weight-loss plan, try to increase it. Without the added physical activity, you probably will not lose much weight. Section 5-3 discusses various types of activities and gives guidelines for becoming more active.

Change Your Eating Habits

Establishing new, more healthful eating habits will also help you reach and maintain a healthy weight. Be sure to follow a sensible eating plan that you enjoy and that allows you to eat a reasonable number of calories a day. You can get a reliable plan from a dietitian.

One key to successful weight management is to monitor your serving sizes. Too much food *of any kind* can result in weight gain. Another key is to eat fewer calories from fat. Remember, fat supplies more than twice as many calories per gram as do carbohydrates or proteins. Therefore, foods high in fat can make you gain weight easier than other foods can. In addition, studies suggest that fats in food are turned into body fat more easily than are excess carbohydrates and proteins.

Eat grains, fruits, vegetables, and other foods naturally low in fat. However, if you eat less fat, but you still consume too many calories, you will not lose weight. Be careful with your portion sizes of low-fat or fat-free potato chips, brownies, or other reduced-fat snacks. Just because fat is removed during processing doesn't mean the snack is a healthful choice.

As you learn to make more sensible food choices, become aware of nutrient-dense foods. They give you the most nutrients for the least number of calories. When consuming meat or dairy products, be sure to choose lean, fat-free, and low-fat varieties.

By moderating portion sizes, eating less fat, and choosing nutrient-dense foods, you may find that you can eat more food instead of less and still lose weight.

INFOLINK

For more specific information on serving sizes according to the Food Guide Pyramid, see Section 3-2. For more on choosing nutrient-dense foods, see Section 3-2.

Serving Sizes

Some people know which foods are healthful, but they forget or have a difficult time determining what a healthy portion is. Here are some fun and simple ways to size up your serving sizes.

Food portion	Compare the size of one serving to . . .
1 medium potato	Computer mouse
½ cup cooked rice	Cupcake wrapper
1 medium piece fruit	Tennis ball
½ cup fruit (chopped)	15 marbles
½ cup vegetables (chopped)	Standard lightbulb
3 oz. meat	Deck of cards
1½ oz. natural cheese	9-volt battery
½ cup or 1 scoop ice cream	Racquetball
1 tsp. butter	Tip of thumb to the first joint

Gaining Needed Weight

Overweight is a serious health problem. So is the flip side of the "weight coin." **Underweight** means weighing 10 percent or more below the standard weight for one's height. A person who is too thin has little body fat as an energy reserve and, possibly, less of the protective nutrients the body stores. This condition makes it harder for the person to fight off infection.

Gaining weight can be just as challenging as losing weight. If you're concerned about being too thin, discuss the matter with a physician. There may be a medical reason for an inability to put on weight.

Here are some hints to help you gain weight without adding fat to your food choices:

◆ Go for larger portions of nutrient-rich foods from the five food groups.

◆ Eat regular meals.

◆ Enjoy nutrient-dense snacks, including yogurt and fresh or dried fruit.

◆ Don't forget to stay active. Exercise can help assure weight gained is muscle, not fat.

Maintaining a Healthy Weight

Whether someone has lost or gained weight, or has always been a healthy weight, maintaining a healthy weight is the goal to meet for better health. Once you achieve a healthy weight, you should have no problem maintaining it as long as you continue to follow sound eating and activity habits. Still, if your weight starts to change, here are some suggestions:

◆ Keep a food record for a few days. Analyze the results to see if you are slipping into a poor eating pattern.

◆ Stay active. If you find your weight going up, increase your activity level.

◆ Keep a list of activities to do as alternatives to eating. If you find you're eating too much or too little because of stress, boredom, or some other reason, look to your list for healthful ways to cope with the situation. Try taking a hot bath, chatting with a friend, going for a walk, or simply brushing your teeth.

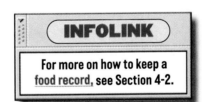

INFOLINK

For more on how to keep a food record, see Section 4-2.

Section 5-2 Review & Activities

1. What are the health risks associated with overweight? With underweight?

2. Name three signs that a weight-loss plan is unsafe.

3. What is behavior modification? How does it relate to weight loss?

4. Analyzing. Why are fad diets popular? What could be done to educate people how to determine when an eating plan may be a fad diet?

5. Synthesizing. Is it possible for someone to gain weight by eating a low-fat diet? Explain.

6. Applying. In newspapers and magazines, find ads for weight-loss methods. Evaluate them on the basis of the information you have read in this section.

Keeping Active

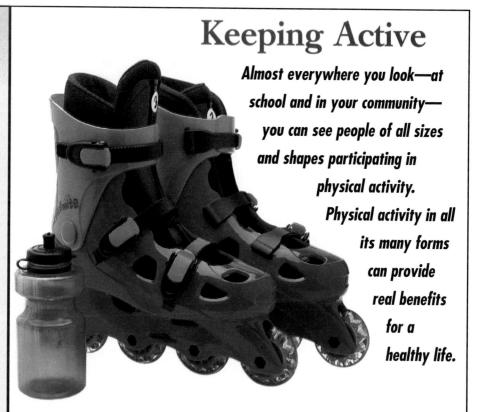

Almost everywhere you look—at school and in your community—you can see people of all sizes and shapes participating in physical activity. Physical activity in all its many forms can provide real benefits for a healthy life.

Objectives

After studying this section, you should be able to:

- Explain the benefits of being active.
- Describe the basic types of exercise.
- Make a plan for an activity program.

Look for These Terms

lifestyle activities

aerobic exercise

anaerobic exercise

Benefits of Activity

You know that staying active is important for weight management. Why else should you be active?

◆ It helps keep your body mobile. If your muscles are not used regularly, they tend to stiffen, and movement eventually becomes painful and difficult. Regular activity can keep your muscles strong and flexible throughout life.

◆ It helps improve psychological health. Regular activity can help you feel better by reducing stress and anxiety. Studies show that active people have a brighter outlook on life.

Types of Activity

You probably already do some physical activity as part of your daily routine, such as biking or playing basketball. Maybe you perform a regular chore at home, such as raking leaves or walking the dog. These are examples of **lifestyle activities**, forms of physical activity that are a normal part of your daily routine or recreation that promote good health throughout a lifetime.

A second type of activity is sports, which usually involve competition and are guided by a set of rules. When you think of sports, you may think of team sports such as football, basketball, and hockey, but other possibilities exist:

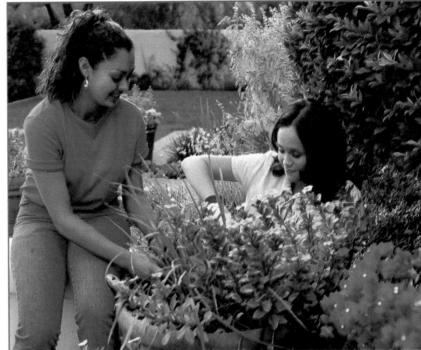

◆ Exercise includes more than running or lifting weights. Hobbies like gardening can reduce stress and increase physical activity. Make a list of leisure activities that you enjoy. Use online or print resources or consult the graphic on page 144 to determine how much energy the activities expend.

◆ **Individual sports.**
Activities you can do by yourself, such as bicycling or golf. Many individual sports also are called lifetime sports because they are more likely than team sports to become part of a person's routine over a lifetime.

◆ **Partner sports.** Activities carried out with one other person. A benefit of partner sports is that they are easier to organize at a moment's notice than are group events, such as a softball game.

◆ **Nature sports.** Activities in which there is some interaction with one of the forces of nature, such as surfing, rock climbing, sailing, orienteering, and swimming. A benefit of nature sports is that they can be relaxing and can promote good mental health.

Safety Check

You may have heard the popular expression, "No pain, no gain." Despite what you may already believe, pain during exercise is a sign that something is not right. If you experience pain, you should modify or stop the exercise you are performing.

Types of Exercise

Virtually all activities work one or more muscle groups and, therefore, include some form of exercise. Some people, including teens, are beginning to rediscover so-called traditional exercises, such as doing crunches or working out with weights.

The many forms of exercise can be divided into two basic types. A well-rounded exercise program includes both.

◆ **Aerobic** (uh-ROH-buhk) **exercise** is vigorous activity in which oxygen is continuously taken in for a period of at least 20 minutes. During this time, the heart rate increases, sending more oxygen to the muscles to be used as energy to do more work. Aerobic exercises include walking, jogging, climbing stairs, bicycling, aerobic dancing, and swimming. A healthy goal is to do aerobic exercise a minimum of three days a week—and for at least 30 minutes total on each of those days.

♦ **Anaerobic** (AN-uh-ROH-buhk) **exercise**, which builds flexibility and endurance, involves intense bursts of activity in which the muscles work so hard that they produce energy without using oxygen. Running the 100-meter dash is an example of an anaerobic activity. Resistance training, another form of anaerobic exercise, builds muscles by requiring them to resist a force. The more work the muscles do, the stronger they become. Resistance can be provided by weights, machines, or your own body weight. Anaerobic exercise should be done at least two times per week—and is especially helpful in combination with aerobic exercise.

Getting the Activity Habit

The first step in starting an exercise or activity program should be to have a medical checkup. Once you get a clean bill of health, you can start planning.

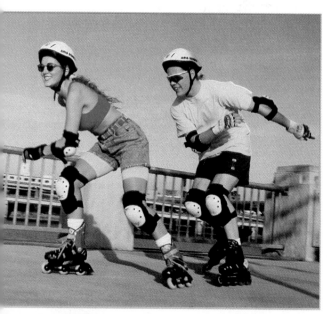

♦ Getting exercise by doing physical activities that you can enjoy with friends is a way of increasing the likelihood of staying with the activity. Give other guidelines for choosing a physical activity that you will want to continue for the exercise benefits.

Finding Your Target Heart Range

Just as eating within a certain fat range is good for the heart, so aerobic exercise needs to be done within a prescribed range for maximum cardiovascular benefit. This range, which differs from person to person, is your *target heart range.* To find your target heart range:

1. First find your *resting heart rate* by sitting quietly for 5 minutes. Then take your pulse by placing two fingers (but not your thumb!) on the side of your neck just under the jawbone.

2. Subtract your age from 220.

3. Subtract your *resting heart rate* (the result of step 1) from the number you arrived at in step 2.

4. Multiply the number you arrived at in step 3 twice—first by 0.85 and again by 0.6.

5. Add each of the numbers you got in step 4 to your *resting heart rate.*

The resulting totals represent your target heart range.

Think About It

1. Do you think your calorie needs will vary if you exercise for 30 minutes at a level below your target heart range? Why or why not?

2. During long bouts of exercise at the target heart range, the body uses glycogen for fuel. What food(s) should be eaten following exercise to replace this reserve fuel?

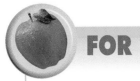

FOR YOUR HEALTH

Act Now!

You can easily work lifestyle physical activity into your everyday schedule. Here are some suggestions:

- Walk rather than ride to school.
- Get up to change the channel instead of using the remote.
- Play upbeat music while doing household chores.
- Plan social activities around physical ones. For example, turn a birthday party into a skating party.

Following Up

1. On the basis of the examples above, think of four ways in which you are currently inactive and four ways of becoming more active. Write your ideas in your Wellness Journal.

2. What would you tell an inactive person about the importance of regular lifestyle physical activity?

Are you already physically active? If not, there is no better time than now to start. Lifestyle activities taken up during the teen years are more likely to become lifelong habits than those acquired later in life. During the teen years, your energy level is also probably higher than it will be at any other period of your life.

What activity or sport should you choose? The possibilities are almost endless. Just be sure to pick something that holds your interest and that you can do—or at least learn to do—well. You're more likely to stick with an activity that you like doing and are good at. In addition, select an activity that fits in with your current lifestyle, including your schedule. If you already belong to several after-school clubs, don't try out for a team sport that holds its practices at the same time. Use the management and decision-making skills you learned about in Chapter 1 to help you make an informed choice.

The benefits of staying active are well worth the time spent. Like good nutrition, regular activity is a habit that gives a lifetime of physical and emotional rewards.

Section 5-3 Review & Activities

1. Name three benefits of exercise.

2. What are the two basic types of activity? Of exercise?

3. What are the steps for getting into the activity habit?

4. Analyzing. Why do you think people are advised to get a medical checkup before beginning a new program of physical activity or exercise?

5. Evaluating. What is your favorite form of activity or exercise? Which of the basic types does it involve?

6. Applying. Make a chart that outlines an exercise plan for the next week. Include at least three exercise sessions and at least two different forms of exercise. Be prepared to explain the benefits of your plan.

Nutrition for Sports and Fitness

When you think of the word athlete, what comes to your mind? Maybe you picture a professional ballplayer. However, an athlete may also be a high school swimmer or a 50-year-old who enjoys her morning run. Regardless of the level of intensity involved, the performance of all athletes can benefit from good nutrition.

Objectives

After studying this section, you should be able to:

- Explain how an athlete's nutrient needs can be met.
- Give suggestions for pregame meals.
- Point out the dangers of using anabolic steroids to build muscles.

Look for These Terms

dehydration

anabolic steroids

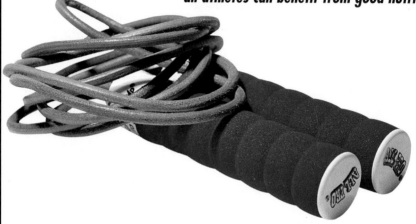

Nutrient Needs of Athletes

Eating right can't improve an athlete's skills—only practice can do that. An athlete's daily food choices, however, can make a difference between a good performance and a poor one.

Generally, an athlete's nutritional needs can be met by following the recommendations in the Food Guide Pyramid. However, the athlete does have two nutritional needs that far exceed those of the average person: the need for energy and the need for water.

Energy Needs

As noted earlier, during digestion, carbohydrates are broken down into the simple sugar glucose, which is used for energy. Extra carbohydrates are turned into a storage form of glucose known as glycogen, which is stored in the liver and muscles.

During vigorous and extended periods of exercise, the body uses glycogen for fuel. When the glycogen is used up, the athlete runs out of energy. Therefore, it's essential for athletes to eat plenty of carbohydrates to build up their glycogen stores.

During training and competition, athletes may need two or three times as much energy as the average person. Complex carbohydrates are the best choice for supplying this additional energy. "Carbohydrate loading," as this eating pattern is called, includes eating foods such as dry beans and peas, breads, cereal, pasta,

◆ **Successful athletes know that performing their best requires good nutrition.** After reading this section, list two do's and don'ts for teen athletes in training.

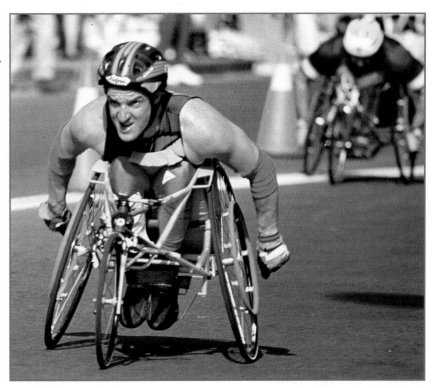

rice, and potatoes. Similar to the nonathlete's calorie needs, about 60 percent of an athlete's calories should come from carbohydrates, about 25 percent from fat, and about 15 percent from protein. Individual needs vary. Note that health experts do not recommend carbohydrate loading for teen athletes.

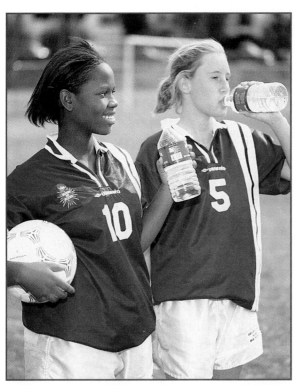

◆ **Be sure to drink additional water whenever you exercise vigorously, even if you don't feel thirsty.** Why is drinking water important?

Liquid Needs

Athletes lose a great deal of water through perspiration—as much as 3 to 5 quarts (3 to 5 L) during a strenuous workout. If the water is not replaced right away, **dehydration** (dee-hy-DRAY-shun), or lack of adequate fluids in the body, can result. This condition can lead to serious health problems.

An athlete who is dehydrated may become weak and confused. The body can become overheated, especially when exercising in hot weather. Heat exhaustion or heat stroke can result. These are serious conditions requiring immediate medical attention.

To prevent dehydration, athletes should drink water before, during (about every 15 minutes), and after an event. They should drink water even if they do not feel thirsty. Thirst is a sign that dehydration has already begun.

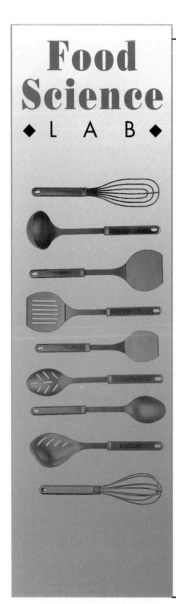

Food Science ◆ L A B ◆

Calories to Burn

You know the expression "Seeing is believing." You are about to see the energy released when food is burned by your system.

Procedure

1. Press the eye of a needle into the narrow end of a cork. Mount a walnut on the point of the needle. Weigh the resulting construction.

2. Remove both ends of a large can and one end of a small can. Punch holes in the large can near the bottom and in the small can near the top (the open end).

3. Pour 100 mL of tap water into the small can. Measure the temperature of the water.

4. Insert a glass rod through the holes in the side of the small can. Use the rod to balance the small can within the large can.

5. Place the nut on a nonflammable surface and light it with a match. Immediately place the large can over the burning nut so that the water can is above the nut. Allow the nut to burn for two minutes or until the flame goes out.

6. Stir the water with the thermometer. Record the water's highest temperature. Weigh the nut/cork/needle construction again, and record the result.

Conclusions

◆ How much did the weight of the nut change?

◆ How much did the temperature change?

◆ Repeat the experiment using a different kind of nut. Do you arrive at a different result? Why or why not?

One good way to gauge the amount of water to drink is to weigh in before and after the event. Loss of water usually shows up as a loss in body weight. For each ½ pound (250 g) lost during exercise, athletes should drink 1 cup (250 mL) of fluid, just as they would do during exercise.

In addition to water, juices and fruit drinks can be used. However, because they are high in sugar, they can cause stomach cramps, diarrhea, and nausea. To cut down on sugar, dilute juices and fruit drinks with an equal amount of water.

Sports drinks are also available. They are valuable mainly to athletes involved in exercise lasting longer than 90 minutes.

Common Myths

Some athletes believe they need extra protein to build muscles. It's true that dietary protein is needed to build body protein. Remember, however, that most Americans eat far more protein than they need. An athlete's protein requirements can be met easily through normal eating. Excess protein does nothing to build up muscles—only physical training can do that.

What about vitamin or mineral supplements? Almost all athletes who eat a wide variety of nutritious foods do not need vitamin or mineral supplements. The same is true of salt tablets. While some salt and potassium are lost through perspiration, these minerals can be easily replaced in well-chosen daily meals.

Timing of Meals

If you eat just before an athletic event, the digestive process competes with your muscles for energy. Instead, eat three to four hours before the event to allow time for proper digestion.

Follow these suggestions to get the most from your pre-event meal:

◆ Choose a meal that is low in fat and protein and high in complex carbohydrates. As you may recall, fat and protein take the longest to digest.

◆ Eat foods you enjoy and have eaten before. A pre-game meal is no time to experiment with a new food.

◆ Choose foods that you know you can digest easily.

◆ Have a reasonably sized meal (not too large) so that the stomach is relatively empty by event time.

◆ Drink large amounts of fluids with the meal.

After an athletic event or a hard workout, you need to refuel your body. In addition to replacing the water you have lost, be sure to eat nutritious food within one to four hours after the event—the sooner the better. Studies indicate that more carbohydrate (as glycogen) can be deposited in the muscles immediately after exercise than hours afterward.

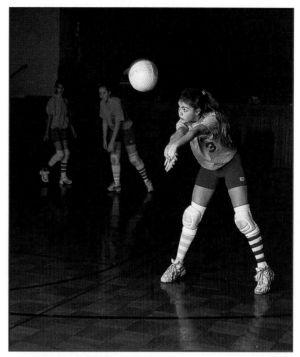

◆ To perform your best, eat a pre-game meal three to four hours before the event starts. Give two other pre-game tips for teen athletes.

Anabolic Steroids

All athletes want to perform well in sports and to have well-developed muscles. Many, however, are in a hurry to build up their muscles. Instead of depending on training alone, they mistakenly resort to taking **anabolic steroids** (AN-uh-bahl-ik STEHR-oydz), prescription medicines used to help build muscle strength in patients with chronic diseases. When used as an illegal drug, anabolic steroids can exact a terrible price on the user in terms of both health and behavior.

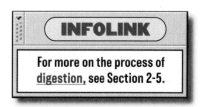

INFOLINK

For more on the process of digestion, see Section 2-5.

Steroids interfere with a person's ability to have children. In teens, they can impair bone growth. When taken over a period of time, they damage the liver, heart, and stomach, and can cause high blood pressure. Other physical side effects of steroid use can include fatigue, muscle cramps, and acne.

Remember that there are no quick fixes to improving athletic performance. Careful training and sound nutrition, practiced every day, are the surest ways to long-lasting top athletic performance.

Safety Check

Creatine, an amino acid that is sold as a supplement, has grown in popularity among athletes hoping to improve performance. Although it's not an anabolic steroid, creatine is not without side effects or concerns. Taking the supplement may cause an electrolyte imbalance that can lead to dehydration and heat-related illness.

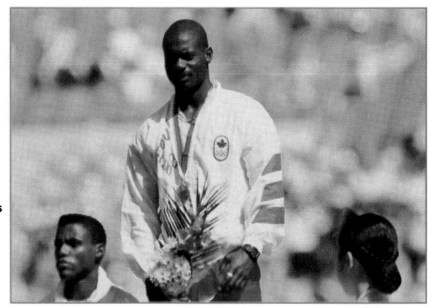

◆ **Canadian sprinter Ben Johnson was stripped of his Olympic medal, and eventually of the right to compete, for illegal use of steroids.** Identify three physical risks and one psychological risk of using these dangerous drugs.

Section 5-4 Review & Activities

1. How do the nutritional needs of athletes differ from those of nonathletes?

2. Give three suggestions for planning meals before an athletic event.

3. What are two negative side effects that can arise from the use of steroids?

4. Synthesizing. How could you persuade a friend of a teammate to avoid using anabolic steroids?

5. Comparing and Contrasting. Jill, an inactive student, and Mina, a swimmer, both weigh 120 pounds (54 kg). How do their protein needs differ?

6. Applying. Use the Food Guide Pyramid and recipe books to plan three meals for an athlete who is in training for a sport of your choice.

CAREER WANTED

Individuals interested in physical fitness and health with strong leadership and management skills.

REQUIRES:

- degree in physical education, sports medicine, or physical therapy
- maintained personal physical fitness program
- training hours under supervision of certified trainer

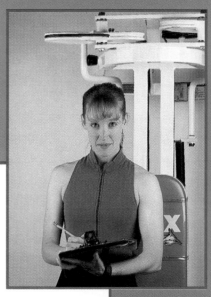

"Fitness training goes a long way beyond sports,"

says Athletic Trainer Jodi Chambers

Q: Jodi, you work at a health club. What are the responsibilities of your position?

A: I teach several exercise classes each day. I also design fitness programs for individual club members that fit their personal needs and goals.

Q: What skills do you need in your line of work?

A: At the very least, a trainer needs a basic knowledge of exercise, conditioning, weight management, nutrition, and injury prevention. You also need to know a lot about anatomy, physiology, kinesiology, and rehabilitation techniques.

Q: What is the greatest challenge of your job?

A: Believe me—this job requires a lot of energy! That's why it is so important that I pay attention to my own nutrition and health.

Q: What's your favorite part of being an athletic trainer?

A: I like being able to make a difference in people's lives as they reach their fitness goals.

Career Research Activity

1. Interview a physical education teacher, team coach, or physician. Ask the person to identify the most important responsibility of an athletic trainer. Share your findings by posting them on a "quote board" in the classroom.

2. Investigate ways in which the public's growing awareness of the need for exercise and good nutrition affects the education and training of paramedics and recreation facility managers. Create a public service announcement that displays your findings.

Related Career Opportunities

Entry Level
- Membership Solicitor
- Volunteer Coach
- Summer Camp Counselor

Technical Level
- Recreation Facility Manager
- Paramedic

Professional Level
- Athletic Trainer
- Sports Recruiter
- Physical Education Teacher

Chapter 5   Review & Activities

--- Summary ---

Section 5-1: Maintaining a Healthful Weight

- It's best to accept your inherited body shape and focus on being fit and healthy.

- Three methods used to evaluate whether a person is at a healthy weight involve determining body mass index, body fat percentage, and waist-to-hip ratio.

Section 5-3: Keeping Active

- Regular physical activity has many physical and psychological benefits.

- Activity takes the form of either lifestyle activities or sports.

- A fitness program that has a variety of enjoyable activities is more likely to be successful.

Section 5-2: Weight Management

- A weight management program can help you achieve and maintain a healthy weight.

- Many popular weight-loss methods are ineffective, and some are dangerous to health.

- The best way to lose weight is through gradual, permanent changes in eating and exercise habits.

Section 5-4: Nutrition for Sports and Fitness

- Athletes should emphasize complex carbohydrates and drink plenty of fluids.

- Pre-event meals should be planned and timed carefully.

- Using unprescribed anabolic steroids is illegal and has dangerous side effects.

Working IN THE Lab

1. **Foods Lab.** Make a list of simple snacks that would be suitable for a person who is changing eating habits to lose weight. The snacks should be easy to prepare, low in fat and calories, and nutritious. Work in groups to prepare the snacks.

2. **Food Preparation.** Plan and prepare a pre-event meal for a group of athletes in your school. Prepare a handout giving facts about nutrition and athletic performance to give to each participant. Interview athletes after their performances to find out how they felt during the events.

Checking Your Knowledge

1. When can the body mass index be an inaccurate measurement of healthy weight?

2. In terms of health, what is the difference between having an apple-shaped figure and a pear-shaped figure?

3. What is an appropriate amount of weight for an adult to lose in one week? Why is this amount suggested as opposed to a higher amount?

4. List three guidelines for setting a reasonable weight-loss goal.

5. Give two suggestions for gaining weight healthfully.

6. Why are flexibility and strength exercises important?

7. What is meant by the term *aerobic exercise*? Give two examples.

8. About what percentage of an athlete's calories should come from carbohydrates?

9. What can happen if an athlete doesn't replace water lost through perspiration?

10. About how long before an athletic event should the pre-event meal be eaten? Why?

Thinking Critically

1. Determining Credibility. Suppose you are interested in losing weight. Several of your friends are following the plan described in a best-selling diet book. Before you decide whether to join them, what information would you want to know about the author? About the diet plan? How will you find the information? How will it influence your decision?

2. Recognizing Bias. Why do you think some children receive more encouragement to participate in exercise and sports than others do? How do you think such encouragement (or lack of it) affects children?

3. Recognizing Fallacies. A basketball coach recommends a special "power supplement," claiming it will improve performance. After using the supplement for a week, several members of the team say that it helped them shoot more accurately. Do you think they are right? Why or why not?

Reinforcing Key Skills

1. Communication. Romy has been instructed by her physician to lose weight. However, she says she already eats the minimum servings suggested by the Food Guide Pyramid. What solutions can you propose to Romy?

2. Leadership. Student athletes are often led to believe that taking anabolic steroids or certain supplements will give them a performance advantage. What steps can be taken to heighten the awareness of the dangers for student-athletes of taking these products?

Making Decisions and Solving Problems

You strain your leg muscle while jogging one day. The doctor tells you to try to stay off your feet for a few weeks. However, you want to continue with some type of exercise during that time.

Making Connections

1. Math. Find the waist-to-hip ratio (rounded to two decimal places) for each of the following adults: (a) female, waist 27 in., hips 36 in.; (b) female, waist 33 in., hips 40 in.; (c) female, waist 35 in., hips 45 in.; (d) male, waist 36 in., hips 35 in.; (e) male, waist 34 in., hips 36 in. Which of the ratios indicate a health risk?

2. Language Arts. Write an article for a newspaper, Web site, or newsletter on one of the following subjects: safe weight loss, planning an exercise program, or nutrition for athletes.

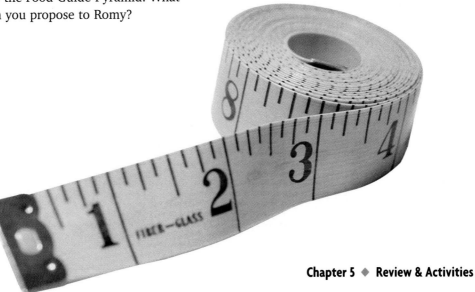

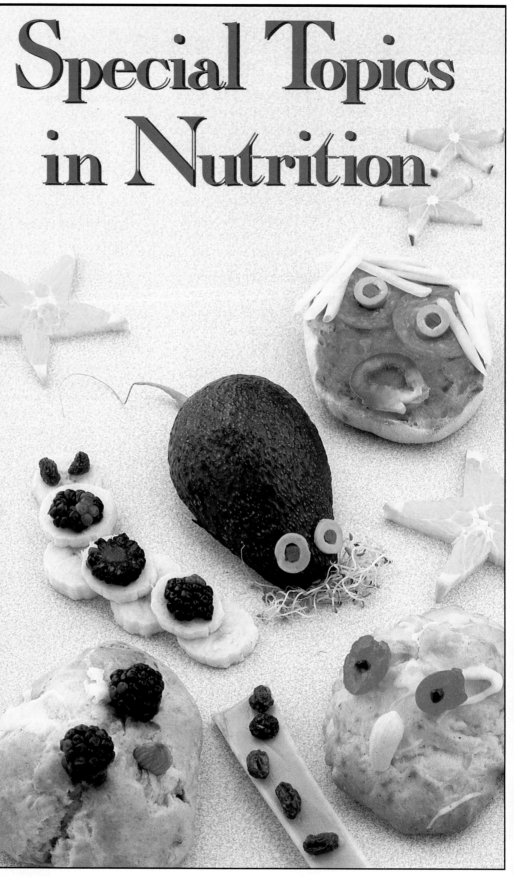

CHAPTER

6

Section 6-1
Food and the Life Span

Section 6-2
Managing Health Conditions

Section 6-3
Eating Disorders

Special Topics in Nutrition

Since Ali was a toddler, people have been telling her that she had her mother's dimples. Like Ali, each of us is the sum of hereditary traits.

Although you cannot control your genetic makeup, you have total control over your behaviors and habits—including the food choices you make.

Food and the Life Span

Life is like a roller coaster—filled with unexpected twists, turns, dips, and steep summits. Just as a roller coaster never stays in the same place for long, so your life consists of a series of changes.

Objectives

After studying this section, you should be able to:

- Identify the varying nutritional needs for each stage of the life span.

- Explain how to encourage healthful eating habits for people in every stage of the life span.

Look for These Terms

life span

fetus

obstetrician

certified nurse midwife

colostrum

pediatrician

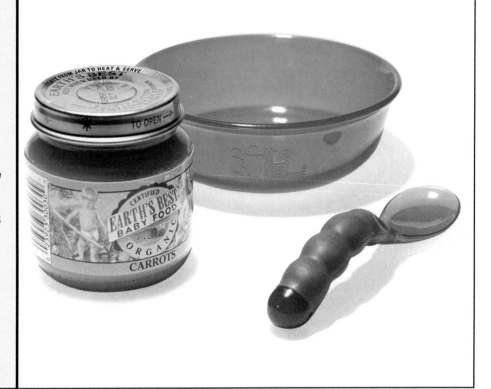

The Life Span

Scientists refer to this constant progression from one stage of development to the next as the **life span**. The human life span is made up essentially of five developmental stages, each with its own growth and nutritional needs. These stages are the prenatal period, infancy, childhood, adolescence, and adulthood.

Prenatal Period

Did you know that each of us begins life as a single cell? During the nine months of a normal pregnancy, this cell divides and multiplies millions of times, ultimately developing into a being able to survive in the outside world. Proper development during the prenatal period depends on the right nutrients. Yet, the **fetus** (FEE-tus)— or unborn baby—is powerless to control its nutrient needs. Responsibility for meeting these needs falls to the mother.

Nutrition During Pregnancy

A woman usually does not learn of her pregnancy until a month or more after she has become pregnant. Meanwhile, the food she has eaten has been the only nourishment for the unborn baby. Therefore, concern about good nutrition should begin before pregnancy. A healthy woman who has good eating habits before her pregnancy begins is more likely to have a safe pregnancy and a healthy baby. Poor eating habits can place the baby at risk for serious health problems.

Teen Pregnancy

Teen pregnancies are particularly at risk because teens need added nutrients for both themselves and the fetus. Poor eating habits can increase the risk of having a baby with a low birth weight (under 5½ pounds, or 2.5 kg) and also with physical or learning problems. Because most teens are not fully developed, they are also more likely to have difficult pregnancies.

Guidelines for Pregnant Women

A female who suspects she is pregnant should see a health professional as soon as possible. Most women see an **obstetrician** (ob-stuh-TRISH-un), a physician who specializes in pregnancy. Increasing numbers of females are opting for the services of a **certified nurse midwife**, an advanced practice nurse who, in addition to providing prenatal care, specializes in the delivery of healthy babies.

Whatever type of health professional is consulted, the expectant mother should follow recommendations for the kinds and amounts of food to be eaten. These generally include the following:

◆ Choose a variety of low-fat, nutrient-dense foods from the Food Guide Pyramid.

◆ Boost calories slightly to supply enough energy for both mother and fetus.

◆ Select at least two daily servings of high-protein foods, such as fish, poultry, meat, eggs, and dry beans.

◆ Have three to four servings of low-fat cheese or yogurt a day (about six servings for pregnant teens).

◆ Opt for foods high in iron, such as meat, poultry, fish, dry beans, and leafy, green vegetables. To help the body better absorb iron, supplement these choices with plenty of citrus fruits and other rich sources of vitamin C.

◆ Pick foods rich in folate, such as enriched breads and cereals, fruits, and dark green vegetables.

◆ Drink eight glasses of water daily, in addition to juices and milk.

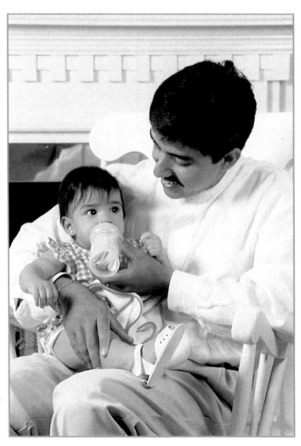

◆ **Eating right is essential throughout a person's life, but nutritional needs vary at different stages of the life cycle.** Write a paragraph explaining why this is true.

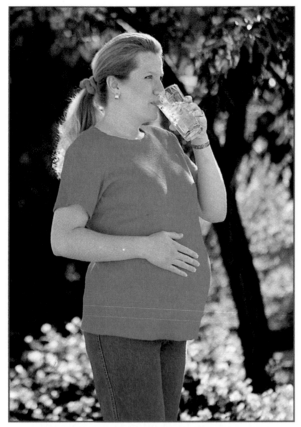

◆ During pregnancy, six to eight glasses of liquid, including water, juices, and milk, are needed daily. **Identify three other specific eating guidelines a mother-to-be needs to follow.**

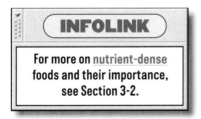

INFOLINK

For more on nutrient-dense foods and their importance, see Section 3-2.

Pregnancy and Weight Gain

Females should expect to gain some weight during pregnancy. A healthy weight gain is usually 25 to 35 pounds (11 to 16 kg). A health professional may recommend a slightly different weight-gain range for underweight or overweight women. Women carrying twins may be advised to gain as much as 35 to 45 pounds (16 to 20 kg).

Pregnant women should not go on weight-loss programs. Limiting food deprives the fetus of much-needed nutrients and can seriously affect the baby's health. Those who have made nutritious food choices should return to their prepregnancy weight within a few months after childbirth.

Infancy

Like the climb up the steepest hill of a roller-coaster, the first years of life are a time of exceptional upward movement. Good nutrition plays a critical role during this period of unparalleled growth and development. The harmful effects of poor nutrition during infancy can last a lifetime.

Feeding Newborns

There are two choices for feeding newborn infants—breast-feeding or bottle-feeding. Both provide all the nutrients the baby needs for the first four to six months.

Breast milk has the right amount and type of fat for a baby. The protein in breast milk is more easily digested and absorbed than the protein in cow's milk.

For the first three days after birth, the mother's breasts produce a special form of milk known as **colostrum** (kuh-LAH-strum). This is a thick, yellowish fluid that is rich in nutrients and antibodies, substances which protect the baby from infection. Later, the colostrum changes to true breast milk.

A woman who is breast-feeding should eat the same kinds of foods recommended during pregnancy and should drink plenty of liquids. The right food choices will ensure that she produces enough milk to keep the baby well fed and healthy. She should not restrict calories while she is breast-feeding.

Bottle-feeding infant formula can also provide good nutrition. Infant formula is usually made of a cow's milk base. Vegetable oils and carbohydrates are added to make it similar to breast milk. Other types of formula are also available. For infants allergic to cow's milk, formulas with a soybean base are often used.

Adding Solid Food

After the first four to six months, the baby will be ready for solid food. The child's **pediatrician**, a physician who cares for infants and children, can offer sound recommendations. A baby's first "solid" foods are

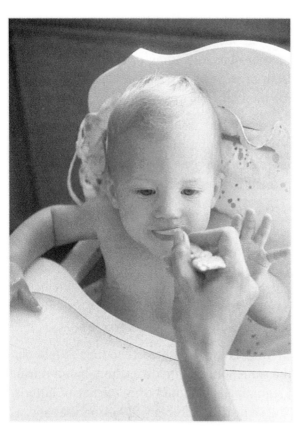

◆ **Introducing solid foods one at a time makes it easier to pinpoint any food allergies.** Which solid food is usually introduced first?

Safety Check

- Cow's milk should not be given to infants because their digestive systems are not fully developed. After 12 months of age, toddlers can be offered about 2 cups (500 mL) of whole milk (in place of breast milk or formula) each day to help assure that calcium needs are met.

- Do not add salt, sugar, fat, or spices to a baby's food. Babies do not need them because their taste buds are more sensitive than an adult's. Added salt, sugar, or fat may also lead to poor eating habits later on.

- Certain foods should not be fed to infants and small children because they can cause choking. These include nuts, seeds, raw carrots, hot dogs, hard candies, whole grapes, popcorn, powdered sugar, and peanut butter.

actually strained foods that are easy to swallow and digest. They should be introduced one at a time. That way, if the baby has a reaction, the cause of the food allergy can be easily identified. The first solid food is usually iron-fortified rice cereal, followed by strained vegetables and fruits. More variety is added later.

During the last half of the first year, infants' eating skills improve. They can be given foods that need some chewing. They begin to learn to pick up some solid foods with their fingers. Healthful finger-food choices include pieces of fruit (without skins), cooked vegetables, cheese, and crackers. Babies also begin to use a spoon for self-feeding.

By the end of the first year, a baby usually can eat the same foods as the rest of the family, but in smaller amounts. Parents or caregivers should not try to limit the amount of fat eaten by children under age two. Babies and toddlers have high energy requirements and, thus, need more fat in their eating plans than do older children and adults.

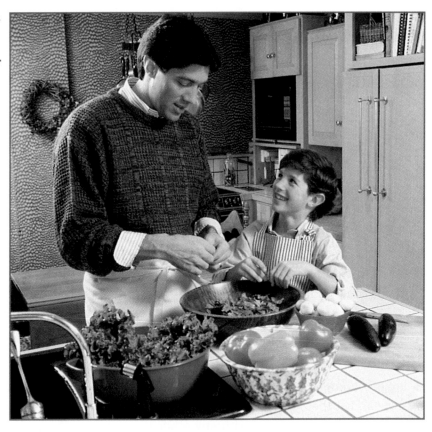

◆ Teaching children to prepare foods by themselves encourages good eating habits. Which areas of skills for food choices does this behavior reflect?

Childhood

Young children are active and growing. So it is essential that they receive a wide selection of nutritious foods from the five food groups in the Food Guide Pyramid.

At meals, food portions should be small. Many experts recommend beginning with 1 tablespoon (15 mL) of a food for each year of the child's life. That means the vegetable serving of a three-year-old should be about 3 tablespoons (45 mL). If the child is still hungry, he or she can be given more. The amount of food needed varies from child to child and from week to week.

During growth spurts—periods of very rapid growth—children may eat more than usual. At other times, they may want less food. Young children sometimes go through phases in which they insist on eating the same food at every meal or they hate a food at one moment and then love it the next. These food jags are usually temporary and don't create long-term nutritional concerns.

Young children need 2 cups (500 mL) of milk each day. It can be served in three or four small portions.

Children have very small stomachs that cannot hold very much food at one time. Therefore, they need between-meal snacks to help supply enough energy and nutrients. Healthful snacks include juice, yogurt, milk, pieces of fruit or vegetables, cooked meat, poultry, or fish, unsweetened cereal, and whole-grain crackers. Nutrient-dense foods should be encouraged.

Promoting Good Eating Habits

Do you have memories from early childhood of trying a food for the first time? Eventually, every child takes a chance with new foods. Introducing a young child to a previously untried food provides an excellent opportunity to add variety to the child's eating plan while simultaneously fostering good eating habits. Here are ways of making the most of that opportunity:

◆ Serve foods that vary in color and texture. If the food has eye appeal, children will be more likely to eat it—and to meet their nutritional needs.

- Eat meals with children, and make the meals enjoyable. Be a role model for good eating habits and behavior.

- Avoid using food as rewards or punishments. This practice gives young children the wrong impression about the purpose of food.

- Don't encourage children to become members of the "clean-your-plate club." Insisting that they finish all their food even after their hunger is satisfied can lead to overeating in later years.

- When possible, let children choose what foods they want to eat for some meals.

- Teach children how to prepare several simple, nutrient-rich foods by and for themselves.

- Invite children to help prepare part of a meal. Let them tear lettuce for a salad, make sandwiches, or aid with any other age-appropriate tasks.

Adolescence

Next to infancy, the second most rapid growth period of life is the one you are going through now—adolescence. Because of the dramatic physical and psychological changes associated with this period, you, as a teen, have an increased need for almost all nutrients.

Many teens don't get enough calcium, zinc, iron, vitamin A, or vitamin C in their eating plans. One easy way to avoid this problem is to be sure you get the minimum number of servings suggested for people your age in the Food Guide Pyramid. If you are highly active or still growing, aim for the maximum number.

As a teen, you are assuming more responsibility for your life, including your food choices. Developing food skills and fitness habits during this period will help set the stage for a healthy and productive future.

Adulthood

Mr. Carstairs, who is 45, has a "spare tire" around his midsection, while his next-door neighbor, who is the same age, does not. The difference relates in part to the fact that Mr. Carstairs eats the same way he did when he was younger, even though most adults require fewer calories.

Despite their decreased need for calories, adults still need their full share of nutrients. They can meet this demand by choosing a variety of low-fat, low-calorie foods from the Food Guide Pyramid. Continuing to get regular physical activity throughout adulthood is important as well.

Many adults don't realize they have slipped into poor eating and exercise habits until they develop a health problem. Developing healthful habits now, while you are in your teen years, may help reduce future health problems. It will also make it easier to continue these habits throughout life.

Older Adults

As people age, they continue to need the same nutrients, although in smaller amounts. If they remain physically active, they can continue to eat as much as younger adults.

With maturity, the body's thirst signal often declines and people don't drink as much water as their bodies require. Older people, like all other adults, need to drink eight cups (2 L) of water daily.

Special Problems for Aging Adults

Some aging adults face special challenges in meeting their nutritional needs. Many live on fixed incomes that are too low to provide enough nutrient-rich food. Those who live alone may dislike preparing a meal just for one—or may be too frail to cook. Some older people have health problems that create nutritional risks.

In many communities, social service programs are available to help aging adults in situations like these. Senior and community centers often offer meals for older citizens at reduced rates. These programs provide nutrient-rich meals as well as an opportunity for socializing.

Living alone or on a limited income can make meal planning challenging for people of any age. In Chapter 11, you will learn helpful suggestions for coping with these challenges.

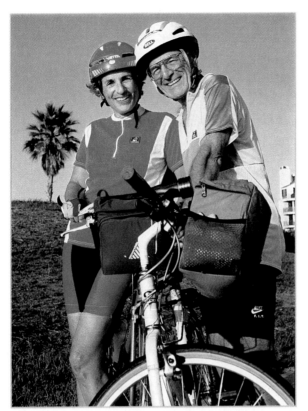

◆ **With proper nutrition and other good health habits, many older adults remain very active.** Interview an older relative, neighbor, or other senior citizen who is active to learn about his or her eating habits.

Section 6-1 Review & Activities

1. Why are good nutrition habits important for a woman even before she knows she is pregnant?

2. Identify three finger foods for infants and three healthy snack foods for young children.

3. How can adults get their full share of nutrients without getting too many calories?

4. Synthesizing. Hugh, a 21-year-old male, grew up learning always to eat everything served to him. What are some potential health problems that could result if he continues this behavior throughout adulthood?

5. Analyzing. Write a paragraph explaining how getting children involved in meal preparation can lead to good eating habits.

6. Applying. Think of a simple food that children can prepare for themselves. Write directions for preparing the food as you would explain it to a child. If possible, share the recipe with a young child in your home or community. Write about the experience in your Wellness Journal.

Managing Health Conditions

Have you ever lost sleep the night before a big exam or had butterflies in your stomach when you had to speak before a large audience? If so, you are not alone. Everyone at one time or another experiences these symptoms.

Objectives

After studying this section, you should be able to:

- Explain the relationship between stress and nutrition.
- Identify the role of nutrition in recovery from illness or injury.
- Identify positive and negative effects of using supplements.
- Give examples of how people with medical conditions or physical impairments can meet their nutritional needs.

Look for These Terms

stress

dietary supplements

megadose

herbal remedies

medical nutrition therapy

diabetes

HIV/AIDS

food allergy

food intolerance

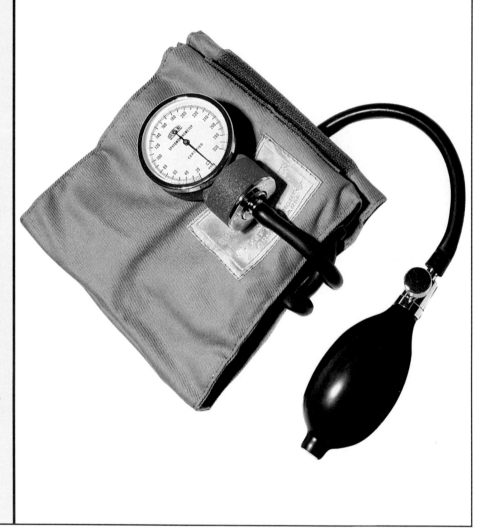

Stress

Physical reactions like the ones described above are symptoms of stress. **Stress** is physical or mental tension triggered by an event or situation in your life.

Not everyone finds the same situations stressful. Some people experience test anxiety, whereas others don't. At school, a teacher will experience types of job stress different from those experienced by a principal or a school counselor. Even going on a date, receiving an

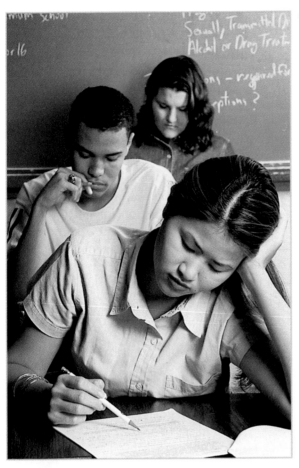

◆ No two people react in quite the same way to what can be a stressful situation. How does your level of stress when taking a test compare with that of a friend?

award, or experiencing some other positive event can be stressful.

Stressful situations are part of life. They can't be avoided. The key is to learn how to cope positively with these situations. When stress is not handled effectively, feelings of worry, fear, or anger can result, leading to depression and lack of energy. Stress may also cause headaches, backaches, or other physical symptoms. It even plays a role in high blood pressure and heart disease.

Nutrition and Stress

The effects of stress on the mind and body can have an impact on personal nutrition. Have you ever been too upset to eat? Negative emotions resulting from stress can cause

heartburn, diarrhea, and other digestive problems. Some people overeat when they are feeling stress; others lose their appetites altogether.

Making poor food choices is not a positive way to deal with stress. It does nothing to help you cope with the actual cause of your stress. Poor eating habits can make you feel worse in the long run—often leading to an unhealthy weight and perhaps serious nutritional or health problems.

In contrast, good nutrition can help reduce stress. Eating right is one way to help prevent stress-related illnesses or manage their symptoms. By reacting to stressful situations in a positive way, you can take control of your life and reduce your risk of illness.

Illness and Recovery

Any type of illness puts a strain on the body. Whether you are fighting off a sore throat or have a broken ankle, a healthy, well-nourished body is better equipped to handle the problem. Even though a person who is ill may lose interest in eating, the body still has to have nutrients—often more of them than during healthy times.

If you are helping care for someone who is ill or recovering from an illness, follow these guidelines:

◆ Encourage fluids. The patient's physician or other health provider may specify how much is needed.

◆ Serve nutritious, eye-catching meals. Varying colors, shapes, textures, and temperatures can spice up any meal.

When the Pressure Is On

It's a vicious cycle that is all too common during the teen years: Pressures—from friends, from teachers, from family members—catch up with you. You begin to eat too much or too little, which takes a toll on your overall health and wellness.

How can you break the chain? Health experts offer a number of stress-busting solutions. Here are a few:

- Learn to manage your time. Keeping a daily planner can help. Be sure to set aside some time for you just to relax and enjoy yourself.

- If you're feeling angry or upset, listen to some calming music, read a funny book, or take your frustrations out by punching a pillow.

- Take positive action to solve a problem if you can. Share your feelings and problems with someone you trust.

- Stress can take the form of negative energy. Turn the negatives into positives. Try physical activity—run, walk, ride a bike, or clean a closet.

- Above all else, take time for eating well. Don't just grab whatever food is in sight. Include breakfast and exercise plans on your agenda for the day. Take care of your health.

Think About It

- In your Wellness Journal, make a list of your activities and responsibilities for a three-day period. As you carry out each task, note in the journal how much time it took. Also keep track of leisure time. At the end of the three days, make a pie graph showing how much time you devoted to each item. If the portion representing time for yourself is too small, think of ways of rearranging your day.

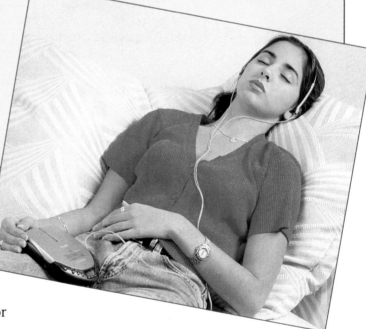

◆ Taking time to relax can help you manage the stress in your life. In your Wellness Journal, list three activities you do or could try to help reduce stress in your life.

◆ Be sure the patient gets enough rest for the healing process.

◆ Ask the physician or pharmacist whether the patient's medication affects the appetite or the way the body uses nutrients.

◆ Use disposable or plastic plates and cups if the patient has an illness that can spread to others.

Nutrients and Disease Prevention

After Vince heard that eating oatmeal might reduce the risk of heart disease, he began having oatmeal each day for breakfast and lunch. Like Vince, many people jump on the bandwagon at the first report of a food or nutrient with supposed disease-fighting properties.

Two such classes of nutrients that have received much attention in the media are dietary supplements and herbal remedies. How can you as a consumer determine if these are for you? For an answer to his question, read on.

Dietary Supplements

Dietary supplements are nutrients people take in addition to the foods they eat. Usually, these supplements take the form of pills, capsules, liquids, or powders.

Dietary supplements may be useful for people taking certain types of medication, pregnant and nursing women, those recovering from illness, older people, and people with special nutritional needs. In such cases, these people may not be able to get enough nutrients from the foods they eat.

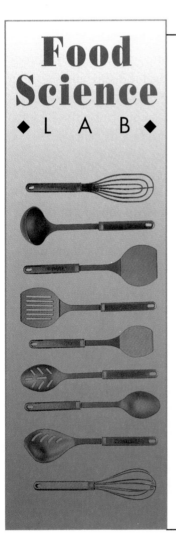

Food Science
◆ L A B ◆

Comparing Antacids

One common food-related health problem facing most people at one time or another is indigestion. In relieving the discomfort of indigestion or heartburn, is one over-the-counter product better than another? You are about to find out.

Procedure
1. Gather several antacid products. Dissolve a standard dose of one of the products in 8 ounces (250 mL) of water. Note the current time to the nearest second.
2. Begin adding vinegar to the cup, an eye dropper full at a time. After each addition, test the acidity of the solution with litmus paper. Keep track of how much vinegar you add.
3. Stop when the solution tests acidic, that is, when the litmus paper turns red.
4. Repeat the procedure for each product.

Conclusions
◆ Did one antacid neutralize the acid more quickly than the others? Did one neutralize more acid than the others?

◆ What ingredient or ingredients listed on the product's label do you think contributed to the antacid's effectiveness?

◆ What conclusions, if any, can you draw about the advertising of products as a whole?

Most people, however, do not need supplements. They can get all the nutrients they need by following a balanced and varied eating plan. People who rely on supplements to make up for poor food choices are only short-changing themselves.

✚ Safety Check

Children often confuse vitamin and mineral pills with candy. They can be harmed by large doses of supplements. In particular, iron supplements are the most common cause of poisoning deaths among children in the United States. If there are children in the home, be sure nutrient supplements are stored in child-resistant packages out of reach of children.

Nutrient Megadoses

Some people believe in taking megadoses (MEH-guh-dohs-es) of vitamins or mineral supplements. A **megadose** is an extra-large amount of a supplement thought to prevent or cure diseases. As noted in Chapter 2, excess amounts of some nutrients can accumulate in the body and cause harm. Excess amounts of those nutrients that are not stored by the body simply pass out of the body unused, making them a waste of money.

Your best choice is to try to get all your nutrients from food. If you decide to take supplements, avoid megadoses. Also, read the list of ingredients on the label of any supplement to be sure you know what you're getting. Avoid unrecognized nutrients.

Herbal Remedies

"Echinacea." "St. John's Wort." "Gingko." Strange and often hard-to-pronounce names like these have become commonplace in magazine and TV ads. You may see these items sold from booths at shopping malls.

They are but a few of hundreds of **herbal remedies**, nonstandardized products containing herbs known to have medicinal-like qualities. They may be advertised as the ultimate cure for illnesses or diseases. Many herbal remedies have been used in Europe and Asia for centuries. Most are just becoming popular in the United States. However, the safety, purity, and effectiveness of herbal products are questionable. Some of them can even cause serious illness or death.

Before experimenting with any herbal product, be sure to use critical thinking and the other food skills covered in Chapter 1. Remember: Scientific evidence has confirmed the benefits of physical activity and healthy eating.

Special Eating Plans

Some people, because of long-term medical conditions, must be especially aware of their food choices. Their physicians may prescribe special eating plans to help manage their medical conditions. A dietitian may need to provide **medical nutrition therapy**, an assessment of the nutritional status of a patient with a condition, an illness, or an injury that puts her or him at risk.

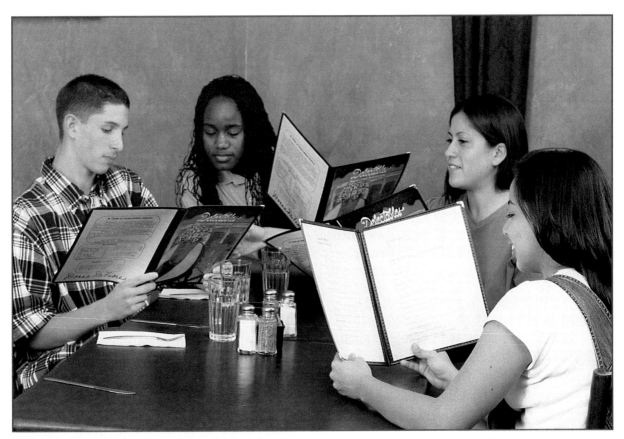

◆ **People with health conditions need to take special care when eating out.** How can a person with diabetes use the skill of communication to ensure that he or she orders wisely from a restaurant menu?

Here are a few conditions that require special eating plans:

◆ **High cholesterol.** People with high cholesterol may develop heart disease. Lowering total fat and saturated fat intake as well as increasing soluble fiber is commonly recommended. Starting the day with oatmeal, strawberries, and nonfat milk would fit well in this plan.

◆ **High blood pressure.** High blood pressure is also a risk factor for heart disease—and other medical conditions. A typical eating plan modification to help lower blood pressure may be to lower fat and sodium (including salt), while increasing potassium and calcium.

◆ **Diabetes. Diabetes** is a condition in which the body cannot control blood sugar levels. Diabetes may cause serious damage to the kidneys, eyes, and heart, as well as other parts of the body. Eating the right balance of food and counting grams of carbohydrate play a role in controlling the blood sugar level. Eating all foods in moderation also helps manage weight, which is very important for many diabetics.

◆ **HIV/AIDS.** For people living with **HIV/AIDS**—a disorder that interferes with the immune system's ability to combat disease-causing pathogens—proper nutrition needs to be a priority every day. Maintaining or improving appetite is vital. Plenty of fluids and regular snacks are important. Often, nutritional supplements are needed.

◆ **Food allergy.** For people afflicted with a **food allergy**, an abnormal, physical response to certain foods by the body's immune system, a single bite of an allergic food can cause symptoms. These range from itching, rash, and hives to abdominal pain, nausea, and even difficulty breathing. For adults, common allergy-causing foods are fish, shellfish, and nuts, especially peanuts. Common allergy-causing foods for children are cow's milk, eggs, peanuts, wheat, and soy. Special tests are used to determine which food or foods are responsible for an allergy.

◆ **Food intolerance.** Another sensitivity, **food intolerance**, is a physical reaction to food not involving the immune system. A food intolerance is most likely to cause digestive problems. One common example is an intolerance for lactose, the sugar found in cow's milk. Substituting lactose-reduced milk or soy milk for cow's milk is a typical solution.

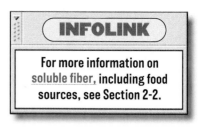

INFOLINK

For more information on soluble fiber, including food sources, see Section 2-2.

Adjusting to a Special Eating Plan

It takes time for people who have been placed on a special eating plan to adjust to a new way of eating. Eating out and shopping for food pose special challenges. When in a restaurant, the person needs to learn to ask questions about how foods are prepared and to request special orders, when necessary. When at the supermarket, the individual needs to read food labels carefully, checking for ingredients to be limited or increased and looking for nutrient-modified products, such as calcium-fortified juice.

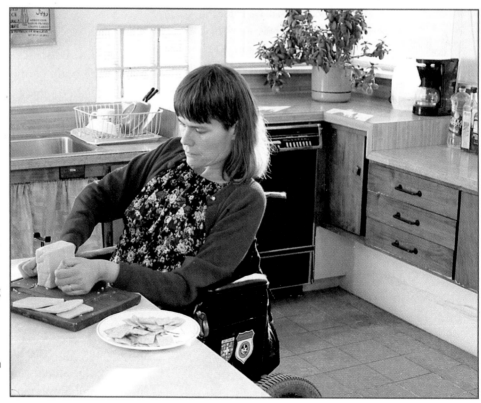

◆ Adapting kitchens for easier use encourages independence and good nutrition among people with physical challenges. What are three differences you see between this specially built kitchen and others you have seen?

People on special eating plans are often surprised at the variety of flavorful foods that can be prepared within the guidelines of their plans. Many are delighted to discover the various herbs and spices that can be pressed into use to make mouth-watering low-fat, low-sodium marinades and sauces. Many medical centers nowadays even offer specialized cooking classes.

If you know of anyone who must follow a special eating plan, offer your support and encouragement. Try to help the person view the special plan as an opportunity to try new foods.

Physical Challenges

Sometimes a physical challenge requires that a person make adaptations in order to meet his or her nutritional needs. Generally, the nutritional needs of such an individual are no different from those of anyone else of similar age, gender, and activity level. However, physical limitations may affect how those needs are met.

People with limited mobility, limited use of the hands, or vision problems may find it difficult to use standard kitchen equipment. In this case, the solution is to adapt the kitchen and its equipment. Design innovations, which are addressed in Chapters 7 and 14, have helped many such people lead independent and self-sufficient lives.

Section 6-2 Review & Activities

1. What is stress? Give three examples of how a negative reaction to stress can affect nutrition.

2. Give three suggestions for planning and preparing meals to fit a medically prescribed special eating plan.

3. In general, how do physical impairments relate to nutritional needs?

4. **Evaluating.** Discuss ways in which good nutrition might help you handle stress more effectively.

5. **Synthesizing.** When Franco complained to his cousin Paul about a lack of energy, Paul told him he needed an herbal remedy to "detoxify" his body. Do you think Franco should follow Paul's advice? Why or why not?

6. **Applying.** Imagine that you are caring for someone who is recovering from surgery. Identify at least six ways that you could make meals more enjoyable for this person.

SECTION
6-3

Objectives

After studying this section, you should be able to:

- Identify the characteristics of anorexia nervosa and bulimia nervosa.
- Describe the effects of eating disorders on health.
- Explain what can be done to help someone with an eating disorder.

Look for These Terms

eating disorder

anorexia nervosa

binge eating disorder

bulimia nervosa

Eating Disorders

When Charlene began to lose excess weight, her friends supported her efforts. As the weeks passed, Charlene reached a healthy weight for her age and height. However, she continued to restrict her calorie intake.

Months later, Charlene had lost so much weight that she looked almost like a skeleton. She was light-headed and felt tired all the time. Concerned, her family scheduled a medical checkup. After a thorough evaluation, Dr. Cho diagnosed Charlene's problem as an eating disorder.

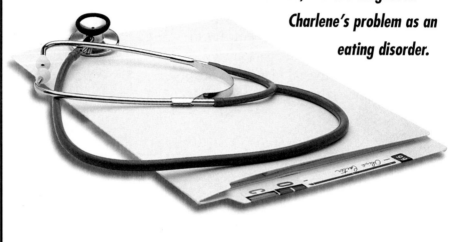

What Are Eating Disorders?

The term **eating disorder** describes an extreme, unhealthful behavior related to food, eating, and weight. Food is not a cause of the disorder but, rather, a symptom. In fact, the causes of eating disorders are not clearly understood, although research continues.

Eating disorders generally occur among teens and young adults, especially females. However, these disorders are occurring increasingly in males, adults, and children as young as eight years old. It is estimated that from 1 to 10 percent of all teens suffer from an eating disorder.

Anorexia Nervosa

Anorexia nervosa (an-uh-REK-see-yuh ner-VOH-suh) is a type of eating disorder that involves an irresistible urge to lose weight through self-starvation and a refusal to maintain a minimally normal body weight. It is often described as "dieting out of control." No matter how thin people with anorexia become, they feel fat. They see themselves as being overweight and show an obsessive fear of gaining weight.

Individuals with anorexia will do just about anything to lose as much weight as possible. They refuse to eat or eat very little. They may use laxatives and diet pills, or force themselves

◆ People with bulimia nervosa have frequent episodes of binge eating of foods high in calories and fat. What are five telltale symptoms of a person with an eating disorder?

to vomit after a meal. In spite of feeling tired, some people with the disorder exercise strenuously every day for long periods of time. Still, most deny they have any problem. They believe their behavior is normal.

Binge Eating Disorder

Binge eating disorder is a type of eating disorder involving a lack of control while eating huge quantities of food at one time, or bingeing. An eating binge, lasting usually under two hours, often occurs when a person is emotionally upset or under severe stress.

Bulimia Nervosa

Bulimia nervosa (byoo-LIM-ee-yuh ner-VOH-suh) is a type of eating disorder that involves episodes of binge eating followed by purging—the use of self-induced vomiting, laxatives, or vigorous activities to prevent weight gain. Like people with anorexia, those with bulimia have a distorted sense of body shape and weight. Unlike people with anorexia, bulimics are usually within 10 to 15 pounds (5 to 8 kg) of a healthy weight.

Individuals with bulimia use secret binges in an attempt to cope with problems such as anger, loneliness, boredom, and frustration. Usually, they binge on high-fat, high-calorie foods that they might normally consider forbidden. A lack of control is typically evident during a binge episode. The foods are eaten in a short time, usually under two hours. It's not unusual for someone with bulimia to eat 3,000 to 5,000 calories at a time. During a day of repeated bingeing, some can eat as many as 20,000 calories. They stop eating only when the stomach hurts, they fall asleep, they run out of food, or someone interrupts them.

After bingeing, individuals with bulimia feel guilty and depressed. Unfortunately, the binge-purge cycle becomes a way of life, with two or more eating binges a week being typical.

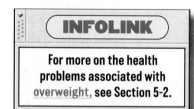

INFOLINK

For more on the health problems associated with overweight, see Section 5-2.

Effects of Eating Disorders

Eating disorders can create serious health problems. Anorexia can result in lowered heart rate and body temperature, constipation, and lowered blood pressure and breathing rate. Heart problems, osteoporosis, and brain damage can develop, too. Teens and children may experience stunted growth. Females stop menstruating. About 10 percent of all individuals with anorexia will die of starvation—a devastating statistic.

Individuals with binge eating disorder gain weight and develop the same health problems as overweight people. They are usually very distressed by their binge eating.

People with bulimia lose fluids as well as potassium, which may result in fatigue, kidney problems, and heart damage—which can be lethal. The vomiting damages the esophagus, teeth, and gums. The salivary glands, located on each side of the neck, enlarge. People with bulimia may rupture the esophagus. Many have sore throats almost all the time.

What Can Be Done?

It is important to realize that a person with an eating disorder has an illness. Most can't stop their self-destructive behaviors on their own. It's often up to others to recognize the problem and encourage the person to get help.

Recognizing Eating Disorders

People with anorexia often exhibit warning signs. In addition to rapidly losing large amounts of weight, eating little, and exercising for hours, they may show sensitivity to cold temperatures and/or seem preoccupied with food and calories. Some anorexics resort to rituals, such as cutting food into very tiny pieces. Spending time alone and avoiding friends is another symptom of the disorder.

Knowing when someone is suffering from binge eating or bulimia is more challenging. Binge eaters and bulimics are often successful in hiding their problems, since both tend to eat in secret.

People with bulimia are aware that they have no control over their unusual eating habits. They are embarrassed by their lack of self-control. Other potential warning signs include:

◆ A preoccupation with food and eating.

◆ Leaving the table immediately after eating (usually to go to the bathroom to purge).

◆ Great fluctuations in weight.

◆ Dependency on laxatives, diuretics (water pills), or diet pills.

◆ Physical changes, such as swollen glands or teeth problems.

Getting Help

Eating disorders stem from complex problems that require professional help. Treatment usually includes nutritional and psychological counseling as well as medical help. Often the person must be hospitalized in an eating disorders clinic.

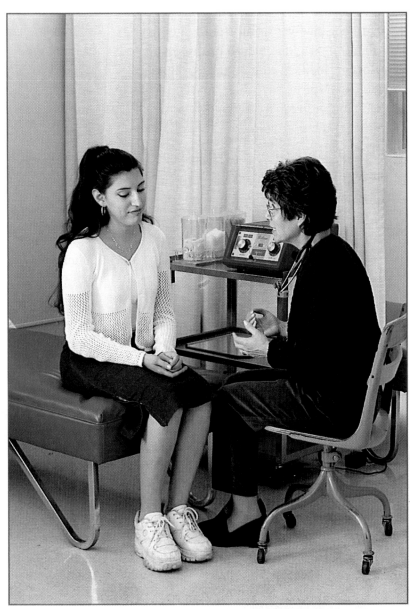

◆ **Professional help is needed to recover from an eating disorder.** Name some of the people and resources to whom an individual with an eating disorder can turn.

People with eating disorders can recover, but the process is very slow. It usually takes at least one or two years of treatment for full recovery to occur. The fact that such people are often resistant to treatment compounds the problem. As with any other illness, support from family and friends is an important part of the recovery process.

Treatment Options

Treatment involves using a team approach. The team may include health professionals to treat specific medical complications, dietitians, behavior therapists, psychotherapists, social workers, and nurses. Treatment options include, but are not limited to, the following:

◆ **Medical nutrition therapy.** Focuses on nutrition education.

◆ **Behavioral therapy.** Focuses on changing eating habits.

◆ **Cognitive behavioral therapy.** Focuses on changing unrealistic thinking.

◆ **Family therapy.** Focuses on developing supportive family attitudes.

◆ **Drug therapy.** May involve antidepressant medication if a patient doesn't respond to other therapies.

In some cases, a combination of therapies is employed. Self-help groups are also available. Your local mental health association and school nurse or counselor may be good initial contacts.

If you know someone who may have an eating disorder, encourage her or him to seek treatment today. Early detection is critical.

Section 6-3 Review & Activities

1. List four characteristics of anorexia nervosa.

2. What types of treatment are available to persons who suffer from eating disorders?

3. Describe two key ways in which bulimia nervosa differs from anorexia nervosa.

4. Comparing and Contrasting. Darla and Monique both eat in secret. Darla is close to a healthy weight, whereas Monique is about 20 pounds overweight. Which eating disorder might each have? What other signs would you look for to confirm your hunches?

5. Analyzing. In recent years, a number of celebrities have admitted to having eating disorders. Do you think such publicity has a positive or negative effect? Explain.

6. Applying. Imagine that Charlene—the teen described in the beginning of the section—is a friend of yours. You have just learned about her eating disorder. Write a journal entry describing the signs that led you to suspect there was a problem. Close by explaining how you plan to give support to Charlene.

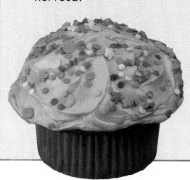

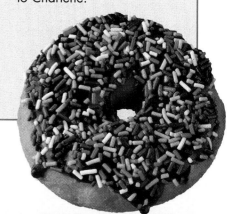

CAREER WANTED

Individuals with excellent writing and research skills who enjoy cooking.

REQUIRES:

- degree in journalism or communication
- track record of meeting deadlines
- fascination with food or cooking

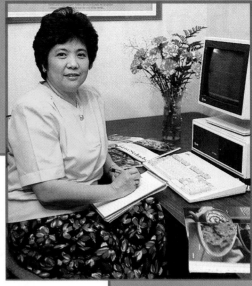

"I love writing as much as eating!"
says Magazine Foods Writer Joyce Nitobe

Q: Joyce, what does being a foods writer for a magazine involve?

A: I'm responsible for producing full-length food and nutrition features, plus creative recipes for each edition of the magazine. I do my own research, interviewing, and arrange to have photos taken.

Q: Do you need to be a good cook to be a good foods writer?

A: Not really, but you do need to enjoy cooking. If I didn't love to cook *and* write, I would not have chosen this career.

Q: Do you ever run out of food ideas to write about?

A: No. I am constantly dreaming up new ideas. Sometimes a food I've eaten at a top-notch restaurant will spark a new idea. The most interesting part is that I'm working six months ahead of the calendar. That means I develop winter holiday food ideas in the summer!

Q: When you develop recipes, do you taste-test them first?

A: I often test recipes on my family. They are pretty good food critics, but I don't have to test them since I'm lucky enough to have an entire test kitchen staff at magazine headquarters.

Career Research Activity

1. Imagine that the above interview with Joyce Nitobe were to take place 50 years from now. Would she be working for a magazine as we now know it? Rewrite the interview as it might appear.

2. Research one of the career opportunities on the right. Write a journal entry as someone in that field looking for work. Title your entry "A Day in the Life of ____." Explain what type of situation you are looking to be placed in and what you bring to the job.

Related Career Opportunities

Entry Level
- Newspaper Stringer
- Salesperson

Technical Level
- Food Web Site Writer
- Test Kitchen Worker
- Dietetic Technician

Professional Level
- Professional Magazine Writer
- Professional Chef
- Consumer Affairs Director

Chapter 6   Review & Activities

Summary

Section 6-1: Food and the Life Span

- At each stage of the life span, people experience changes in nutritional needs.

- Good nutrition during pregnancy is essential for the health of the baby.

- Infants and children need the right kinds of foods for health and growth.

- Children should be encouraged to develop good eating habits.

- Through adolescence and adulthood, changing energy needs are a consideration.

- Some older people face special challenges regarding nutrition needs.

Section 6-2: Managing Health Conditions

- Good nutrition is important in preventing and managing stress-related illnesses.

- Along with rest, nutritious food helps the body heal itself during illness and recovery.

- Most people can meet their nutritional needs without taking dietary supplements.

- The purity, safety, and effectiveness of herbal products are questionable.

- Some people have long-term medical conditions requiring medical nutrition therapy.

- Physical impairments sometimes require that a person make adaptations in order to meet nutritional needs.

Section 6-3: Eating Disorders

- Anorexia nervosa involves losing weight through self-starvation.

- Bulimia nervosa involves bingeing and purging.

- Binge eating disorder involves eating huge quantities of food at one time.

- All eating disorders can cause health complications—some of which are serious.

- Warning signs may indicate a problem.

- People with eating disorders need professional help.

Checking Your Knowledge

1. Why is nutrition of particular concern for pregnant teens?

2. Name three healthful finger foods a toddler might be given.

3. Why do people often tend to put on weight as they move from the teen years to adulthood?

4. Name two factors that may keep some older people from eating nutritious meals.

5. Name two ways in which stress and nutrition are related.

6. What dangers are associated with megadoses of dietary supplements?

7. What is the main difference between a food allergy and a food intolerance?

8. In which groups of people do eating disorders occur most often?

9. Describe the binge-purge cycle characteristic of bulimia nervosa.

10. Why is bulimia nervosa usually more difficult to recognize than anorexia nervosa?

Thinking Critically

1. Identifying Cause and Effect. The text states that using food to reward or punish children can lead to poor eating habits. Give some examples to show how this might happen.

2. Determining Accuracy. Some people believe that certain foods can help cure certain illnesses—for example, that chicken soup helps cure a cold. Do you think there is any truth to such beliefs? Why or why not? How might a scientist try to test such theories?

Working IN THE Lab

1. Foods Lab. List ideas for making nutritious foods that would appeal to young children. Consider using unusual colors, animal shapes, funny faces, and so on. Prepare samples of the foods. Serve them to classmates or to a group of young children, if possible.

2. Foods Lab. Find and prepare a simple recipe designed for a modified eating plan, such as a low-sodium or wheat-free plan. Rate the food for appearance, texture, and flavor.

3. Foods Lab. Prepare a simple meal, such as soup and a sandwich. Place it on a tray as if you were serving it to someone who was in bed recovering from an illness. Show how you would make the meal attractive as well as easy to eat.

Reinforcing Key Skills

1. Leadership. Many teens choose foods that don't provide enough calcium, zinc, iron, or vitamins A and C. What steps can be taken within a school cafeteria environment to heighten the awareness of these important nutrients?

2. Directed Thinking. What social influences exist that cause some teens to take supplements in place of food, to purge, and/or to eat very little?

Making Decisions and Solving Problems

Your 75-year-old neighbor has poor vision and no longer drives a car. He does his grocery shopping only when someone is available to drive him to the supermarket. You are worried that he isn't getting regular, nutritious meals.

Making Connections

1. Science. Using library or Internet sources, research the connection between herbs and health. Possible topics: What effect does echinacea have on colds? What effect does ginseng have on energy? Are there any herbs that help lower high blood pressure? Report your findings to the class. Reports need to include positive and negative uses of the herbs, in addition to your overall evaluation.

2. Language Arts. Work in groups to write, illustrate, and produce a pamphlet discussing the warning signs of eating disorders. Distribute the pamphlet in your school or community.

UNIT
2

Workspace,

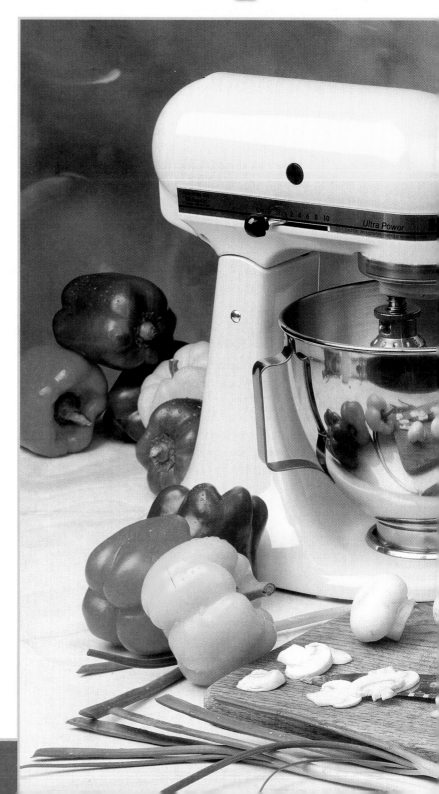

Tools, and Techniques

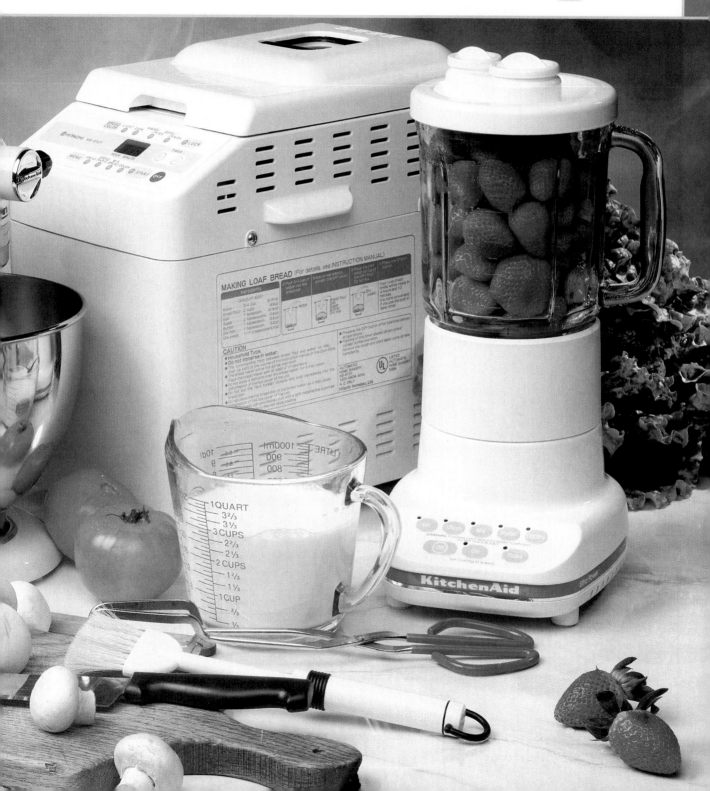

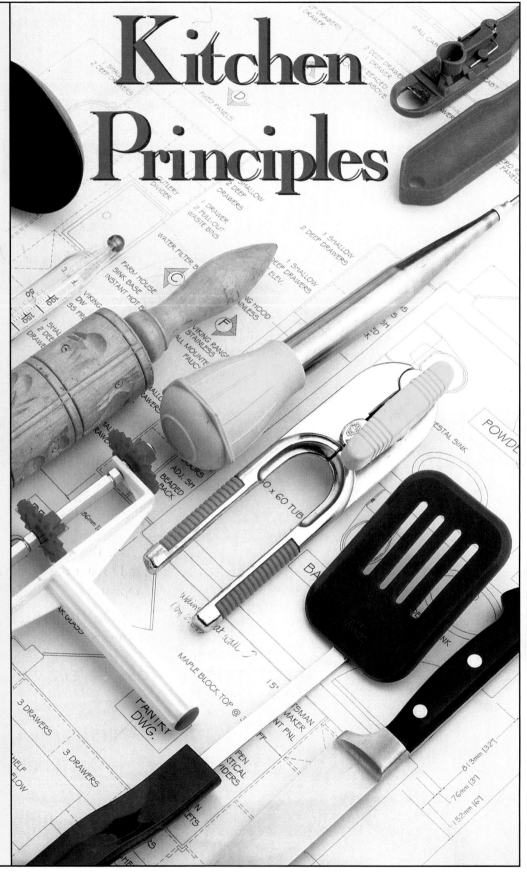

Kitchen Principles

Section 7-1
Introduction to the Kitchen

Section 7-2
Preventing Kitchen Accidents

Section 7-3
Keeping Food Safe to Eat

Section 7-4
Storing Food

Section 7-5
Conserving Natural Resources

Working in the kitchen is more than just putting on a good show. It involves knowing rules of safety, including safe ways of storing food. After reading this chapter, you will know all about these topics.

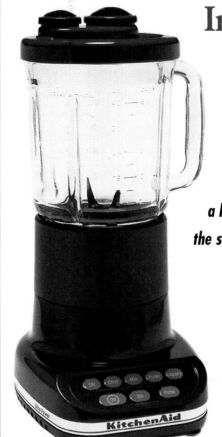

Objectives

After studying this section, you should be able to:

- Define and give examples of major appliances, small appliances, and utensils.

- Explain what a work center is and identify the three basic kitchen work centers.

Look for These Terms

major appliance

small appliance

utensils

work center

Introduction to the Kitchen

Food preparation involves many tasks and many tools. This section introduces you to the equipment and work centers you will find in a kitchen, whether at home or in the school foods lab.

Types of Kitchen Equipment

Kitchens contain three basic kinds of equipment: major appliances, small appliances, and utensils.

A **major appliance** is a large device that gets its energy from electricity or gas. Most kitchens have at least two major appliances: a refrigerator-freezer for cold storage and a range for cooking. Some kitchens have a separate cooktop and oven instead of a single range unit. Many kitchens also have a microwave oven and a dishwasher.

A **small appliance** is a small electrical household device used to perform simple

tasks. The mixer, food processor, blender, and toaster are examples of small kitchen appliances.

Utensils are kitchen tools, such as measuring cups, knives, and peelers. Other kitchen utensils include pots, pans, and other cookware.

⊕ Safety Check

As any cook who has ever shorted out a microwave oven or burned a pot can tell you, appliances and utensils require careful use and regular care. Before using or cleaning any appliance, read the owner's manual.

Kitchen Work Centers

You wouldn't store videotapes or CDs in a different location from the VCR or CD player. The same principle applies to kitchen organization. Organizing a kitchen efficiently can save time and energy by reducing the steps you need to take to carry out a task.

Most home kitchens and school foods labs are organized around work centers. A **work center** is an area designed for specific kitchen tasks. A well-designed work center has the equipment you need for a task, sufficient storage space, and a safe, convenient work space.

Technological advances are making kitchen designs more user-friendly. One example is an adjustable range cooktop that can be raised or lowered to a convenient height.

Basic Work Centers

The refrigerator-freezer, sink, and range—and the counters and cabinets around them—form the three basic kitchen centers.

◆ **Cold storage center.** The refrigerator-freezer is the focus of this center. Items stored nearby might include plastic storage bags, food wraps, and containers for leftover foods.

◆ **Sink center.** This center is the main source of water. It is used for a variety of tasks, including washing fresh fruits and vegetables, draining foods, and washing dishes. Dishpans and other cleanup supplies should be kept handy.

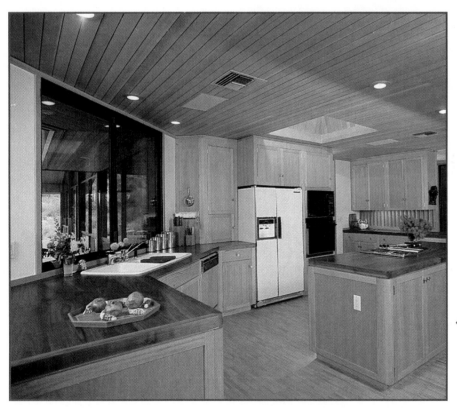

◆ **The overall design of a kitchen depends on lifestyle and budget.** Which of the kitchen work centers can be seen in the kitchen shown here?

◆ **Cooking center.** This center includes the range and related items, such as cooking tools, pots and pans, and pot-holders. Small cooking appliances might be kept near the range. Some canned and packaged foods might also be stored here.

Sometimes there is more than one logical place for equipment. For instance, a microwave oven may be part of the cooking center. However, it could also be placed near the refrigerator-freezer for quick heating of left-overs and frozen food. José's family keeps the microwave oven on a sturdy rolling cart so that it can be moved to wherever it's needed.

Other Work Centers

Some kitchens contain additional, separate work centers.

◆ **Mixing center.** This area is used for preparing and mixing foods. Measuring cups, bowls, mixing spoons, and an electric mixer are commonly stored here, along with foods such as flour and spices. In a small kitchen, this center might be combined with one of the others.

◆ **Planning center.** Some home kitchens include a planning center with space to store cookbooks, recipes, and coupons. A desk provides a convenient place for writing out meal plans and shopping lists. Other useful features are a calendar, a bulletin board, a telephone, and perhaps even a computer.

A well-organized and well-equipped kitchen is a place where good food can be prepared quickly, easily, and safely.

Section 7-1 Review & Activities

1. What is a major appliance? A small appliance? A utensil?

2. What is a kitchen work center?

3. Name three major work centers of the kitchen.

4. Why is it important to organize a kitchen around work centers?

5. **Analyzing.** Which of the three kinds of kitchen equipment do you think you could most easily get along without—major appliances, small appliances, or utensils? Explain your answer.

6. **Evaluating.** The Ameslers are designing a new kitchen. The family does a lot of baking. Identify which work centers they should plan their kitchen around. Explain your answers.

7. **Applying.** Draw a rough floor plan of your school foods lab kitchen. Show the location of the sink, major appliances, cabinets, and counters. Circle and label each work center. Identify the location of at least two small appliances and three kinds of utensils.

Preventing Kitchen Accidents

As Kaneesha cracked eggs for an omelet, some egg white fell on the floor. "I'll clean that up later," she thought. Minutes later the telephone rang. As Kaneesha turned to answer it, she felt something slick underfoot. "The egg white!" she thought, as her foot slid out from under her.

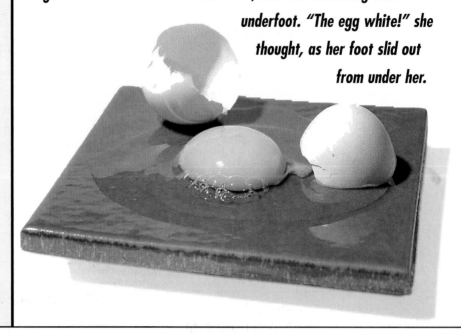

Objectives

After studying this section, you should be able to:

- Identify ways to prevent common kitchen accidents.
- Discuss special safety needs.
- Describe what to do if a kitchen accident results in injury.

Look for These Terms

polarized plugs

Heimlich maneuver

CPR

An Accident-Free Kitchen

A kitchen should be a place to prepare enjoyable food. Yet, just a few seconds of carelessness can turn the kitchen into an accident waiting to happen. Falls, electrical shocks, cuts, burns, and poisoning are all kitchen hazards. The keys to preventing kitchen accidents are careful kitchen management and proper work habits.

General Safety Guidelines

Your work habits are vital to your safety in the kitchen. Here are some general guidelines:

- Don't let hair, jewelry, sleeves, or apron strings dangle. They could catch on fire or become tangled in appliances.

- Keep your mind on what you're doing.

- Prevent clutter. Put items back where they belong as you finish with them or after you've washed them.

- Close drawers and doors completely after you open them. You could be seriously hurt if you bump into an open door or drawer.

- Use the right tool for the job. Don't use a knife to pry off a jar cover, for example. Take the time to find the tool you need.

- Store heavy or bulky items, such as cookware, on low shelves so that you can reach them easily.

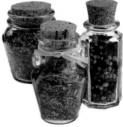

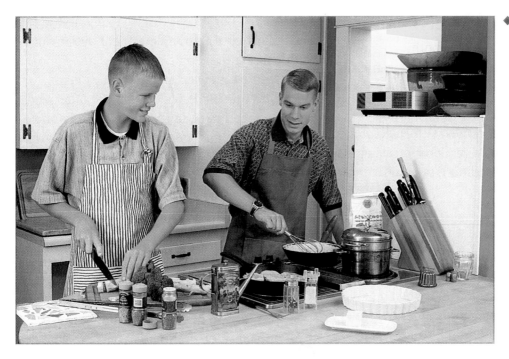

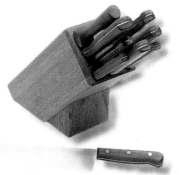

♦ Accident prevention in the kitchen begins with dressing appropriately. How might the saying "An ounce of prevention is worth a pound of cure" apply to work in the kitchen?

Preventing Falls

As Kaneesha learned, spills on the floor can cause accidents. To prevent falls, keep the floor clean and clear of clutter. Wipe up spills, spatters, and peelings so that no one will slip on them. Eliminate other hazards, such as slippery throw rugs, and replace damaged or worn flooring. Don't wear untied shoes, floppy slippers, or long clothing that could cause you to trip.

To reach higher shelves, use a firm step-stool. If you use a chair or a box, you could fall and be injured.

Preventing Cuts

Cuts are an everyday hazard for the cook. Here are some safety guidelines for handling knives, other sharp tools, and broken glass:

♦ Keep knives sharp and use them properly. You'll learn how in Section 8-4.

♦ Use a drawer divider, knife block, or knife rack for storing sharp cutting tools.

♦ Don't try to catch a falling knife—you might grab the blade instead of the handle. Step aside and let it fall.

♦ Don't soak knives or other sharp-edged utensils in a sink or dishpan with water in it. When you reach into the water, you could cut yourself.

♦ Sweep up broken glass from the floor immediately with a broom and dustpan. If you need to pick up pieces by hand, use a wet paper towel instead of bare fingers. Seal the broken glass in a paper or plastic bag; then place the bag in the wastebasket. Take out the trash as soon as possible.

♦ Storing knives in a block or special rack helps prevent cuts. Identify two other precautions to take when using knives.

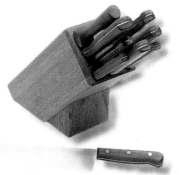

Using Electricity Safely

Electrical appliances save both time and work in the kitchen. However, they can also be a source of shocks, burns, and other injuries.

To avoid accidents, carefully read the owner's manual that comes with each kitchen appliance. Follow the directions for using the appliance safely. In addition, remember these basic guidelines:

◆ **Water and electricity don't mix.** Never use an electric appliance when your hands are wet or when you are standing on a wet floor. Keep small electric appliances away from the water when you use them. Don't run cords around a sink. If an electric appliance falls into water or becomes wet, unplug it immediately without touching the appliance itself. Don't put small appliances in water for cleaning unless the owner's manual says it's safe to do so.

◆ **Avoid damage to electrical cords.** Even a single exposed wire could start a fire or produce a shock. To keep from damaging cords, don't run them over a hot surface or try to staple or nail them in place. Never disconnect an appliance by tugging on the cord. Instead, grasp the plug at the electrical outlet to remove it.

◆ **Use outlets properly.** Plugging too many cords into an electrical outlet can cause a fire. Some appliances are equipped with **polarized plugs**—plugs made with one blade wider than the other and designed to fit in the outlet in only one way. You may not be able to fit a polarized plug into an older outlet. If that's the case, don't try to force the plug in or change the shape of the plug. Instead, have the outlet replaced, or buy an adapter.

◆ **Use care with any plugged-in appliance.** Never put your fingers or a kitchen tool inside an appliance that is plugged in. You might touch parts that could shock you, or you might accidentally turn the appliance on and injure yourself. Don't let the cords dangle off the counter—an appliance could accidentally be pulled off while in use. Turn off small appliances as soon as you are through with them.

◆ **Watch for problems.** Don't try to use a damaged appliance or one that gives you a shock. Have it repaired before you use it again. If an appliance starts to burn, unplug it immediately.

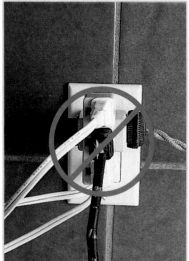 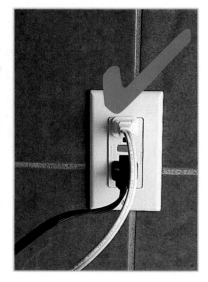

◆ Exercising electrical safety can help prevent a kitchen disaster. In what way is the situation on the left an accident waiting to happen?

Hazardous Chemicals

Hazardous chemicals are not limited to use in industries. Many can be found under most kitchen sinks. Hazardous household chemicals include oven cleaners, lighter fluid, drain cleaners, pesticides, and polishes. Some of these chemicals can cause burns, breathing difficulties, and poisoning.

Before you buy any household chemical, read the label carefully to be sure you understand the directions. You'll find important information about adequate ventilation, ways to protect yourself, and proper disposal of any unused product. You will also learn what to do if the product is accidentally swallowed or inhaled. Here are some additional tips:

◆ Never transfer a hazardous product to another container. You'll need the directions that appear on the original container each time you use the product.

◆ Never mix different chemical products. They could combine to give off poisonous fumes.

◆ With spray products, be sure you're pointing the spray nozzle where the product is supposed to go. Never point it at yourself or anyone else.

FOR YOUR HEALTH

Safe Cleaning Substitutes

Before reaching for a potentially hazardous cleaning product, consider using a safe substitute. The following cleaning solutions were used before household chemicals turned up on supermarket shelves.

Cleaning Product	Safe Substitute
Dishwashing liquid	Use a combination of soap flakes and vinegar.
Dishwasher detergent	Use equal parts borax and washing soda (hydrated sodium carbonate).
Oven cleaner	Use a paste of baking soda, salt, and hot water, or sprinkle baking soda on the soiled area and scrub it with a damp cloth after about five minutes. Be sure not to let the baking soda touch the heating elements.
Drain cleaner	Pour ¼ cup baking soda followed by ½ cup white vinegar in the drain. Cover the drain until the fizzing stops. Then flush by running hot water in the drain.
Window cleaner	Use alcohol to remove the residues. When the glass is dry, spray it with a mixture of equal parts white vinegar and water. You can recycle newspaper by drying the window with a crumpled page.

Following Up

1. Check the contents labels of three household cleaners you use regularly. Use a dictionary to check unfamiliar ingredients. How many of the ingredients are toxic?

2. Read the warnings on the labels for several cleaning products. How safe do you feel using these products? What effect could they have on the environment after being washed down household drains?

- Store hazardous chemical products away from food. Be sure children can't reach them. Flammable products, such as kerosene, lighter fluid, and aerosol sprays, must be stored away from any source of heat.

- Avoid using hazardous chemicals unnecessarily. Whenever you can, substitute simple, safe cleaners, such as lemon juice, vinegar, soap flakes, baking soda, washing soda, or borax.

Preventing Range and Microwave Accidents

The range is the most likely place for fires and burns to occur. The microwave oven also presents some hazards. Here are some rules for using these appliances safely:

- Use potholders or oven mitts when picking up or uncovering hot pots and pans.

- When uncovering a pot or pan, lift up the far edge of the cover first so that the steam will flow away from you. Otherwise, it could burn your face and hands.

- Use only pots and pans in good condition. A loose handle or warped bottom could cause an accident.

- Keep pan handles turned toward the back or middle of the range top. Otherwise, someone might bump into a handle, causing a spill, and possibly be burned by a hot liquid.

- Keep flammable items, such as paper towels, away from the range. A draft could blow them onto the range and start a fire. For the same reason, do not put curtains on a window that is close to the range.

- Do not use plastic items near the range except for those made of heatproof plastic, such as plastic turners and spoons for nonstick pans. Some plastics are highly flammable and give off poisonous fumes when they burn.

- Arrange oven racks properly before you start the oven. You risk being burned if you have to reposition them once the oven is hot.

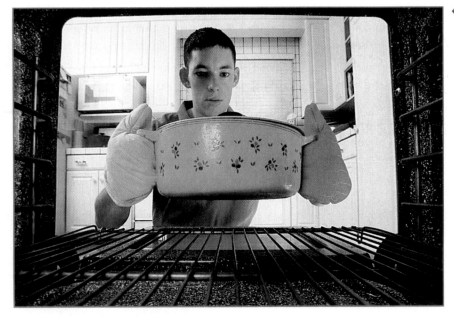

- **Oven mitts provide more protection than potholders.** Explain why both should be inspected from time to time.

- Stand to the side when you open the oven door. The heat rushing from the oven could burn your face.

- Don't reach into a hot oven. Pull out the rack first, using a potholder or an oven mitt.

- Clean up spills and crumbs after the oven has cooled. If allowed to build up in the oven, they could catch fire.

- Be sure cooktop and oven/broiler controls are turned off when not in use.

- Keep a fire extinguisher handy, and be sure everyone knows how to use it.

Safety Check

Be sure to inspect oven mitts and potholders for wear and tear from time to time. Worn or scorched spots will not protect you from getting burned by hot pots and pans.

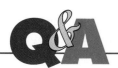

Q What should I do if I smell gas in the kitchen?

A First check to see whether the pilot light on the range has gone out. If it has, light the match first; then turn on the burner and light it. Turning on the burner first will cause gas to accumulate, a condition that could lead to an explosion. If you still smell gas, turn off all controls and open the windows for ventilation. Alert others and leave the building immediately. Call your gas company from another location.

If a Fire Starts

You've followed all the proper safety procedures, but suddenly there's a fire in your kitchen. What should you do? What to do depends on where the fire occurs.

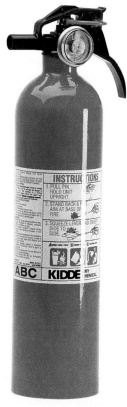

- **Range top or electric skillet.** Turn off the heat. Put the cover on the pan, or pour salt or baking soda on the flames. Never use water—the grease will splatter and spread the fire, and it could burn you. Don't use baking powder— it could make the fire worse.

◆ No kitchen should be without a fire extinguisher. Do you know how to use one correctly?

- **Oven, broiler, microwave, toaster oven.** Turn off or disconnect the appliance. Keep the oven door closed until the fire goes out.

Never attempt to carry a pan with burning contents. You could cause an injury or a bigger fire. If you can't immediately put out a fire, go outdoors and call the fire department.

Special Needs for Accident Prevention

As a rule, anything you could do to prevent accidents will benefit the entire family. The very young and old, however, may need special consideration.

Children

Small children like to be where adults are—especially the kitchen. They want to watch you and do what you're doing. If your household includes young children, follow these guidelines for accident prevention:

◆ Never leave young children alone in the kitchen, even for a few seconds.

◆ Protect toddlers by using safety latches on drawers and cabinet doors.

◆ If children want to help you work, set up a child-size table or a safe stepstool. Provide small utensils they can use easily for simple tasks such as mixing and mashing. Don't let young children use knives or work near the range. Supervise them at all times.

◆ Model safe work habits for children. Use the accident prevention skills you have learned. If you practice safe work habits in the kitchen, they will too.

Aging Adults and People with Disabilities

Kitchen safety is an important issue for those with physical challenges, such as poor eyesight or arthritis. Changes in the work space or equipment may be needed so that people with special needs can use the kitchen safely. Ask for their suggestions. What kitchen tasks are hard for them? How could the kitchen be reorganized to make jobs easier and safer? Here are some ideas for creating a barrier-free kitchen:

◆ Keep a magnifying glass in the kitchen to aid with reading small print.

◆ Relabel items in larger letters, if necessary, using stick-on labels and a marking pen.

◆ Add more or better lighting.

◆ Store frequently used equipment and foods in easy-to-reach places.

◆ Add a cart with wheels to the kitchen to make it easier to move food and equipment from place to place.

◆ Use nonbreakable dishes and glassware.

◆ Replace hard-to-open cabinet hardware with U-shaped or pull handles.

◆ Provide tongs or grippers to grab items that would otherwise be out of reach.

◆ Put mixing bowls on a damp dishcloth or a rubber disk jar opener to keep them from sliding on a slippery countertop during mixing.

◆ Use rubber disk jar openers for gripping appliance knobs.

◆ Provide a stool or tall chair so that the person can sit while working at the counter.

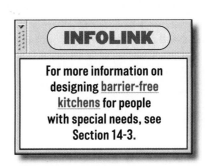

INFOLINK

For more information on designing barrier-free kitchens for people with special needs, see Section 14-3.

In Case of Accident

In spite of all your precautions, an accident may happen when you are working in the kitchen. If you have practiced the management skills discussed in Chapter 1, you will be prepared for that possibility. You will have a list of emergency numbers next to the phone and a first aid kit in a handy location. If you don't know how to administer first aid, contact your local chapter of the American Red Cross to find out about training.

One first aid technique everyone should know is administering the **Heimlich maneuver**—a technique used to rescue victims of choking. The technique can even be performed on yourself. Another vital technique is **CPR**, or cardiopulmonary resuscitation (KARD-ee-oh-PULL-muh-nare-ee ree-SUSS-uh-TAY-shun), a technique used to revive a person whose breathing and heartbeat have stopped. Knowing these techniques can save a life.

If an accident does occur, stay calm. Panic will only keep you from thinking clearly. If necessary, take a few deep breaths to get yourself under control.

Never hesitate to call for help, whether for yourself or someone else. It is better to summon help, even though you may not need it, than to try to handle the accident yourself.

Section 7-2 Review & Activities

1. Name three ways to prevent falls.

2. Give three suggestions that might improve kitchen safety for an older person with special needs.

3. Name two things you should do in case an accident does occur in the kitchen.

4. **Analyzing.** What is the most serious kitchen accident you have ever had? Why did it happen? How could it have been prevented?

5. **Evaluating.** Some people are in the habit of unplugging toasters and other small kitchen appliances after every use. Besides being overly cautious, how might this practice actually lead to an accident situation?

6. **Applying.** Make a mini-poster for the school foods lab to remind class members of one of the accident prevention pointers discussed in this section. Compose a slogan that will help people remember the tip. Set aside one wall of the classroom to display posters.

Keeping Food Safe to Eat

Manuel checked the chicken sizzling on the grill. "It's done!" he called to his aunt. "I'll bring it in." He started to reach for the platter he had used to carry the raw chicken outside when his aunt stopped him. "Don't use that! It hasn't been washed. I'll get you a clean plate."

Objectives

After studying this section, you should be able to:

- Discuss the causes of foodborne illness.
- Explain how proper food handling practices can prevent foodborne illness.

Look for These Terms

food safety

microorganisms

toxins

cross-contamination

spores

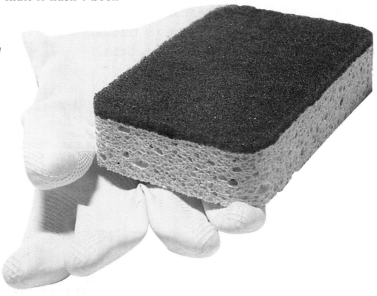

Food Safety

Manuel almost forgot an important rule of food safety. **Food safety** means following practices that help prevent foodborne illness and keep food safe to eat.

It's estimated that up to 80 million Americans suffer from foodborne illness, also known as food poisoning, every year. The illness may be mild, lasting just a day or two, or severe enough to require hospitalization. In some cases it can even result in death. Children, females who are pregnant, aging adults, and people with chronic illness are most at risk.

Most cases of foodborne illness can be traced to harmful **microorganisms**—tiny living creatures visible only through a microscope. In another sense, however, people are to blame. Improper food handling practices allow harmful microorganisms to grow and spread. It's up to you to handle food properly to prevent illness.

> **INFOLINK**
>
> For more on prevention of foodborne illness and other health risks associated with outdoor grilling, see Section 24-4.

Harmful Microorganisms

Most harmful microorganisms associated with foodborne illness are bacteria—and they're everywhere. Bacteria are carried by people, animals, insects, and objects. Many bacteria are harmless, but others can cause illness. Sometimes the illness is not caused by the bacteria themselves but by the **toxins**, or poisons, they produce.

Most harmful bacteria can be tolerated by the human body in small amounts. When the amounts multiply to dangerous levels, however, they create a health hazard. Bacteria reproduce quickly in the presence of food, moisture, and warmth. In just a few hours, one bacterium can multiply into thousands. You can't tell whether food contains harmful bacteria. The food generally looks, smells, and tastes normal.

The chart below describes some bacteria that cause foodborne illness and where that bacteria are found.

Bacteria That Cause Foodborne Illness

Bacteria	Where Bacteria Are Found
E. coli	Contaminated water, raw or rare ground beef, unpasteurized milk or apple juice.
Listeria monocytogenes	Contaminated soil and water; meat and dairy products; ready-to-eat foods such as hot dogs, luncheon meats, cold cuts, dry sausages, and deli-style meats and poultry.
Salmonella	Raw or undercooked foods, such as poultry, eggs, and meat; unpasteurized milk.
Clostridium botulinum	Improperly processed canned foods, garlic in oils, vacuum-packed or tightly wrapped food—environments where there is little or no oxygen.
Campylobacter jejuni	Contaminated water, unpasteurized milk, or undercooked meat or poultry; on human skin, in nose, and in throat.
Staphylococcus aureus	On human skin, in nose, and in throat—spread by improper food handling.
Clostridium perfringens	Environments where there is little or no oxygen; spores can survive cooking; often called the "cafeteria germ" because it most often strikes food served in quantity and left for long periods on a steam table or at room temperature.

Cleanliness in the Kitchen

Cleanliness is one of the keys to food safety. Whenever you work with food, be sure to keep yourself and the kitchen clean.

Personal Hygiene

When you're handling food, you don't have to scrub as surgeons do before operating. Remember, however, that keeping clean is important. Here are suggestions for minimizing the risk of introducing harmful microorganisms when you are working in the kitchen:

◆ Wear clean clothes and cover them with a clean apron. Spots and stains can harbor bacteria.

◆ Remove dangling jewelry, roll up long sleeves, and tie back long hair. That will help keep them out of food.

◆ Using soap and warm water, scrub your hands for 20 seconds before you begin to handle food. Use a brush to clean under and around your fingernails.

◆ Wear rubber or plastic gloves if you have an open wound on your hands. Because gloves can pick up bacteria, wash gloved hands as often as you wash bare hands.

◆ Scrub your hands immediately after using the toilet or blowing your nose.

◆ Do not sneeze or cough into food.

◆ Do not touch your face, your hair, or any other part of your body while working with food. If you do, stop working and scrub your hands.

Work Methods for Food Safety

In addition to keeping yourself clean, remember to follow these important guidelines:

◆ Be sure that work areas and equipment are clean before you start preparing food.

◆ Avoid **cross-contamination**—letting microorganisms from one food get into another. For example, the juices from raw meat, poultry, and fish and other seafood contain harmful microorganisms. A knife used to cut raw meat could contaminate raw vegetables. After you have handled raw meat, poultry, or seafood, wash everything that came in contact with those foods. This includes tools, work surfaces, and your hands.

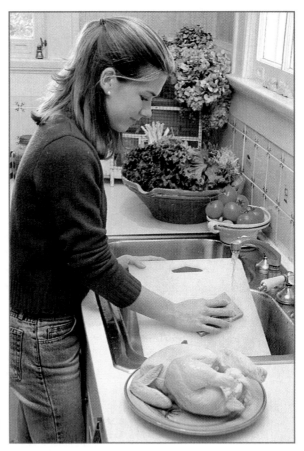

◆ **Washing cutting boards and other equipment in between uses can prevent cross-contamination of foods.** Explain why juices from raw meat, poultry, or seafood should not come in contact with other foods.

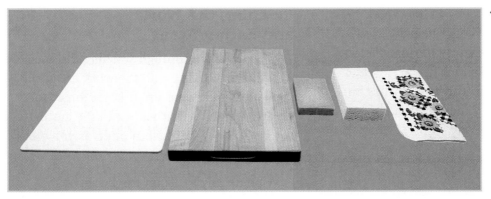

◆ The kitchen items pictured here all have some potential risk as breeding grounds for microorganisms. Which of the items have the highest degree of risk?

◆ If possible, avoid using cutting boards made of porous materials, such as soft wood. Such materials provide a breeding ground for harmful bacteria.

◆ Wash the top of a can before opening it to keep dirt from getting into the food.

◆ If you use a spoon to taste food during preparation, wash it after each use to avoid transferring harmful bacteria from your mouth to the food you're preparing.

◆ Keep pets out of the kitchen.

◆ Keep two towels handy in the kitchen— one for wiping hands and a second one for drying dishes.

◆ Dishcloths and sponges can harbor harmful bacteria. Use a clean dishcloth each day. Wash sponges at the end of the day and allow them to air-dry before reuse.

Cleanup Time

After food has been prepared and eaten, it's time to clean up. A clean kitchen has no food particles and spills to encourage bacterial growth or to attract insects or rodents.

Using Cleanup Appliances

Many kitchens are equipped with a food waste disposal and a dishwasher to help speed cleanup. A food waste disposal system grinds food waste and flushes it down the drain. Always run plenty of cold water when grinding food. Don't overfill the disposal. Instead, grind small bunches at a time. To avoid clogging the disposal, don't put fibrous food, such as onion skins and corn husks, in it.

When using an automatic dishwasher, follow the instructions in the owner's manual. Be sure the dishwasher is full before running it. Small loads waste water and energy.

Washing Dishes by Hand

Washing dishes can go faster and more easily if you're well organized. The following suggestions can help you with this task.

Rinse soiled dishes and place them on one side of the sink. Group like items and arrange them in this order: glasses, flatware, plates, kitchen tools, and cookware. Keep sharp knives separate. If food is stuck to cookware, presoak it. Pour a little dish detergent in, add hot water, and let the pan stand for a while.

Fill a dishpan or sink with soapy water— hot enough to remove grease but not hot enough to burn your hands. Using a sponge or dishcloth, wash the dishes in the order you grouped them. Wash glasses first and greasy cookware last. When necessary, refill the sink or dishpan with clean, hot, soapy water.

Rinse dishes thoroughly in hot water. Be sure the insides of containers are well rinsed. A safe and easy way to rinse the outsides is to put the dish rack in the sink and let hot water run over it. Let the dishes air-dry in the rack, or dry them with a clean, dry towel.

Safety Check

What if a glass or dish breaks in a sink full of water? Using a paper towel to protect your fingers, carefully reach into the sink and open up the drain. After the water has drained, use the wet paper towel to pick up the broken pieces. Remember to dispose of broken glass properly.

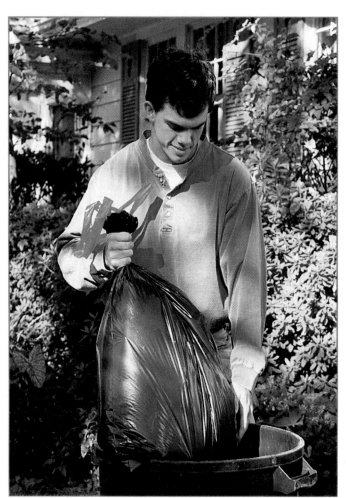

Cleaning the Work and Eating Areas

When you are through washing dishes, wipe the table. Clean all the work areas and appliances that were used. Don't forget to wash the can opener blade and the cutting board. Rinse the dishcloth often as you work, using hot, soapy water.

Wipe up any spills on the floor. Wash the sink to remove grease and food particles. If the kitchen is equipped with a disposal, run it a final time.

Finally, put any garbage in a plastic bag, close the bag tightly, and put it in the garbage can outside. Wash garbage cans regularly so that they don't attract insects and rodents.

Controlling Pests

Insects can bring disease into the kitchen. However, chemical insecticides can be hazardous to humans and the environment. Here are some ways to control household insects without using insecticides:

◆ Repair holes in walls and screens. Caulk cracks and crevices.

◆ Keep the kitchen and other areas clean.

◆ Sprinkle chili powder, paprika, or dried peppermint across ant trails.

◆ To control roaches, dust borax lightly around the refrigerator and range.

◆ **Be sure to wrap garbage tightly and store it outside the home.** Name two other precautions to take to reduce the risk of foodborne illness.

Proper Food Temperatures

Temperature is one of the most important factors in food safety. Keeping food at proper temperatures can be critical to preventing foodborne illness.

How Temperatures Affect Microorganisms

Bacteria multiply rapidly at temperatures between 60°F and 140°F (16°C to 60°C). Note that this range includes room temperatures.

Most foodborne illnesses are caused by bacteria that thrive in these temperatures.

High food temperatures, from 160°F to 212°F (71°C to 100°C), kill most harmful bacteria. These temperatures are normally reached during cooking. However, some bacteria produce **spores**, cells that will develop into bacteria if conditions are right. Spores can survive cooking heat.

Cold refrigerator temperatures, below 40°F (4°C), slow down the growth of some bacteria but do not kill them.

If food is frozen at 0°F (–18°C), bacteria stop growing. Bacteria or spores already present in food, however, will not be killed. When the food is thawed, bacteria will start to grow again.

The diagram on the left shows you the proper temperatures for storing and cooking food. Red is the danger zone—where bacteria grow rapidly. Bacteria also grow in the orange zone, but more slowly than in the red zone.

As you have learned, foodborne illness can also be caused by toxins. Some types of toxins are destroyed by heat. Others remain unchanged even after food is cooked.

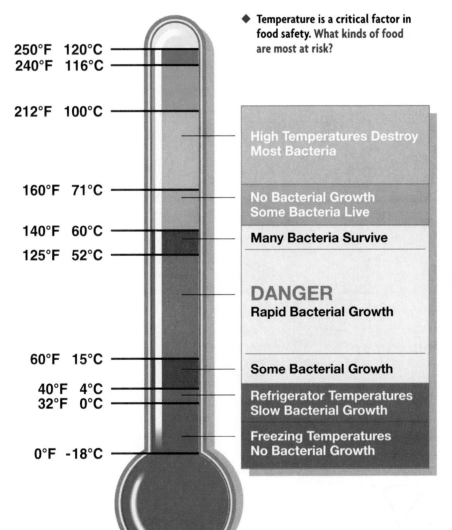

◆ Temperature is a critical factor in food safety. What kinds of food are most at risk?

250°F	120°C
240°F	116°C
212°F	100°C
160°F	71°C
140°F	60°C
125°F	52°C
60°F	15°C
40°F	4°C
32°F	0°C
0°F	-18°C

High Temperatures Destroy Most Bacteria

No Bacterial Growth
Some Bacteria Live

Many Bacteria Survive

DANGER
Rapid Bacterial Growth

Some Bacterial Growth

Refrigerator Temperatures
Slow Bacterial Growth

Freezing Temperatures
No Bacterial Growth

Food Handling Guidelines

Many foods require special care to keep them out of the danger zone. Meat, poultry, fish and other seafood, eggs, and dairy products are some of these foods.

When cooking and serving food, follow these guidelines:

◆ Cook food to the proper internal temperature or until thoroughly cooked. Avoid partial cooking—cook the food completely at one time.

◆ Taste foods containing ingredients from animal sources only after they are fully cooked. Do not taste them when they are raw or during cooking.

◆ When microwaving, take steps to ensure even, thorough cooking.

◆ Do not leave food out more than two hours at room temperature or more than one hour if the temperature is above 90°F (32°C).

◆ Keep extra quantities of food either hot—on the range or in another cooking appliance—or cold—in the refrigerator.

◆ Do not add more food to a serving dish of food that has been out for a while. Instead, use a clean dish.

◆ Discard foods that have been held at room temperature for more than two hours.

◆ Refrigerate food in shallow containers. Large, deep containers keep the food from cooling rapidly and evenly.

◆ When reheating food that has been refrigerated, bring it to an internal temperature of 165°F (74°C) or higher to kill any bacteria. Keep in mind that if the food has not been properly stored, it can't be made safe just by reheating.

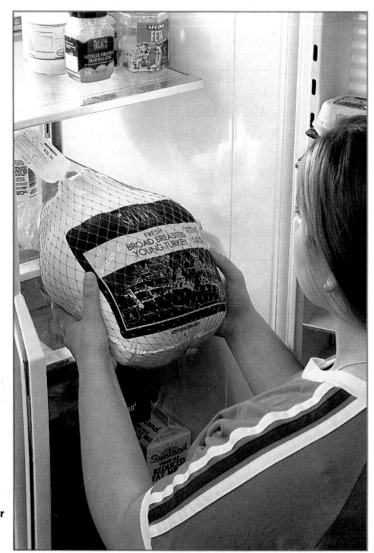

◆ Thawing food at proper temperatures is another important safeguard. How would you thaw a frozen turkey safely?

Thawing Food Safely

Anita was about to leave a package of frozen chicken on the counter to thaw when she remembered what she had learned in foods lab: Never thaw food at room temperature. Quickly, she placed the package in the refrigerator to thaw.

When food is thawed at room temperature, the outside of the item may contain millions of harmful bacteria by the time the inside is thawed. To thaw food safely, use one of these methods:

◆ Place food in the refrigerator where it will thaw slowly. Be sure packages of thawing food do not leak onto other foods.

◆ For faster thawing, put the package in a watertight plastic bag and submerge it in cold water. Change the water every 30 minutes. The cold slows down the growth of bacteria as the food thaws.

◆ Use a microwave for quick, safe defrosting. Follow the manufacturer's directions. Foods thawed this way should be cooked immediately.

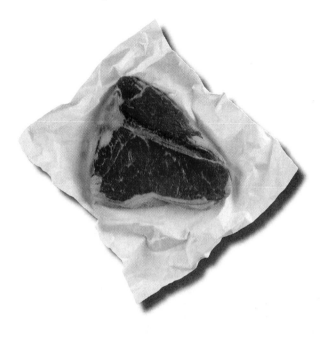

Section 7-3 Review & Activities

1. Identify three ways in which bacteria are spread.

2. Name five instances when you should wash your hands while working with food.

3. What temperature range is considered the "danger zone"? Why?

4. **Analyzing.** Why do you think so many Americans suffer from foodborne illness each year?

5. **Evaluating.** In Morocco, as well as other African countries, people traditionally eat food with their hands directly from a large communal bowl. It is customary for the host to bring a pitcher of water and a basin to the table and to pour the water as the guests wash their hands both before and after the meal. What makes this a good cleanliness practice? What other meaning might this custom convey?

6. **Applying.** Write at least six slogans or rhymes that could help you and your classmates remember important rules for keeping foods safe.

Storing Food

"The bread's moldy again!" Noelle exclaimed. "Why doesn't it keep longer?" One of the most common answers to Noelle's question is improper storage.

Objectives

After studying this section, you should be able to:

- Identify causes and signs of food spoilage.

- Give examples of foods that are stored at room temperature and in cold storage.

- Give guidelines for each type of storage.

Look for These Terms

shelf life

shelf-stable

freezer burn

inventory

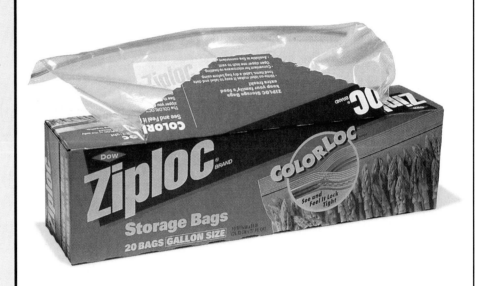

Spoilage and Nutrient Loss

When food is not properly stored, it begins to lose quality and nutrients. Eventually, it will spoil. Spoiled food often develops bad tastes and odors and must be thrown out. Some types of spoilage can cause foodborne illness.

What causes spoilage? Under the right conditions, harmful bacteria, yeasts, and molds can spoil food. Spoilage can also be caused by natural chemical changes within the cells of the food. Yet another cause is conditions in the environment, which can cause or speed up nutrient loss and spoilage.

- **Heat.** Heat speeds up chemical reactions that cause spoilage.

- **Air.** Exposure to oxygen can destroy some nutrients, such as vitamins C and E. It can also cause oils to become rancid and develop an unpleasant flavor.

- **Moisture.** Moisture is a double-edged sword. Too little moisture can cause fresh foods to dry out, wilt, and lose nutrients. Too much moisture can provide a breeding ground for bacteria and molds.

- **Light.** Light can destroy nutrients, especially vitamin C and riboflavin.

- **Dirt.** Dirt contains harmful microorganisms.

◆ **Damage to food or packaging.**
Both these conditions make spoilage by
microorganisms more likely. Be alert for
signs of spoilage in packaging, such as
bulging cans, liquids that spurt when you
open the container, or liquids that are
cloudy when they should be clear.

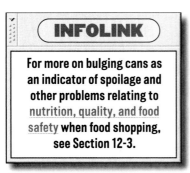

INFOLINK

For more on bulging cans as
an indicator of spoilage and
other problems relating to
nutrition, quality, and food
safety when food shopping,
see Section 12-3.

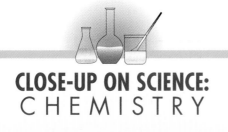

CLOSE-UP ON SCIENCE:
CHEMISTRY

Enzymes in Food

The cells of living things contain *enzymes,*
protein substances that cause chemical
changes to occur. When a plant or animal is
processed into a food, some of the enzymes
remain active. Unless foods are heated to
destroy the enzymes, chemical changes
continue—destroying the cells and causing
the food to spoil.

When Food Is Spoiled

How do you know when food is starting to
spoil? Some fresh foods, such as apples and
celery, may wilt, get wrinkled, or turn brown.
Some foods become slimy, a sign that decay
has started. Other signs of spoilage are spots
of fuzzy mold; damage such as holes, tears,
and bruises; bad flavors; and bad odors.

Spoiled foods should be discarded.
Those that have turned moldy require special
handling because mold gives off spores,
which can easily spread. Very gently wrap
the moldy food, or place it in a bag before
discarding it. Examine other foods that may
have been in contact with the moldy food.
Clean the container that held the moldy food,
and if necessary, wash out the refrigerator.

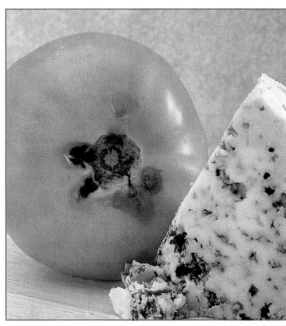

◆ **Blue cheese gets its flavor from a special type of mold.
However, most foods with mold must be thrown out.**
Name two ways of retarding the formation of mold in
the foods you store.

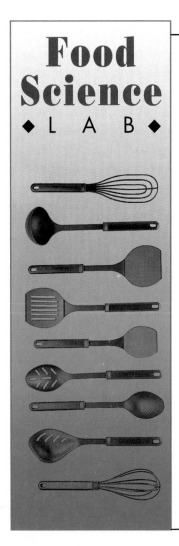

Food Science ◆ L A B ◆

Growing Microorganisms

You can't see a single microorganism, but you can see colonies of microorganisms, called *cultures*. In this experiment, you'll discover just how widespread microorganisms really are.

Procedure

1. With a felt-tip pen, divide into quarters a Petri dish coated with nutrient agar. Number the quarters 1 to 4.

2. Touch the end of a 4-inch (10-cm) strip of cellophane tape to a doorknob, and press it into area 1 of the Petri dish. Touch another tape strip to a clean dish and a third strip to your hair, and press these into areas 2 and 3.

3. Touch a fourth piece of tape to the agar without letting it touch any other surface, including your fingers.

4. Leave the Petri dish at room temperature for three days. Observe it each day, and describe any growths that have appeared.

Conclusions

◆ Were any of the surfaces you tested free of microorganisms? Was the tape itself free of microorganisms?

◆ Which surfaces produced the most bacterial growth? Why do you think this occurred?

◆ What changes in your food preparation practices might you consider making as a result of this experiment?

Basic Storage Principles

No food can be stored indefinitely. Each food has a **shelf life,** the length of time it can be stored and still retain its quality. Shelf life depends on the type of food, packaging, and storage temperature, as well as how the food is handled.

To avoid loss of quality in stored food, follow these guidelines:

◆ Buy only what you need.

◆ Follow the principle of "first in, first out." Store new food behind the same kind of older food. Use up the older food first.

◆ Look for "sell by" or "use by" dates on the containers. If there are none, you may want to write the purchase dates on the containers before storing them. Use canned food within a year.

◆ Clean storage areas regularly. Throw out food that has started to spoil or containers that have been damaged. Wash and dry surfaces thoroughly.

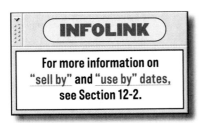

INFOLINK

For more information on "sell by" and "use by" dates, see Section 12-2.

Room Temperature Storage

Many canned, bottled, and packaged foods are **shelf-stable,** which means they are able to last for weeks or even months at room temperatures below 85°F (30°C). Examples are most unopened canned foods, dry beans and peas, oils and shortening, and many grain products (except whole grains). In general, foods that you find on grocery shelves can be stored at room temperature when you bring them home.

Kitchen cabinets are used for most room temperature storage. They should be clean and dry, with doors to keep out light and dirt. Temperatures should be no higher than 85°F (30°C) and no lower than freezing, 32°F (0°C). Do not store food on shelves near or above heat sources, such as a range, toaster, refrigerator, or radiator. Also avoid areas that may be wet, such as cabinets under the sink.

Once packages or containers have been opened, storage requirements differ. Some shelf-stable foods, including most canned goods, must be refrigerated after opening. Others, such as a bag of dry beans or a box of cereal, can remain at room temperature. Reseal the package if possible. Otherwise, transfer the contents to a storage container with a tight-fitting cover. Do the same with the foods you buy in bulk.

Safety Check

If you have to stack items to store them, put the lightest on top so that you'll be less likely to accidentally knock over heavy items that could cause injury. Boxes of dried soup mix, for example, can be stored on top of canned soups.

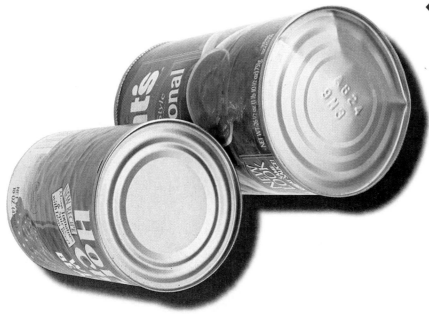

◆ **Shelf-stable foods may be stored at normal room temperature.** Which of the two foods shown has telltale signs of possible bacterial contamination?

Cold Storage

Perishable foods spoil quickly at room temperature. They require cold storage in the refrigerator or freezer, depending on the kind of food and how long you want to store it. The package may give instructions for storage. The chart below and on the next page gives you a general timetable for keeping foods in cold storage.

Refrigerator Storage

Foods normally refrigerated include:

♦ Foods that were refrigerated in the store, such as dairy products, eggs, delicatessen foods, and fresh meat, poultry, and fish and other seafood.

♦ Most fresh fruits and vegetables. Exceptions are onions, potatoes, and sweet potatoes, which should be stored in a cool, dry area.

♦ Whole-grain products, seeds, and nuts. They contain oils that can spoil and give foods an off-flavor.

♦ Leftover cooked foods.

♦ Baked goods with fruit or cream fillings.

♦ Any foods that according to label directions must be refrigerated after opening.

Cold Storage Chart

NOTE: —— means food should not be stored in that area.

Type of Food	Refrigerator Storage 40°F (4°C)	Freezer Storage 0°F (–18°C)
Meats, Poultry, Fish		
Beef, lamb, pork, or veal chops, steaks, roast	3-5 days	4-12 months
Chicken or turkey, whole	1-2 days	1 year
Chicken or turkey, pieces	1-2 days	9 months
Ground meats or poultry	1-2 days	3-4 months
Lean fish (cod)	1-2 days	6 months
Fatty fish (salmon)	1-2 days	2-3 months
Shellfish (shrimp)	1-2 days	3-6 months
Dairy Products		
Fresh milk, cream	7 days	3 months
Butter, margarine	1-3 months	6-9 months
Buttermilk	2 weeks	3 months
Sour cream	1-3 weeks	——
Yogurt, plain or flavored	1-2 weeks	1-2 months
Cottage cheese	1 week	——
Hard cheese (cheddar), opened	3-4 weeks	6 months
Hard cheese, unopened	6 months	6 months
Ice cream, sherbet	——	2-4 months

Cold Storage Chart (cont'd)

NOTE: —— means food should not be stored in that area.

Type of Food	Refrigerator Storage 40°F (4°C)	Freezer Storage 0°F (−18°C)
Miscellaneous Foods		
Bread	7-14 days	3 months
Cakes, pies (not cream-filled)	7 days	2-3 months
Cream pies	1-2 days	——
Fresh eggs, in shell	3 weeks	——
Raw yolks, whites	2-4 days	1 year
Hard-cooked eggs	1 week	——
Egg substitutes, opened	3 days	——
Egg substitutes, unopened	10 days	——
Mayonnaise, opened	2 months	——
Salad dressing, opened	3 months	——
Salsa, opened	3 months	——
Cookies	2 months	8-12 months
Cooked Foods, Leftovers		
Cooked meats, meat dishes	3-4 days	2-3 months
Fried chicken	3-4 days	4 months
Poultry covered in broth	3-4 days	6 months
Fish stews, soups (not creamed)	3-4 days	4-6 months
Cured Meats		
Hot dogs, opened	1 week	1-2 months
Lunch meats, opened	3-5 days	1-2 months
Hot dogs, lunch meats, unopened	2 weeks	1-2 months
Bacon	7 days	1 month
Smoked sausage (beef, pork, turkey)	7 days	1-2 months
Hard sausage (pepperoni)	2-3 weeks	1-2 months
Ham, canned (refrigerated, unopened)	6-9 months	——
Ham, fully cooked, whole	7 days	1-2 months
Ham, fully cooked, half or slices	3-5 days	1-2 months

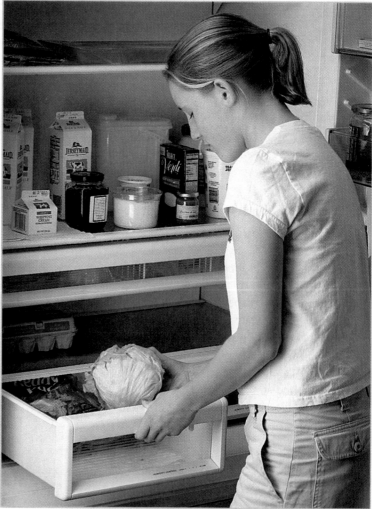

◆ **Not all areas of the refrigerator have the same temperature.** Which areas offer the coldest storage? Which foods should be stored in the door?

Refrigeration Guidelines

Avoid overloading the refrigerator when storing foods. If the cold air can't circulate well, some areas may become too warm to store perishables safely. Be sure, also, that foods are tightly covered. This will keep them from drying out and will also prevent odors from being picked up by other foods. Opened canned foods may pick up an off-flavor from the can, so transfer them to another storage container.

Store meat, poultry, and seafood in the store wrap in a plastic bag to prevent leakage. Leaking foods can contaminate other stored foods.

When storing fruits and vegetables, wash them only if necessary to remove dirt. Wipe hard-skinned fruits and vegetables dry, and drain others well.

Leftovers require special care. To ensure thorough chilling, use shallow containers. Large, deep containers keep food from cooling rapidly and evenly. Cut large pieces of meat into smaller ones so that they cool quickly. Close the containers tightly, and label them with the current date. Be sure to use the food within a few days. (Remember that some foods can be frozen for longer storage.) You may want to keep all leftovers on the same shelf so that none get overlooked.

Every refrigerator has a temperature control or coldness setting. To promote freshness and retard spoilage of stored foods, follow the manufacturer's recommended settings. Do not let the temperature fall to a point where frost or ice forms. Foods with a high water content, such as lettuce, may freeze and be damaged.

Freezer Storage

Freezing allows long-term storage of many foods. At temperatures of 0°F (–18°C) or below, foods keep from one month to a year, depending on the type of food and proper packaging.

Foods purchased frozen should be stored promptly in the home freezer. Many other foods can also be frozen to increase shelf life. These include fresh meats, poultry, and fish; baked goods such as breads and rolls; and many leftovers.

Some foods don't freeze well. Examples are fresh vegetables that are to be eaten raw, cooked or whole raw eggs, products made with mayonnaise, meat and poultry stuffing, cream- or egg-based sauces, custards, baked goods with cream filling, and many cheeses.

To freeze foods at home, you need a two-door refrigerator-freezer or a separate freezer unit. Separate freezer units generally maintain food quality longer than refrigerator-freezers.

Some refrigerators have only one outside door and a small freezer compartment inside. The freezer compartment maintains a temperature of 10°F to 15°F (–12°C to –10°C). It can be used for storing already frozen food for several weeks. However, it is not cold enough to freeze fresh or leftover food satisfactorily.

A freezer functions best when fairly full. Some freezers need regular defrosting.

Packaging and Freezing Foods

Foods that are purchased already frozen can be stored in their original packaging. However, foods frozen at home must be specially packaged to avoid freezer burn. **Freezer burn** is a condition that results when food is improperly packaged or stored in the freezer too long. The food dries out and loses flavor and texture.

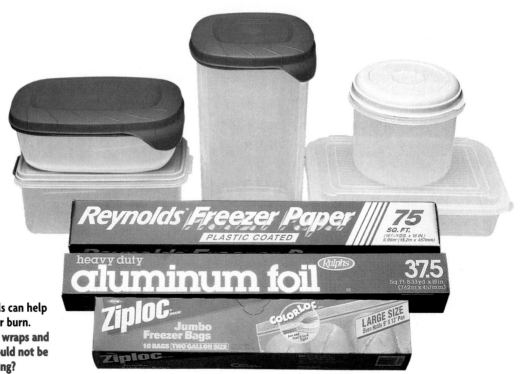

◆ These materials can help prevent freezer burn. What types of wraps and containers should not be used for freezing?

Packaging materials for freezing must be vapor- and moisture-resistant. Plastic containers with tight-fitting covers, heavy-duty plastic freezer bags, and wraps such as heavy-duty foil and freezer wrap are recommended. Don't use regular refrigerator storage bags or plastic tubs from foods such as margarine and yogurt. They do not provide enough protection. Fresh meat, poultry, and fish need additional wrap for freezing because the lightweight store wrapping does not provide sufficient protection.

When wrapping solid foods, such as meat, squeeze out as much air as possible to prevent freezer burn. Seal packages with freezer tape. When filling storage containers, leave enough space for food to expand as it freezes—about 1 inch (2.5 cm) in a quart (or liter) container. Then seal the container tightly. Label all packages and containers with the contents, amount (or number of servings), date frozen, and any special instructions.

For best quality, freeze food quickly. Spread the packages out so that they touch the coils or sides of the freezer. Leave enough space between packages for air to circulate. When the food is frozen (at least 24 hours later), you can stack it according to the kind of food.

Keep an **inventory**, or ongoing record, of the food in the freezer. Include the food, date frozen, and quantity. As you remove food, change the quantity on the inventory so that you know how much is left.

Power Outages

When the power goes off or the refrigerator-freezer breaks down, the food inside is in danger of spoiling. In general, avoid opening the door of the freezer or refrigerator. This will help maintain cold temperatures longer.

Keeping Frozen Foods Safe

A full freezer will keep food frozen for about two days after losing power. A half-full freezer will keep food frozen for about one day. If the freezer is not full, stack packages closely together so that they will stay cold. Separate frozen meat, poultry, and fish from other foods. That way, if they begin to thaw, their juices will not get into other foods.

If the power will be off longer than two days, you can put dry ice (frozen carbon dioxide) in the freezer. Be careful! Never touch dry ice with bare hands or breathe its vapors in an enclosed area. Carbon dioxide gas in high concentration is poisonous.

When the freezer is working again, follow these guidelines to decide what to do with the food:

◆ If ice crystals are still visible or the food feels as cold as if it were refrigerated, it's safe to refreeze. Some foods may lose quality, but they can still be eaten.

◆ Discard any food that thawed or was held above 40°F (4°C) for more than two hours. Discard any food that has a strange odor.

Once the freezer is working again, wash up any food spills and wipe surfaces dry. If odors remain, wash again with a solution of 2 tablespoons (30 mL) baking soda dissolved in 1 quart (1 L) warm water. Leave an open box of baking soda inside the freezer to absorb odors.

Keeping Refrigerated Foods Safe

During a power outage, food will usually keep in the refrigerator for four to six hours, depending on the temperature of the room. If the power will be out for a long time, you can place a block of ice in the refrigerator.

When the refrigerator is working again, follow these guidelines to decide what to do with the food:

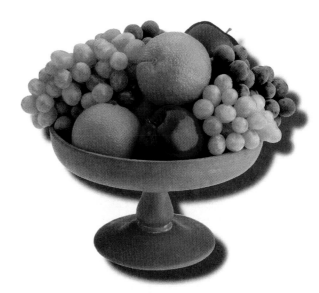

♦ Discard fresh meats, poultry, fish, lunch meats, hot dogs, eggs, milk, soft cheeses, and cooked foods if they have been held above 40°F (4°C) for more than two hours.

♦ Keep butter or margarine if it has not melted and does not have a rancid odor.

♦ Other foods, including fresh fruits and vegetables, are safe if they show no signs of mold or sliminess and do not have a bad odor.

Once the refrigerator is working again, clean it as described for the freezer.

Section 7-4 Review & Activities

1. What is the difference between shelf-stable foods and perishable foods?

2. What is the ideal temperature range for room temperature storage? Refrigerator storage? Freezer storage?

3. Describe how you would wrap a package of fresh ground meat for freezing.

4. Analyzing. Most people have to throw away spoiled food now and then. What do you think is the major reason?

5. Extending. What guidelines could you suggest for determining whether a food should be stored in the refrigerator or the freezer?

6. Applying. Use a refrigerator-freezer thermometer to check cold storage temperatures at home or in the school foods lab. Are the temperatures at safe levels?

Objectives

After studying this section, you should be able to:

- Explain the importance of conservation.
- Identify ways to conserve resources when working in the kitchen.

Look for These Terms

conservation

recycling

Conserving Natural Resources

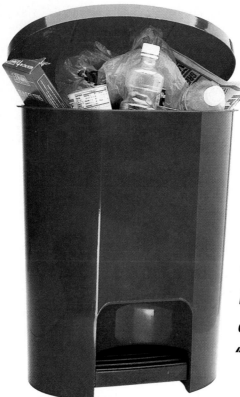

Marcus was studying in the kitchen. He could hear the kitchen radio vaguely in the background—something about the environment. "Conserve natural resources. . . . Don't waste or pollute." Marcus went back to his homework. "I'm just one person," he said to himself. "There's not much I can do."

Conserve Energy

Ironically, the room in which Marcus was sitting—the kitchen—is a major producer of trash that threatens to choke the environment. It is also an energy-guzzler, filled with appliances that liberally use natural gas, electricity, and water. By failing to turn off the radio when he wasn't listening to it, Marcus missed a chance to help conserve energy. **Conservation** is concern about, and action taken to ensure, the preservation of the environment.

What can you as a consumer do to save energy? For starters, remember to turn off lights and appliances when they are not in use. Cook as many foods as possible when using the oven, and freeze the extra for future meals. Here are some other tips:

- Use small appliances or a microwave oven when cooking small amounts of food. They use less energy than the range.

- Match the pan size to the size of the burner or heating unit for top-of-range cooking so that less energy will be lost.

- Decide what you want to eat before opening the refrigerator door. The air in the refrigerator warms up if you leave the door open. Then more energy is needed to cool it down.

- Keep the refrigerator and freezer well organized so that you can find food easily.

- Don't run the dishwasher unless it's full.

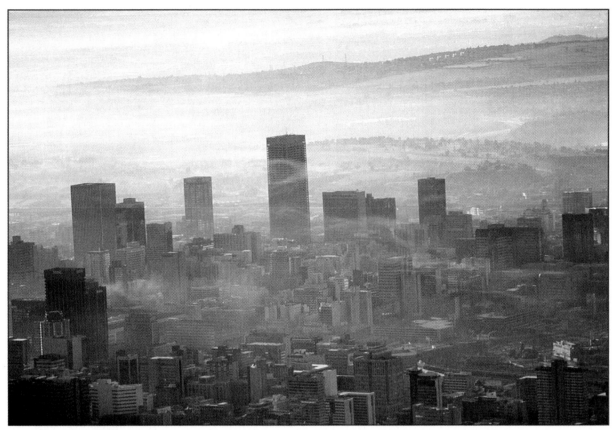

◆ **Pollution is a global problem. What decisions can you make to decrease its severity? What actions can you take to alert others to this problem?**

Never try to save energy by letting hot food cool to room temperature before refrigerating it. Remember, harmful bacteria grow quickly at room temperature.

Conserve Water

Clean, safe water is scarce in many areas. Water use may be restricted because of a shortage. Learn more about the water situation in your area. By conserving water in your home, you can help preserve this precious resource for all.

Look for ways to use less water during food preparation. For example, don't let tap water run unnecessarily as you pare vegetables.

Cleanup takes lots of water, but it is also possible to conserve in this task. When hand-washing dishes, don't keep the water running. Wash all the dishes first; then rinse them at the same time, as quickly as possible.

Be sure to repair dripping faucets immediately. Water dripping from a kitchen or other faucet at the rate of a drop a second can waste about 700 gallons (2,800 L) a year.

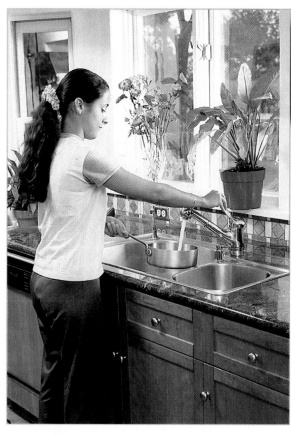

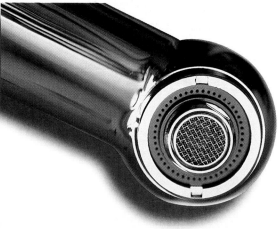

◆ **Installing aerators on faucets cuts down on water waste.** Identify three other regular habits that can help with this problem.

Reduce Trash

Picture a four-lane highway running from Boston to Los Angeles, filled with trash about 6 feet (3 m) deep. That's about the amount of trash Americans create in one year. The trash usually ends up in landfills, which can pollute soil and water. Communities are running out of landfill space.

You can help minimize the trash problem. Start by remembering three key words: *reduce, reuse,* and *recycle.*

Reduce

One way to cut down on trash is to reduce food waste. Studies of residential garbage cans show that a significant percentage of all food an American family buys (not including bones and other inedible parts) gets thrown

away. Reducing food waste will save you money. It will also help the environment. How can proper storage help reduce food waste?

Another way to cut down on trash is to reduce the use of disposable products. For example, use dishcloths instead of paper towels to wipe up spills. Use cloth napkins instead of paper ones. Buy or make cloth bags to carry groceries. Choose items in reusable or recyclable containers rather than disposable ones.

Reuse

Reusing gives second life to materials. Find creative ways to reuse items that might otherwise be thrown away. In the kitchen, you might:

◆ Wash plastic tubs from margarine, yogurt, and cottage cheese, and use them to refrigerate leftovers. Do not use them for freezing—they aren't heavy enough and food will dry out.

- Turn glass jars and bottles with tight-fitting covers into storage containers. Use them for foods such as rice, pasta, and dry beans. Wash the jars and covers carefully; then let them dry out for at least 24 hours to remove odors.

- Reuse plastic or paper grocery bags as trash bags.

Recycle

We could not live without water and many other resources the earth has provided for us. Recycling is a chance to give something back to the planet. **Recycling** is the treating of waste so that it can be reused, as well as an awareness of such practices.

The kinds of materials that are recycled can vary from community to community. Generally, newspapers, aluminum cans and foil, glass bottles, and some plastic containers are recycled. Learn about and cooperate with recycling efforts in your community.

Some communities have curbside pickup for recycled materials. In others, the items must be brought to the collection centers. Many supermarkets collect plastic shopping bags for recycling.

Precycling

You can do your part in the recycling effort before you even get your products home. Do you know how? The answer is *precycling*—

Connecting Food and Language Arts

Rachel Carson Speaks Out

Few writers or scientists have spoken out on the plight of the environment as eloquently as Rachel Carson, a pioneer of the modern ecology movement. Carson authored several best sellers, including *The Sea Around Us* and *Silent Spring,* and fought a lifelong crusade against the use of chemical pesticides.

In a speech, she voiced her concern about the use of pesticides, noting, "We are subjecting whole populations to exposure to chemicals which . . . have proved to be extremely poisonous and in many cases cumulative in their effect. These exposures now begin at or before birth and—unless we change our methods—will continue through the lifetime of those now living." Although her concerns have since echoed through the halls of government, prompting legislative action, during her life they

met with frequent opposition—especially from the chemical industry, which she criticized in *Silent Spring* for feeding the public "little . . . pills of half-truths. We urgently need an end to these false assurances, to the sugar-coating of unpalatable facts."

Think About It

1. Imagine that you had written to Rachel Carson during her lifetime for her views on reducing household trash, including hazardous household wastes. In a level of language equivalent to that of the quotes in the above passage, write what you believe her reply would have been.

2. What do you think she was referring to in the phrase "sugar-coating of unpalatable facts"? Can you identify present-day food safety issues in which manufacturers in the private sector are attempting to sugar-coat unpalatable facts?

choosing packaging and products that can ultimately be reused. Here are some tips:

◆ Avoid products packaged in plastic—a material that cannot be recycled—or polystyrene, which releases harmful chemicals into the atmosphere.

◆ Avoid items that you use once and throw away, such as disposable razors and paper cups and plates.

◆ Buy in bulk. Bulk quantities use less packaging than small or single-serving sizes.

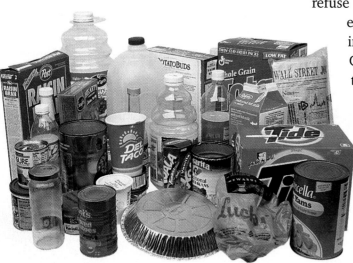

Show Your Concern

Some people, like Marcus, believe they can't do much to help solve environmental problems. Yet conservation begins with the individual. If each person does his or her share, waste and pollution can be reduced.

Some people blame business, industry, and government for environmental problems. Even in those areas, individual consumers have a voice. Every time you buy a product or use a service, you "vote" for it and for the policies of the company that sells it. If you refuse to buy items or services that waste energy or pollute, the producers will improve them or develop new ones. Consumer power is an effective way to conserve natural resources.

By making the right choices and cooperating with community programs, you can do your share to help conserve natural resources.

◆ Many materials can be recycled and used again. Find out what steps your community has taken to recycle waste.

Section 7-5 Review & Activities

1. Why is it important for individuals to conserve resources?

2. Name five ways to conserve energy in the home.

3. Name three keys to reducing trash, and give an example of each.

4. Extending. Describe some ways you can influence business, industry, and government to conserve natural resources.

5. Synthesizing. How might you convince someone who doesn't recycle to start recycling?

6. Applying. Develop a plan to reduce, reuse, and recycle at home. Where can you start? How can you proceed? How might you persuade family members to take part in your plan?

CAREER WANTED

Individuals able to follow procedures, uphold laws, and pay keen attention to detail.

REQUIRES:

- training program in inspection procedures
- certification by county or other locality

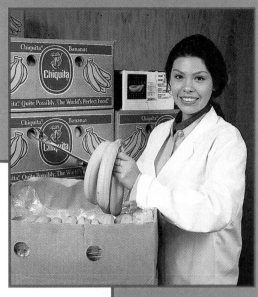

"Cleanliness is more than meets the eye,"

says Local Health Inspector Sasha Rafidi

Q: In a nutshell, what is a local health inspector's job?

A: We identify and document conditions in area food service establishments that may lead to foodborne illness. This includes a thorough inspection of the premises, including all work areas and refrigeration compartments.

Q: What is the biggest misconception people have of local health inspectors?

A: Most people think that this is a job anyone can do without any education or training beyond high school. The requirements do vary from one community to another. However, a background in either chemistry or microbiology enables you to do your job easily and well.

Q: How accurate are your findings?

A: Very accurate. To measure food temperature, for example, we use a thermocouple. It is a black box connected to a very sensitive thermometer, which precisely measures food temperature and gives a digital readout.

Q: What do you like best about your job?

A: I am good at detail work. Being a local health inspector allows me to do that type of work and help people avoid getting sick at the same time.

Career Research Activity

1. Investigate the different requirements for OSHA Inspectors and Local Health Inspectors in your community. Note the salary range and advancement opportunities for each. Create a poster of your findings.

2. Create a guide to the available education and training institutions in your area that offer the courses needed to pursue three of the careers above. Compare the course requirements and tuition at each institution for those careers. Publish your findings on the bulletin board.

Related Career Opportunities

Entry Level
- Restaurant Grader
- Legal Assistant

Technical Level
- OSHA Inspector
- Local Health Inspector
- Food & Beverage Manager

Professional Level
- Public Health Educator
- Nematologist
- Chemist

Chapter 7 Review & Activities

Summary

Section 7-1: Introduction to the Kitchen

- Kitchens are equipped with major appliances, small appliances, and utensils.
- Kitchens are organized around work centers; the three basic ones are the cold storage, sink, and cooking centers.

Section 7-4: Storing Food

- Proper food storage prevents spoilage and nutrient loss.
- Shelf-stable foods may be stored at room temperature.
- Store perishable foods in the freezer or in the refrigerator.
- Frozen and refrigerated foods require special handling after a power outage.

Section 7-2: Preventing Kitchen Accidents

- Good management and safe work habits are the keys to kitchen safety.
- Common kitchen hazards include falls, cuts, shock, and burns.
- People with special needs require special safety measures.
- Learn first aid, including the Heimlich maneuver and CPR.

Section 7-5: Conserving Natural Resources

- Conservation begins with the individual.
- Consider measures for saving energy and conserving water.
- To reduce trash, identify ways to reduce, reuse, and recycle.

Section 7-3: Keeping Food Safe to Eat

- If food is handled improperly, microorganisms can multiply and cause foodborne illness.
- Prevent illness by practicing good personal hygiene, using sanitary work methods, keeping the kitchen clean, and keeping food at proper temperatures.

Working IN THE Lab

1. **Food Preparation.** Prepare a food using a recipe that requires the use of the three basic kitchen work centers. Analyze how organizing a kitchen by work centers helped ease and speed this food preparation task.

2. **Food Science.** Observe spoilage in fresh fruits with this experiment. Label small samples of fresh fruits with the type of fruit and the date. Leave the samples out at room temperature (along with a sign warning "Do Not Eat"). Each day, record changes in appearance and smell.

Checking Your Knowledge

1. Name three items that might be found at each of the three basic kitchen work centers.

2. List two knife safety rules.

3. Give three guidelines for storing hazardous household chemicals.

4. How can you help children learn safe kitchen work habits?

5. List two personal hygiene habits that can help prevent foodborne illness.

6. What is cross-contamination? How can you prevent it?

7. Describe two procedures for thawing food safely.

8. What is shelf life?

9. Name two ways to keep frozen foods safe when the power goes off.

10. Give three alternatives to using disposable items.

Thinking Critically

1. Recognizing Assumptions. Elaine's mother uses a toaster with a damaged wire. She says that the toaster still works and refuses to have it fixed or buy a new one. What assumption is she making? Is it a correct one? Explain your answer.

2. Distinguishing Between Fact and Opinion. Analyze this statement: "I use up leftovers, even if they smell a little spoiled. After all, if I boil food long enough, it can't make people sick." Which of these sentences is a fact? Which is an opinion? Defend your answer and suggest possible consequences of this attitude.

3. Analyzing Behavior. Think about or observe your family's everyday habits over the space of several days. Make a checklist of habits you observe (for example, water usage), and consider the impact of each on the environment (for example, older brother leaves water running while he shaves). Using the information from the chapter, make a list of recommendations for alternatives that can help reduce, reuse, and recycle the products your family uses. Share your recommendations with family members.

Reinforcing Key Skills

1. Leadership. It seems that whenever Tanya needs a utensil to prepare a dish, she can't find it. Things are thrown into drawers in a haphazard fashion by whoever empties the dishwasher. Covers might be at the opposite end of the kitchen from pots. How can Tanya work with her family to solve this problem?

2. Communication. Rick has noticed that the school cafeteria does not practice recycling. All trash, including recyclable cans and glass jars, goes into the same dumpster. What steps would you suggest to Rick to bring this problem and possible solutions to the attention of the school community?

Making Decisions and Solving Problems

Kim's family has a hard time functioning in the kitchen on weekday mornings. Some family members are making bag lunches while others are preparing a quick breakfast. As family members get in each other's way, accidents and spills sometimes occur. What could Kim's family do?

Making Connections

1. Health. Working with a partner, use library or online resources to investigate treatment for the foodborne illnesses caused by the bacteria in the chart on page 199. Gather statistics on how many people have become victims of each illness and what steps safety officials are taking to curb each problem. Share your findings in a report.

2. Social Studies. Create a timeline showing how contaminated water represented a life-threatening problem in earlier periods of civilization, how efforts in the early twentieth century helped clean up the water supply, and how carelessness in the second half of the twentieth century reintroduced the problem. Project the timeline into the future with your own ideas and innovations for how water pollution can be stopped permanently.

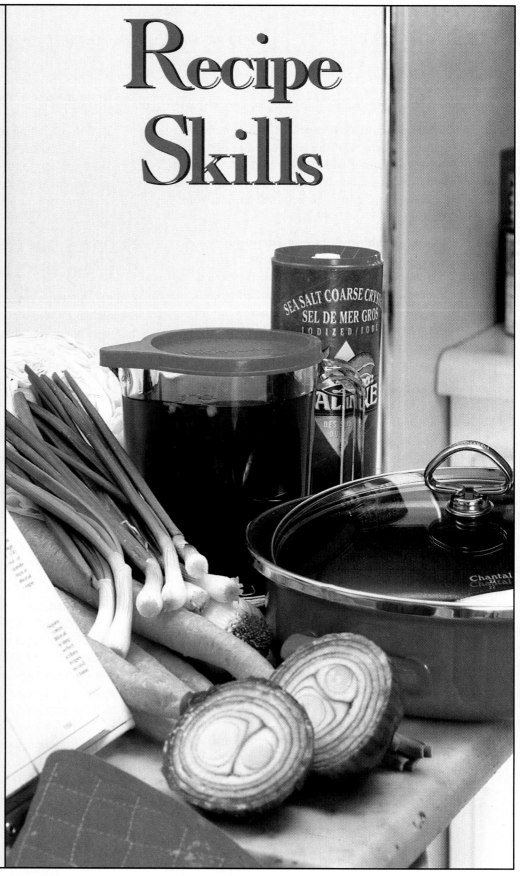

CHAPTER
8

Recipe Skills

Debra tried a cake recipe she saw on a TV cooking show. Her cake was heavy and coarse and didn't look like the one on TV.

Why did Debra get different results using the same recipe? This chapter will explain the possible answers.

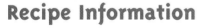

SECTION
8-1

Objectives
After studying this section, you should be able to:
- List the kinds of information a good recipe provides.
- Give guidelines for evaluating and collecting recipes.

Look for These Terms
recipe

yield

assembly directions

Recipe Basics

You've seen the phrase "Handle with Care" on packages with fragile contents. A case could be made for including these words at the beginning of every printed recipe. When you choose and handle recipes carefully, you're more likely to get good results.

Recipe Information

A **recipe** is a set of directions for making a food or beverage. Success with a recipe depends not only on the cook's skill but also on the recipe itself. Here are the components of a well-written and complete recipe:

◆ **Ingredients.** The ingredients should be listed in the order in which they are used. This makes it easier to follow the recipe and not omit an ingredient. Amounts of ingredients are also given.

◆ **Yield.** The **yield** is the number of servings or amount the recipe makes. The yield of a recipe can be increased or decreased, as necessary. You will learn more about this in Section 8-3.

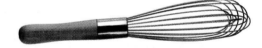

◆ **Information about temperature, time, and equipment.** This may include pan size and type, oven temperature or power, and cooking time. A well-written recipe will also tell you if a conventional oven needs to be preheated.

◆ **Step-by-step directions.** The directions should be clear and easy to follow. Steps may be numbered so that you won't skip any or lose your place. Some recipes include more than one set of directions, such as a conventional method and a microwave method.

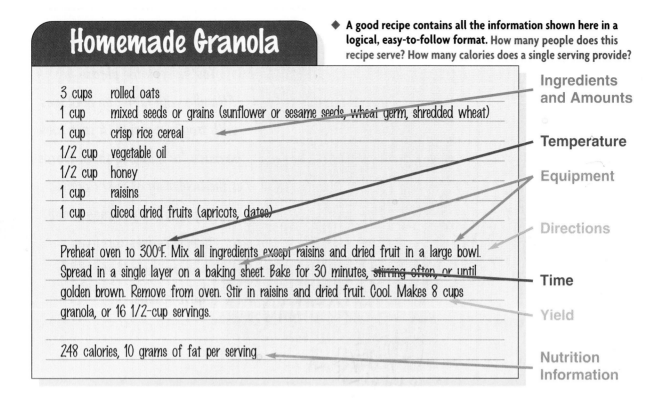

◆ **A good recipe contains all the information shown here in a logical, easy-to-follow format.** How many people does this recipe serve? How many calories does a single serving provide?

Homemade Granola

3 cups	rolled oats
1 cup	mixed seeds or grains (sunflower or sesame seeds, wheat germ, shredded wheat)
1 cup	crisp rice cereal
1/2 cup	vegetable oil
1/2 cup	honey
1 cup	raisins
1 cup	diced dried fruits (apricots, dates)

Preheat oven to 300°F. Mix all ingredients except raisins and dried fruit in a large bowl. Spread in a single layer on a baking sheet. Bake for 30 minutes, stirring often, or until golden brown. Remove from oven. Stir in raisins and dried fruit. Cool. Makes 8 cups granola, or 16 1/2-cup servings.

248 calories, 10 grams of fat per serving

Ingredients and Amounts

Temperature

Equipment

Directions

Time

Yield

Nutrition Information

◆ **Nutrition information.** This information is not essential, but it can be useful in helping you choose recipes that provide vital nutrients and that fit in with your eating plan. Typical nutrition information tells you the number of calories and the amount of fat and sodium for each serving of food. Some recipes also include information about carbohydrates, fiber, protein, cholesterol, both saturated and unsaturated fats, vitamins, and minerals.

Recipe Formats

The standard, or most common, format for a recipe lists the ingredients first, followed by the **assembly directions**, the step-by-step procedure that explains how to combine the ingredients in a recipe. Recipes in this book are in the standard format.

A less common recipe format combines the ingredients and assembly directions. You may

see a recipe written this way on a food package, for example. This format takes less space than the standard format.

Collecting Recipes

A reliable recipe source is a basic cookbook that gives standard recipes for common foods. You probably have several in your classroom or school library. If you don't find one you like, ask your teacher for recommendations. Other reliable recipe sources are magazines, newspapers, package labels, and Web sites.

How can you tell if a recipe is accurate and complete? When you first read a recipe, analyze it. Are basic ingredients missing? Are descriptions of ingredients clear? Is a direction included for each ingredient? Do you have all the information needed to prepare the recipe? If the answer to any of these questions is no, look for another recipe.

Once you have a reliable recipe source, you can expand a recipe collection in whatever direction you choose, depending on the kinds of food you enjoy. Why not start a collection of recipes that are tasty, healthful, and easy to prepare? After trying a particular recipe, decide whether to add it to your list of favorites. If you plan to use a new recipe on a special occasion, try it ahead of time first and evaluate the results.

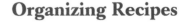

Organizing Recipes

Organizing recipes in your collection can help you find them when you need them. You can paste your recipes on index cards and use a card file box for storage. If you have access to a computer, you can use a word processor file or cookbook software to save recipes. You can then print a particular recipe any time you need it. Use whatever system of organization works best for you.

Section 8-1 Review & Activities

1. What basic information should be found in a well-written recipe?

2. What information does the yield of a recipe give?

3. Identify three things to look for when evaluating a new recipe.

4. **Evaluating.** Discuss the characteristics that make it difficult or easy to follow a recipe.

5. **Extending.** Antonia wants to make a low-fat recipe that she has found in a weekly newspaper in her community. The recipe is complete except for the nutrition information. What would you advise Antonia to do?

6. **Applying.** Find a recipe on a food package or in a magazine or newspaper. Use the guidelines given in this section to determine whether you would want to try it. Write down any questions you have about the recipe. What are some ways this recipe could be improved?

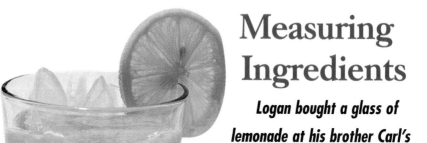

<table>
</table>

Measuring Ingredients

SECTION 8-2

Objectives

After studying this section, you should be able to:

- Identify customary and metric units of measure.

- Identify measuring tools.

- Describe the proper procedures for measuring various types of ingredients.

Look for These Terms

volume

equivalents

Logan bought a glass of lemonade at his brother Carl's lemonade stand.

"How much sugar did you put in this?" Dom asked, after one sip of the very sweet drink.

"The directions said 1 cup," Carl replied, "and that's what I used." He held up an oversized coffee mug. As Carl found out, measuring properly is very important.

Units of Measurement

In a recipe, amounts of ingredients can be given in several ways. Most ingredients are measured by **volume**, the amount of space an ingredient takes up. For instance, a pasta salad recipe might list "1 cup cooked pasta." Some ingredients are measured by weight: 1 pound of shrimp and 8 ounces of baking chocolate are examples. A few ingredients may be measured by the number of items, such as one medium banana or two eggs.

Customary Units

Units of measure may be expressed in one of two ways—customary or metric. The customary system is the system of weights and measures used in the United States. Following are the most common customary units found in recipes, with their abbreviations in parentheses.

- **Volume:** teaspoon (tsp.), tablespoon (Tbsp.), cup (c.), fluid ounce (fl. oz.), pint (pt.), quart (qt.), gallon (gal.).

- **Weight:** ounce (oz.), pound (lb.).

- **Temperature:** degrees Fahrenheit (°F).

- **Length:** inches (in.).

Notice that *ounce* is used to express both volume (in fluid ounces) and weight. The two are not the same. To understand the difference, imagine a cup of popcorn and a cup of water. Both take up the same amount of space, but the popcorn is mostly air and, therefore, is much lighter. To find out how much each *weighs*, you would use a scale, not a measuring cup.

Metric Units

The metric system is based on multiples of ten. For instance, just as there are 100 pennies in one dollar, there are 100 centimeters in one meter. Once you become familiar with it, the metric system is easier to use than the customary system.

Here are the metric units and symbols most often found in recipes.

◆ **Volume:** milliliter (mL), liter (L).

◆ **Weight:** milligram (mg), gram (g), kilogram (kg).

◆ **Temperature:** degrees Celsius (°C).

◆ **Length:** centimeter (cm).

Equivalents

You can express the same amount in different ways by using **equivalents**, different units of equal measure. For instance, 4 tablespoons of flour is the same amount as ¼ cup of flour, or about 50 milliliters. The chart on page 230 shows equivalents for food preparation.

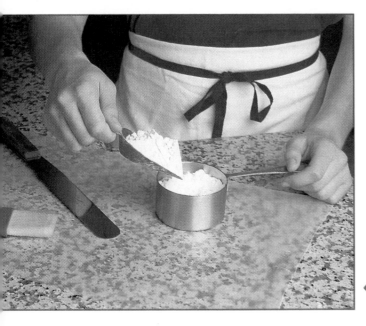

Connecting Food and Math

Converting Temperatures

Most customary-to-metric conversions are fairly straightforward. One that is not is temperature. The table of equivalents on page 230 gives you some general temperature conversion guidelines, but you may need to use an oven temperature that is not listed. What would you do if a recipe specified setting your oven to 145°C? A simple solution is to use the following formula:

$$1.8 \times {}°C + 32 = {}°F$$

Doing the computation for the above example reveals that the correct Fahrenheit setting is 300°F (1.8 × 145 = 261; 261 + 32 = 293, which can be rounded to 300).

To convert from Fahrenheit to Celsius is just as easy. The formula is:

$$({}°F - 32) \times 0.56 = {}°C$$

Think About It

• Paula is sending a recipe to her cousin Esteban, who lives in Spain. The recipe contains this instruction: "Bake at 375°F for 15 minutes." At what temperature should Paula instruct her cousin to set his oven?

◆ **Accurate measurements are the key to successful food preparation.** Why is accuracy important when cooking?

Equivalents

Customary Measure	Customary Equivalent	Approximate Metric Equivalent
Volume		
1 tsp.		5 mL
1 Tbsp.	3 tsp.	15 mL
1 fl. oz.	2 Tbsp.	30 mL
¼ cup		50 mL
⅓ cup		75 mL
½ cup		125 mL
⅔ cup		150 mL
¾ cup		175 mL
1 cup	8 fl. oz. or 16 Tbsp.	250 mL
1 pt.	2 cup or 16 fl. oz.	500 mL
1 qt.	2 pt. or 4 cup or 32 fl. oz.	1000 mL or 1 L
1 gal.	4 qt.	4 L
Weight		
1 oz.		28 g
1 lb.	16 oz.	500 g
2 lb.	32 oz.	1,000 g or 1 kg
Temperatures		
0°F		−18°C
32°F		0°C
350°F		180°C
400°F		200°C

Equipment for Measuring

Now that you understand the different units for measuring ingredients, you'll want to be sure you have the right tools for measuring. A well-equipped kitchen includes the following measuring tools. Each has specific uses, as you will learn.

◆ **Dry measuring cups** usually come in a set of several sizes. A typical customary set includes ¼-cup, ⅓-cup, ½-cup, and 1-cup measures. A metric set includes 50-mL, 125-mL, and 250-mL measures.

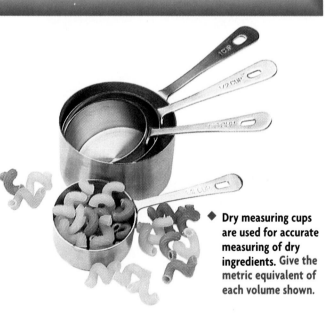

◆ Dry measuring cups are used for accurate measuring of dry ingredients. Give the metric equivalent of each volume shown.

- **Liquid measuring cups** are transparent and have measurement markings on the side. They are typically marked in fractions of a cup, fluid ounces, and milliliters. A head space of about ¼ inch above the top marking makes it easier to move a filled cup without spilling. A spout makes pouring easier. Common sizes are 1-cup (25-mL) and 2-cup (500-mL).

- **Measuring spoons** generally come in sets of four or five. Most customary sets, as you'll notice in the photo on the right, include these four sizes: ¼-teaspoon, ½-teaspoon, 1-teaspoon, and 1-tablespoon. Metric sets include these five: 1-mL, 2-mL, 5-mL, 15-mL, and 25-mL measures.

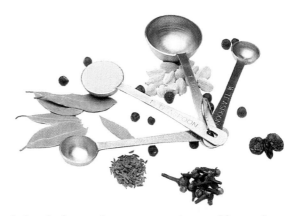

- **Standard measuring spoons come in sets of four as shown here. Metric spoons come in sets of five.** How many ½ tsp. measures would you need to make up the volume of 1 Tbsp.?

Always use standard measuring cups and spoons. A standard 1-cup measuring cup, no matter how it is shaped or designed, always holds the same amount. Coffee mugs, beverage glasses, soup spoons, and other nonstandard items used for serving or eating food vary in size.

Other helpful measuring tools are a straightedge spatula for leveling off dry ingredients, a rubber scraper for removing ingredients from measuring cups, and a food scale for measuring ingredients by weight.

Using Combinations of Measures

What happens if you need a dry measurement but lack a measuring cup or spoon for that exact amount? The answer is to use a combination approach. For instance, if you need ¾ cup flour, use the ½-cup and ¼-cup measures. For ⅔ cup, measure ⅓ cup twice.

Sometimes you may need to measure unusual amounts of an ingredient, such as ⅝ cup. How would you measure such an amount? First, measure out the closest amount you can with a standard-size measure. For example, the closest measure to ⅝ cup is ½ cup (since ½ = ⁴⁄₈). This leaves you with ⅛ cup left to measure. Since ⅛ cup is a small amount, you will need to use measuring spoons. Here is where equivalents come in handy. Using the equivalents chart on page 230, you'll note there are 16 tablespoons in one cup. Therefore, ⅛ cup equals 2 tablespoons (⅛ × 16 = ¹⁶⁄₈ = 2). You would add 2 tablespoons to ½ cup to get ⅝ cup.

You can also remove small amounts from a measuring cup to get the exact amount called for in a recipe. To get ⅞ cup milk, you would first measure one cup and then remove 2 tablespoons (⅛ cup). How would you measure ⅜ cup?

Techniques for Measuring

In addition to the correct tools, the proper procedures are essential to accurate measuring and a successful recipe. The guidelines that follow will help you.

Banana Citrus Smoothie

When a big thirst strikes, a refreshing smoothie can be the perfect answer. As you prepare this recipe, note the various measuring tools and methods called for.

Customary	Ingredients	Metric
1 cup	orange juice	250 mL
⅓ cup	plain nonfat yogurt	75 mL
½ cup	crushed ice	125 mL
½ cup	nonfat dry milk	125 mL
½ medium	banana	½ medium
¼ cup	powdered sugar	50 mL

Yield: Three servings, each 8 fl. oz. (250 mL)

Directions

1. Place all ingredients in blender container.
2. Cover and blend until smooth.
3. Pour into glasses and serve immediately.

Nutrition Information

Per serving (approximate): 139 calories, 6 g protein, 29 g carbohydrate, trace fat, 2 mg cholesterol, 83 mg sodium
Good source of: potassium, vitamin C, B vitamins, calcium, phosphorus

Food for Thought

• For which ingredient(s) would you use a liquid measuring cup? A dry measuring cup? Measuring spoons?
• What should be done to the powdered sugar before measuring it?

Measuring Liquids

Liquid measuring cups are used to measure all liquids, including oils and syrups. To measure liquids, follow these steps:

1. Set the cup on a level surface. If you try to hold it in your hand, you may tip it and get an inaccurate reading.

2. Carefully pour the liquid into the measuring cup.

3. Bend down to check the measurement at eye level for an accurate reading.

4. Add more liquid or pour off excess, if needed, until the top of the liquid is at the desired measurement mark.

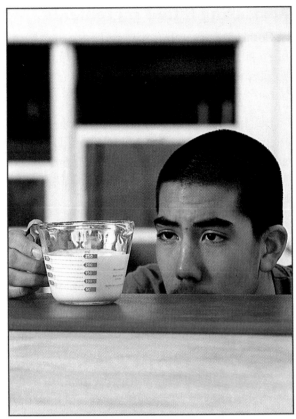

◆ Check the measurement of liquids at eye level. Explain why this is important.

Measuring Dry Ingredients

Dry measuring cups are used to measure flour, sugar, dry beans, and other dry ingredients. They can also be used for foods such as diced meat, chopped vegetables, and yogurt. Here are the steps to take when measuring dry ingredients:

1. Put a piece of waxed paper under the measuring cup to catch any extra ingredient. Don't measure an ingredient while holding the cup over the bowl in which you are mixing.

2. Fill the cup with the ingredient. Some ingredients must be spooned into the cup lightly. Others can be packed down if specified in the recipe.

3. Level off the top of the cup using the straight edge of a spatula. Let the excess fall on the waxed paper. Put the excess back into the original container.

4. Pour the ingredient into the mixture. With semisolid foods, such as yogurt, use a rubber scraper to be sure the entire ingredient has been emptied out of the cup.

5. Pour the ingredient into the mixing container. If needed, use a rubber scraper to empty the cup completely.

For small amounts of liquids, use measuring spoons. To measure ⅛ teaspoon of a liquid ingredient, dribble it into the ¼-teaspoon measure until it looks half full.

◆ Carefully level off the measure of dry ingredients with a straight-edged instrument, such as a spatula. Why has this teen set waxed paper on his work space?

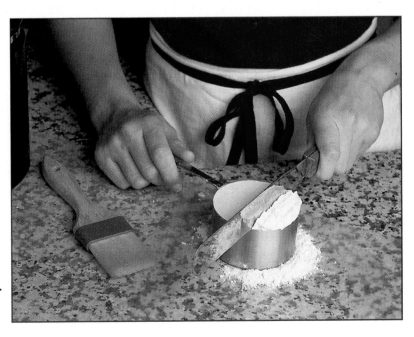

As a general rule, spoon flour and sugar into the measuring cup lightly. If you shake the cup or pack it down, you will measure too much of the ingredient. Brown sugar contains moisture and tends to be fluffy, so pack it down with a spoon. When you empty the cup, the sugar should hold its shape.

Measuring Small Amounts

For amounts smaller than ¼ cup or 50 mL, use measuring spoons. Dry ingredients are usually measured by leveling them off evenly at the rim of the spoon. Sometimes, however, a recipe calls for a "heaping" teaspoon or tablespoon. In that case, do not level off the ingredient. A heaping spoonful will give almost twice the amount you would get in a leveled-off spoon.

If you need ⅛ teaspoon of a dry ingredient, fill the ¼ teaspoon measure and level it off. Then, using the tip of a straightedge spatula or a table knife, remove half the ingredient.

Still smaller amounts of dry ingredients are measured as a dash or a pinch, the amount that can be held between the thumb and finger. These amounts are generally used for herbs, spices, and other seasonings.

Measuring Sifted Ingredients

Some recipes call for ingredients that have been sifted. Flour is an ingredient that is sometimes, though not always, sifted before use.

Be sure to sift ingredients *before* measuring them. Never sift whole-grain flours, which are too coarse to go through the sifter. Instead, stir whole-grain flour with a spoon before measuring.

Sift powdered sugar before you measure it. Granulated sugar can be sifted to remove lumps, if needed.

Measuring Fats

Fats, such as margarine or shortening, can be measured in several ways:

◆ **Stick method.** Use this method for fat that comes in ¼-pound sticks, such as butter or margarine. The wrapper is marked in tablespoons and in fractions of a cup. Simply cut off the amount you need.

◆ **Dry measuring cup method.** Pack the fat down into the cup, pressing firmly to fill in all spaces. Level off the top. Using a rubber scraper, empty as much of the fat as possible. Use the same technique when using measuring spoons to measure fat.

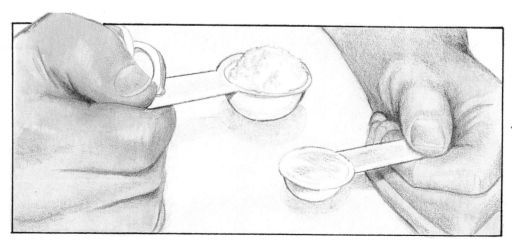

◆ Unless a recipe specifies a heaping spoonful, level off the measuring spoon. In what way could not doing this affect your recipe?

◆ **Water displacement method.**
This method, which requires some math, involves combining fat with water in a liquid measuring cup. First, subtract the amount of fat to be measured from one cup. The difference is the amount of water to pour into the measuring cup. (For example, to measure ⅔ cup of shortening, use ⅓ cup of water.) After pouring in the water, spoon the fat into the cup, making sure it is completely below the level of the water. When the water reaches the 1-cup level, you have the right amount of fat. Pour off the water, and remove the fat with a rubber scraper.

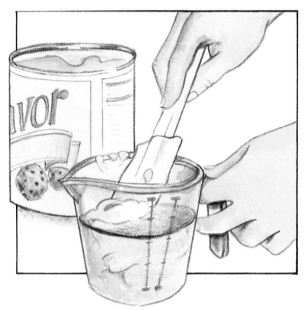

◆ **The water displacement method is a way of measuring fats accurately. What other technique could be used to measure fats?**

Measuring by Weight

As you have read, the amounts of some recipe ingredients may be given by weight. Sometimes you can buy the exact weight of food you need, such as an 8-ounce package of spaghetti. If that's not practical, a food scale, also known as a "portion scale," comes in handy.

To use a food scale:

1. Decide what container you will put the food in. Place the empty container on the scale.

2. Adjust the scale until it reads zero. Usually this is done by turning a knob.

3. Add the food to the container until the scale shows the desired amount.

Section 8-2 Review & Activities

1. One cup is equivalent to how many fluid ounces? How many tablespoons? How many milliliters?

2. How does a liquid measuring cup differ from a dry measuring cup?

3. Describe three ways to measure fats.

4. Analyzing. Why is accuracy so important when measuring ingredients?

5. Applying. Find a recipe with at least ten ingredients. List all the measuring tools you would need to measure the ingredients. Describe any special techniques needed.

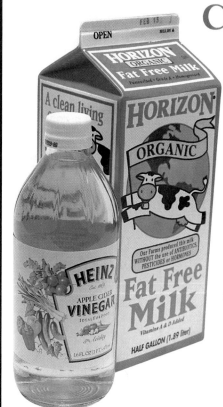

Changing a Recipe

Heather was getting ready to make drop biscuits for dinner when she realized that she did not have any buttermilk. That didn't stop her. She knew she could substitute a mixture of fat-free milk and vinegar and the recipe would come out fine.

Objectives

After studying this section, you should be able to:

- Explain how to increase or decrease recipe yield.
- Give basic strategies for changing a recipe to decrease fat and sodium.
- Describe how high altitudes affect the cooking process.

Look for This Term

desired yield

Why Change a Recipe?

From time to time, you may find that, like Heather, you have to change a recipe. Perhaps you don't have one of the ingredients and can't take the time to go out to buy it. You might want to substitute a more healthful or less expensive ingredient for one in the recipe. You might want to increase or decrease the recipe yield.

Changes are more likely to be successful in some recipes than in others. Mixtures such as salads, stir-fried foods, soups, and stews can usually be changed easily.

On the other hand, recipes for baked products such as muffins and custards are like chemical formulas. Because each ingredient does a job in the recipe, the ingredients must be used in specific amounts in relation to each other. If one amount is changed or one ingredient is omitted, you risk having the recipe not turn out right.

When you change the ingredients in mixtures, you may notice a difference in flavor and texture. For instance, Paige sometimes substitutes cooked turkey for beef when making tacos. How might this change affect the flavor and texture of the dish?

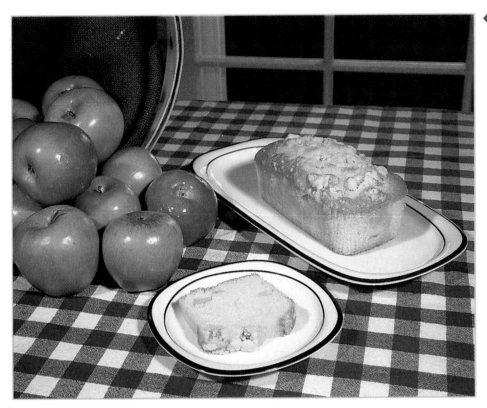

◆ **The success of a recipe depends on choosing appropriate substitutes and measuring them carefully.** What might be used in place of the apples in this loaf cake?

Changing the Yield

Recipes may need to be changed if the yield is not what you need. Most recipes, even those for baked goods, can be successfully doubled. Remember that larger equipment may be needed for mixing and cooking, and cooking times often need adjustment. For baked goods, it is best to use two baking pans of the original size rather than one larger one.

Many recipes for mixtures such as casseroles and soups can be not only doubled, but halved, tripled, and so on. The same process is used for both increasing and decreasing.

1. *Determine the desired yield.* The **desired yield** represents the number of servings you need.

2. *Use the formula.* To adjust the yield of a recipe, multiply the amount of each ingredient in the same number. That number is determined by using a simple formula:

desired yield ÷ regular yield = number to multiply by

Example: Your chili recipe serves eight and you need to serve only four: 4 ÷ 8 = 0.5.

3. *Multiply each ingredient amount by that number.* This keeps all the ingredients in the same proportion as in the original recipe.

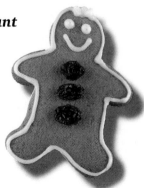

4. Convert measurements into logical, easy-to-manage amounts. Suppose that you want to make 6 times the standard yield of a recipe that normally calls for 2 tablespoons of flour. Rather than measure out 12 tablespoons (6 × 2), use a more workable unit of measurement, ¾ cup. Review the equivalents chart on page 230.

5. Make any necessary adjustments to equipment, temperature, and time. The depth of a pan affects how fast the food in it cooks. Use pans that are the right size for the amount of food, not too large or too small.

Making Ingredient Substitutions

If you don't have an ingredient you need for a recipe, you may be able to substitute another. The chart on the next page gives some common substitutions.

People who are concerned about healthful eating may have another reason to make substitutions. They want to reduce the fat and sodium in their eating plans.

Substitutions that Reduce Fat

Most recipes can be modified to reduce fat content. Changes in the ingredients used or the amounts of ingredients can make a significant difference. A change in the cooking method can sometimes also reduce the amount of fat.

Tony decided to try to reduce the fat in his favorite spaghetti sauce. First, he reduced the amount of beef from 1½ pounds to 1 pound. He also chose lean ground beef instead of the regular ground beef because it has less fat. Instead of cooking the onion and garlic in 2 tablespoons of oil, he used a nonstick pan and cooking spray. He enjoyed the flavor and didn't miss the fat. He is still experimenting.

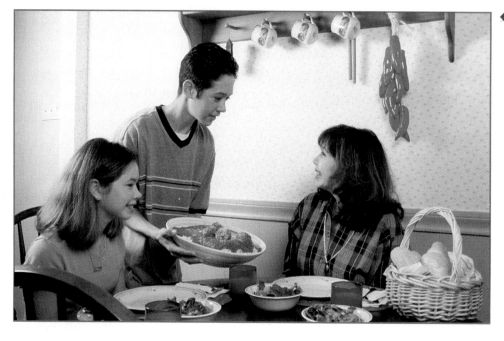

◆ **Ground turkey meat was substituted for ground beef in this recipe.** What lower-fat substitution could you recommend for sour cream?

Ingredient Substitutions

When you don't have . . .	Substitute . . .
Baking chocolate, unsweetened, 1 oz.	3 Tbsp. cocoa + 1 Tbsp. butter or margarine
Buttermilk, 1 cup	1 Tbsp. lemon juice or vinegar + enough fat-free milk to measure 1 cup—or—1 cup plain, nonfat yogurt
Cake flour, 1 cup	⅞ cup (¾ cup + 2 Tbsp.) sifted all-purpose flour
Garlic, 1 clove	⅛ tsp. garlic powder
Herbs, 1 Tbsp. fresh, chopped	Herbs, 1 tsp. dried, crushed
Lemon juice	Equal amount vinegar
Milk, fat-free, 1 cup	¼ cup nonfat dry milk powder + ⅞ cup of water
Mustard, dry, 1 tsp.	1 Tbsp. prepared mustard
Onion, 1 small	1 Tbsp. minced dried onion or 1 tsp. onion powder
Sugar, powdered, 1 cup	1 cup plus 1 Tbsp. granulated sugar
(Thickening) Cornstarch, 1 Tbsp.	2 Tbsp. flour
Worcestershire sauce, 1 Tbsp.	1 Tbsp. soy sauce + dash red pepper sauce

Tips for Reducing Fat

Here are some other suggestions that will help you cut the fat in recipes:

◆ Compare similar recipes and choose the ones with the least fat in their nutritional breakdown.

◆ Use fat-free or low-fat dairy products in place of all or part of high-fat dairy products. Instead of straight mayonnaise, try a mixture of half mayonnaise, half nonfat yogurt.

◆ Substitute chicken or turkey for high-fat cuts of meat. Use fresh, ground, skinless turkey breast in place of ground beef for meat loaf, for instance. You may want to increase the seasonings in the recipe because of the difference in flavor.

◆ Use lemon juice, flavored vinegar, or fruit juice instead of salad dressings that contain oil.

◆ Substitute two egg whites for a whole egg or use egg substitutes.

Substitutions that Reduce Sodium

Most people take in far more sodium than the body needs. This excess can have harmful effects. Here are some ideas for reducing sodium in recipes:

◆ When shopping, reach for the lower-sodium versions of canned broth, soy sauce, and similar products.

◆ Use herbs, spices, lemon juice, or vinegar to enhance food flavors.

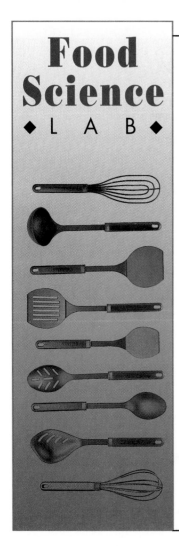

Taste-Testing a Reduced-Fat Product

According to an old saying, the proof is in the eating. You are about to test the truth of this saying by conducting a taste test of a full-fat dairy product and a lower-fat version made in the food lab.

Procedure

1. Place 8 ounces (250 mL) of low-fat small-curd cottage cheese in a blender. Blend until smooth. Add 1 tablespoon (5 mL) of lemon juice and blend again.

2. Force the cottage cheese through a strainer. Remove as much of the solid contents as possible.

3. Have classmates taste small samples of both this cottage cheese blend and full-fat sour cream. Record their reactions in a chart.

4. Add commercial onion soup mix to both foods to make dips. Repeat step 3.

Conclusions

◆ How did the subjects rate the cottage cheese blend in comparison with the sour cream? Did all the subjects have the same reaction to the two samples? If not, explain.

◆ Did the results of the experiment differ when you added the onion soup mix? If so, how? What can you infer?

◆ How can the results of this food science lab help you use recipes in the future?

High-Altitude Cooking

Unless otherwise indicated, recipes are intended to be used at altitudes of 3,000 feet (about 1,000 m) or below. If used at higher altitudes, they may not turn out right. Why? As the altitude gets higher, the air pressure gets lower. This affects food preparation in two main ways.

First, water boils at a lower temperature. This means that foods that are boiled, such as pasta, take longer to cook. Second, when the air pressure is low, bubbles of gas that form in liquids escape into the atmosphere more readily. As a result, baked goods are likely to rise less and be heavy. Sometimes reducing the amount of baking powder or soda and sugar and increasing the liquid can help.

People who live in high-altitude areas often can get helpful information about adapting recipes from their local utility company, newspapers, or nearest cooperative extension office. Many packaged foods include special directions for preparation at high altitudes.

FOR YOUR HEALTH

Adding by Subtracting

According to a mathematical principle, subtracting one amount from another yields a lower number. Nutritionists, however, are discovering that it is possible to *add* to the flavor of a recipe *and increase* its nutritional value, *while cutting down* on certain ingredients. Here are some examples of this new food math:

- Toast nuts before using them in dishes. That way, you can use fewer nuts to get the same nutty flavor.

- Add a pinch of cinnamon, nutmeg, or other sweet spice to a recipe and use less sugar.

- Add dried fruits or pureed dried fruits to a sweet recipe. They will pack in more nutrition while allowing you to cut down on the amount of sugar called for.

- Subtract heavy, fatty sauces on meats, vegetables, and other foods. In their place, add light, tangy salsas instead. You will be surprised at the boost in flavor.

Following Up

- Think of at least two ways to add flavor to foods while subtracting ingredients high in sodium, such as salt and ketchup. Be creative.

Section 8-3 Review & Activities

1. Name three reasons to change a recipe.

2. List the basic steps in changing recipe yield.

3. Name three changes that can be made to a recipe for health reasons.

4. Synthesizing. What are some other ways Tony might modify the spaghetti sauce to make it healthful while maintaining its good flavor?

5. Comparing and Contrasting. What are the pros and cons of modifying favorite recipes to lower their fat content as compared with buying a cookbook with low-fat recipes?

6. Applying. Find a simple recipe that makes 4 servings. Show how you would change the ingredient amounts to make 12 servings or 2 servings.

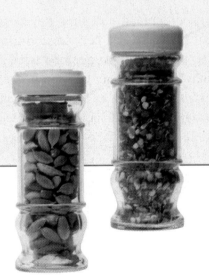

Preparation Tasks

If you were lost in a foreign country, you would need to know the language in order to ask directions. In the same way, success with a recipe depends on the ability to navigate through the directions, which may include terms that are "foreign" to a new cook. In this section, you will learn about these terms.

Objectives

After studying this section, you should be able to:

- Describe the techniques that correspond with common recipe terms.
- Identify the kitchen equipment used for each technique.

Look for These Terms

sharpening steel

pare

serrated

score

whisk

folding

purée

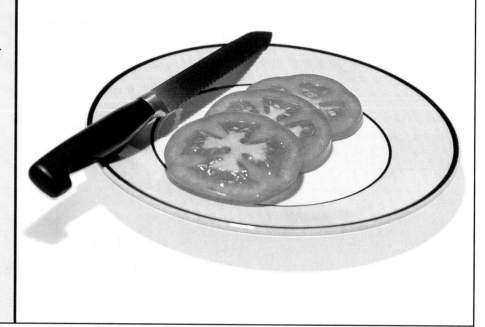

Cutting Foods

Food preparation often involves a variety of cutting tasks. You may need to trim unwanted parts from food or cut food to the desired size. With practice, you can become a cutting expert. Knowing how to use cutting tools properly is the first step to succeeding in the kitchen as well as to preventing accidents.

Equipment for Cutting

Two key cutting tools for a well-equipped kitchen do no actual cutting. One of these is a cutting board, a specially-designed surface to help protect kitchen counters. To reduce the risk of foodborne illness, choose a cutting board made of a nonporous material.

The second cutting tool, a **sharpening steel**, is a long, steel rod on a handle used to help keep knives sharp. Regular and correct use of a sharpening steel is an essential skill to learn. Here is what to do (reverse the directions if you are left-handed):

1. Hold the handle of the steel in your left hand. Place the point straight down, very firmly, on a cutting board. In your right hand, hold the knife by the handle, blade down.

2. Place the knife blade against the right side of the steel. The knife blade and steel should touch near the handles. Tip the knife away from the steel at a 20-degree angle.

3. Draw the blade down the steel and toward you, keeping it at a 20-degree angle to the steel. Use gentle pressure.

4. When the tip of the knife reaches the tip of the steel, repeat the process, holding the knife against the steel on the left. Draw the blade down along the steel four or five times, alternating right and left sides.

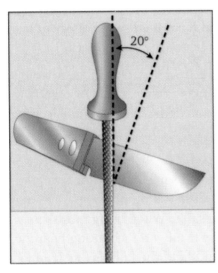

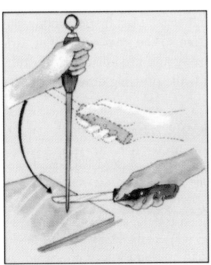

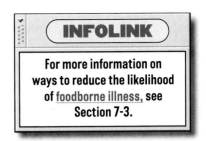

INFOLINK

For more information on ways to reduce the likelihood of foodborne illness, see Section 7-3.

Knives

Many cutting tasks require the use of a knife. The basic types of knives include:

- **Chef's knife.** Also called a French knife. Has a large, triangular blade. Ideal for slicing, chopping, and dicing.

- **Slicing knife.** Used for cutting large foods, such as meat and poultry.

- **Utility knife.** Similar in shape to a slicing knife but smaller. Used for cutting smaller food items, such as tomatoes and apples.

- **Paring knife.** Used to **pare**—cut a very thin layer of peel or outer coating from—fruits and vegetables.

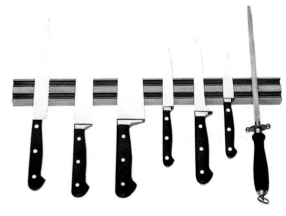

- From left to right: bread knife, slicing knife, chef's knife, utility knife, boning knife, paring knife, sharpening steel. Identify the task you would perform with a utility knife.

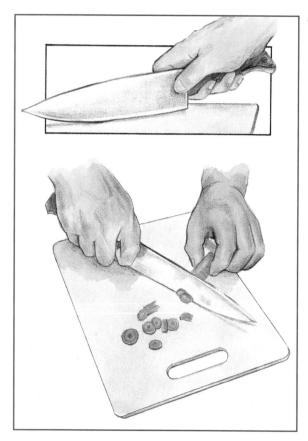

Alternative Cutting Tools

Other simpler cutting tools and their uses include:

◆ **Vegetable peeler.** Has blade that swivels. Perfect for paring fruits and vegetables.

◆ **Poultry shears.** Scissors-like tool, capable of cutting through bone. May also be used for snipping, trimming, or cutting dried fruit, pastry, or fresh herbs.

◆ **Food chopper.** Ranges in size from small hand-held nut chopper to large chopper with several blades.

◆ **Food grinder.** Grinds meat, poultry, nuts, and many other foods. Also good for grating, shredding, and other fine cutting needs.

Techniques for Cutting

Although some cutting tools require you only to push a button, using knives requires specific skills. When using most knives, hold the food firmly on the cutting board with one hand and hold the knife by its handle with the other. For rounded foods, such as some fruits and vegetables, first cut a thin slice from the bottom so the item will sit flat. Grip the knife firmly and use a back-and-forth, sawing motion while pressing down gently.

◆ **Boning knife.** Has a thin, angled blade, well suited to removing the bones from meat, poultry, and fish. May also be used to trim fat from meat.

◆ **Bread knife.** Has a **serrated**, or sawtooth-patterned, blade for slicing through coarse-grained breads.

Small Appliances

With its many speed settings, an electric blender can be used to cut, grind, and mix. A food processor is similar to a blender, but is often more powerful and versatile. This heavy-duty cutting machine comes with an assortment of blade attachments for various jobs such as slicing and grinding meats. Some food processors may have a blade for kneading bread dough.

✛ Safety Check

Keep knives sharp. A dull knife is much more likely to slip and cut you because you will have to exert more pressure.

When using a knife, keep your fingers away from the sharp edge of the blade. Be sure the fingertips of the hand holding the food are curled under. Never hold the food in your hand while cutting, and never cut with the blade facing your body.

Common Cutting Tasks

Recipes often use terms such as *cube, grate,* or *score* to indicate how foods are to be cut. To prepare food successfully and prevent accidents, you need to know what each term means and how to perform the technique correctly. Here is a guide to some common cutting tasks.

Look and Learn:

What are the safety precautions being taken in each of these diagrams?

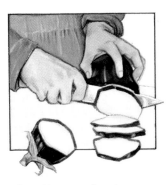

Slice. To cut a food in large, thin pieces.

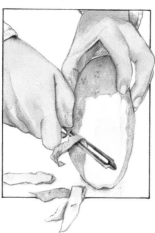

Pare. To cut off a very thin layer of peel. A peeler or paring knife works best.

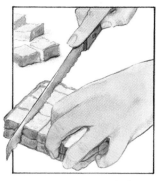

Cube and dice. Both these terms refer to cutting food into small, squared pieces. Make the pieces about ½ inch (1.3 cm) on each side when cubing and ⅛ to ¼ inch (3 to 6 mm) when dicing.

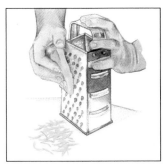

Grate. Cut food into smaller pieces or shreds by pressing and rubbing the food against the rough surface of a grater.

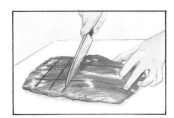

Score. To **score** means to make shallow, straight cuts in the surface of a food, such as a flank steak. Scoring helps tenderize meat. A slicing knife is most often used to score meats.

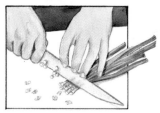

Chop and mince. Both these terms refer to cutting food into small irregular pieces. Minced pieces are smaller than chopped pieces. To use a chef's knife to chop or mince, hold the knife handle with one hand, pressing the tip against the cutting board. The other hand should rest lightly on the back of the blade, near the tip, as in the picture. Rock or pump the knife handle up and down, keeping the tip of the blade on the board so that the blade chops through the food.

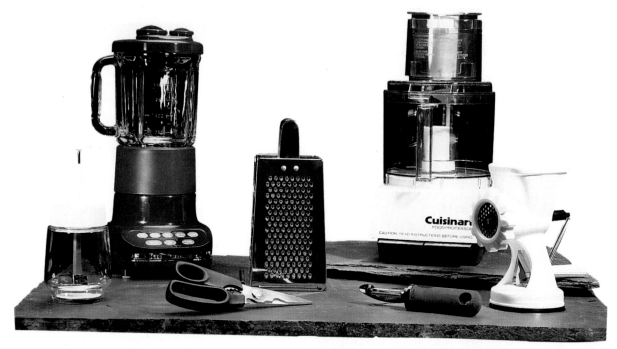

Mixing Foods

Another common recipe task is combining ingredients through mixing. You can use different mixing tools and techniques, depending on the food and the desired results.

Equipment for Mixing

Many kinds of mixing tools, from small hand-held utensils to electrical appliances, are used for mixing tasks. Two mixing appliances, the blender and food processor, were mentioned earlier in connection with cutting.

Other tools commonly used when mixing include:

- **Electric mixer.** Used to blend, beat, and whip ingredients. Lightweight, hand-held models are convenient. Heavy-duty models are attached permanently to a stand.

- **Rotary beater.** Used to mix and whip foods more quickly and easily than can be done with a spoon or whisk. Often used to beat egg whites.

- **Mixing bowls.** Come in many different sizes. May be of stainless steel, glass, pottery, or plastic.

- **Mixing spoon.** Used for many mixing tasks. Different sizes and shapes are available.

- **Sifter.** A container with a fine wire screen at the bottom and a blade that forces dry ingredients through the screen.

- **Wire whisk.** A **whisk** is a balloon-shaped device made of wire loops held together by a handle. Used for mixing, stirring, beating, and whipping.

- **Rubber scraper.** Used to scrape food from bowls, pans, and other containers. Helpful in moving thick ingredients from the sides of the bowl to the middle while mixing. Also used for folding, which is described on page 247.

Techniques for Mixing

As with cutting, the techniques of mixing have a vocabulary all their own. Some of these terms found in recipes will be readily familiar to you. Others will not.

Look and Learn:

Name one recipe in which you would use each of the following mixing techniques.

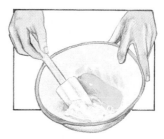

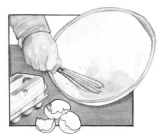

Mix, combine, blend. To thoroughly incorporate one ingredient into another, using a wooden spoon, wire whisk, rotary beater, electric mixer, or electric blender.

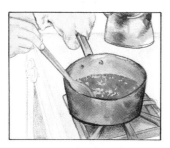

Stir. To mix by hand, using a wooden spoon or wire whisk in a circular motion. Can also be done while cooking to keep food from sticking to the pan and to distribute heat throughout foods.

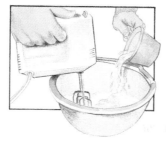

Beat. To thoroughly mix foods using a vigorous over-and-over motion. Egg whites may be beaten to add air to them.

Cream. To beat together ingredients, such as shortening and sugar, until soft and creamy.

Whip. To incorporate air into a mixture to make it light and fluffy.

Fold. **Folding** is a technique used to gently mix delicate ingredients, usually with a rubber scraper or wooden spoon. The technique involves cutting down through the mixture, moving the utensil across the bottom of the bowl, and bringing it back up to the surface along with some of the mixture from the bottom. The utensil is never lifted out of the mixture.

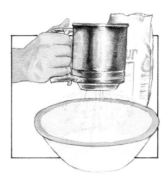

Sift. To force one or more dry ingredients—for example, flour—through a sifter or strainer to add air, remove small lumps, or mix two ingredients.

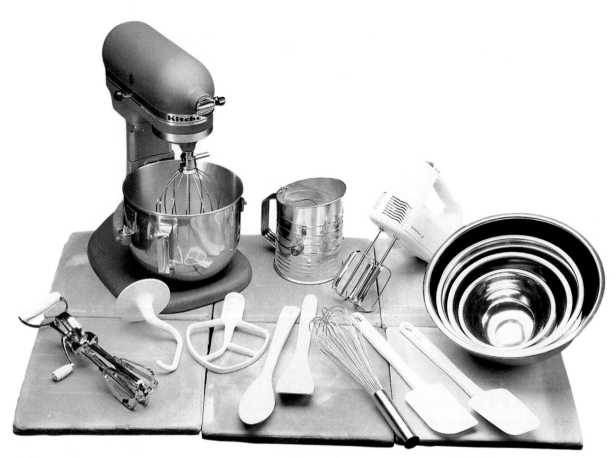

◆ These are common mixing tools. In back (left to right): electric mixer (with extra attachments), sifter, hand-held electric mixer, mixing bowls; in front: rotary beater, wooden spoons, wire whisk, rubber scrapers. Why are rubber scrapers such an important tool to have when cooking or baking?

Other Tasks

A variety of other tools and techniques are used in food preparation. Here are some additional terms you may find in recipes:

◆ **Strain.** To separate solid particles from a liquid, such as broth or juice. The liquid is poured through a bowl-shaped fine screen called a strainer or sieve (SIV).

◆ **Drain.** To drain from a solid food, such as fruits, vegetables, or cooked pasta. This is done by putting the food in a colander—a bowl with small holes in the bottom—or a large strainer.

◆ **Purée (pyoo-RAY). Purée** means to make food smooth and thick by putting it through a strainer, blender, or food processor.

◆ **Baste.** To brush or pour a liquid over a food as it cooks.

◆ **Dredge.** To coat a food with a dry ingredient, such as flour or crumbs.

Many heating and cooking tasks are also involved in food preparation. These techniques and the equipment needed are explored in the next chapter.

◆ A colander (left) is used for draining foods. A strainer is used for the same purpose as well as for straining. What types of uncooked and cooked foods require draining? What types of foods might require straining?

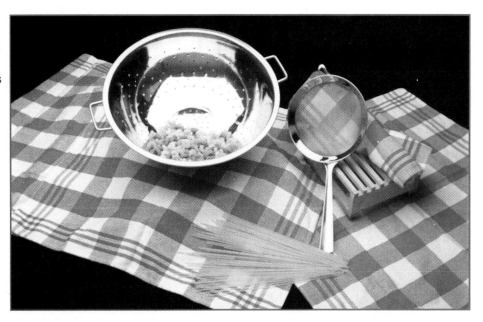

Section 8-4 Review & Activities

1. Describe the differences between a paring knife, a boning knife, and a chef's knife.

2. What does *beating* mean when used to describe a mixing technique? Name three tools that could be used to beat a mixture.

3. Name two small electrical appliances that are useful for both cutting and mixing tasks.

4. Analyzing. Charles and his dad are pricing kitchen equipment to replace devices that have worn out. Some of the cutting tools are beyond their budget. What recommendation could you make to the family to help them fully equip their kitchen while staying within their budget?

5. Evaluating. What might happen if you tried to follow a recipe without understanding the meaning of food preparation terms?

6. Applying. Develop a checklist for use in your school foods lab on which cutting equipment to use with which foods. Post your checklist on a wall in the classroom.

Easy English Trifle

This recipe can be a light, refreshing dessert. Try using a variety of canned, frozen, or fresh fruits to create your own combinations.

Customary	Ingredients	Metric
1	Angel food cake*	1
20-oz. can	Fruit cocktail packed in juice	567-gram can
3-oz. package	Instant vanilla pudding and pie filling mix	95-gram package
2 cup	Fat-free milk	500 mL
4-oz. carton	Light, nondairy whipped topping, thawed	112-gram carton

Yield: 8-10 servings

* May be either made from a packaged mix or bought already baked.

Directions

1. Cut the cake into slabs about 1 inch (2.5 cm) thick. Use the slabs to line the inside of a large serving bowl.

2. Spoon half the fruit cocktail and all the juice over the cake.

3. Prepare the pudding mix according to the package directions, using the 2 cups (500 mL) of milk.

4. Fold in half the thawed whipped topping. Spoon the mixture over the cake and fruit. Add the remaining fruit.

5. Spread the remaining whipped topping over all. Refrigerate for at least 2 hours before serving.

Nutrition Information

Per serving (approximate): 160 calories, 7 g protein, 31 g carbohydrate, 1 g fat, 0 mg cholesterol, 85 mg sodium

Good source of: vitamin E, B vitamins, calcium, phosphorus

Food for Thought

• How many different mixing tools mentioned in the text could you use to prepare the pudding mix?

• Why does the recipe instruct you to "fold in," rather than merely blend in, the whipped topping?

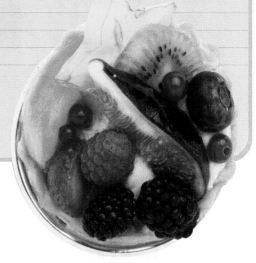

Time Management and Teamwork

Objectives

After studying this section, you should be able to:

- Describe a work plan and a schedule, and explain the usefulness of each.
- Give examples of efficient work techniques.
- Give guidelines for working cooperatively in the school foods lab or at home.

Look for These Terms

work plan

pre-preparation

dovetail

Whenever you are preparing food, either in the school foods lab or for your family's dinner, time is likely to be a concern. At such times, management, communication, and critical thinking can help you meet your deadlines.

Time Management in the Kitchen

Winning a race takes strategy, speed, and skill. These same properties are the keys to time management in the kitchen.

Strategy: A Work Plan

Food preparation involves more than choosing a recipe and starting to work. Rather, it involves mapping out all the procedures and tasks that play a part in your recipe or meal. Do you have the ingredients and equipment you need? Are you familiar with the cooking techniques called for in the recipes? Can you complete the food preparation and cleanup in the time available?

A smart strategy is to always start with a **work plan**. Basically, this is a list of all the tasks required to complete the recipe and an estimate of how long each task will take.

Developing a Work Plan

Recipes and package directions often provide help in estimating time. The directions on a spaghetti package, for example, may tell you that the product requires 9 minutes to cook. As an effective manager, however, you will need to draw on your ability to think critically to help you identify other tasks and find or estimate the time each requires—for example, boiling water for the pasta, chopping vegetables for the sauce, and cleaning salad greens. A good rule of thumb for beginning cooks is to allow more time than you think you will need. As your skills improve, you will be able to work faster and make more accurate time estimates.

Look at the recipe for "Pizza Snacks" below and the work plan Naomi made for it on the next page. Note that some of the first steps on the work plan come from the list of ingredients, not the assembly directions. Naomi saw from this list that the tasks would include halving the English muffins, shredding the cheese, and chopping and slicing the toppings.

Even before these steps comes the **pre-preparation**, tasks done before actual recipe preparation. In Naomi's case, these tasks included washing the green pepper and onion and measuring out the other ingredients.

A successful work plan might even include important tasks like washing your hands and setting the oven temperature. Including such steps ensures that a new cook won't forget to do them.

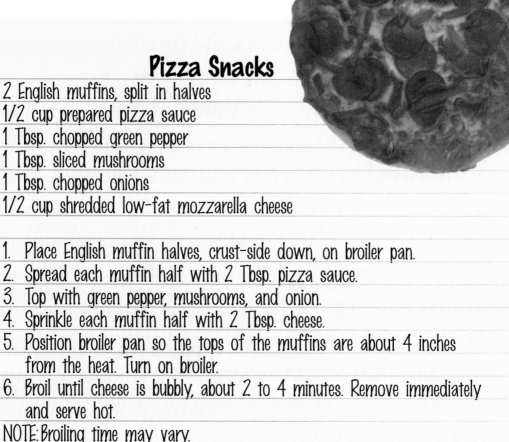

Pizza Snacks

2 English muffins, split in halves
1/2 cup prepared pizza sauce
1 Tbsp. chopped green pepper
1 Tbsp. sliced mushrooms
1 Tbsp. chopped onions
1/2 cup shredded low-fat mozzarella cheese

1. Place English muffin halves, crust-side down, on broiler pan.
2. Spread each muffin half with 2 Tbsp. pizza sauce.
3. Top with green pepper, mushrooms, and onion.
4. Sprinkle each muffin half with 2 Tbsp. cheese.
5. Position broiler pan so the tops of the muffins are about 4 inches from the heat. Turn on broiler.
6. Broil until cheese is bubbly, about 2 to 4 minutes. Remove immediately and serve hot.
NOTE: Broiling time may vary.

Yield: 4 small pizzas

Work Plan-Pizza Snacks

Task	Approx. Time
Gather ingredients and equipment. Scrub hands.	8 min.
Split English muffins in half.	2 min.
Chop green pepper and onion. Slice mushrooms.	7 min.
Shred cheese.	3 min.
Put muffins on broiler pan and put on toppings.	3 min.
Broil until cheese is bubbly.	6 min.
Prepare to serve.	1 min.
	Total: 30 min.

Speed: A Schedule

Once you have a work plan, you can use it to make a schedule that shows when each task must be started. If you have developed a sound work plan, making a schedule should be a snap. Simply do the following:

1. Consult your work plan for the estimated time each task will take to complete.

2. Add these times to find the total preparation time.

3. Subtract the total preparation time from the time you want the food to be ready. This step tells you what time to start.

Naomi's estimated total preparation time is 30 minutes. She plans to serve the pizzas at 6:30, so she needs to start at 6:00. To keep to her schedule, Naomi decides to chop and slice the vegetables first, shred the cheese next, and then split the English muffins. For this recipe, the remaining tasks match the order of the recipe directions.

When you are learning to prepare food, it's a good idea to make a work plan and schedule every time. Eventually, you may need to do so only when you prepare a new dish or plan a special meal.

Schedule-Pizza Snacks

6:00	Get ready.
6:08	Split English muffins.
6:10	Chop and slice vegetables.
6:17	Shred cheese.
6:20	Assemble pizzas.
6:23	Broil pizzas.
6:29	Prepare to serve.
6:30	Serve pizzas.

Skill: Working Efficiently

As you gain food preparation experience, you will notice an obvious improvement in your skills. You'll be able to complete some tasks in half the time they once took. Yet there is more to efficiency than just experience. Even a beginner can be efficient by knowing how to save time and energy. Here are some keys to efficiency:

◆ **Organize the kitchen.** Always store items in the same place so that you won't waste time looking for them.

◆ **Learn to use equipment properly.** Take the time to read the owner's manuals for the small and large appliances in the kitchen. Besides learning to use them safely, you may find they can be helpful in ways you didn't realize. Practice using your tools until you are comfortable with them.

◆ **Look for ways to simplify.** Could a different piece of equipment complete a task more quickly? Would a different cooking method be more efficient? Thinking through your options can help you save time and energy.

◆ **Gather all equipment and ingredients first.** Assembling everything you will need before you start has several advantages. First, you won't discover halfway through a recipe that you are out of an ingredient you need. Second, it will be easier to check whether you used every ingredient. Third, and perhaps most important, you will have everything you need right at your fingertips.

◆ **Dovetail tasks.** To **dovetail** means to fit different tasks together smoothly. Not every preparation step needs your undivided attention. You could, for example, make a tossed salad while chicken pieces are roasting. Dovetailing is especially important when you are preparing a whole meal. If you plan to dovetail tasks, be sure to adjust your time schedule.

◆ **Clean up as you work.** Before you start work, fill the sink or a dishpan with hot, sudsy water. Whenever you have a few free moments, wash the equipment you have finished using. Also keep a clean, wet dishcloth handy to wipe up spills as they happen. Put away ingredients as you finish with them. Your final cleanup will take much less time.

Teamwork in the School Kitchen

In the foods lab at school, you work as part of a team. You also work against the clock. Every lab activity needs to be completed—including cleanup and evaluation—within a limited period of time. Success depends on organization and cooperation.

◆ **Organizing the job.** As a team, you and your classmates need to start with a basic work plan. When you plan your schedule, decide not only when each task should start, but also who will do it. With every team member working, several tasks can be accomplished at the same time. You may want to use a schedule that has five-minute blocks of time down the left and columns with each person's name across the top. That way, the schedule shows what each person should be doing throughout the lab period. Be sure to consider work space and equipment as you plan your schedule.

- **Working together.** Foods labs, like many school and work situations, depend on everyone doing his or her job. Be responsible for the tasks you have agreed to take on. Work quickly and efficiently. Remember that accuracy is essential. If you have a question or a problem, ask another team member for help. Be willing to help out when someone else falls behind or makes a mistake. Keeping a sense of humor will help the work go more smoothly.

- **Cleaning up.** Cleaning as you go will make end-of-class cleanup easier and faster. Be sure all equipment is clean and dry. Most important, return everything to its proper place. Otherwise, you will slow down the next team using the kitchen. Be sure all work surfaces and appliances are clean and that you have disposed of waste properly.

- **Evaluating the results.** Labs usually involve the evaluation of both the finished product and the preparation process. Thoughtfulness and honesty are important for both. This is especially true if the food did not turn out as expected, if you experienced preparation problems, or if your team did not work together well. Think about what you learned from the experience and what you might do differently the next time.

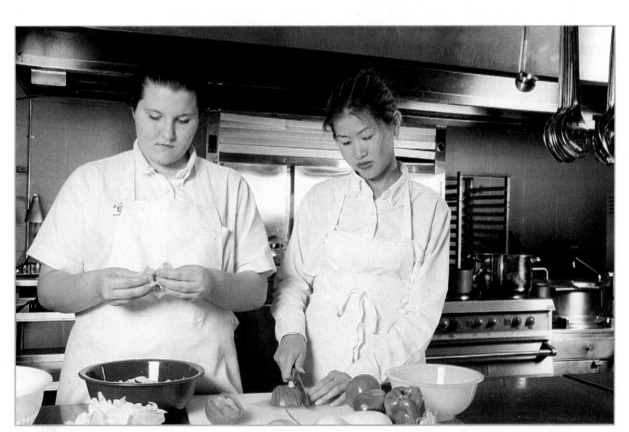

◆ Dovetailing tasks—for example, preparing a salad while boiling water to cook spaghetti—can help you streamline the preparation of a meal. What skill for food choices comes into play when you prepare a meal in this fashion?

Teamwork at Home

In many ways, teamwork in your kitchen at home is as important as it is in the foods lab. Organization, cooperation, and cleanup are again the watchwords of a successful effort.

Whether you are responsible for helping prepare family meals on a regular basis or just occasionally, you need to remember that these can be fun times. You might help a younger brother or sister learn a new cooking skill or just take time to talk with a family member. When you have more time, try out a new recipe together. Daily food preparation can be a chore or an opportunity to build togetherness. It all depends on your attitude.

Section 8-5 Review & Activities

1. What is a work plan? How can it help you manage time when preparing food?

2. Give three examples of ways to work efficiently in your kitchen or the school foods lab.

3. What should you think about when evaluating a completed foods lab?

4. Synthesize. What are some specific problems that can occur in the kitchen or foods lab if you don't work efficiently?

5. Analyze. Imagine that you are preparing a dinner of salad (chopped tomato, shredded lettuce, French dressing) and sandwiches (turkey, cheese, sliced tomatoes, whole wheat bread, deli mustard). Explain how you could dovetail tasks in the preparation of these foods.

6. Applying. Working in groups, design a work plan and schedule form that could be used when planning school foods labs. Use the forms in the next foods lab and evaluate how much more or less efficiently your group worked in the lab. If necessary, redesign the forms.

CAREER WANTED

Individuals who can work with others to find answers to complex problems.

REQUIRES:

- associate degree in food science or related field
- previous laboratory experience

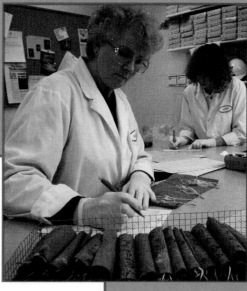

"Putting food on the world's table is my goal,"

says Research Lab Technician Freda Cisco

Q: Freda, how did you end up working for the U.S. Department of Agriculture?

A: I held several jobs as a lab technician with private-sector food manufacturers before coming to the USDA. I liked my work, but I wanted my research to help the general public.

Q: What kinds of projects have you been involved with at the USDA?

A: Most projects have focused on efforts to increase the world's food supply. For example, by making heartier species of produce that can survive adverse weather conditions, we can feed people year round. We grow hydroponic trees that yield significantly larger quantities of fruit than a normal fruit tree.

Q: Do you head up the projects you work on?

A: No. Projects are overseen by a senior research chemist. These people "design" the research and guide the protocols of our experiments.

Q: Do you have aspirations to move up to be a senior chemist?

A: I enjoy solving problems and think I could learn to design research. I would have to go back to college. That position requires more education as well as increased responsibility.

Career Research Activity

1. Working in teams, create a "Guide to Government-affiliated Food and Nutrition Careers." Gather information by visiting the USDA and FDA web sites. Print out your guide on the computer before turning it in.

2. Find out what an environmental engineering technician does and whether or not it could lead to a career as a cytotechnologist. Write a report explaining what you discovered and answer why you would, or would not, be interested in either career.

Related Career Opportunities

Entry Level
- Commodity Grader
- Lab Assistant

Technical Level
- Research Lab Technician
- Environmental Engineering Technician
- Preservationist

Professional Level
- Senior Food Chemist
- USDA Department Administrator
- Cytotechnologist

Chapter 8   Review & Activities

Summary

Section 8-1: Recipe Basics

- Before using a recipe, check to be sure it includes certain basic information and is clearly written.
- Recipes are available from many sources.
- A well-organized recipe collection is easy to use.

Section 8-4: Preparation Tasks

- To follow a recipe, you need to understand the meaning of the terms used.
- You need to know which utensil or appliance to use and the correct technique.

Section 8-2: Measuring Ingredients

- Recipes include weight and volume measurements in customary or metric units.
- For accurate measurements, select the right tools and follow the correct procedures.

Section 8-5: Time Management and Teamwork

- A work plan helps you identify the tasks that must be done.
- A schedule tells you when to do the tasks.
- Look for ways to make the job easier and more efficient.
- Teamwork is essential when working in the kitchen.

Section 8-3: Changing a Recipe

- You can alter the yield of a recipe by changing the amounts of ingredients.
- To make a recipe healthier, you can change ingredients, modify the way food is prepared, or reduce portion sizes.
- High-altitude cooking may require changes in cooking time or ingredients.

Checking Your Knowledge

1. What are important features of step-by-step directions?

2. In measuring, what is an equivalent? Give an example.

3. Describe how to measure liquids accurately.

4. What type of recipe is difficult to alter? Why?

5. When changing the yield of a recipe, by what number do you multiply or divide each ingredient?

6. Define *score* and *pare*. What do *mince* and *grate* mean?

7. What is the difference between straining and draining? What equipment is used for each purpose?

8. Describe the technique for folding one ingredient into another.

9. Why should you clean up as you work in the foods lab?

10. Describe how a work plan for a team differs from a work plan for an individual.

Working IN THE Lab

1. **Food Preparation.** Choose a recipe from a cookbook or use one provided by your teacher. Make at least one ingredient substitution to lower the fat or improve the nutrient content. Evaluate the results.

2. **Food Preparation.** Pare a raw potato. Cut it into slices ½ inch (1.3 cm) thick. Set two slices aside; then cube the rest. Set some of the cubed pieces aside; then dice the rest. Have your teacher check your work.

Review & Activities Chapter 8

Thinking Critically

1. Analyzing Decisions. Peggy looked through several cookbooks trying to find a recipe for a special meal for her friends in the chess club, who had just won a state championship. Some of the recipes she examined were complex, involving many steps and techniques, while others were less so. In the end, Peggy decided to make a dish she had prepared many times before. Do you think Peggy's decision was a wise one? Explain your answer.

2. Recognizing Assumptions. Part way through preparing a batch of banana pudding, Dana discovered that she had only four bananas, instead of the six called for in the recipe. She decided to subtract two from every ingredient listed. Do you think the recipe will turn out well? Why or why not?

3. Identifying Evidence. Some people may believe that it's not worth spending the time to make a work plan and schedule. Why might they feel this way? What could you say to change their opinion?

Reinforcing Key Skills

1. Directed Thinking. It is Portia's turn to cook the family's dinner. She would like to do something different. While looking through the kitchen cookbook collection, she finds a recipe for fish in a hand-stapled batch of recipes. Before gathering ingredients for the dish, what questions about this recipe source does Portia need to ask?

2. Communication. Manto is planning a dinner party to help celebrate his aunt and uncle's wedding anniversary. While preparing his work plan, he finds that one of the foods he is using—an imported grain product—does not list a cooking time on the package. What would you advise Manto to do?

Making Decisions and Solving Problems

You've found a recipe for a casserole that you want to try. The ingredients list includes shredded cheese, but the directions do not tell you what to do with it. What would you do?

Making Connections

1. Math. Find a recipe that makes twelve or more servings. Change the recipe so that it yields four servings.

2. Social Studies. Using the library or other resources, find information about food preparation in colonial America or another historical period. Describe at least three tools that were commonly used for food preparation tasks. How did the tools differ from what is used today?

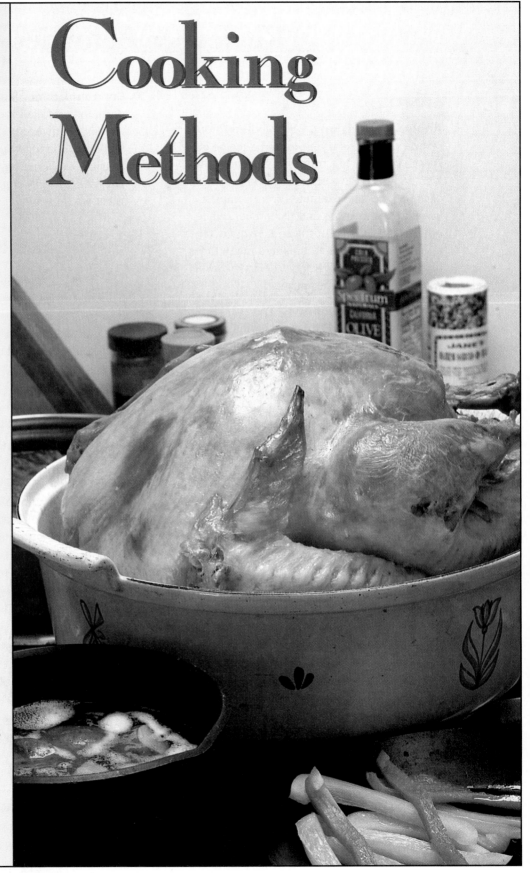

CHAPTER 9

Cooking Methods

Lisa stared at the package of pork chops thawing in the refrigerator. She had never cooked pork chops and wondered how to cook them for her family's dinner.

What should Lisa do? This chapter describes different types of cooking equipment and techniques.

SECTION 9-1

Equipment for Cooking

Look around any kitchen, and you'll find many kinds of equipment designed for cooking. These include major appliances, small appliances, and a variety of utensils.

Objectives

After studying this section, you should be able to:

- Describe how cooktops and conventional, convection, and microwave ovens work.
- Identify small cooking appliances and describe their uses.
- Identify cookware, bakeware, and cooking tools.

Look for These Terms

heating units

cookware

bakeware

Major Cooking Appliances

The major appliances used for cooking are the conventional range, the convection oven, and the microwave oven. At least one of the first two appliances is found in almost every kitchen. Some kitchens have all three.

The Range

A range usually consists of a cooktop, an oven, and a broiler. The cooktop has either dials or push buttons to control the heat. The heat is generated by **heating units**—energy sources in ranges used to heat foods. Ovens have thermostatic controls so that you can set precise temperatures. Oven temperature settings vary from "warm"—below 200°F (93°C)—to "broil," which is generally about 500°F (260°C). The broiler cooks food by direct heat from a heating unit located in the top of the compartment.

Instead of a freestanding range, some kitchens have separate cooktop and oven units built into cabinets. Other kitchens have a portable oven that can be placed on a countertop or cart.

Ranges use either gas or electricity for heat. The two types of ranges have slightly different features.

Gas Range

In a gas range, the oven and broiler are often in separate compartments. The broiler is generally located below the oven. When you're broiling in a gas range, keep the compartment door closed.

The heating units in a gas range are called *burners*. The burners in gas cooktops heat with a flame that is easily regulated. The change in heat level is almost immediate. Some gas ranges have sealed burners that show no visible flame.

In most newer ranges, when a burner is turned on, gas flows through and is ignited by an electronic spark. Older ranges contain pilot lights—small gas flames that burn continuously. When the burner is turned on, the pilot light ignites the gas. Sometimes, however, the pilot light goes out and must be relighted. This should be done by lighting a match and *then* turning on the burner. If the burner is turned on first, gas will accumulate and could cause an explosion when you strike the match.

Air flow is needed for burning gas, so take care not to block the vents in a gas range (by, for example, lining the burner bowls with foil). If air flow is blocked, the gas will not burn properly, resulting in the release of carbon monoxide, a deadly gas.

Electric Range

The heating units in electric ranges are called *elements*. Electricity passes through the element, causing it to heat up.

The oven and broiler in an electric range are in the same compartment. The compartment has two heating elements, one at the top and one at the bottom. The bottom element heats the compartment for all cooking purposes except broiling. For broiling, only the top element comes on. When you're broiling food in an electric range, leave the door slightly open.

There are two main cooktops available in electric ranges, each with unique characteristics:

◆ **Coil elements.** Elements heat up and cool down relatively quickly, although more slowly than gas burners. Coils may vary in size to fit smaller and larger cooking containers.

◆ **Induction cooktops.** A glass-ceramic top covers the heating elements, making this cooktop very easy to keep clean. With induction cooktops, heat is produced when a ferrous metal pan—such as stainless steel or cast iron—is placed on the element. The magnetic attraction between the pan and the heating element produces heat. This cooktop stays cool, except for any heat transferred from the pan.

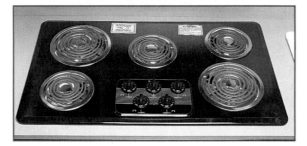

◆ **The two most common types of cooktops for electric ranges are coil elements (below) and induction.** Name two things that might make an induction cooktop preferable to one with coil elements.

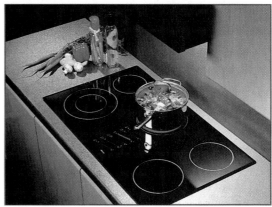

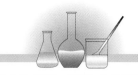

CLOSE-UP ON SCIENCE:
P H Y S I C S

Electrical Resistance and Heat

As electricity passes through a material, its flow is interrupted by a characteristic of the material called *resistance*. The result is that the material heats up. The greater the current flow and the higher the resistance of the material, the greater the heat produced. Cooktop elements have high resistance to produce the heat needed for cooking.

The Convection Oven

A convection oven is similar to a conventional oven except that a fan circulates the heated air. This speeds up cooking time and keeps temperatures even throughout the oven. As a result, foods brown more evenly than in a conventional oven. A convection oven cooks more quickly than a conventional oven, but not as quickly as a microwave oven.

A convection oven can be combined with either a conventional or a microwave oven. The combination oven has more advantages than any single type.

The Microwave Oven

Microwaves are a form of energy that travels like radio waves. In a microwave oven, a magnetron (MAG-nuh-trahn) tube turns electricity into microwaves. The microwaves are distributed throughout the oven by a stirrer blade, a fanlike device. The microwaves bounce off the oven's walls and floor until they are absorbed by the food. Microwave energy is reflected from metal but passes through glass, paper, and plastic to get to food.

Microwaves make food molecules vibrate against each other, producing friction. This friction produces heat that cooks the food. Microwave ovens cook many foods in one-fourth the time that it takes to cook them conventionally, making this an energy-efficient way to cook.

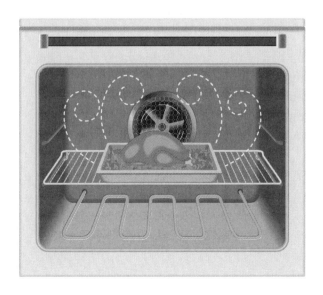

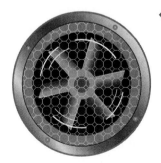

◆ **Convection ovens use a built-in fan to circulate hot air in the oven compartment.** Explain the advantages of this method of cooking.

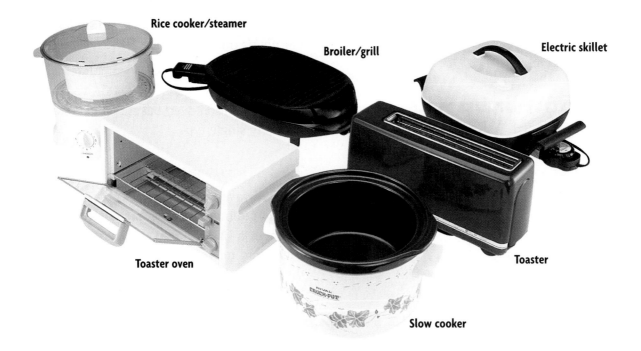

Rice cooker/steamer

Broiler/grill

Electric skillet

Toaster oven

Toaster

Slow cooker

Small Cooking Appliances

Many small appliances are available to help you perform certain cooking tasks quickly and easily. Here are some basic ones:

◆ **Toaster.** Browns bread products on both sides at the same time. You set the controls for the degree of browning. Two- and four-slice models are available.

◆ **Toaster oven.** Toasts bread, heats up foods, and bakes small amounts of many foods. Some toaster ovens can broil food.

◆ **Electric skillet.** A thermostat controls the temperature of the skillet. This appliance is useful for frying, roasting, steaming, and baking.

◆ **Portable electric burner.** A small appliance that works like the cooktop on a range.

◆ **Slow cooker.** A deep pot with a heating element in the base that allows food to cook slowly over many hours. It's a convenient way to cook one-dish meals such as stews.

◆ **Broiler/grill.** A small, portable electric grill used to broil or grill food indoors.

◆ **Rice cooker/steamer.** Used to cook large quantities of rice or to steam vegetables. The controlled heat cooks all types of rice perfectly.

Cookware and Bakeware

Cookware is equipment for cooking food on top of the range. **Bakeware** is equipment for cooking food in an oven. Both cookware and bakeware are available in a variety of materials. Microwave ovens have special requirements for cooking containers.

As a general rule, all types of cookware and bakeware should be washed in hot water with dish detergent. To remove baked-on food, soak pans in hot water with a little detergent prior to washing them.

Cookware

If you were packing for an overnight trip, you'd use a lightweight travel bag, not a huge trunk. In much the same way, you can choose cookware, which comes in many shapes and sizes, depending on how you plan to use it. Here is a guide to some common items:

◆ **Saucepans.** Saucepans have one long handle and often come with a cover. Some types have a small handle on the opposite side as well. Sizes range from ½ quart to 4 quarts (500 mL to 4 L). Saucepans are usually made of metal or heatproof glass.

◆ **Pots.** Larger and heavier than saucepans, pots range in size from 3 to 20 quarts (3 to 20 L). Pots have two small handles, one on either side, which make it easier to lift a heavy pot. Most pots come with covers.

◆ **Skillets.** Sometimes called "frypans" or "frying pans," skillets are used for browning and frying foods. They vary in size and often have matching covers.

◆ **Double boiler.** A double boiler consists of two saucepans—a smaller one fitting into a larger one—and a cover. Boiling water in the bottom pan gently heats the food in the upper pan. This type of cookware is used for heating foods that scorch easily, such as milk, chocolate, sauces, and cereal.

◆ **Dutch oven.** This is a heavy-gauge pot with a close-fitting cover. This type of pot may be used on top of the range or in the oven. Some Dutch ovens come with a rack to keep meat and poultry from sticking to the bottom.

◆ **Steamer.** This basketlike container is placed inside a saucepan containing a small amount of boiling water. Holes in the steamer allow steam to pass through and cook the food.

◆ **Pressure cooker.** This heavy pot has a locked-on cover and steam gauge. Steam builds up inside the pot, causing very high cooking temperatures that cook food more quickly than in an ordinary pot.

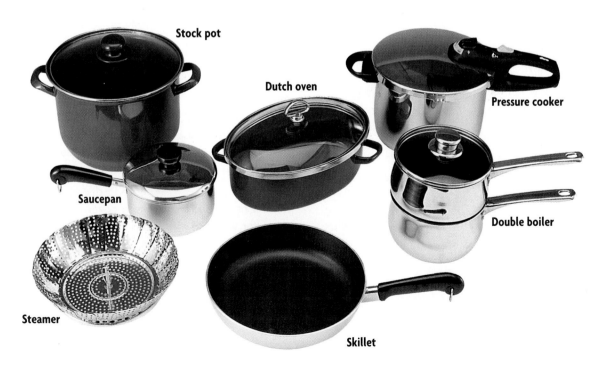

Stock pot

Dutch oven

Pressure cooker

Saucepan

Double boiler

Steamer

Skillet

Materials Used for Cookware

Material	Advantages	Disadvantages	Use and Care
Aluminum	• Conducts heat quickly, evenly. • Lightweight. • Durable. • Comes in a variety of finishes.	• Warps, dents, and scratches easily. • Darkens and stains, especially in dishwasher. • Pits if used to store salty or acid foods.	• Cool before washing to prevent warping. • Avoid sharp tools like knives and beaters. • Do not use to store salty or acid foods.
Anodized Aluminum	• Maintains an even, consistent cooking temperature. • Durable. • Will never peel, chip, or crack. • Resists sticking and scratching.	• Heavy. • Can be expensive.	• Use nonabrasive cleaners and nylon scrubbers.
Stainless Steel	• Durable, tough, hard. • Will not dent easily. • Attractive.	• Conducts heat unevenly. • Stains when over-heated or from starchy foods. • Can develop hot spots. • Pits if used to store salty or acid foods.	• Use nonabrasive cleaners and nylon scrubbers. • Use stainless steel cleaner to remove stains. • Do not use to store salty or acid foods.
Copper	• Excellent heat conductor. • Attractive.	• Discolors easily. • Discolors food and may create toxic compounds. Inside must be lined with tin or stainless steel.	• Dry after washing. • Do not scour inside —the thin lining may be worn away. • Polish with copper cleaner or mixture of flour and vinegar.
Cast Iron	• Distributes heat evenly. • Retains heat well.	• Heavy. • Rusts if not wiped dry after washing.	• Store in dry place. • Store cover separately—pan may rust if stored covered.

Materials Used for Cookware (cont'd)

Material	Advantages	Disadvantages	Use and Care
Glass	• Attractive; can be used for cooking and serving. • Easy to clean.	• Breaks easily, especially if exposed to extreme temperature changes. • Some can be used only on the cooktop; others only in the oven. • Holds heat, but does not conduct heat well.	• May need a wire grid if used on an electric cooktop. • Use nonabrasive cleaners and nylon scrubbers. • Do not plunge hot pan into cold water or put into the refrigerator.
Glass-Ceramic	• Goes from freezer to oven or cooktop. • Durable, heat-resistant, attractive. • Used for roasting, broiling, and baking in conventional or microwave ovens.	• May break if dropped. • Holds heat well—reduce oven temperatures by 25°F (14°C) for baked goods.	• Use nonabrasive cleaners and nylon scrubbers. • Dishwasher-safe. • Use manufacturer's care instructions.
Stoneware	• Attractive; can be used for cooking and serving. • Retains heat.	• Breaks easily.	• Dishwasher-safe. • Use nonabrasive cleaners and nylon scrubbers.
Enamel (glass baked on metal)	• Attractive; can be used to cook and serve.	• Chips easily.	• Dishwasher-safe. • Use nonabrasive cleaners and nylon scrubbers.
Microwave-safe Plastic	• Durable. • Stain-resistant. • Easy to clean.	• Some cannot be used in conventional ovens. • Can be scratched by sharp kitchen tools.	• Dishwasher-safe. • Use nonabrasive cleaners and nylon scrubbers.
Nonstick Finishes	• Keeps food from sticking to pans—fat may not be necessary for browning, sautéing, or frying.	• Easily scratched by metal kitchen tools or abrasive cleaners. • High heat may stain finish or warp pan.	• Follow manufacturer's directions for use and care. Some cannot be washed in dishwasher. • Use nonmetal tools to prevent scratching.

Safety Check

Don't use copper cookware if it's unlined or if the lining wears out. Acidic foods can cause copper to be released into food. Too much copper in the body can cause nausea, vomiting, and diarrhea.

Bakeware

Most bakeware consists of pans of different sizes and shapes. Light-colored pans transfer oven heat to food quickly and give baked products a light, delicate crust. Dark pans absorb more heat from the oven and can produce thick brown crusts in baked products, though not in other foods.

Glass pans absorb more heat than metal bakeware does. If you use a glass pan for baking, reduce the oven temperature by 25°F (14°C).

Here are some basic types of bakeware:

- **Loaf pan.** A deep, narrow, rectangular pan used for baking breads and meat loaf.

- **Cookie sheet.** A flat, rectangular pan designed for baking cookies and biscuits. A cookie sheet has two or three open sides.

- **Baking sheet.** Similar to a cookie sheet, except with four shallow sides about 1 inch (2.5 cm) deep. Baking sheets are used for baking sheet cakes, pizza, chicken pieces, and fish.

- **Cake pans.** Available in assorted sizes and shapes.

- **Tube pan.** A variation on the standard cake pan with a central tube to help trap added air in angel food and sponge cakes.

- **Pie pans.** Shallow, round pans with slanted sides. Pie pans are used for pies, tarts, and quiches.

- **Muffin pans.** Used for baking muffins, rolls, and cupcakes. These pans are available in 6- and 12-cup capacities.

- **Roasting pans.** Large, heavy pans, oval or rectangular in shape, and used for roasting meats and poultry. Roasting pans may be covered or uncovered.

- **Casserole.** A covered or uncovered pan used for baking and serving main dishes and desserts. Various sizes are available.

- **Aluminum foil pans.** Disposable pans made of foil. These pans are useful for special, one-of-a-kind occasions and can be recycled.

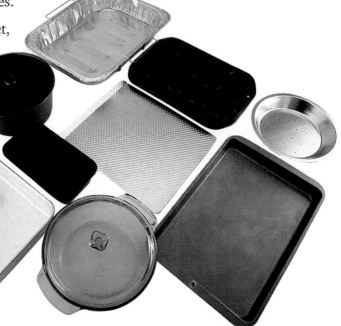

◆ A variety of bakeware is available. **Compare and contrast the results achieved by cooking with shiny vs. darker metal pans.**

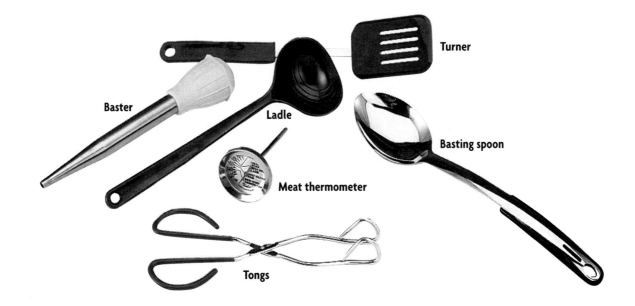

Baster

Ladle

Turner

Basting spoon

Meat thermometer

Tongs

Cooking Tools

A variety of tools are available for the many different cooking tasks. Here are some you might find helpful:

◆ **Turner.** Used to lift and turn flat foods such as hamburgers and pancakes.

◆ **Tongs.** Used to grip and lift hot, bulky foods, such as broccoli spears.

◆ **Basting spoon.** Used to stir and baste foods during cooking.

◆ **Baster.** A long tube with a bulb on the end used for suctioning up juices for basting.

◆ **Ladle.** Has a small bowl and a long handle for dipping hot liquids from a pan.

◆ **Pastry brush.** Used to brush hot foods with sauce or pastry with a glaze.

◆ **Skewers.** Long rods made of metal or bamboo, with one pointed end. Pieces of food are threaded onto skewers for cooking or serving.

◆ **Oven meat thermometer.** Used to measure the internal temperature of meat and poultry as it roasts in the oven. This type of thermometer cannot be used with thin food or in a microwave oven.

◆ **Instant-read thermometer.** Used to measure the internal temperature of food at the end of cooking time, including foods prepared in a microwave or conventional oven. This type of thermometer cannot be used while food is cooking in the oven. To gauge the internal temperature of thin foods, insert the thermometer sideways. Both digital and analog models of instant-read thermometers are sold, with the digital version being easier to read.

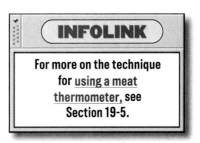

INFOLINK

For more on the technique for <u>using a meat thermometer</u>, see Section 19-5.

◆ **Wire cooling racks.** Used for holding baked goods during cooling or hot pans when they are removed from the heat.

◆ **Potholders, oven mitts.** Thick cloth pads used to protect hands while handling hot containers.

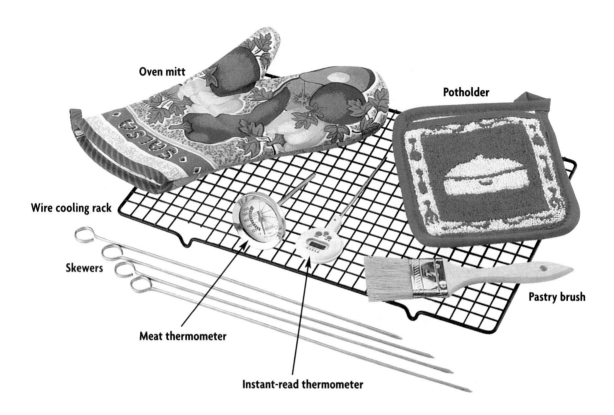

Oven mitt

Potholder

Wire cooling rack

Skewers

Meat thermometer

Instant-read thermometer

Pastry brush

Section 9-1 Review & Activities

1. Name four small appliances for cooking foods.

2. What are the key differences between a saucepan and a pot? Between a cookie sheet and a baking sheet?

3. What is the difference between cookware and bakeware?

4. How are conventional, convection, and microwave ovens alike? How are they different?

5. Extending. Explain the following quote as it applies to the information in this section: "Technology helps us keep in touch with the past by reinventing it."

6. Synthesizing. Bret's family is on a limited budget. What small cooking appliances might you advise them to buy or not to buy? Explain your answer.

7. Applying. Working in groups, identify the cooking equipment found in the foods lab kitchen and note where it is located. Be prepared to report orally to your teacher.

Heat and Cooking

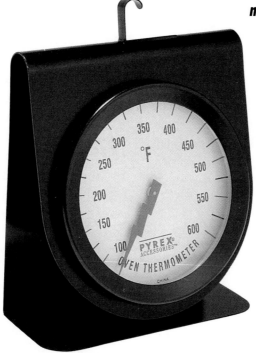

Wonderful things happen in the kitchen. A mixture of vegetables, meat, and water becomes a savory stew. A turkey browning in the oven or soup simmering on top of the range creates delicious aromas. These are just a few of the delightful changes that result from applying heat to food.

Objectives

After studying this section, you should be able to:

- Explain how heat is transferred by conduction, convection, and radiation.
- Describe some changes in food brought about by cooking.

Look for These Terms

conduction

convection

convection current

radiation

Methods of Heat Transfer

When any material—metal, glass, or a food—is heated, its molecules vibrate. The greater the heat, the higher the vibration. Depending on the heat source, these vibrations can come from different forms of energy. The three types of energy transfer central to all cooking are *conduction, convection,* and *radiation.*

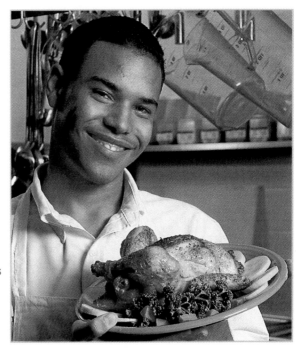

◆ **Heat affects the flavor of foods.** Name two other senses besides taste to which browned foods might appeal.

Conduction

Think of a pancake cooking in a skillet. Heat from the cooktop heating unit is conducted into the skillet, which in turn passes the heat along to the bottom of the pancake and finally to the inside of the food. This heat transfer by direct contact is known as **conduction**.

As molecules are heated, they pass the heat on to neighboring molecules. In this way, heat can travel within an object and to other objects that are in direct contact. To cook the top of the pancake, you flip it over. Can you see why?

Convection

Transfer of heat by the movement of air or liquid is called **convection**. As air or liquid is heated, the hotter portions rise above the colder ones. This creates a **convection current**— a circular flow of air or liquid resulting from uneven heating. Imagine a saucepan of water heating on the cooktop. The water nearest the bottom of the saucepan gets warm and rises through the colder water to the surface. The colder water on the surface is forced down to the saucepan bottom. As the cold water on the bottom of the saucepan warms up, it rises to the surface. This process continually repeats, creating a convection current. This same process also occurs with heated air in an oven.

◆ Conduction and convection are alternative methods of transferring heat to food. Write a brief paragraph that explains how each method works.

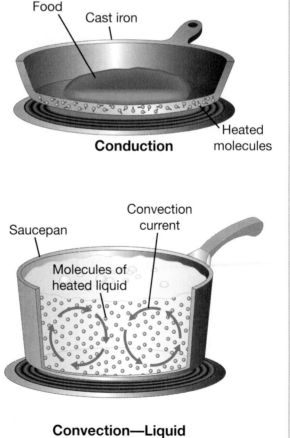

Food

Cast iron

Conduction

Heated molecules

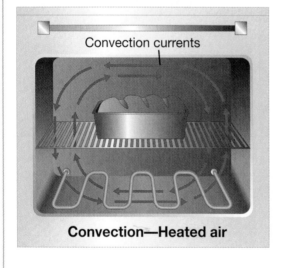

Conventional oven

Convection currents

Convection—Heated air

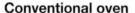

Saucepan

Convection current

Molecules of heated liquid

Convection—Liquid

Radiation

The sun radiates heat to warm the earth. In a similar way, radiant heat from a broiler strikes and warms the food below. This type of heat transfer method that uses infrared rays to strike and warm an object is called **radiation**.

Most cooking techniques use a combination of some or all the heat transfer processes described here. For example, a broiler heats the surface of a food by radiation. The heat then travels through the food by conduction.

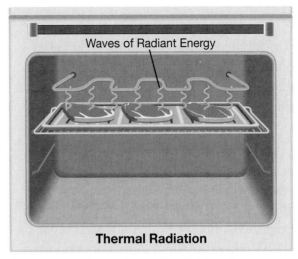

Waves of Radiant Energy

Thermal Radiation

◆ Heat can also be transferred through infrared rays. Name two cooking methods that use these rays.

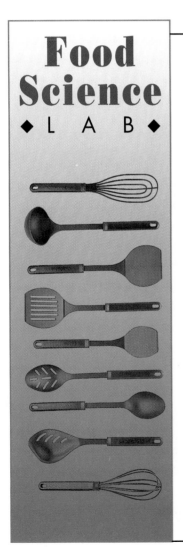

Food Science
◆ L A B ◆

How Does Heat Affect Aroma?

Some experts claim that as much as 85 percent of what we call "taste" is actually smell. How much of a role does heat play in the aroma of foods and whether those aromas are pleasant?

Procedure

1. Ask several classmates to serve as aroma testers. Have them stand 6 feet or more from your work area.

2. Slice half a large onion. Have the aroma testers begin walking toward you. They should stop when they can detect an aroma. Have the testers rate the aroma in terms of how pleasant they found it. Note their responses. Remove the onion and have the testers return to their original positions.

3. Slice the other half of the onion. Place it in the microwave oven and cook it for 3 minutes at 100 percent power. Again, have the testers walk toward you and stop when they detect an aroma. Record their ratings as before.

4. Repeat steps 2 and 3, using celery ribs and bacon strips.

Conclusions

◆ How did the before and after ratings compare? How do you account for any differences?

◆ What generalization can you make about the effects of heat on foods that require cooking as opposed to those that can be eaten cooked or raw? How can you test this generalization?

How Heat Affects Food

As Matt removed a loaf of freshly baked bread from the oven, he breathed in its delicious aroma. Heat waves rose from the crisp brown crust. He could hardly wait to cut himself a slice.

The oven's heat brought out the aroma of the bread and baked its crust to a golden brown. These are two ways in which heat affects food. Heat releases flavor and aroma from foods. Cooking different foods together allows flavors to mingle, creating a pleasing combination. Heat also changes the color of foods. Some foods become darker when cooked and some become lighter. Heat brightens the color of some foods.

Heat also changes the texture of foods. Some foods become harder, some softer, some crispy, and some tender. In addition, heat has an effect on nutrients.

How Cooking Affects Nutrients

One of the goals of food preparation is to retain nutrients such as vitamins and minerals. You've already learned that proper storage helps retain nutrients. Another key is to choose cooking methods that minimize nutrient loss and to use those methods properly.

Some nutrients can be destroyed by cooking heat. These include vitamin C, thiamin, and folate.

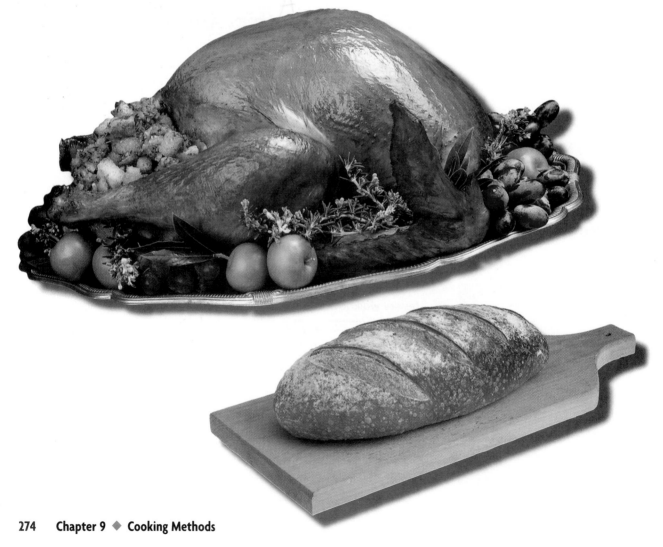

When foods are cooked in liquid, water-soluble vitamins and some minerals dissolve into the liquid. Unless the cooking liquid is consumed, these nutrients are lost. Some minerals and fat-soluble vitamins may be lost as fats and juices drip from meat, poultry, and fish.

Although very little protein is lost during cooking, animal proteins are sensitive to high temperatures. Overcooking in dry heat toughens them, making them unpleasant to eat.

The exact effect of heat on food depends on both the food and the cooking method. In the next section you will learn more about various cooking methods, as well as ways to retain vitamins and minerals and to reduce fat.

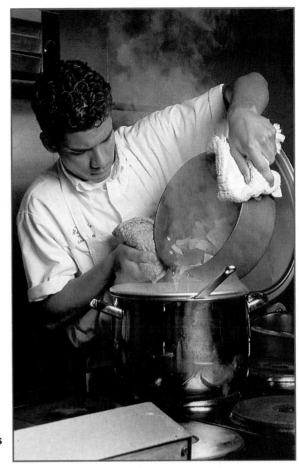

◆ Adding the cooking liquid from simmered vegetables to soup is one way of conserving nutrients. What are some others?

Section 9-2 Review & Activities

1. Briefly describe the three ways heat can be transferred to food during cooking.

2. Name three general ways heat can affect food.

3. Name ways in which nutrients such as vitamins and minerals can be lost during cooking.

4. **Synthesizing.** How might understanding heat transfer processes help you in using appliances to cook food?

5. **Extending.** Explain the effect of heating on vitamin C, thiamin, and folate. Suggest ways to prevent loss of these vitamins during cooking.

6. **Applying.** Prepare a lesson plan for teaching young children about safety in and around kitchen ranges. Include a definition of the term *heating unit*, as well as original pictures of heating units that transfer energy visibly, such as gas, and those where the heat is invisible—radiation, for example. If possible, teach your lesson to an elementary school class in your community.

Conventional Cooking Techniques

Kristie wanted to try something new, so she bought and cooked a chuck roast for her family. She cooked it the way her mother always cooked roasts—in an open pan in the oven. The roast turned out so tough and dry that it was barely edible.

Objectives

After studying this section, you should be able to:

- Explain basic differences between moist-heat cooking, dry-heat cooking, and frying.
- Identify specific types of moist-heat cooking, dry-heat cooking, and frying, as well as combination methods.
- Give guidelines for conventional cooking.

Look for These Terms

moist-heat cooking

stewing

poaching

dry-heat cooking

preheating

hot spot

frying

sauté

smoking point

wok

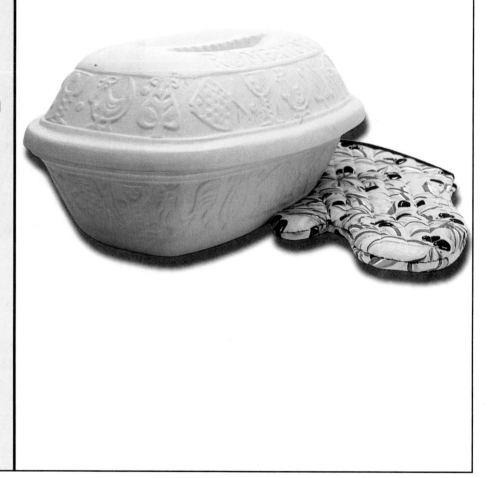

Moist-heat Methods

Cooking methods vary depending on the kind of food being cooked and the results desired. **Moist-heat cooking** includes methods in which food is cooked in hot liquid, steam, or a combination of the two. Moist heat may be used for a number of reasons. Long, slow moist-heat cooking can help tenderize meat. Some foods, such as rice or dry beans, must absorb liquid as they cook.

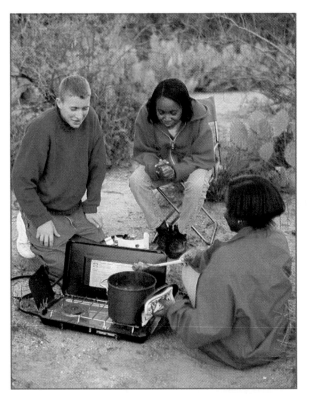

◆ **Moist-heat cooking can produce tender, flavorful one-dish meals.** What other types of foods are best cooked with moist heat?

Sometimes cooking foods together in broth or a sauce helps blend their flavors.

Many cooking appliances, including the microwave and slow cooker, use moist heat. When using a conventional range, you can choose any of these moist-heat methods: boiling, simmering, steaming, and pressure cooking.

Boiling

When a liquid reaches boiling temperature, it forms large bubbles that rise to the surface and break. Water boils at 212°F (100°C). Boiling is suitable for only a few foods, such as corn on the cob and pasta. Many other foods tend to overcook easily or break apart when boiled. Nutrient loss is higher with boiling than with other methods.

Boiling also toughens foods high in protein, such as eggs.

When boiling foods, be sure to use a saucepan or pot large enough to hold the food and the boiling liquid. Bring the liquid to the boiling point; then add the food. Be sure the liquid continues boiling as the food cooks.

Boiling is also useful when you want liquid to evaporate quickly. For instance, you might boil a sauce to thicken it or boil a soup to concentrate the flavor.

Simmering

Simmering differs from boiling in that bubbles in the liquid rise gently and just begin to break the surface. Water simmers at about 186°F to 210°F (86°C to 99°C). Simmering is used to cook many types of food, including fruits, vegetables, and less tender cuts of meat and poultry. Some foods that would break apart or toughen if boiled can be successfully simmered. As with boiling, some nutrients, especially water-soluble vitamins, are lost during simmering. For this reason, it is wise to use the cooking liquid from simmered foods, such as vegetables and dry beans, whenever possible.

To simmer food, bring the liquid to a boil and then add the food. After the liquid returns to a boil, reduce the heat so that the food simmers. A slow cooker can also be used to simmer some foods, such as meats and dry beans.

Safety Check

When adding food to boiling liquid, use tongs or a long-handled spoon to hold the food just above the surface of the liquid. Then ease the food in. Dropping the food from high above the liquid can cause the liquid to splash up, resulting in burns.

FOR YOUR HEALTH

Full Steam Ahead

Steaming not only locks in flavor and nutrients but also is a simple way of cooking certain foods, such as rice, which can become sticky when simmered. Here are some healthful steaming suggestions:

- Steam chunks of boneless chicken breast with broccoli florets, carrot strips, and slices of onion, for a nutrient-rich alternative to stir-frying.

- When steaming vegetables or rice, steam them over seasoned, canned chicken or vegetable broth instead of water. This method adds flavor without adding fat.

Following Up

- Experiment with steaming foods that you ordinarily enjoy cooked by other methods. Try different vegetables and vegetable combinations. Introduce any pleasant discoveries to members of your household and ask for their reactions. Write about the experience in your Wellness Journal.

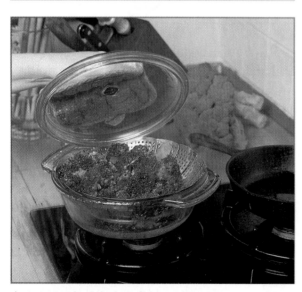

◆ **Steaming foods locks in flavor and nutrients. Can you explain why?**

Two special cooking techniques that make use of simmering are stewing and poaching. **Stewing** involves covering small pieces of food with liquid and then simmering until done. **Poaching** refers to simmering whole foods in a small amount of liquid until done. Eggs, fish, and whole fruits can be poached.

Steaming

Steaming is a method of cooking food over, but not in, boiling water. The food is usually placed in a steamer basket that fits inside a saucepan. Steam is created by a small amount of boiling water in the bottom of the pan. The boiling water does not come in contact with the food. The pan is covered during cooking to trap the steam. You can also use an electric steamer to cook food.

Many foods can be cooked in steam, including vegetables and fish. Foods retain their color, shape, and flavor well when steamed. Few nutrients are lost. Cooking time is longer with steaming than with boiling or simmering.

Pressure Cooking

A pressure cooker cooks food in steam under pressure. Because pressure makes temperatures above 212°F (100°C) possible, the food cooks 3 to 10 times faster than with other methods.

A pressure cooker is best used with foods that take a long time to cook. Examples are less tender cuts of meat and poultry, dry beans, soups, one-dish meals, and vegetables. This method has all the advantages of steaming plus faster cooking times. Follow the manufacturer's directions and accident prevention guidelines carefully. The food in a pressure cooker is superheated and under high pressure.

Dry-heat Methods

Dry-heat cooking means cooking food uncovered without added liquid or fat. Dry-heat methods include roasting and baking, broiling, and pan-broiling.

Roasting and Baking

Roasting and baking both involve cooking food uncovered in a conventional or convection oven. *Roasting* generally refers to cooking large, tender cuts of meat or poultry. *Baking* is the term used with foods such as breads, cookies, vegetables, and casseroles, though some meat, poultry, and fish preparations are also baked. Baked ham and baked chicken are examples.

Roasting gives tender meat and poultry a flavorful, crispy, brown crust. Use a shallow, uncovered roasting pan with a rack. The roasting rack allows fat to drain away from the food—a real benefit for those trying to reduce their fat intake.

For baked goods such as breads, cookies, and cakes, preheating is important. **Preheating** means turning the oven on about 10 minutes before using it so that it will be at the desired temperature when the food is placed inside.

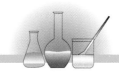

CLOSE-UP ON SCIENCE: CHEMISTRY

The Maillard Reaction

Food cooked in dry heat or in fat goes through a browning process. As food browns, the color, flavor, and texture are altered as the result of complex chemical changes. One of these changes is the Maillard reaction. It occurs when carbohydrates (either sugar or starch) and amino acids combine on the surface of a food such as roasting meat. The reaction occurs only at temperatures over 300°F (150°C). The surface of the food cooked in dry heat or in fat reaches that temperature. With moist heat, the cooking temperature is limited to the boiling point of water, 212°F (100°C). That is why foods cooked in moist heat don't brown.

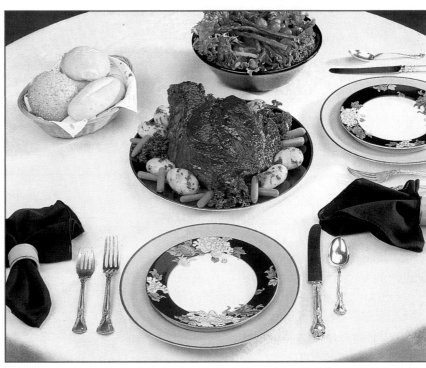

◆ Roasting and baking are dry-heat cooking methods. Name two more foods that would be cooked using these methods.

Pan Placement in the Oven

When baking, placement and spacing of pans are important. The pans must be placed so the hot air in the oven can circulate freely. If pans touch each other or the oven walls, they create a hot spot—an area of concentrated heat. The food overcooks in these areas. When baking several pans of food at one time, place them diagonally opposite one another, as shown here.

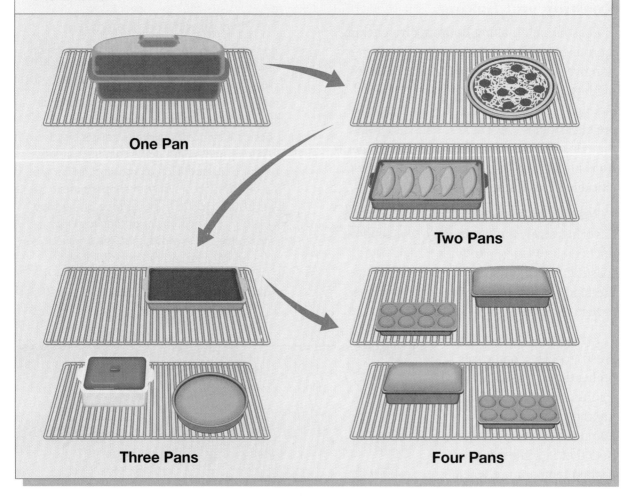

One Pan

Two Pans

Three Pans

Four Pans

It is also important to place pans in such a way that the hot air in the oven can circulate freely. If pans touch each other or the oven walls, they create a **hot spot**—an area of concentrated heat—that can cause the food to overcook. When baking several pans of food at one time, place them diagonally opposite one another.

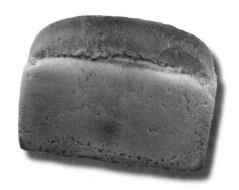

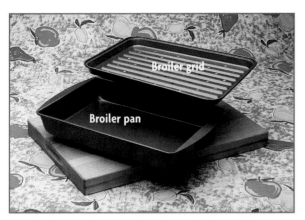
◆ A broiler pan consists of two parts that fit together. What makes broiling a low-fat cooking method?

cooking, you can vary the distance of the pan from the heat source and the cooking time. For thicker foods, position the pan farther from the heat and increase the cooking time. This allows the food to cook all the way through without burning on the outside. Check a cookbook for guidelines about positioning specific foods for broiling.

Outdoor cooking on a grill or spit is similar to broiling except that the heat source is below the food. The food is placed on a wire grid.

Broiling

Broiling refers to cooking food under direct heat. The broiler pan is placed below a burner or heating element. The heat radiates down onto the food, cooking it quickly.

Broiling works well with tender cuts of meat and poultry as well as fish, fruits, and some vegetables. Foods that are already cooked may be broiled for a short time to brown them. Broiling may also be used to melt cheese toppings.

A broiler pan has two parts. A slotted grid holds the food. The grid fits on top of a shallow pan that catches drippings. This allows fat to drain away during cooking.

For broiling in most ranges, set the oven control on "broil." You can't control the broiling temperature. To control the

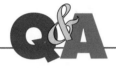

Q What are some tips to help me broil successfully?

A Pat meat and poultry dry. Moisture can keep food from becoming brown and crisp. Don't salt foods before broiling. Salt draws moisture from foods, causing them to dry out. Brush fish, fruit, and vegetables lightly with oil or melted butter or margarine to keep them from charring. To prevent foods from sticking, always start with a cold broiler pan. Use tongs, not a fork. The fork pierces the food, making holes that allow juices to escape.

Safety Check

Never cover the broiler grid with foil. Foil keeps drippings from falling through, which could cause a grease fire.

Never put your hands into the broiler compartment to turn or remove food. The intense heat can cause severe burns. Instead, take the broiler pan from the compartment first. Remember to use potholders or oven mitts. Put the pan on a heatproof surface or wire rack; then turn or remove the food.

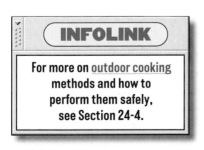

INFOLINK

For more on outdoor cooking methods and how to perform them safely, see Section 24-4.

Pan-Broiling

Pan-broiling is a range-top method of dry-heat cooking. Foods such as hamburgers, tender cuts of steak, and some cuts of pork may be pan-broiled. The food cooks quickly and retains a minimum amount of fat.

To pan-broil, cook the food in a heavy skillet over medium heat. Don't add fat. As fat accumulates in the pan during cooking, pour it off or remove it with a baster.

Frying

Frying involves cooking food in oil or melted fat. Here are several different methods:

◆ **Sautéing.** To **sauté** (saw-TAY) means to brown or cook foods in a skillet with a small amount of fat. Low to medium heat is used. This method is often used for chopped vegetables, such as onions and peppers, and small pieces of meat and fish.

◆ **Pan-frying.** Pan-frying is similar to sautéing but usually involves larger pieces of meat, poultry, or fish. The food may need to be turned several times during the cooking process for complete, even cooking. Pan-frying is often used to brown meat before cooking it in moist heat.

◆ **Deep-fat frying.** This method is also called "french frying." Food is immersed in hot fat and cooked until done. This method is used for tender foods, such as vegetables, and some breads, such as doughnuts. For best deep-fat frying results, use a deep-fat thermometer to keep the fat at the correct temperature.

Note that every fat has a **smoking point**— a temperature at which fats begin to give off irritating smoke and break down chemically. Oil that has reached its smoking point is no longer good for cooking. Animal fats, such as butter and lard, have low smoking points. Safflower, soybean, corn, and peanut oils have relatively high smoking points. They make the best choices for frying.

Combination Methods

Sometimes the best way to cook a food is by a combination of methods. Braising and stir-frying are two popular cooking methods that combine dry-heat and moist-heat cooking.

Braising

Braising combines browning food (frying) with a long period of simmering to tenderize the food and enhance the flavor. It is often used for large, less tender cuts of meat and poultry.

Use a Dutch oven or other heavy pot with a tight-fitting cover. Brown the food first on all sides. Then add seasonings and a small amount of liquid to the food and cover the pot. The cooking may be completed in the oven (usually at 350°F or 180°C) or on top of the range. Vegetables are sometimes added to braised meat or poultry near the end of the cooking time.

Safety Check

When frying, don't overheat the fat or oil. It could catch fire.

Be sure the food to be fried is dry. Moisture could cause the fat or oil to spatter and burn you. Be prepared to act quickly in case of a grease fire. Have a fire extinguisher handy.

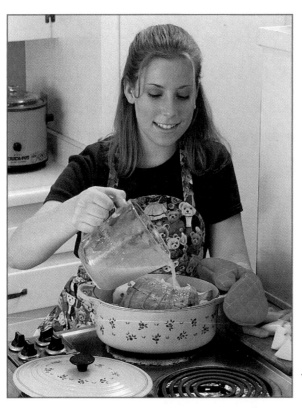

Stir-Frying

Stir-frying also combines frying and moist-heat cooking. In this method, small pieces of food are fried quickly in a small amount of oil at high heat. Stir the food constantly to keep it from sticking to the pan. During the last few minutes of cooking, add a small amount of liquid to the food and cover the pan, allowing the food to steam briefly.

Stir-frying, which began in Asia, is most often used for cooking mixtures of vegetables and other foods. A special bowl-shaped pan called a **wok** is traditionally used, but a skillet also works well.

◆ Braising combines frying and moist-heat cooking. What is another combination method of cooking?

Section 9-3 Review & Activities

1. What are three basic categories of cooking methods? Which could you use to make meat more tender? Which could you use to brown meat?

2. List the methods of dry-heat cooking.

3. Name and describe three methods of frying.

4. Rank these cooking methods according to how well they retain nutrients in food: frying, simmering, pressure cooking, roasting, boiling, steaming.

5. Evaluating. Woks, commonly used in Eastern cultures, have become very popular with cooks in the West in recent decades. Explain this from both a cultural and nutritional standpoint.

6. Synthesizing. Raina would like to cut down on the amount of fat in the foods her family eats but hesitates to give up on cooking the fried foods the family enjoys. What recommendations can you make for a healthy compromise?

7. Applying. Find several recipes for the following: eggs for breakfast, a vegetable side dish, a ground beef dish, soup, and chicken. What basic cooking method does each recipe use?

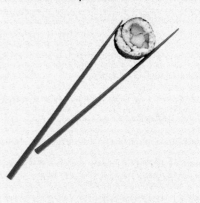

Microwave Cooking Techniques

Objectives

After studying this section, you should be able to:

- Explain why the choice of power setting, foods for cooking, and cookware are important in microwave cooking.
- Describe the techniques necessary for successful microwaving.
- Identify safety precautions for microwave oven use.

Look for These Terms

watts

arcing

standing time

Tori put a dish of leftovers in the microwave and punched in the time and power setting. In two minutes she had a hot, nutritious meal. "What did people do before the microwave was invented?" she said to herself as she sat down to eat.

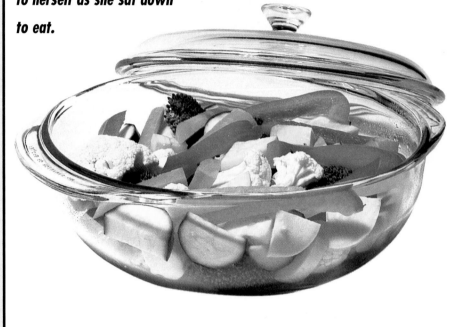

Microwave Oven Basics

Microwaving is a fast, healthful way to cook. Food cooks quickly with less fat and liquid than in most conventional methods. That means more of the water-soluble vitamins are retained, and fewer vitamins are destroyed by heat.

Microwave cooking isn't complicated, but it is different from conventional cooking methods. Start by reading the owner's manual. It will give specific directions for using your microwave oven. It will also help you understand how the microwave power settings work, the kinds of foods that can be microwaved, and the proper equipment to use.

Power Settings

When you cook foods in a microwave oven, you have to choose the power setting. The equation between power setting and the speed with which you get your food to the table is a simple one: The higher the power setting, the faster the cooking.

On some microwave ovens the power setting is identified as a percentage, such as 50 or 100 percent power. On others it is a description—for example, "low" or "medium." The chart below gives typical equivalents for these two kinds of power settings. Because microwave ovens do differ, be sure to check your owner's manual for information on power settings.

Microwave Power Levels

Description	Percentage of Power
High	100
Medium-High	70
Medium	50
Medium-Low	30
Low	10

Safety Check

Standards for microwave ovens require at least two independent interlock systems. Each of these systems stops the production of microwaves the moment the latch is released or the door is opened. If an interlock system fails, a monitoring system stops the oven. Don't operate the oven if the door is bent, the latches are broken or loosened, or the door seals are damaged.

Microwave ovens vary in the amount of microwaves they produce at each setting because they have different power ratings. These ratings are based on units of electrical power called **watts**. The higher the oven wattage, the more microwaves it produces at various settings. Compact models produce about 600 to 700 watts. Midsize and large models produce between 800 and 1,000 watts. You'll usually find the wattage rating on the back of the oven, along with the serial and model numbers.

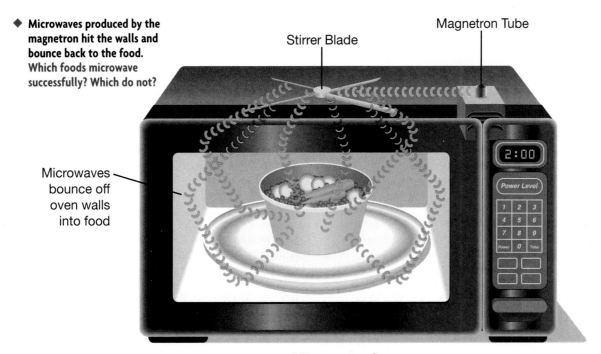

◆ Microwaves produced by the magnetron hit the walls and bounce back to the food. Which foods microwave successfully? Which do not?

Stirrer Blade

Magnetron Tube

Microwaves bounce off oven walls into food

2:00

Power Level

Microwave Oven

How Microwaves Cook

Microwaves cook by making food molecules vibrate. The microwaves penetrate food to a depth of about 1½ inches (3.8 cm). There, they agitate food molecules and produce heat. If the food is thicker, conduction moves the heat deeper into the food and eventually cooks it throughout.

Microwave cooking is a better choice for some foods than others. Generally, the best choices are foods that are moist to begin with or that can be cooked in moist heat.

Food Composition

A food's composition—what it is made of—affects the way it cooks in the microwave. Foods high in water, such as vegetables, will cook faster than foods with a lower water content, such as meat.

Fat, sugar, and salt also attract microwaves; however, you must be careful when heating these items. Concentrations of fat or sugar can create hot spots when exposed to microwaves. If you microwave a jelly doughnut, for example, the jelly will be superheated while the doughnut itself is only warm. Serious burns on the skin or mouth could result. Food under salted areas will cook faster than that under unsalted areas. Therefore, don't sprinkle salt on food before microwaving—wait until after cooking.

Some foods—pasta and rice, for example—need time to absorb liquids as they cook. As a result, no real time is saved when cooking such foods in the microwave. Other foods, such as potatoes and winter squash, have a tough skin that keeps moisture from evaporating. Steam can build up inside the skin and cause the food to burst. Pierce foods like these with a fork to allow steam to escape. For the same reason, do not cook eggs in the shell in the microwave oven—they will burst.

Other Factors

Here are some additional principles to guide you in microwave cooking:

◆ **Food density.** The heavier a food feels for its size, the more dense it is. For example, a slice of bread is less dense than a slice of meat the same size. The denser a food, the longer the cooking time.

◆ **Shape and size of food.** Foods of a uniform thickness cook most evenly. If foods are unevenly shaped, the thinner parts will cook through before the thicker parts. Small pieces cook faster than large ones.

◆ **Starting temperature of food.** The colder the food is to start with, the longer it will take to cook. Thaw most frozen foods, except vegetables, before microwaving. For commercially frozen foods, follow package directions.

◆ **Amount of food.** The more food you're cooking, the longer it will take. The same number of microwaves are produced no matter how much food you put in the oven. One potato cooks quickly, but cooking four potatoes takes longer because they must share the microwaves.

Microwave Cookware

Microwaves are reflected by metal but pass through glass, plastic, and paper materials. These characteristics are important to remember when choosing and using containers for microwave cooking.

Metal and foil are not generally used in microwave ovens. They can cause **arcing**, electrical sparks that can damage the oven or start a fire. Use metal and foil only if your owner's manual specifies. Never leave metal tools, such as a spoon, in any food being microwaved.

Some general guidelines for choosing containers for microwave cooking follow. Some containers that cannot withstand high cooking temperatures are safe for heating foods at lower temperatures.

◆ **Glass and glass-ceramic.** Use oven-proof glass and glass-ceramic for cooking. Regular glass may be suitable for heating.

◆ **Stoneware, china, and pottery.** Most items are suitable for cooking unless they have metal trim. Avoid pottery with metallic glazes.

◆ **Plastic.** For cooking, use only plastic items that are marked "microwave-safe." Some special plastics can be used both in the microwave and at low to moderate temperatures in conventional ovens.

◆ **Paper.** Use paper plates only if they are firm enough to hold food. Choose paper towels labeled "microwave-safe." Avoid products containing recycled paper. They may contain metal fragments or chemicals that could catch fire.

The size and shape of microwave cookware also affects the way food cooks and the cooking time. Pans should be shallow with straight sides. Round pans allow for even cooking. Square and rectangular pans should have rounded corners.

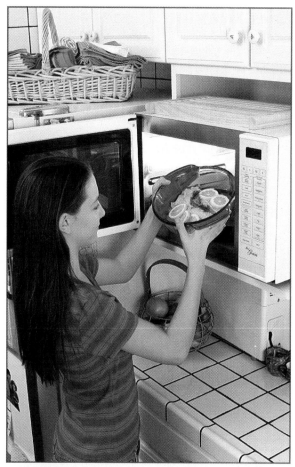

◆ Be sure to choose cookware that can safely be used in a microwave oven. What are some types that would not be suitable?

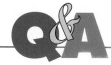

Q If a glass or pottery container isn't marked "microwave-safe," how can I tell whether or not I can use it for microwave cooking?

A Here's a simple test: Fill a glass measuring cup with water and place it in the oven next to the empty container you're testing. Heat for 2 minutes at 100 percent power. If the empty container is too hot to touch, don't use it in the microwave oven.

Microwaving Successfully

A few special techniques are needed in microwave cooking. They involve placing food in the oven and in the pan, covering, stirring, rotating, turning, and timing.

Food Placement

When he's in a hurry for a meal, Beau usually tosses a few leftovers into the microwave. He's often annoyed to find that one or more of the foods hasn't heated through. How you place food in a microwave is a factor in successful heating and cooking.

The best arrangement of food for microwaving is a ring shape. This allows microwaves to enter food from as many sides as possible.

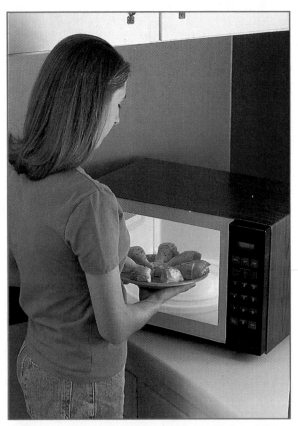

◆ For even cooking, arrange foods for microwaving with the thickest or toughest parts toward the outside. **Explain the reasons for this instruction.**

A meatloaf can be shaped into a ring in a pan or cooked in a ring mold.

When possible, leave space between pieces of food to allow better microwave penetration.

When cooking foods of uneven thickness, use the characteristics of microwave patterns to your advantage. Food in the center of the oven cooks more slowly. Arrange food like the spokes of a wheel, with the thickest or toughest parts toward the outside and the thinnest or most tender parts toward the center. With broccoli spears, for example, place the tops toward the center and the stalks toward the outside.

Covering Food

A cover holds in steam, keeps foods moist, and shortens cooking time. It also keeps food from spattering in the oven.

Foods you would cover for conventional cooking are usually covered for microwave cooking. If you want foods to steam, cover them tightly. For drier foods, cover loosely.

Foods may be covered with microwave-safe glass or plastic covers. An inverted plate is another option. Here are still other options:

◆ **Waxed paper and cooking parchment.** Waxed paper and cooking parchment prevent spatters and allow some steam and moisture to escape. Use them on foods such as casseroles.

◆ **Paper towels.** Paper towels absorb excess moisture and prevent spatters. Wrap rolls, breads, and sandwiches in paper towels before microwaving to keep them from becoming soggy.

When you remove covers or inverted plates, use a potholder or an oven mitt. Tilt the cover away from you to prevent the escaping steam from causing burns.

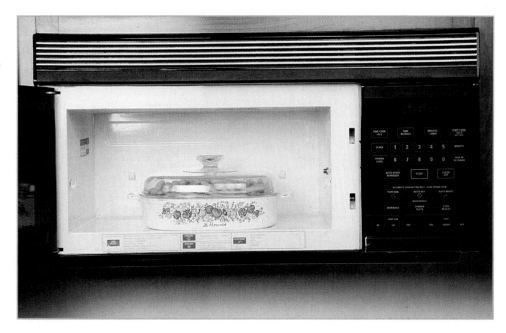

◆ In microwaves not equipped with turntables, it is important to rotate foods a half turn so they cook more evenly. What other measures can you take to ensure that microwave foods cook evenly?

Stirring, Rotating, and Turning

Microwaves may not be distributed evenly throughout the oven, especially in older models. To be sure that food cooks as evenly as possible, stir, rotate, or turn it during cooking. Unless directed otherwise, stir or turn foods after half the cooking time.

Stirring helps foods cook evenly. If the food can't be stirred, rotate the pan. To rotate, use a potholder to grasp the pan and give it a half turn. Dense foods such as meat and poultry should also be turned over. Use tongs to turn foods over.

Most newer ovens have turntables that rotate the food as it cooks. Follow directions in the owner's manual.

Determining Cooking Time

Microwave cooking has two parts. The first part occurs when the oven is on and microwaves are being produced. After the oven turns off, the heat trapped inside the food continues cooking it. This period during which heat buildup in a microwaved food completes its cooking is called **standing time**. Microwave recipes give directions for both cooking and standing time. If you cooked the food uncovered, cover it during standing time to retain heat.

Check a food's progress as it cooks. Test food for doneness after the standing time, not before. Avoid overcooking. Foods overcooked in the microwave oven become hard and tough.

Food will cook slightly faster in higher-wattage ovens. Some ovens have sensors that will turn the oven off when the food is done.

Even with turntables, microwave ovens may not cook evenly. To be sure microwaved foods such as meat, poultry, fish, and casseroles are thoroughly cooked, use an instant-read thermometer at the end of cooking and standing times. Insert the thermometer in several different areas to be sure the food is evenly done.

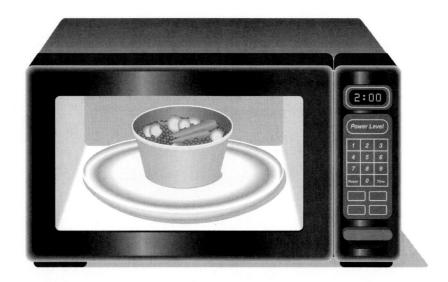

Microwave Recipes

Amanda has a favorite recipe for chicken with orange sauce, but it takes so long to prepare that she seldom uses it. She'd love to be able to use the microwave instead of a conventional oven.

Adapting a standard recipe for cooking in the microwave oven works best if you can find a similar microwave recipe. A basic microwave cookbook can help you ease into microwave cooking successfully. With experience, you can begin experimenting.

A well-written microwave recipe has the same features as a conventional recipe. In addition, it specifies:

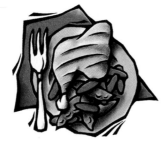

◆ The size and shape of the cooking container.

◆ How to arrange food for even cooking.

◆ Whether or not to cover the dish.

◆ A range of cooking and standing times.

Microwave Care and Accident Prevention

Accident prevention rules for conventional cooking also apply to microwave cooking. Here are some additional microwave accident prevention rules:

◆ Never turn on the oven unless there's food in it. You could damage the oven.

◆ Follow the manufacturer's directions for preparing commercially frozen foods in the microwave oven. Don't eat the food if the package turns brown. Don't reuse containers.

◆ Loosen tight-fitting covers or caps before microwaving. Otherwise, a buildup of steam pressure could cause the container to explode.

◆ Never attach kitchen magnets to the microwave oven. They can affect the electronic controls.

◆ Have your microwave oven tested by an authorized repairperson if you're concerned about microwaves leaking from the oven. Microwave leakage meters available for home use are often not reliable.

Cleaning the Microwave Oven

Clean spots and spills after every use. If allowed to build up, they will absorb microwaves and cut down on the cooking power. Keep the door seal clean. Spilled food also allows bacteria to grow.

To clean the interior of the oven, wipe it with a clean, wet dishcloth. Dry it thoroughly. Don't use abrasive cleaners.

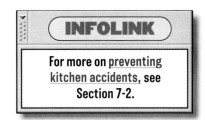

INFOLINK

For more on <u>preventing kitchen accidents,</u> see Section 7-2.

Section 9-4 Review & Activities

1. Describe the factors involved in the choice of power setting, foods for cooking, and cookware.

2. What is the purpose of stirring, rotating, and turning food during cooking?

3. Give three guidelines for accident prevention when using a microwave oven.

4. Synthesizing. Many families limit their use of microwave ovens to thawing frozen foods and heating leftovers. Why do you think more people don't use the microwave oven for other types of cooking?

5. Analyzing. You have been asked to create an advertising campaign for a line of microwave ovens. Write three persuasive facts about microwave cooking that might lead a consumer to consider buying a microwave oven.

6. Applying. Check plastic containers, tools, and cookware in the foods lab. Which items are marked "microwave-safe"?

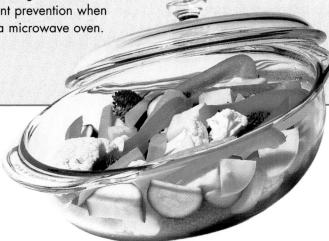

Recipe File

Chicken Quesadillas

This zesty recipe is great for lunch, along with a tossed salad and fresh fruit.

Customary	Ingredients	Metric
1	Boneless, skinless chicken breast, cooked and shredded	1
2	12-in. flour tortillas	2
1	Tomato, diced	1
Dash	Ground cumin	Dash
1 tsp.	Chili powder	5 mL
½ cup	Shredded low-fat Monterey jack or cheddar cheese	125 mL

Yield: Two servings

Equipment: Microwave-safe tray or large plate
Power level: 100%

Directions
1. Place the tortillas on a microwave-safe tray or large plate. Distribute half the shredded chicken on each tortilla.
2. In a small bowl, combine the diced tomato, cumin, and chili powder. Gently toss to mix.
3. Spread half the seasoned tomato on each tortilla. Top each with half the cheese.
4. Microwave at 100% power for 30 seconds to 1 minute. Let stand 1 minute.
5. Fold each quesadilla in half. Serve hot.

Nutrition Information
Per serving (approximate), based on use of boneless, skinless, roasted chicken breast: 337 calories, 39 g protein, 22 g carbohydrate, 10 g fat, 87 mg cholesterol, 150 mg sodium
Good source of: potassium, magnesium, iron, vitamin C, phosphorus, B vitamins

Food for Thought
- What kitchen tool would you use to dice the tomato? To shred the cheese if it came in a block?
- What substitutions could you make for the chicken? What adjustments, if any, would you need to make to the power setting or cooking time?

CAREER WANTED

Individuals with strong interpersonal skills and a good head for business.

REQUIRES:

- degree or certificate from a cooking school
- food service and business management courses

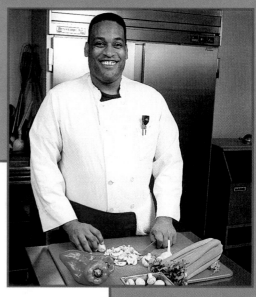

"I earn money doing what I love—cooking!"

says Caterer Storey Peak, Jr.

Q: Storey, what does being a caterer involve?

A: I specialize in providing food for parties and receptions. This entails meeting with clients and discussing menus, preparing the food, delivering and serving it, and cleaning up afterwards.

Q: What skills are needed in your line of work?

A: Cooking, of course. It also helps to be personable, since you're dealing with clients on a one-to-one basis. You also need a lot of organizational and management skills to be successful.

Q: What is a typical day like for you?

A: Each day is different. Some are spent meeting with potential clients, while others are spent in the kitchen or working on the financial paperwork.

Q: What's your favorite part of being a caterer?

A: The flexibility of owning my own business is a real plus. I also get a lot of satisfaction from hearing my clients say what a great time their guests had and ask whether I'd be available to do another event for them next month.

Career Research Activity

1. Arrange to interview a caterer in your community or via the web. Try to learn at least five new details about this career. Write up your findings as "Five Reasons You Should (or Should Not) Become a Caterer."

2. Compare and contrast the skills used to be a Fruit & Vegetable Grader, a Shopping Investigator, and a Hospital Food Service Supervisor. Place your findings on a "Satisfaction Barometer," a graphic that tells what level of professional satisfaction each of these careers could bring.

Related Career Opportunities

Entry Level
- Produce Department Manager
- Fruit & Vegetable Grader

Technical Level
- Caterer
- Shopping Investigator

Professional Level
- Nutritionist
- Professional Chef
- Hospital Food Service Supervisor

Chapter 9   Review & Activities

Summary

Section 9-1: Equipment for Cooking

- Major cooking appliances include gas and electric ranges and convection and microwave ovens. Each is different.

- Small cooking appliances are useful for specialized tasks.

- Cookware and bakeware items have specific uses and come in a range of materials.

- A variety of small tools are used in cooking.

Section 9-3: Conventional Cooking Techniques

- The three basic types of cooking methods—moist-heat, dry-heat, and frying—affect food differently.

- Braising and stir-frying are cooking techniques that combine two basic methods.

Section 9-2: Heat and Cooking

- Heat travels by conduction, convection, or radiation.

- When food is heated, the color, flavor, aroma, and texture are all affected.

- Take steps to minimize nutrient losses during cooking.

Section 9-4: Microwave Cooking Techniques

- Microwave cooking requires an understanding of the power settings and how microwaves affect different foods and materials.

- Follow instructions for arranging, covering, stirring, rotating, turning, and timing foods.

- Use guidelines for preventing accidents when using the oven, and care for it properly.

Working IN THE Lab

1. **Presentation.** Collect several cookware and bakeware items. Give a presentation explaining how the differences in size, shape, materials, and handle placement make each item helpful for particular kinds of cooking tasks.

2. **Food Science.** Cook potato slices by baking, simmering, boiling, and frying. Compare the flavors and textures.

Checking Your Knowledge

1. Where is the broiler in a gas range? In an electric range?

2. What is a double boiler used for?

3. List four cooking tools and tell what they are used for.

4. What is convection? How is it different from conduction?

5. Name three possible reasons for using moist heat in certain situations.

6. What is the difference between stewing and poaching?

7. What kinds of foods can you roast successfully?

8. How is pan-broiling different from broiling?

9. What happens when you change the power setting of a microwave oven from high to medium? How does this affect the cooking time?

10. Name four specific materials suitable for microwave cooking.

Thinking Critically

1. Recognizing Values. Imagine that you saw an advertisement for a microwave oven that specified the product as "ideal for the modern American family." Identify the value that you believe this ad is addressing. In what way is the value you have identified responsible for the popularity of microwave ovens and similar appliances?

2. Identifying Cause and Effect. Soo-Kim used a recipe that she cut out of a magazine to braise a mixture of meat and vegetables. When the cooking time ended, she was upset when she found the food dried out and charred on the bottom. What might have caused this? What advice can you give Soo-Kim for the future?

Reinforcing Key Skills

1. Communication. Julio knows that he needs to reduce fat and calories in his eating plan. He loves to cook, and pan-fried steak and french fries are two of his specialties. What changes in cooking methods can you suggest to Julio that would help him prepare his favorite foods in a more healthful way?

2. Management. You are a member of a group of students who have taken on the task of preparing a guidebook to accident prevention in the foods lab kitchen. List the procedure you would suggest the group follow in accomplishing this task.

Making Decisions and Solving Problems

Your family is packing for a week's vacation at a lakeside cabin that has a small gas range. Your parents have asked you to choose the cookware, bakeware, and kitchen tools to pack. You can take only as much as you can fit in a small cardboard box. How would you use management skills to help you solve this problem?

Making Connections

1. Science. Place a long, all-metal kitchen tool, such as a ladle, in a saucepan of boiling water. Using a watch with a second hand, time how long it takes for the handle to become hot to the touch at the midpoint and at the end. What kind of heat transfer is involved in the movement of heat through the metal handle?

2. Art. Develop a diagram that shows how to arrange fresh broccoli in a casserole for microwaving. Indicate how the microwaves will be absorbed by the food.

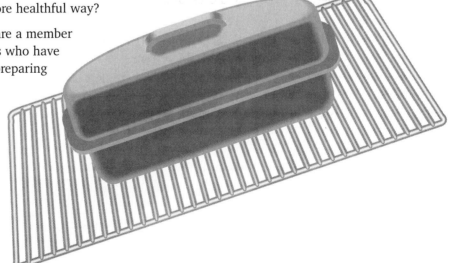

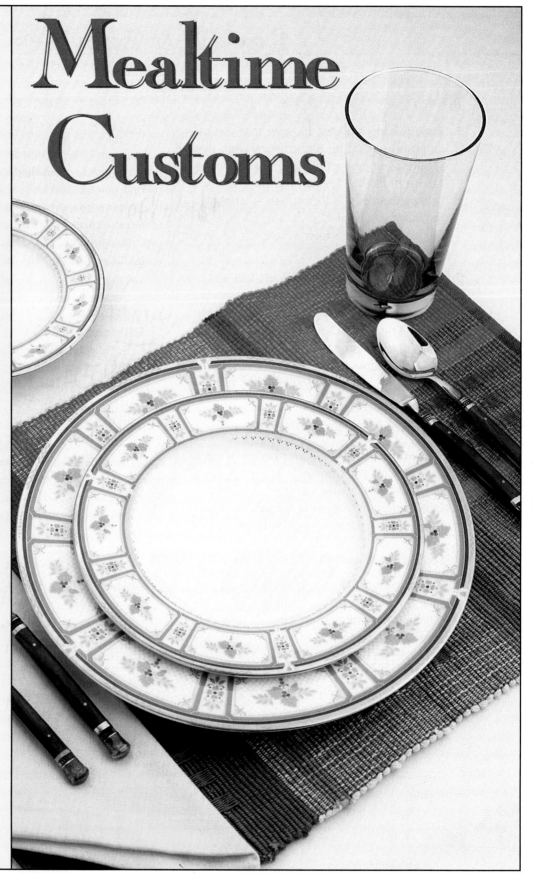

CHAPTER

10

Section 10-1
Serving Family Meals

Section 10-2
Mealtime Etiquette

Mealtime Customs

Mealtime customs may vary, but the purposes of sharing meals with others are generally the same—to enjoy food, to socialize, or to conduct business. Meals give families a chance to spend time together and strengthen the family as a unit. In this chapter, you'll learn strategies for making family meals and other mealtimes a success.

Serving Family Meals

"I won't be home for dinner, Mom—my debate team meets tonight."

"I'll be working late. I'll pick something up on the way home."

Does this sound familiar? In this section, you will learn about the importance of having meals together as a family.

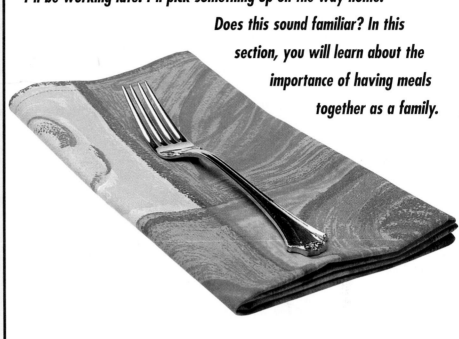

Objectives

After studying this section, you should be able to:

- Explain why meals together can be important to the family.
- Demonstrate how to arrange tableware for a simple family meal.
- Describe family service and plate service.

Look for These Terms

tableware

place setting

serving pieces

cover

Family Meals

In today's fast-paced society, finding time to sit down and enjoy a meal as a family can be a challenge. The good news is that more and more families are meeting this challenge. Whether it is only once a week for dinner or each day at breakfast, eating together is important to a family's social health. Family meals are a time when everyone can relax, enjoy food, talk with one another, catch up on family news, and just have fun.

To make the most of family meals, you need to follow a few simple guidelines. These include keeping a positive mealtime atmosphere and paying attention to the table's appearance.

Mealtime Atmosphere

Sierra's family keeps the TV on during dinner. Dinner at Mark's house often erupts into complaints and accusations involving Mark, his sister, and their parents. What is wrong with these scenarios? Both families do not realize the importance of a positive mealtime atmosphere. An upbeat atmosphere can be as essential to your family's health as nutritious food. Mealtime isn't the time to complain, criticize, or air the day's problems. Keep family meals fun. Focus on the pleasure of eating and of each other's company. What interesting topics can you think of to discuss with your family?

Even when you are eating alone, it is important to sit down and take time to enjoy yourself and your food. People who read or watch television as they eat pay little attention to what and how much they eat. They often eat more than they would if they relaxed, concentrated on the food, and enjoyed the meal.

Setting the Table

How the table looks at mealtime can be as significant as how the people around it behave. Start by making the eating area easy on the eye. Be sure the table is free of papers and other clutter. Place a simple decoration on or near the table—for example, a vase with a single garden flower or a few interesting seashells.

Table settings include the following components:

◆ **Tableware. Tableware** includes any items used for serving and eating food. Types of tableware are dinnerware (plates, bowls, and cups), flatware (knives, forks, and spoons), glassware, and "linens" (anything from a cloth tablecloth and napkins to wipe-clean placemats).

◆ **Place setting.** The pieces of tableware used by one person to eat a meal are called a **place setting**.

◆ **Serving pieces.** Platters, large bowls, and other tableware used for serving food are known as **serving pieces**.

◆ **Cover.** The arrangement of a place setting for one person is called a **cover**. The rules for this arrangement are based on both tradition and practicality.

Table-Setting Basics

Knowing how to set a table will help you serve family meals, entertain guests, and feel comfortable when you eat out.

The cover is usually on the table before people sit down to eat. The plate goes in the center of the cover, about 1 inch (2.5 cm) from the edge of the table.

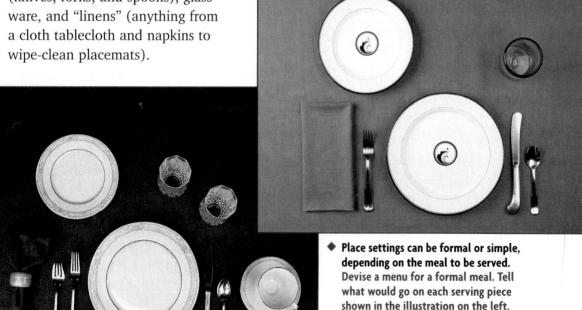

◆ Place settings can be formal or simple, depending on the meal to be served. Devise a menu for a formal meal. Tell what would go on each serving piece shown in the illustration on the left.

Arrange flatware in the order in which it is used, starting at the outside and working in toward the center. Forks go to the left of the plate, knives to the right. Place spoons to the right of the knives. If you have both a soup spoon and a teaspoon, you'd probably use the soup spoon first. Place it to the right of the teaspoon.

Place a beverage glass just above the tip of the dinner knife. The cup and saucer or mug go to the right of the spoon, about 1 inch (2.5 cm) from the edge of the table. The napkin is usually placed to the left of the fork.

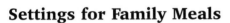

Settings for Family Meals

Most families choose simple table settings for everyday meals. For most meals, you need at least a dinner plate, fork, knife, teaspoon, and beverage glass. Add a cup and saucer or a mug if a hot beverage is being served. If salad is on the menu, add a salad plate or bowl. For soup, you'll need a bowl and a soup spoon.

At home, the same fork can be used to eat both a salad and the main dish. For a formal meal, separate forks would be used.

Serving Family Meals

In Ray's family, serving bowls are passed around the table, and everyone takes whatever she or he wants. Julie's dad prefers to dish food onto plates at the range. These two most common styles of serving food are known as *family service* and *plate service*.

Family Service

In family service, the cover is set with the necessary tableware. The food is placed in serving dishes and passed around the table, with people helping themselves. It's less confusing if all the foods are passed in the same direction, generally to the right.

Sometimes, if a serving plate is too hot or a roast or ham is sliced at the table, a family member serves the food at the table. In that case, the dinner plates are stacked in front of the server. The food is placed on a plate and passed along to the diners, who then help themselves to other foods in the meal.

The main advantage of family service is that people can serve themselves the amount they want. This is especially helpful for those who are limited in the kinds or amounts of food they can eat. There are, however, several disadvantages. The hot food left on the table in serving dishes may cool to room temperature quickly. This allows harmful bacteria to multiply. Family service also makes it difficult to practice portion control, which can lead to overeating. A third disadvantage is that excess food left on a plate must be thrown away, which wastes food and money.

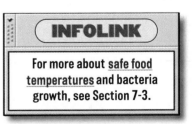

INFOLINK

For more about **safe food temperatures** and bacteria growth, see Section 7-3.

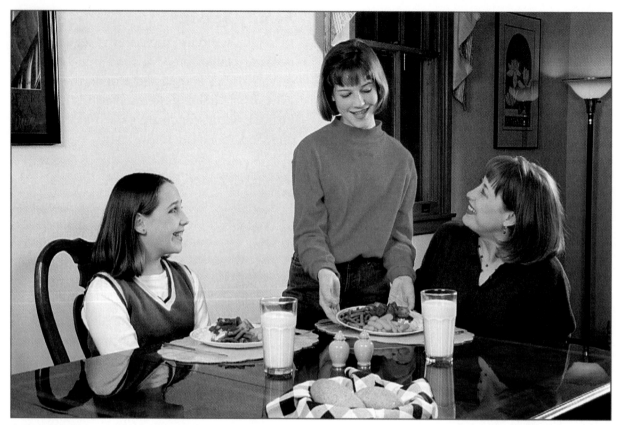

◆ **Some families use plate service at home.** How is plate service different from other ways of serving family meals?

Plate Service

Plate service is generally used for family meals and in restaurants. The table is set without dinner plates, though space is left on each cover for the plate (and salad bowl if a salad is to be served). Food is placed on the plates directly from the containers in which it was cooked, and the plates are then brought to the table. The food remaining in pans can be kept hot on the range or in the oven. The only exception is salad. This may be passed around the table in a serving bowl so that people can help themselves.

Besides cutting down on waste and bacteria buildup, and discouraging the tendency to overeat, plate service saves cleanup time. Because no serving dishes are used, there are none to wash.

General Guidelines

Place breads and rolls on a plate or in a basket, and pass it around the table. If a basket is used, line it with a napkin. Diners can place bread or rolls on the edge of their dinner plates. At more formal meals, provide a small bread-and-butter plate above the forks.

Serve salads either in individual bowls at each place setting or in a serving bowl to be passed around the table. If possible, serve salad dressing separately so that people can use the amount they want.

Serve dessert after the dinner plates, salad bowls, and serving dishes have been cleared from the table. If forks or spoons are needed, bring them to the table with the dessert.

Remembrances of Meals Past

Do you recall the best meal you ever had? As the following passage from Charles Dickens's *A Christmas Carol* reveals, size is not the only measure of a meal's success.

"At last the dishes were set on, and . . . [followed] by a breathless pause as Mrs. Cratchit, looking slowly all along the carving-knife, prepared to plunge it in the breast [of the goose]; but when she did, and when the long-expected gush of stuffing issued forth, one murmur of delight arose all [a]round. . . .

"There never was such a goose. . . . Its tenderness and flavour, size and cheapness, were the themes of universal admiration. Eked out by apple-sauce and mashed potatoes, it was a sufficient dinner for the whole family; indeed, as Mrs. Cratchit said with great delight (surveying one small atom of a bone upon the dish), they hadn't ate it all at last! Yet every one had had enough, and the youngest Cratchits in particular, were steeped in sage and onion to the eyebrows!"

Think About It

1. What does the server do to make the meal one that the whole family will remember for years to come? What word or phrase in the passage clues you in to the fact that this practice is probably a family tradition?

2. Write your own story describing a meal (real or imagined) you found memorable and really enjoyed. Include specific details that show how the presentation of the meal made it special.

Section 10-1 Review & Activities

1. Identify two benefits of a pleasant mealtime atmosphere.

2. Name the items included in a simple, everyday table setting.

3. Traditionally, how is flatware arranged with respect to the dinner plate?

4. Compare and contrast family service and plate service.

5. **Analyzing.** With several classmates, brainstorm obstacles a family can face in planning meals together. Devise strategies for overcoming each problem. Share your findings with the class.

6. **Extending.** Plate service can cut down on the tendency to overeat. Identify other factors of meal service that can help cut down on this tendency.

7. **Applying.** Set a cover incorrectly. Challenge a classmate to identify and correct the errors in the setting.

Mealtime Etiquette

"You should have seen the game!" Aaron shouted with his mouth full. "We really creamed Central." He reached across the table for the salsa.

His twin sister Kayla swallowed, then quietly asked, "Would someone please pass the tortillas?"

Objectives

After studying this section, you should be able to:

- Explain the importance of knowing simple table etiquette.
- Describe basic etiquette guidelines.

Look for These Terms

table etiquette

reservation

gratuity

Table Etiquette

Aaron and Kayla are twins, but there is one important difference between them: table etiquette. **Table etiquette** is the courtesy shown by using good manners at meals.

Good table manners help put you at ease in social situations. They can also be an asset in the working world. Many business transactions take place over meals. Often, when companies consider an applicant for a job, the interview may include a meal. This gives the interviewer a chance to observe how the applicant would act during similar business situations.

Basic Etiquette

Here are some general etiquette guidelines:

Before Eating

- Place the napkin on your lap before you start eating. Don't tuck it into a belt or under your chin.

- If there are six or fewer people at the table, wait until everyone is served before you begin to eat. If there are more, wait until two or three have been served.

- You may reach for serving dishes as long as you don't have to lean across your neighbor. If you can't reach the food easily, politely ask the person nearest the food to pass it to you.

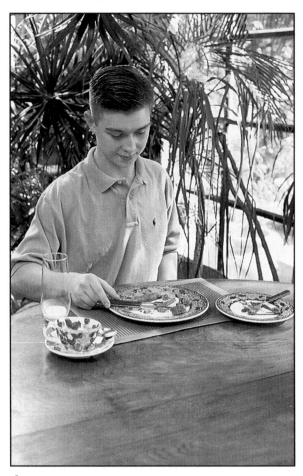

While Eating

♦ Don't talk with your mouth full. Finish chewing, swallow the food, and then talk.

♦ If you're having problems getting foods (such as peas) onto your fork, push them on with a piece of bread. If you have no bread, use the tip of your dinner knife to push the food onto the fork.

♦ Break bread into smaller pieces before buttering or eating it.

♦ If you're dining at someone's home and aren't sure what to do, use your host's actions as a guide.

♦ Cut food into small pieces for eating. If you try to eat large pieces, you may have difficulty chewing and may choke.

♦ **At the end of the meal, place your knife and fork on your plate as shown. Give two other do's and don'ts of table etiquette.**

♦ Sit up straight when you eat, and don't lean on your elbows.

♦ If you must cough or sneeze, cover your mouth and nose with a handkerchief or a napkin. If your coughing continues, excuse yourself and leave the table.

After Eating

♦ Never comb your hair or apply makeup while at the table.

♦ Don't leave a spoon in your cup. You might knock the cup over if your hand accidentally hits the spoon.

♦ When you have finished eating, place your fork and knife on your plate, pointing toward the center.

Finally, remember that people from other countries and cultures have table manners that may be different from yours. Respect and accept people with other customs.

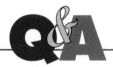

Q Is it all right to eat fried chicken with my fingers?

A That depends. When you're at home or in a fast-food restaurant, feel free to eat fried chicken with your fingers. When in someone else's home, follow the lead of your host. In fine restaurants, eat all meat except crisp bacon with a knife and fork. Note that some foods—namely breads, celery, olives, carrot sticks, pickles, and most sandwiches—are normally eaten with the fingers regardless of where you are eating.

Restaurant Etiquette

Restaurant etiquette involves the same good manners that you use anywhere else. Still, there are a few basic guidelines that deal with situations found only in restaurants.

When You Arrive

When you enter a restaurant, you may be asked whether you have a reservation. A **reservation** is an arrangement made ahead of time for a table at a restaurant. When calling, give your name, the number of people in your group, and the time you plan to arrive. If you will be late or decide not to go, call and ask to change or cancel the reservation.

Near the entrance, you may see a check-room. If you do, leave coats, umbrellas, packages, books, and briefcases. You are expected to tip the attendant.

Unless a sign states otherwise, never seat yourself. A restaurant employee will direct you and your group to a table.

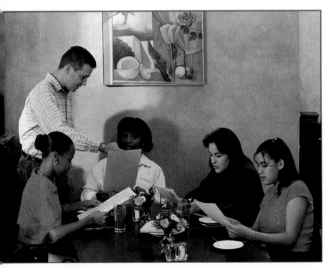

◆ When eating at a restaurant, be sure and look at the menu carefully and ask any questions before placing an order. What types of questions might be good to ask?

FOR YOUR HEALTH

Safe Practices = Safe Food

Personal hygiene and sanitation practices are just as important when you are serving and eating food as when you are preparing it. For example, if hand-washing practices are not followed, bacteria on your skin can be transferred to the food. Regardless of these precautions, many bacteria remain. Whether you are eating in a restaurant or at home, or are a guest in someone else's home, follow these safety guidelines when you serve yourself:

- Never touch food that someone else will be eating.

- If a dip is served, dip a piece of food in the dip mixture just once. Try to take enough dip for the whole piece. If you need more dip for the piece you've already bitten, use a serving spoon and put some on a small, individual plate.

- Don't use your fingers to pick up and taste food as you make your selections.

Following Up

- What might you provide along with finger foods that people could use to safely transfer food to their own plates? What precautions should you take when you are preparing food and need to taste it for seasonings from time to time?

The Meal

Jorge was puzzled by the term *á la carte* on his restaurant menu. Instead of ordering and possibly making a mistake and not getting what he wanted, he asked his server to explain it.

◆ If the server takes care of the payment of the check, the money or credit card should be given to the server. Name two ways the tip can be handled in this situation.

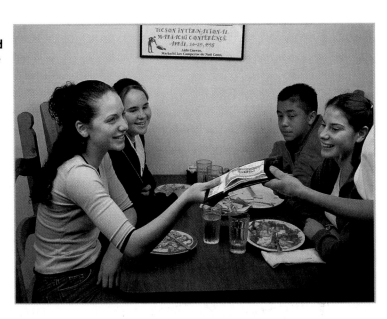

When dining out, don't be afraid to ask a few questions. This can be especially important when it comes to the restaurant's pricing policy. Sometimes the price of the entrée, or main dish, includes side dishes such as vegetables and salad. Other restaurants price each item individually. Knowing the policy can help you avoid an embarrassing and uncomfortable situation.

On occasion, each person in a group will want to pay for his or her own meal. If the group is small, ask the server for separate checks before you order. Alternatively—or if the restaurant's policy is to make out only one check for each table—you might ask the server to figure out the cost for each person.

Restaurants may serve more food than some people can eat. If you have leftover food, such as part of a steak or chicken, ask to have it wrapped up so that you can take it home. Most restaurants have special containers and supply them for diners. This does not apply to all-you-can-eat buffets or salad bars.

In fast-food restaurants, self-serve restaurants, and some delicatessens, customers are expected to clear their own tables after they've eaten. Trays and disposables are deposited in specified containers.

Communicating with Servers

Be polite to servers, whether in a fast-food or an elegant restaurant. Remember, they're working hard to serve you and a number of other people at the same time. Be considerate and patient, especially during busy periods.

To call your server, catch his or her attention by calmly raising your hand. If necessary, ask one of the other servers to get your server. Never call out or disturb other diners.

Paying the Check

At the meal's end, the server will bring you the check. In some restaurants you pay your server. In others you take the check to the cashier for payment. If you're not sure what to do, ask the server.

Look over the check carefully and add up the items. If there is a mistake, quietly point it out to the server. The server should correct any mistake or explain why the amount shown is right.

In most restaurants you are expected to leave a **gratuity** (grah-TOO-uh-tee). Also known as a "tip," this is extra money given to the server in appreciation for good service. Servers rely on tips as an important part of their pay. Sometimes the tip has been added in on the check. A standard amount to tip is 15 percent of the pretax food bill. The chart on the next page shows how much to leave depending on the type of restaurant and other circumstances.

How Much to Tip

Average	15 percent—more if service was exceptionally good.
Fancy restaurants	20 percent
Coffee shops	• No less than 25 cents if just a beverage was ordered. • If food is ordered, 15 percent of the bill or at least 50 cents, whichever amount is greater.
Buffet-type restaurant	10 percent if a server filled water glasses, brought beverages, and cleared the table.
Fast-food restaurants	No tip required.

Methods of Payment

When paying for a meal in cash, leave the money, including the tip, on the table or in the tray on which the check was presented. If you use a credit card, the server or cashier will process the card and hand you the credit card slip. Again, go over the math to be sure the totals are correct. The slip has a space for a tip. Fill in the amount, add the final total, sign the slip, and hand it back to the server or cashier. Be sure to get your copy of the credit card slip for your records—and don't forget the credit card.

Complaints and Compliments

If you have any complaints about the food, tell the server. If nothing is done, complain to the manager. You can also complain to the manager if the service was poor.

While people rarely hesitate to voice their complaints, few remember to express their appreciation for exceptional food and service. Compliments are just as important to the management as are complaints.

Section 10-2 Review & Activities

1. What is the importance of using good table manners?

2. Explain two ways of solving the problem of getting food onto your fork.

3. Describe two polite ways of calling your server to the table.

4. Analyzing. Why do you think a meal is part of many job interviews? What might an employer learn about a job applicant by his or her dining etiquette?

5. Evaluating. Which points covered in the lesson could help a person avoid an awkward or embarrassing situation? Explain.

6. Applying. With one or two classmates, write and perform a skit demonstrating at least three dining etiquette errors. Have the rest of the class identify the errors and offer suggestions to correct them.

CAREER WANTED

Individuals who communicate well and feel comfortable in a variety of social settings.

REQUIRES:

- degree in communications or human relations
- travel abroad

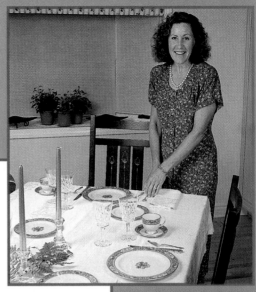

"Proper social behavior does make a difference,"

says Etiquette Consultant Terrie Tilghman

Q: Terrie, who hires an etiquette consultant?

A: Many businesses hire me to conduct workshops for their employees who travel abroad on business. They learn about proper table manners and dining customs in other cultures.

Q: What skills must someone have in order to provide this service?

A: It helps to be friendly and self-motivated, but the most important thing is being able to communicate with people in a tactful way. I remember how difficult it was when I first started out. Once I offended someone to whom I was trying to teach proper manners!

Q: How did you get started in this field?

A: I worked for six years in the human resources department of a large firm, where I fine-tuned my interpersonal communication skills. When the company was sold, I was laid off. My former supervisor suggested that I start my own business.

Career Research Activity

1. Find out more about the work done by an etiquette consultant. Then work in teams to role-play a training session among executives of an international company that has hired one of you as its etiquette consultant. Demonstrate the appropriate skills and methods used.

2. Search the classified ads of a local newspaper for openings that match any of the careers listed on the right. How many jobs are there? What is the salary range? Are any similar careers posted? How are they different? Does that impact the salary range?

Related Career Opportunities

Entry Level
- Restaurant Host or Hostess
- Recreation Leader

Technical Level
- Etiquette Consultant
- Travel Agent
- Personnel Director

Professional Level
- Family & Consumer Sciences Teacher
- Dietetics Researcher
- Foreign Diplomat

Chapter 10 Review & Activities

Summary

Section 10-1: Serving Family Meals

• Family meals are important for strengthening family bonds.

• Creating a pleasant mealtime atmosphere, including the table setting, helps make meals more enjoyable.

• A basic cover includes a dinner plate, fork, knife, teaspoon, and beverage glass. The items are arranged in a specific way based on tradition and convenience.

• Meals may be served using either family service or plate service.

Section 10-2: Mealtime Etiquette

• The purpose of table manners is to make eating a pleasant experience for everyone at the table.

• Rules of etiquette involve common sense and consideration for others.

• When dining in a restaurant, follow the accepted etiquette for making reservations, ordering and paying for the meal, and leaving a tip.

• Be courteous to food servers, and offer your compliments for good food service.

Checking Your Knowledge

1. Give three general guidelines for creating a pleasant mealtime atmosphere.

2. In what way are the components of a place setting for a formal meal different from those for an informal family meal?

3. Describe how to arrange a cover.

4. What are the advantages of plate service?

5. Name one advantage and one disadvantage of family service.

6. When dining with others, when may you begin to eat?

7. Give five examples of acceptable finger foods.

8. Explain the procedure for paying the bill and leaving a tip when paying with cash and by credit card.

9. How much should you tip food servers in an elegant restaurant? A buffet-style restaurant? A coffee shop?

10. If your food or service was poor, how should you register your complaint?

Working IN THE Lab

1. *Presentation.* Design and carry out a table setting, using items available in the foods lab or brought from home. Choose a specific meal and theme. Include table linens and decoration as well as all necessary tableware items in their proper places.

2. *Simulation.* Simulate a family meal using either family service or plate service. Include the proper arrangement of tableware, the rules of mealtime etiquette, and conversation that would contribute to a pleasant dining atmosphere.

3. *Demonstration.* Demonstrate rules of restaurant etiquette for one of the following situations: arriving at the restaurant and being seated; ordering and eating the meal; paying the bill and leaving the tip; registering a complaint or compliment with the manager.

Thinking Critically

1. **Identifying Cause and Effect.** How might eating family meals together affect family members' attitudes toward food and nutrition?

2. **Analyzing Behavior.** Suppose you and a friend are at a restaurant and see someone eating food in a manner that seems strange to you. Your friend thinks that person is either uneducated or deliberately rude. Is this a fair judgment? What are some possible explanations for the person's behavior?

Reinforcing Key Skills

1. **Communication.** Although your family often eats meals together, there is little conversation at the table. You would like to encourage family members to be more open and sharing at mealtime. How can you use your own communication skills to improve communication among family members?

2. **Leadership.** A friend is eating dinner with your family. She has made some etiquette mistakes that are embarrassing to her and your family. What steps can you take to put everyone at ease?

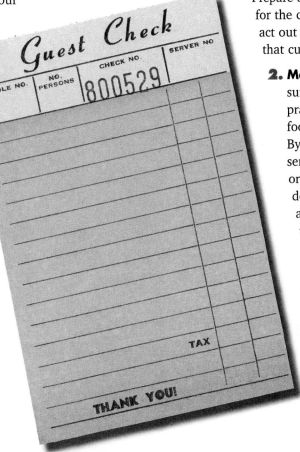

Making Decisions and Solving Problems

You are being considered for a job that you want very much. Your potential employer has asked you to lunch at a fancy restaurant. You are worried about making a good impression.

Making Connections

1. **Social Studies.** Use library resources to find information about table settings and mealtime etiquette in another culture. How are meals served? What is the proper way to eat the meal? Prepare a brief presentation for the class in which you act out a typical meal in that culture.

2. **Math.** Conduct a survey of tipping practices in local food establishments. By questioning servers, cashiers, or other personnel, determine the average percentage of tip that is left in each type of establishment. Create a bar graph comparing these percentages with the percentages suggested in this chapter.

UNIT
3

Consumer

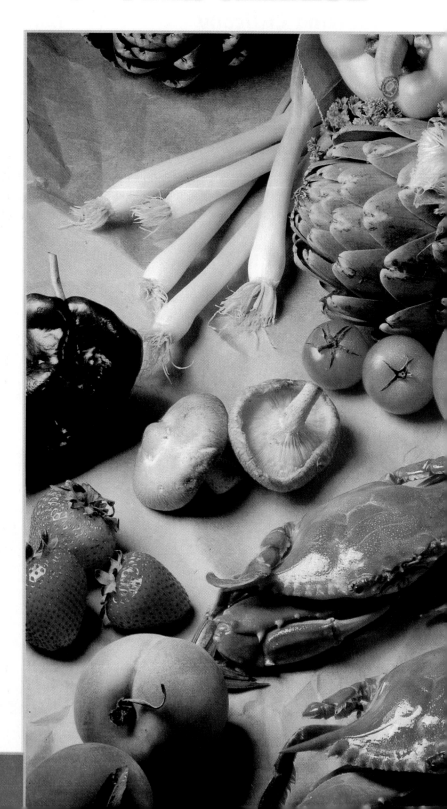

Decisions

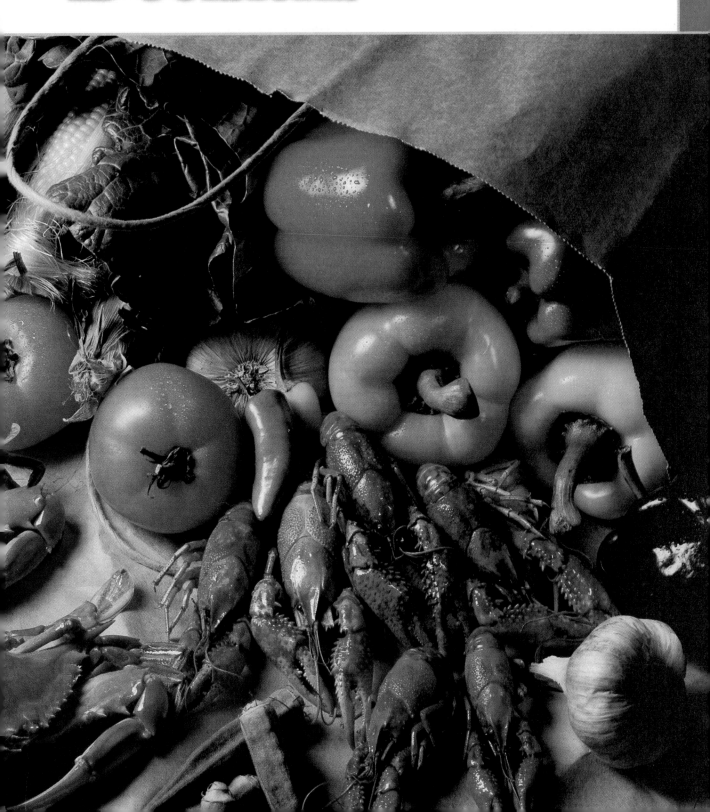

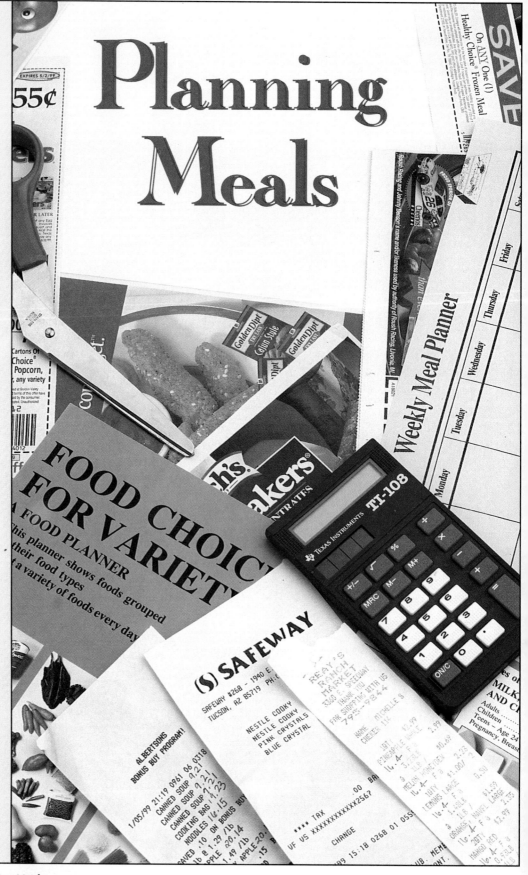

CHAPTER 11

Planning Meals

It was Li's turn to make dinner. With notepad in hand, she mapped out an ingredients list, a work plan, and a schedule. Within minutes, Li had built the foundation for a nutritious and delicious meal.

After reading this chapter, you—like Li—will know how to plan and produce healthful and delicious meals within a budget.

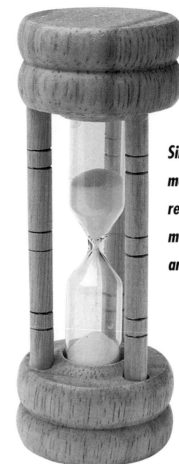

Objectives

After studying this section, you should be able to:

- Identify factors that affect meal planning.
- Describe characteristics that make meals appealing.
- Explain how to coordinate a work plan and schedule for preparing a meal.
- Discuss the benefits of weekly meal planning.

Look for These Terms

meal appeal

texture

Basic Meal Planning

Before you can play ice hockey, you must know how to skate. Similarly, before you can plan an entire meal, you need to know how to plan a recipe. Many of the skills involved in meal planning and recipe planning are the same.

Factors to Consider

Planning a meal involves making decisions about what foods to include and how to prepare them. As you begin to plan, keep in mind a number of factors. One is nutrition. Use what you have learned about the Dietary Guidelines and the Food Guide Pyramid to create healthful menus.

Another factor is how the meal fits in with the day's eating pattern. You might choose different foods for the main meal of the day than you would for a light lunch or supper. A third factor to think about is the people who will be eating the meal. What are their individual nutrition needs? What foods do they like and dislike? Are there certain foods that must be avoided for medical or other reasons? Finally, consider your resources. Good meal planning makes use of resource management.

```
┌─────────────────────────────┐
│        INFOLINK             │
├─────────────────────────────┤
│    For specific nutrition   │
│  recommendations found in   │
│   the Dietary Guidelines and│
│   Food Guide Pyramid, see   │
│     Sections 3-1 and 3-2.   │
└─────────────────────────────┘
```

Resources for Meals

What resources are involved in meal planning and preparation?

◆ **Time and energy.** If time or energy for meal preparation is limited, plan a meal that's simple to fix. You might look for a quick and easy recipe or think about using convenience foods along with fresh ones.

◆ **Food choices and availability.** Supermarkets offer an amazing variety of food. Still, your choices may be limited. Some foods are seasonal, especially fresh fruits. Your food store may not carry the items needed to prepare a special recipe. You might have to substitute an ingredient or choose another recipe.

◆ **Money.** Most people have a limited food budget. With careful planning, however, you can stretch your food dollars. You'll find helpful suggestions in Sections 11-3 and 12-3.

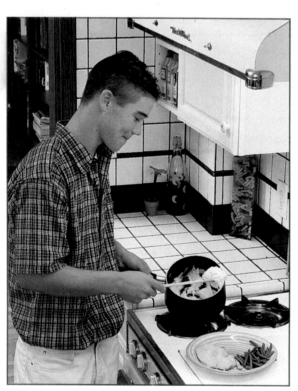

◆ **Preparation skills.** If you are just learning to cook, choose simple recipes that you can prepare with confidence. As you develop your skills, you can choose more complex recipes.

◆ **Equipment.** When you find a new recipe you think you might like, consider whether you have the necessary tools and equipment. If you don't, think about other items you might substitute. For example, a chicken stir-fry dish could be cooked in a skillet instead of a wok.

Using resources wisely often means making trade-offs. For instance, a microwave oven lets you use one resource (equipment) to save another (time). Cooking with convenience foods also saves time but may cost more than cooking meals from scratch. You must decide which is most important to you, time or money.

Meal Appeal

Usually, meal planning begins with choosing a main course. Then you add side dishes that will complement it.

When selecting a main course, think about **meal appeal**—the characteristics that make a meal appetizing and enjoyable. In particular, consider:

◆ **Color.** Think of your dinner plate as an artist's palette. Plan meals that include an array of colors. Colorful fruits and vegetables, for example, can help brighten any meal.

◆ **Shape and size.** Food is most appealing when the shapes and sizes vary. For example, cut carrots into strips and tomatoes into quarters. To vary the shape, chop, dice, cube, serve whole, or cut food with decorative cutters.

◆ With practice, you can plan meals that are simple and delicious. Identify two factors to think about when planning a meal.

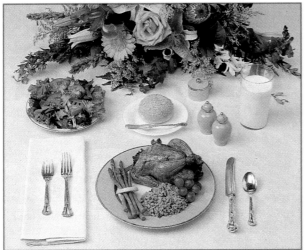
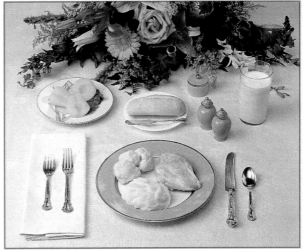

◆ **Planning for eye appeal is critical. Which of these two meals would you rather eat?**

◆ **Flavor and aroma.** Try to avoid using foods with similar flavors or aromas in one meal. If all the foods are strongly flavored—for example, spicy chili with garlic bread—the combination can clash. What type of bread would be better suited to this dish? Why?

◆ **Texture. Texture** is the way food feels when you chew it—for example, soft or hard, crisp or chewy. A meal should include a variety of textures. For example, with a soft main dish, such as pasta, you might serve a crisp tossed salad.

◆ **Temperature.** If you were planning lunch for a cold winter day, steaming hot soup would be more welcome than a chilled salad. Keep meal appeal in mind when you serve the food, too. Hot foods should be piping hot and cold foods crisply chilled. To be sure they stay that way, serve hot and cold foods on separate plates.

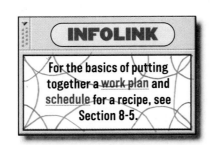

INFOLINK

For the basics of putting together a work plan and schedule for a recipe, see Section 8-5.

Planning a Meal

Drew's plan—to make a surprise Sunday brunch to celebrate his parents' wedding anniversary—started off well. In a magazine, he found a delicious-sounding recipe for French toast with a cherry topping. When his parents entered the kitchen, however, they found Drew fuming over burned food, an empty coffee pot, and still-frozen orange juice.

What went wrong? Drew didn't prepare a work plan and schedule. After deciding on his menu, Drew should have listed the basic steps in preparing each item. He should then have estimated the preparation and cooking time needed for each step, including the time needed for general tasks such as getting ready to cook and setting the table. Finally, Drew should have considered the best way to combine the separate tasks for each food into one plan for the meal by noting which tasks would take the most time.

As you make your work plan, remember to allow time for:

• Washing utensils and work surfaces to prevent cross-contamination.

• Returning perishable foods to the refrigerator or freezer.

• Cooking or chilling foods thoroughly.

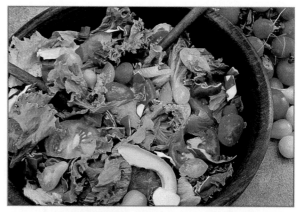

◆ **A tossed salad can be made ahead and refrigerated until mealtime. What other foods might be prepared in advance?**

Food Science ◆ L A B ◆

The Role of the Senses in Meal Appeal

What role do your senses play in your enjoyment of a meal? As you will see, the solution involves using not just your eyes, nose, and mouth but also your mind.

Procedure

1. Arrange nine different foods on a table. Ask each of three groups of volunteers to select three foods. Foods used in the experiment should range from fairly bland and colorless (for example, cottage cheese) to fairly spicy and bold (such as salsa).

2. Invite each group to arrange its three foods on a plate as attractively as possible. Then ask each group to smell the combined foods and, finally, to taste them.

3. Ask each group to rate the combinations from 1 to 5 in terms of sight, taste, and smell. Record the reactions.

Conclusions

◆ Which sense—sight, smell, or taste—appeared to play the greatest role in a group's reaction?

◆ Was variety a factor in the results? Explain.

◆ Repeat the experiment. This time carefully choose combinations for each group that have meal appeal. How, if at all, did the ratings differ?

A Meal Work Plan

A basic principle in any meal work plan is to start with the food that takes the longest time to prepare. Suppose you plan to bake chicken pieces in the oven for an hour. If the other foods will take less time, plan to get the chicken ready to bake first. Then you can work on other parts of the meal while the chicken is in the oven.

To cut down on last-minute tasks, consider whether foods can safely be prepared early. For instance, you could assemble a tossed salad (except for the dressing) and then put it in the refrigerator. Setting the table can also be done ahead of time, or you might plan on asking a helper to do it for you.

After you've decided on the sequence of steps in your work plan, figure out the total time needed. If the meal will take too long to prepare, think about changes that would help. For example, would chicken pieces cook faster than a whole chicken? Would changing to a different cooking method cut down on time?

A Meal Schedule

When you're satisfied with the work plan, you can use it to make a schedule for meal preparation. Decide what time you want to serve the meal. Count backward from that time to determine when you need to start preparation.

The work plan and schedule on page 318 show how the planning process could have prevented Drew's surprise brunch from turning into a catastrophe.

Weekly Meal Planning

Most people find it helpful to plan meals for a week or more at a time. Long-range planning has several advantages. It cuts down on anxiety and time spent on deciding what to serve every day. It promotes a greater variety of meals and helps you get the most for your food dollar. It decreases unneeded trips to the supermarket for forgotten items. It also makes food preparation more organized and efficient.

When planning a week's worth of meals, use what you have already learned about planning menus. Here are some additional tips:

- Aim for balanced nutrition and variety in meals and snacks over the course of the week. Check to see that the menus for each day provide enough servings from the Food Guide Pyramid.

- Set aside a regular time and place for meal planning.

- Ask family members about their plans for the week. Knowing when family members need to eat early, late, or away from home can affect the menus and recipes you choose.

- Check the refrigerator, freezer, and kitchen cabinets to see what foods you have on hand. Think of ways to use these foods (especially perishables, such as leftovers and fresh fruits and vegetables).

- Check newspaper ads to see what foods are on sale.

- Plan nutritious snacks as well as meals.

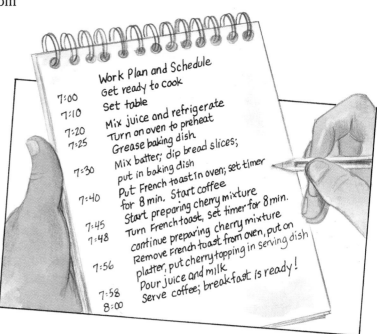

Work Plan and Schedule

7:00	Get ready to cook
	Set table
7:10	Mix juice and refrigerate
7:20	Turn on oven to preheat
7:25	Grease baking dish
	Mix batter; dip bread slices;
7:30	put in baking dish
	Put French toast in oven; set timer
7:40	for 8 min. Start coffee
	Start preparing cherry mixture
7:45	Turn French toast, set timer for 8 min.
7:48	continue preparing cherry mixture
	Remove French toast from oven, put on
7:56	platter; put cherry topping in serving dish
	Pour juice and milk
7:58	Serve coffee; breakfast is ready!
8:00	

Work Plan and Schedule

Task	Preparation Time	Cooking Time
General Tasks:		
Get ready to cook.	10 min.	
Set table.	10 min.	
Oven French Toast:		
Preheat oven.		15 min.
Grease baking dish.	5 min.	
Mix egg batter; dip bread slices in batter; put in baking dish.	10 min.	
Bake on first side.		8 min.
Turn and bake on other side.		8 min.
Glazed Cherry Topping:		
Open canned cherries; put in saucepan; mix cornstarch and water and add to cherries.	5 min.	
Cook cherry mixture as directed in recipe.		4-6 min.
Orange Juice:		
Mix frozen concentrate in pitcher; refrigerate.	5 min.	
Coffee:		
Prepare in coffeemaker.	5 min.	15 min.
Serving Tasks:		
Put food in serving dishes.	2 min.	
Pour beverages.	2 min.	

Time	Task
9:00	Get ready to cook.
9:10	Set table.
9:20	Mix juice and refrigerate.
9:25	Turn on oven to preheat. Grease baking dish.
9:30	Mix batter; dip bread slices; put in baking dish.
9:40	Put French toast in oven; set timer for 8 min. Start coffee.
9:45	Start preparing cherry mixture.
9:48	Turn French toast; set timer for 8 min. Continue preparing cherry mixture.
9:56	Remove French toast from oven; put on platter; put cherry topping in serving dish.
9:58	Pour juice and milk.
10:00	Serve coffee; brunch is ready!

Once you have the menus for the week, you can use them to make your shopping list. As you will learn in Chapter 12, a shopping list can help you manage money as well as time.

When you first try it, planning a week's worth of meals may seem time-consuming. However, it becomes easier with practice. Once you have planned meals for several months, you can use them over and over again. In the long run, weekly planning is well worth the initial investment of time.

Sample Weekly Menu Plan

	Breakfast	Lunch	Dinner	Snacks	Memos

MONDAY	Bran Cereal
	Sliced Bananas
	Rye Toast
	Milk/Coffee
		(Packed)
		Turkey
		  Sandwich
		Carrot/Celery
		  Sticks
		Pretzels
		Apple
		Milk (buy)
			Spaghetti and
			  Meatballs
			Tossed Salad
			Garlic Bread
			Milk/Coffee
			Italian Ice
				Fresh Fruits or
				  Vegetables
				Trail Mix
				Cranberry Juice
					Krystal—not
					home for
					dinner, swim
					team banquet.

TUESDAY	French Toast
	Kiwi Halves
	Milk/Coffee
		(Packed)
		Peanut
		  Butter–Whole
		  Wheat
		  Sandwich
		Broccoli/Carrots
		Pear
		Milk (buy)
			Beans and Rice
			Corn Tortillas
			Spinach Salad
			Milk/Coffee
			Sliced Fruit
				Fresh Fruits or
				  Vegetables
				Popcorn
				Vegetable Juice
					Everyone home
					for dinner.

WEDNESDAY	Bagels with
	  Nonfat
	  Cream
	  Cheese
	Orange Slices
	Milk/Coffee
		Mom and
		  Dad—lunch
		  out
		Jason and
		  Krystal—
		  school lunch
			Baked Chicken
			Brown Rice
			Broccoli Spears
			Whole Wheat
			  Rolls
			Coleslaw
			Milk/Coffee
				Fresh Fruits or
				  Vegetables
				Pretzels
					Dad—late for
					dinner, grocery
					shopping after
					work.

THURSDAY	Oatmeal with
	  Raisins
	Whole Wheat
	  Toast
	Milk/Coffee
		(Packed)
		Leftover
		  Chicken
		  Sandwiches
		Carrot/Celery
		  Sticks
		Banana
		Milk (buy)
			Spicy Chili with
			  Beans
			Cornbread
			Tossed Salad
			Milk
				Popcorn
				Strawberry
				  Frozen
				  Yogurt
					Jason's
					basketball
					game—eat
					early.

Sample Weekly Menu Plan (cont'd)

	Breakfast	Lunch	Dinner	Snacks	Memos
FRIDAY	Assorted Cereals Bananas Whole Wheat Toast with Fruit Spread Milk/Coffee	(Packed) Leftover Chili Red and Green Pepper Sticks Corn Chips Mixed Fruit Cup Milk (buy)	Take-out Pizza Tossed Salad Mixed Fruit Juice	Fresh Fruits with Plain Yogurt Brownie	Jason—eating out with friends.
SATURDAY	Scrambled Eggs Bacon Whole Wheat Toast Orange Juice Milk/Coffee	Hearty Vegetable Soup Corn Muffin Fruit Milk	Grilled Burgers with Buns Potato Salad Sliced Tomatoes Milk/Coffee	Popcorn Flavored Yogurt Mixed Fruit Juice	Rob and Kara coming over for dinner.
SUNDAY	Bran Muffins Grapefruit Milk/Coffee	Baked Ham Sweet Potatoes Broccoli Fruit Salad Milk Angel Food Cake	Sandwiches or Leftover Pizza Coleslaw	Fresh Fruits or Vegetables Rice Cakes	Plan next week's menus.

Section 11-1 Review & Activities

1. Identify six factors that affect your decisions when planning meals.

2. What is meal appeal?

3. What is the first step in making a work plan for a meal?

4. Evaluating. Do you think it is necessary to make a work plan and schedule for every meal? Why or why not? What are the pros and cons of doing so?

5. Comparing and Contrasting. Make a Venn diagram showing how energy, time, and money management are related in meal planning.

6. Applying. Plan a basic meal for you and your family. Develop a work plan and schedule for preparing this meal. If possible, proceed with the preparation; then write about the experience in your Wellness Journal.

Challenges in Meal Planning

Serena's mother has a full-time job and her brother plays several school sports. With Serena's own busy schedule, it is anyone's guess which family members will be home for dinner!

Situations like this one are a real challenge to meal planning. A busy lifestyle, however, does not have to interfere with enjoying nutritious, tasty foods. In this section, you will learn about ways of dealing with the challenges of meal planning.

Objectives

After studying this section, you should be able to:

- Identify meal planning strategies for families with busy schedules.
- Give suggestions for planning meals for one person.
- Discuss ways to handle unexpected changes in mealtime plans.

Look for This Term

versatility

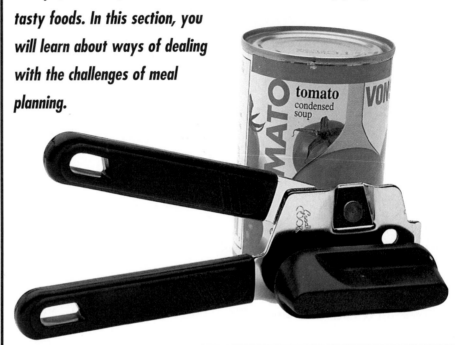

Busy Schedules

"There's no time to cook—but I'm tired of frozen dinners and take-out food!" Does this sound familiar? When everyone is busy with work, school, and other activities, finding time for home-prepared meals may seem difficult. With planning and ingenuity, however, you can find ways to solve this problem.

Start by holding a family meeting to decide who will be responsible for food tasks such as planning, shopping, cooking, and cleaning up. You may want to rotate these responsibilities from week to week. If family schedules are

hectic but predictable, planning at least a week's worth of meals at a time can also help.

Here are some additional suggestions:

- Start a collection of healthful, quick recipes that fit your busy lifestyle. Put them where they can be found easily.

- Learn more about the microwave oven. It can be used for much more than heating leftovers and convenience foods.

- Make use of one-dish meals, which are often easier to prepare than a main dish with separate side dishes.

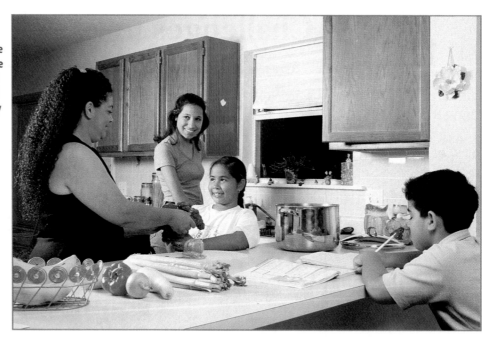

◆ **A busy lifestyle can influence a person's cooking style.** What are some ways in which the skills of teamwork and leadership can be used to help organize family chores in the kitchen?

◆ Look for ways to combine convenience foods with fresh foods in recipes and meals.

◆ Learn how to "cook for the freezer." When preparing a recipe, double or triple it and freeze the extra. Some families make cooking for the freezer a weekend project.

◆ Look for recipes with **versatility**—the capability of being adapted to many uses. For instance, Janice has a recipe for a basic seasoned meat-and-bean mixture, which can be used in a variety of recipes, such as chili, burritos, and taco salad. She prepares a large amount of the mixture and freezes it in recipe-size quantities to use in different ways.

➕ Safety Check

Freezing extra portions of food is a good idea for people with busy schedules. Be careful, however, when thawing frozen food. The safest way to thaw it is slowly in the refrigerator. If you need the item in a hurry, thaw it in the microwave and cook it immediately.

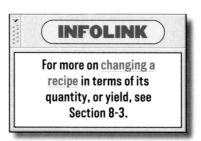

INFOLINK

For more on changing a recipe in terms of its quantity, or yield, see Section 8-3.

Unpredictable Schedules

When family members have varied schedules, it's not always possible for everyone to sit down to a meal together. Here are some ideas for flexible meals:

◆ Plan meals that can be cooked early and refrigerated or frozen. Include instructions on how to assemble or reheat.

◆ Prepare one-dish meals in a slow cooker. Family members can help themselves as time permits.

◆ Set up a "breakfast bar" near the refrigerator with assorted cereals, bowls, spoons, and glasses. Keep milk, juice, and fresh fruit on one refrigerator shelf within easy reach.

Meals for One

Shopping for food and preparing meals for one person is another challenge that requires thought, planning, and creativity. Most recipes provide four, six, or even eight servings, and not all can be decreased easily. Small sizes of packaged foods may be hard to find or expensive. Buying and preparing large quantities of food can result in a person eating the same food day after day.

One suggestion for getting around this problem is buying bulk foods in just the quantity needed. Another option is sharing large food packages—or even meals—with a friend. Still another is storing as many foods as possible in single-serving packages. For example, a pound of ground meat might be divided into four patties that can be separately wrapped and frozen.

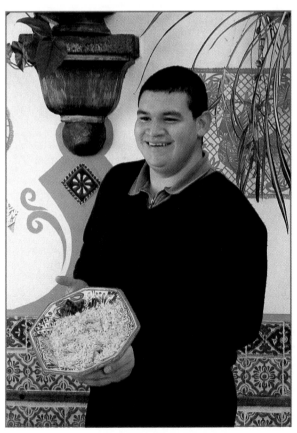

FOR YOUR HEALTH

Table for One

With increasing numbers of people marrying later or not marrying at all, more and more Americans are living "the single life." Is it possible to plan and prepare healthful meals for one person? The answer is yes. Here are some strategies for eating well and alone:

- To ensure that the foods you buy stay fresh, ask store managers for small packages of produce and meat items. For example, a whole watermelon could be cut in half or quarters.

- Consider buying small portions of salad ingredients at the supermarket salad bar if one is available. This option may seem more costly, but you'll have less waste.

Following Up

- Which of the strategies recommended above would also help a single person avoid the tendency to overeat? Explain your answer.

Some singles slip into poor eating habits because they neglect to plan for and prepare nutritious meals. Cooking and cleaning up a meal may not seem worth the effort for just one person. Here again, management skills can help. The suggestions already given for busy lifestyles can help make meal preparation easier for single people, too.

Even when dining alone, singles should attempt to make mealtime special. Setting an attractive table and enjoying a relaxing meal can be a satisfying and healthful end to a busy day.

◆ Simple one-dish meals such as arroz con pollo—a flavorful blend of seasoned rice and chicken—can save time. What are four other ways of working preparation into a busy schedule?

When Plans Must Change

Life can be unpredictable. Sometimes it becomes necessary to change plans. You may not get home in time to prepare the meal you had planned. Illness or last-minute schedule changes can also disrupt meals.

To prepare for these times, keep a supply of "backup" foods on hand. Stock up on nutritious, quick-to-prepare foods that are shelf-stable or freezer-ready. Some basic items to consider are nonfat dry milk; canned chicken, tuna, and salmon; canned beans; and frozen portions of cooked dry beans, rice, and pasta. Set aside a few recipes or menus planned around your backup foods. If the unexpected happens, you'll be prepared.

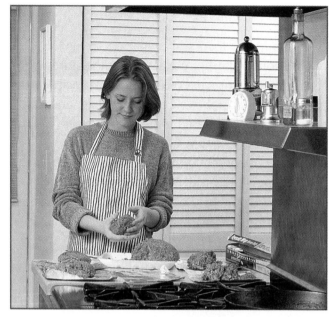

◆ Larger packages of meat, which are often more economical, can be divided into single-serving portions and stored in the freezer. Give two other suggestions that people cooking for one might use to plan meals.

INFOLINK

For more on shelf-stable foods and how to store them, see Section 7-4.

Section 11-2 Review & Activities

1. What is meant by "cooking for the freezer"? How can it help families whose members lead busy lives?

2. Give three suggestions singles can use to plan and prepare meals.

3. Analyzing. Suppose a cousin of yours has just started living on her own. Which of the suggestions in this section might be most helpful to her? Why?

4. Extending. Johnna doesn't like to cook, but her mother told her to prepare her own dinner two nights a week. Offer suggestions to Johnna for meals she could prepare that would be enjoyable to make and to eat.

5. Applying. Plan an "emergency" meal for you and your family using foods that can be kept on hand. Evaluate the meal for nutrition and appeal.

RECIPE FILE

Fresh 'n' Fast Fried Rice

This tasty recipe combines fresh and convenience foods for families in a hurry.

Customary	Ingredients	Metric
3	Eggs	3
2 tsp.	Vegetable oil	10 mL
2 tsp.	Vegetable oil	10 mL
4 cups	Cooked rice, chilled	1 L
1 cup	Reduced-sodium chicken broth	250 mL
1 cup	Frozen green peas, thawed	250 mL
⅓ cup	Diced red pepper	75 mL
1 cup	Canned bean sprouts, drained	250 mL
⅓ cup	Chopped green onions	75 mL

Yield: Six 1-cup (250-ml) servings

Directions

1. In a small bowl, beat the eggs until well combined.
2. In a large, nonstick skillet or wok, heat 2 tsp. vegetable oil over medium heat. Add the eggs and cook, stirring occasionally, for 2 to 5 minutes or until eggs are set. Remove eggs to a bowl and set it aside.
3. Heat the remaining 2 tsp. oil over medium-high heat. Add the rice and stir-fry 5 minutes.
4. Add the remaining ingredients and the cooked eggs, and stir-fry a final 2 minutes.
5. Season as desired, or serve with sodium-reduced soy sauce.

Nutrition Information

Per serving (approximate): 207 calories, 8 g protein, 29 g carbohydrate, 6 g fat, 106 mg cholesterol, 188 mg sodium, 2 g fiber
Good source of: iron, vitamin E, vitamin C, B vitamins

Food for Thought

- Could you prepare this recipe for one person? Which ingredients would be the most difficult to divide by 6?
- Name at least two time-saving suggestions for preparing this recipe.

Food Costs and Budgeting

One day at the supermarket, Myra overheard a couple talking about the price of food. "Food has gotten so expensive. Many of the foods our family likes just cost too much anymore." Myra started to wonder how the cost of food fits into her own family's food budget.

Objectives

After studying this section, you should be able to:

- Identify reasons food spending varies from family to family.

- Describe how using a food budget can help control spending on food.

- Identify programs that offer food assistance to individuals and families in need.

Look for These Terms

budget

WIC program

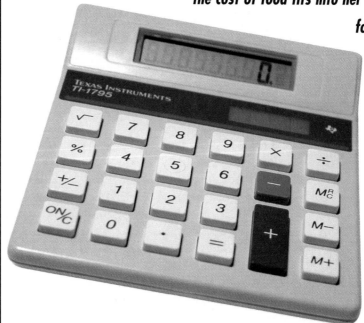

Why Budget?

A **budget** is a plan for managing your money in order to cover the costs of life's necessities. Budgeting involves looking at your income and deciding how much money to set aside for food, housing, clothing, transportation, health care, savings, and other uses.

Food expenses make up a significant portion of most family and personal budgets. For example, an average middle-income family spends about 15 percent of the family income on food. A lower-income family may spend a greater percentage on food simply because the total income amount is less. The challenge for any family is meeting nutrient needs without spending more than the budget allows.

Factors Affecting Food Expenditures

The amount of money spent on food varies according to your personal or family resources, goals, and priorities. Other factors that affect the amount of money a family spends on food include:

- Total family income.

- The number of family members. The larger a family is, the more it will need to spend.

- The age of family members. It costs more to feed growing teens than other members. By the same token, it costs less to feed aging relatives who may be part of the household.

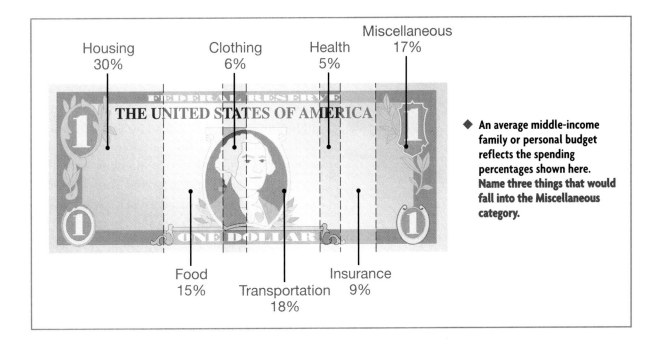

Housing
30%

Clothing
6%

Health
5%

Miscellaneous
17%

THE UNITED STATES OF AMERICA

◆ An average middle-income family or personal budget reflects the spending percentages shown here. Name three things that would fall into the Miscellaneous category.

Food
15%

Transportation
18%

Insurance 9%

◆ Food prices in your area at various times of the year.

◆ The amount of food eaten away from home.

◆ Time and skills available for food preparation.

◆ The amount of food wasted. Food waste may occur if a food was not stored or prepared properly.

If someone in your family enjoys cooking, you might spend less money by eating more home-prepared meals. However, if busy schedules make convenience a family priority, you may spend more money on convenience foods. Every family has different priorities, so food budgets will vary.

Using a Food Budget

Whether you spend a little or a lot, you can benefit from following a food budget. It can show you whether you may be wasting money—or spending it wisely. It can also help you think about your food choices and determine whether they are wise ones.

Keeping a Spending Record

Setting up a food budget is simple. To begin, analyze how much you spend on food now. Keep a record of all the food you buy for two typical weeks. Divide your record into food bought at the food store and food eaten out. Food eaten out includes take-out food, delivered food, and foods bought from vending machines. Do not include nonfood supplies in your list, such as paper products, even if you buy them at the supermarket.

Add up the expenses for groceries and foods eaten out for the two weeks. Divide the total by two to get the average you spend per week.

Setting a Budget Amount

Use the information from your spending record when you plan your budget. What percentage of your income are you spending on food? Are you comfortable with the amount you are currently spending? If so, plan to spend a similar amount in future weeks. If you want to plan on spending less, set an amount that's slightly lower. Be realistic. If you set an amount

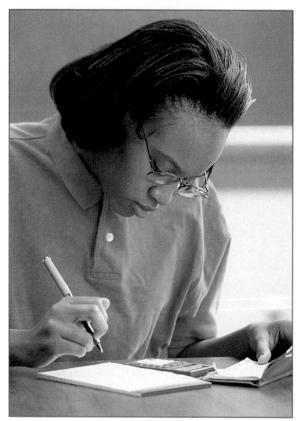

◆ Keeping track of your food spending for a period of time helps you decide on a realistic amount for your food budget. **Why is it important to set a realistic food budget?**

that's unrealistically low, you'll find it hard to stay within your budget.

Sticking with Your Budget

Once you've set an amount for your food budget, stay within those guidelines. Continue keeping records of how much you spend on groceries and foods eaten out. You will likely spend more some weeks than others, such as when you buy staples or special items. If you have any money left over, keep it as a reserve in your food budget for emergencies.

Evaluating the Food Budget

After you have used your budget for several weeks, take a look at what you've spent. On the

average, were you able to stay within your budget? If you were not, you have two options —increase the amount budgeted or reduce your spending.

Use your spending record to evaluate your food purchases. If you made only basic purchases—with no "frills"—and you haven't eaten out, you may not be allowing enough money for food. Take a look at your budget again. Perhaps you can cut back in some other spending category to allow more money for food.

On the other hand, you may decide that you are spending more than you would like on food. If so, planning and money management can help you reduce your spending.

Reducing Your Spending

You can save money even before you begin spending it by planning your meals with your budget in mind. Here are some helpful tips to guide you:

◆ **Look for supermarket advertisements.** Newspaper ads and flyers can tell you about special prices on nutritious foods that your family can enjoy. Compare prices among stores.

◆ **Choose economical main dishes.** Meat can be an expensive part of a meal. You can save money by serving more beans with grains and other plant-based protein foods. If you want to include meat, fish, or poultry in meals, use a smaller amount in combination with vegetables, grains, and fruits.

◆ **Reduce food waste.** As you plan meals, think about how much your family eats. Prepare appropriate amounts of food for each meal. Safely store any leftovers for future use. Practice portion control when serving the food.

- **Prepare simple meals at home more often.** Homemade meals can cost less than convenience meals or food eaten out. Your family may find it worthwhile to take the extra time needed to prepare meals at home. Sharing meal preparation tasks can cut down on preparation time and bring family members closer together.

- **Allow some flexibility in meal planning.** Be ready to take advantage of good prices on items such as seasonal fresh fruits and vegetables. When it's in season, fresh produce is often less expensive—and may taste better.

- **Choose less expensive forms of food.** Compare prices between different forms of foods (fresh, frozen, canned, dried) to find the best buy. Lower cost doesn't mean lower nutritional value or less flavor.

Careful shoppers find ways of getting more for less. In Chapter 12, you will learn more about shopping practices and techniques that can save you money when you shop for food.

Food Assistance Programs

Some people may not have enough money to pay for the necessities of life, including food. They may be retired or living on a low or limited income. They may be too ill to work or unable to find a job.

Help is available from a variety of valuable sources. Federal, state, and local governments, along with many private organizations, have food assistance programs for those who cannot afford to buy enough food.

- **Aid for low-income families.** Depending on income and family size, some low-income households qualify for assistance in the form of food stamps or an Electronic Benefits Transfer (EBT) card. Both are issued by the USDA. These forms of assistance are limited to essential food purchases. They cannot be used for non-food items, tobacco, or alcohol. They also can't be used for restaurant meals, take-out foods, and pet foods.

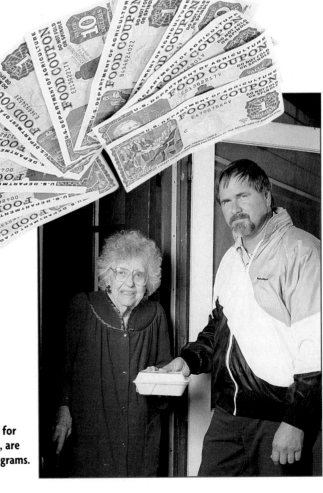

- Food stamps and nutrition programs for the elderly, such as meals-on-wheels, are two examples of food assistance programs. Name two others.

- **National School Lunch Program.**
  Low-income students may qualify to receive free or reduced-price meals. Some schools also offer school breakfast programs. Nonprofit food services in elementary schools, secondary schools, and residential child care centers receive government surplus foods and some cash to provide for children in need. In some areas, the Summer Food Service Program provides breakfast and lunch during summer vacation.

- **Child and Adult Care Food Program.**
  Cash and food assistance are provided to child and adult care centers and family day care homes. The program operates similarly to the National School Lunch Program.

- **WIC Program.** The **WIC** (Women, Infants, and Children) **program** is a government-sponsored program designed to improve the health of low-income pregnant and breast-feeding women, infants, and children up to five years of age. Supplemental foods, nutrition education, and access to health services are provided. Participants receive vouchers that can be used at retail food stores for specified nutrient-rich foods.

- **Elderly Nutrition Program (ENP).**
  This program provides grant money for meals served to aging citizens. Meals are served to the homes of qualifying individuals, community centers, and care facilities for the aging population.

- **Soup kitchens and food banks.** These services—run by religious groups as well as private organizations—provide food for people in need of meals or food assistance.

If you know of anyone in need of food assistance, let him or her know of the food programs available in your area. You can get details by calling local government agencies, such as social services and public health nursing services. While you're collecting information, ask about any opportunities for volunteering. Helping at a soup kitchen or food bank can be a rewarding experience.

Section 11-3 Review & Activities

1. Identify four factors that affect how much families spend on food.

2. What is the benefit of keeping a food budget?

3. Give five suggestions for reducing food spending through wise meal planning.

4. Interpreting. What factors do you think account for people spending more for food than they would like to spend?

5. Analyzing. Shannon's husband was laid off from his job three months ago, and the family of five is having trouble affording food. Shannon has told her husband about food assistance programs in their community, but he says he is "too proud to take charity." Identify three points Shannon can make to persuade her husband to change his mind.

6. Applying. Imagine that you have only $5 to spend on a meal for a family of four. Choosing foods from newspaper ads and store flyers, plan the meal and compute the cost.

CAREER WANTED

Individuals who listen well, are full of compassion, and desire to help a wide range of people.

REQUIRES:
- degree in social work, psychology, or related field
- prior experience in field of social work

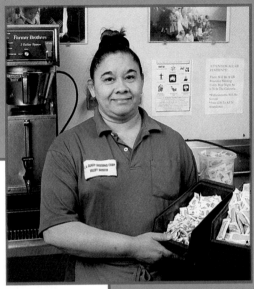

"No one should go to bed hungry,"
says Social Services Worker Marilyn Lakota

Q: What is your biggest challenge as a social services worker in an urban area?

A: I suppose it's managing my emotions. Some of my cases are heartbreaking. I see children who look as though they haven't eaten in weeks. I also find it tough dealing with pregnant teens who have run away from home.

Q: What is your biggest responsibility?

A: Keeping aware of changes in state and federal funding guidelines is challenging. I am lucky to have prior job experience with government agencies.

Q: What is a typical day like for you at work?

A: There is no typical day. That's what I like so much about my work. I spend some time in the office, where I supervise staff and meet with a wide range of clients with different needs. I also teach classes on nutrition for pregnant women at a nearby community college.

Q: Do you find your job satisfying?

A: It is particularly satisfying to me. I can help a baby get a better start in life by teaching his mother about good nutrition. My job is actually my mission in life—to help people.

Career Research Activity

1. Research one career from each of the levels listed on the right. Then write an original short story about someone who has moved along that particular career pathway. Your story should contain factual information about each career.

2. Contact the local American Red Cross to find out about career opportunities involving community social work. Write a poem, song, or short essay about why you would or would not be interested in a career in social services.

Related Career Opportunities

Entry Level
- Administrative Assistant
- Social Services Aide
- Candystriper

Technical Level
- Licensed Practical Nurse
- Legislative Reporter

Professional Level
- Social Services Worker
- Welfare Director
- Penologist

Chapter 11 Review & Activities

Summary

Section 11-1: Basic Meal Planning

- When you plan meals, consider nutrition, eating patterns, individual needs and preferences, and your resources.

- Meals should appeal to all the senses.

- Having a work plan and schedule for preparing a meal allows you to have all the foods ready at the same time. Good management skills are also important.

- Weekly meal planning can help you use your resources wisely.

Section 11-2: Challenges in Meal Planning

- Many individuals and families in today's fast-paced society face challenges in meal planning.

- A variety of solutions are available for meeting the challenges of preparing meals for families with busy schedules or for one person.

- On days when plans change at the last minute, a supply of "backup" foods can be helpful.

Section 11-3: Food Costs and Budgeting

- Food expenses make up a significant portion of most family and personal budgets.

- The amount of money spent on food depends on the family's situation and composition.

- A spending record and food budget can help you determine whether you are making wise food-buying choices.

- Planning and money management can help reduce food spending.

- A number of food assistance programs are available to help people with low or limited incomes.

Checking Your Knowledge

1. How do food choices and availability affect meal planning?

2. Name four elements of meal appeal.

3. Give two suggestions for deciding the sequence in which to prepare the foods in a meal.

4. Name three things you should find out before preparing a weekly meal plan.

5. Give three suggestions to help families with busy schedules plan meals.

6. List two suggestions to help single people avoid buying larger quantities than they need.

7. Give three examples of foods to keep on hand for meals when plans change at the last minute.

8. What is the first step in setting up a food budget?

9. How can flexibility in meal planning help you save money?

10. What services are provided by the WIC Program? For whom are they provided?

Thinking Critically

1. Determining Accuracy. Gilberto is planning to buy his aunt a cookbook for her birthday. In the cookbook section of a bookstore, he sees a book with a colorful, eye-catching cover and the title *The Anything Goes Guide to Cooking*. The preface to the book states that "Cooking should first and foremost be fun. Forget all that stodgy advice about shopping lists and preliminaries. Just go into the kitchen and let your creativity be your guide! That's what the best chefs do." What would you advise Gilberto to do before he decides whether or not to buy this book? Explain.

2. Recognizing Stereotypes. You overhear a student in your school saying that people who use food assistance programs are simply too lazy or stupid to get decent jobs to support themselves. How do you respond?

Working IN THE Lab

1. *Foods Lab.* Prepare a work plan and schedule for a simple meal. Use them when preparing the meal in the foods lab. Evaluate how well your schedule worked. What would you change before preparing the same meal again?

2. *Foods Lab.* Write the menu for a meal that you might purchase from a restaurant or supermarket deli. Find or create recipes to prepare these foods yourself. Estimate the price difference between the purchased meal and the homemade meal. If possible, prepare the meal and compare it with the purchased version.

Reinforcing Key Skills

1. Management. The main ingredients of your family's favorite chicken-rice casserole are cooked rice, diced chicken, cream soup, and shredded Swiss cheese. Usually it is served with dinner rolls and with pie for dessert. You want to increase the meal's nutritional value and appeal. Before you can adapt the meal, what information would you need to have?

2. Communication. Delaine and her parents do most of the family's meal planning and preparation. She would like to get her seven-year-old brother and ten-year-old sister interested and involved as well. What solutions can you propose to Delaine?

Making Decisions and Solving Problems

You know that one family in your neighborhood is on a very strict budget and has been skimping on food to make ends meet. You would like to help, but you don't want to offend them.

Making Connections

1. Social Studies. Using library or online resources, prepare a report on meal planning in other cultures, such as Asian or Middle Eastern. How do cultural differences (family structure, tradition, available foods, and so on) affect how and when meals are prepared and served?

2. Math. Keep a record of your spending for one week. Figure out what percentage of your weekly spending goes toward food. Combine your findings with those of your classmates to find the average percentage for the class.

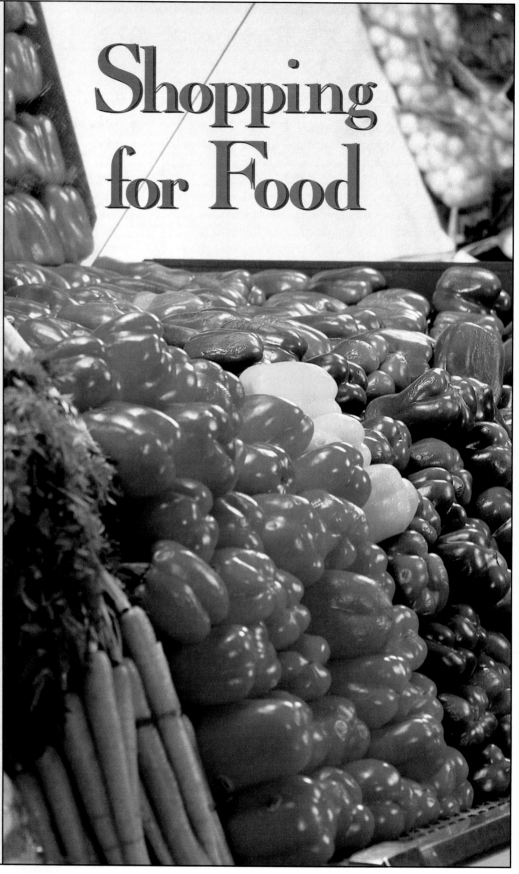

The food you buy is the foundation for the meals you prepare. Wise food shopping can save time and money and ensure nutritious meals.

In this chapter, you will learn how to be a successful food shopper. Learning the basic logic behind food labels, as you will discover, is one of the keys.

Objectives

After studying this section, you should be able to:

- Give guidelines for planning where and when to shop.
- Explain the benefits of preparing a shopping list.
- Discuss ways to make the best use of coupons.

Look for These Terms

food cooperatives

impulse buying

staples

rebate

Before You Shop

Like many other activities, successful food shopping begins with planning. As an informed consumer, you need to ask yourself these questions: Where should I shop? When is the best time to go? Should I make a shopping list? Although these questions may seem basic and obvious, answering them, as you will see, is an important decision-making process.

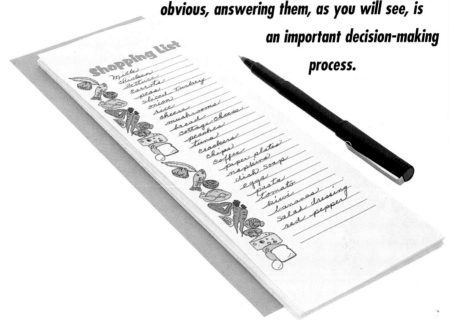

Where to Shop

You can buy food at several kinds of food stores. Each has its pluses and minuses. Your choice will depend on your own needs and wants.

♦ **Supermarkets.** Large stores that sell not only food but also many other items and services. Some have as many as 20,000 different food items. Most supermarkets offer a variety of customer services. In a large, busy supermarket, you may find it difficult to buy just a few items in a hurry.

♦ **Warehouse stores.** Offer basic items with few customer services. As a result, prices are lower than in most supermarkets. Although most warehouse stores are large, they have a limited variety of items. Items are usually displayed in cartons rather than on shelves. Shoppers must bag their own groceries and carry them out.

♦ **Food cooperatives.** Another low-cost option. **Food cooperatives** are food distribution organizations mutually owned and operated by a group of people. Members buy food in quantity and do the sorting, unloading, and other work themselves.

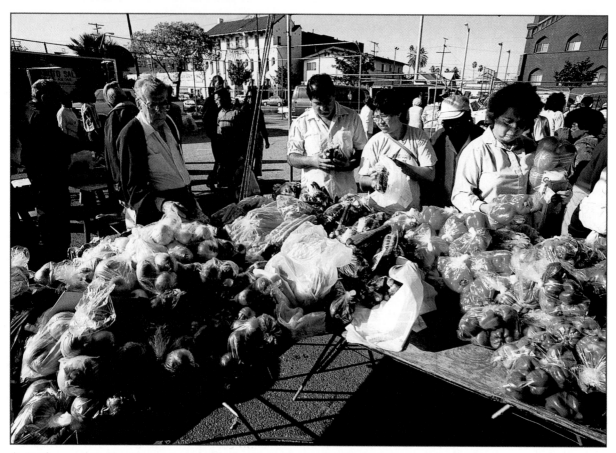

◆ Outdoor markets like this one are cost-effective alternatives to shopping in more conventional settings. What priorities besides cost need to be considered when shopping for food?

Doing these things helps keep costs down. Some cooperatives are licensed to sell to the public as well as to members.

◆ **Health food stores.** Offer a wide range of foods, including items seldom found elsewhere. Foods are likely to be more expensive, however, than in other stores.

◆ **Specialty stores.** Limited to specific items, such as fish, meat, baked goods, delicatessen foods, or ethnic foods. Prices are usually higher than in supermarkets. In return, customers may get personal attention and fast service. Specialty stores may also carry food items, such as ethnic staples, not readily found elsewhere.

◆ **Convenience stores.** Give fast service and usually open early and close late. Some stay open around the clock. Their small size makes it easy to shop quickly, but they do not carry a full line of groceries. Prices are generally higher than in supermarkets.

◆ **Farmer's markets.** Also known as greengrocers. Specialize in fresh fruits and vegetables. The selection depends on the area and the season. You may find locally grown foods that are fresher and less expensive than those in the supermarket. Some markets are closed during cold-weather months.

How to Decide

What should you consider when choosing a place to shop? First, be sure the store is clean. Next, consider your priorities. What kinds of food do you shop for most often? How far will you travel to shop? Are you willing to give up some services in exchange for lower prices?

If time is a priority, you may want to do most of your shopping at one store. That way, you can become familiar with the location of the items and spend less time shopping.

Some stores use promotions, such as giveaways, special prices, or discount clubs for frequent shoppers, to attract customers. When choosing a place to shop, consider whether these promotions will actually save you money. You may find you can save as much or more by shopping at a store with low everyday prices.

Safety Check

A safe shopping experience begins with a clean store. Here are some important qualities to consider:

- Check for cleanliness not just on the floor but also on the grocery shelves, in display cases, and in the checkout aisles.
- Self-serve areas, including bulk bins and salad bars, should be clean and, in some cases, covered.
- Fresh produce should look fresh—a sign of quality.
- Raw meat, poultry, and fish should look fresh, too. If you detect an odor when you pass by the seafood section, something's "fishy" about the freshness.
- Cold foods should be cold. Freezer sections should house solidly frozen foods, without signs of ice crystal formation or thawing.

When to Shop

The issue of when to shop involves answering three questions:

◆ **How often should you shop?**
The answer depends on several factors. One is the storage space you have, including the size of your refrigerator-freezer. Over half of all American families do their shopping once a week.

◆ **Which days should you shop?**
Be aware that many stores advertise in newspapers on Wednesdays. Special prices may start on Thursdays and be valid through the weekend. The days may vary depending on the area.

◆ **What time of day should you shop?**
One time of day *not* to shop is right before mealtimes (or any time you are hungry). Studies show that people spend as much as 15 percent more on food when they shop on empty stomachs. Other times to steer clear of are early evenings and weekends—when stores are generally the most crowded. Shopping when the store is free of crowds can save you time. You are also more likely to make better choices when you are not feeling pressured.

A Shopping List

A well-thought-out shopping list can save you both time and money. It helps you speed up your shopping time and saves you from making special trips for forgotten items. A shopping list can also help you avoid **impulse buying**—buying items you didn't plan on purchasing and don't really need. Impulse buying can ruin any food budget.

Making a Shopping List

Once you get in the habit of making a shopping list, you'll find it can be done quickly and easily. The first step is to plan the meals you will serve for that shopping period. Be sure to check the newspaper ads to see what's on sale—perhaps you can include some of those items in your meal plan.

Next, check your menus and recipes to see what ingredients you need to purchase. Be sure to include the amount or quantity of each item needed, increasing the number if you plan to cook for the freezer.

From time to time you will want to check your supply of these basic items:

- **Staples**, items you use on a regular basis, such as flour, honey, and nonfat dry milk.

- Foods you keep on hand for emergencies: frozen dinners, canned foods, and other shelf-stable items.

- Cleaning supplies and paper products.

Many people keep a shopping reminder list handy in the kitchen. Whenever they notice that items are running low, they jot down a reminder to add those items to the shopping list.

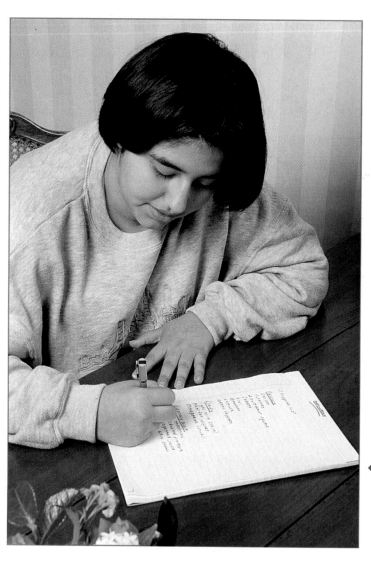

INFOLINK

To learn more about the steps involved in <u>meal planning</u> and <u>cooking for the freezer</u>, see Sections 11-1 and 11-2.
For more on <u>shelf-stable foods</u> and <u>methods for proper storage</u>, see Section 7-4.

◆ A well-organized shopping list makes it easier to find needed items once you get to the store. What is the most logical order in which to shop for groceries? Explain your answer.

◆ **Coupons can save money if used wisely. Name three types of information that should be looked at carefully before using a coupon.**

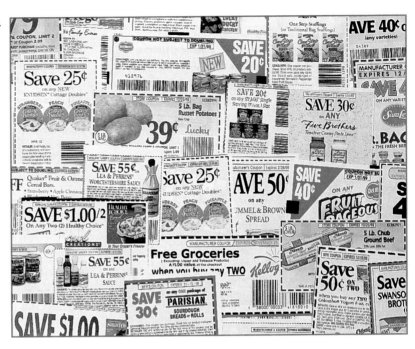

Organizing Your List

Organizing your list will help you shop more efficiently. When writing out your list, group items that are found in the same area of the store, such as dairy foods, meats, and frozen foods. This will help you avoid making several trips to the same area.

If you shop at one store regularly, make out your shopping list according to the way the store is arranged. Some stores provide a map or directory sheet showing which items are found in each aisle. Most have overhead signs above each aisle telling which foods are found there.

Some people keep copies of a basic shopping list that has the items they usually buy, arranged in the order those items are found in the store. Each week, they circle or check off the basic items they need and add any others. Alicia has her mother's basic shopping list stored in her computer. When her mother finishes the week's menus, Alicia adds the needed foods to the basic list and prints out the final one.

Coupons

Another consideration before you go shopping is whether you will use coupons. Coupons offer savings on the price of a specific product. Coupons are found in newspapers,

magazines, product packages, and mailed advertisements. In some stores, a checkout computer automatically prints out coupons for future use on the basis of the purchases you have just made.

There are two basic types of coupons:

◆ **Cents-off coupons.** These offer reduced prices on specific items. You present the coupon to the cashier when you make the purchase. The face value is subtracted from the total price of your purchases. Some stores will double or triple the amount of some coupons.

◆ **Rebate coupons.** A **rebate** is a partial refund from the manufacturer of a purchased good. You pay the regular price at the store. Later you fill out the rebate coupon and mail it, along with the required proof of purchase, to a specified address. The proof of purchase might be part of the package or a cash register receipt or both. A check for the coupon's face value is mailed to you.

Using Coupons

Clipping and sorting coupons takes time. For some people, the savings are well worth the effort. Others may find that they can save just as much by buying less expensive products without coupons.

Here are some suggestions for using coupons:

◆ Be choosy. Collect coupons only for items you usually buy or want to try. Otherwise, you may be tempted to buy an unnecessary item just because you have a coupon.

◆ Read coupons carefully. Some are good only on a certain size of a product or only in a specific store. Most coupons have a time limit. Stores cannot accept coupons after the expiration date printed on them.

◆ Organize coupons so that they are easy to find and use. For example, you might sort them alphabetically, by store aisle, or by food groups.

◆ Swap coupons. Some families and friends have coupon exchanges—they exchange coupons of food items they won't use for ones they will.

◆ Go through your coupon collection regularly. Pull out ones that expire soon so that you'll remember to use them. Throw away outdated ones.

Ready to Shop

Now that you've planned your shopping, you're ready to go to the store. Take along your shopping list and your coupons. Remember the environment, too. If you use cloth shopping bags or have paper or plastic bags to return to the store, take those with you.

Consider any errands you might want to do during your shopping trip. Do them before you shop for food. That way, you can bring food home immediately so that it can be properly stored.

◆ **Cloth shopping bags conserve resources because they are reusable. Which items should you take to the store with you?**

Section 12-1 Review & Activities

1. What is an advantage of shopping in a warehouse store? Name two drawbacks.

2. Give two guidelines for choosing a time of day to shop.

3. How can preparing a shopping list help you save money?

4. Analyzing. Angelina clips every coupon in the Sunday paper and then tries to use them all. What might be some drawbacks of this approach?

5. Evaluating. Is it always wrong to buy on impulse? When is it most likely to be a problem?

6. Applying. Identify three to five places to buy food in or near your community. Note the type of shopping establishment for each one. Record your findings in a "Shopping Guide" that also contains recommendations from this section. Publish your guide on the classroom computer.

Food Labels

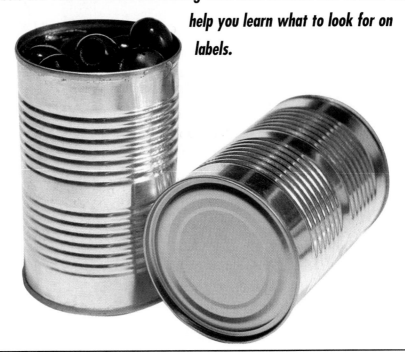

SECTION
12-2

Objectives

After studying this section, you should be able to:

- Identify types of information found on food labels.
- Explain how to interpret nutrition information found on food labels.
- Explain what is meant by product dating.

Look for These Terms

net weight

Daily Value (DV)

open dating

code dating

UPC

Imagine going to the supermarket and discovering that none of the packaged foods has labels. What kinds of important information would be missing?

In addition to helping you identify the contents of the package, food labels are valuable tools for making wise food choices. This section will help you learn what to look for on labels.

Basic Information

You may not be able to tell a book by its cover, but you can tell what's in a food product by its label. Certain basic information found on all food labels answers these questions:

◆ What food is in the container? Does it contain baked beans or chicken pot pie?

◆ How much food is in the container? The amount may be given as a volume measurement, such as 2 liters, or as a **net weight**, the weight of the food itself, not including the package. Net weight includes the liquid in canned food.

◆ Who manufactured, packed, or distributed the food? Where is the company located?

◆ What ingredients are in the food (assuming the food has more than one ingredient)? The ingredients are listed in order from largest to smallest amount by weight. To avoid certain ingredients, such as a food substance you are allergic to, read the ingredients list carefully.

Nutrition Information

In addition to basic information, food labels are sources of helpful nutrition information. Nearly all packaged foods carry a standardized "Nutrition Facts" panel like the one shown below. Each panel contains the same types of information in a standard format, making it easy to find what you need. The information includes serving size, calories, nutrient amounts, and percent of Daily Values.

◆ Food labels provide a variety of helpful information. What is the net weight of the canned item expressed in metric terms?

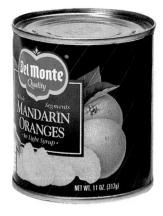

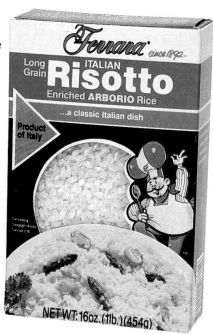

Serving Size

Near the top of the panel, you will see "Serving Size" and "Servings Per Container." The serving size is based on the amount of food customarily eaten at one time. The FDA has established standard amounts for various types of food.

The rest of the nutrition label information, including calories and nutrient amounts, is based on one serving size. If you eat a larger or smaller serving than is listed on the label,

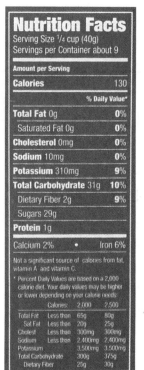

you need to take that into account when reading the rest of the nutrition panel. For example, if you normally eat twice as much as the serving size shown on the label, you would need to double the amounts shown for calories and nutrients.

Calories

The label lists total calories per serving as well as the number of calories from fat per serving. You can use this information to keep track of the number of total calories and calories from fat you eat throughout the day. It also helps you determine fairly quickly which foods derive the recommended one-third or less of their calories from fat.

◆ The Nutrition Facts panel provides easy-to-read nutrition information on the spot. How many calories are contained in this product?

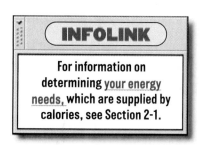

INFOLINK

For information on determining your energy needs, which are supplied by calories, see Section 2-1.

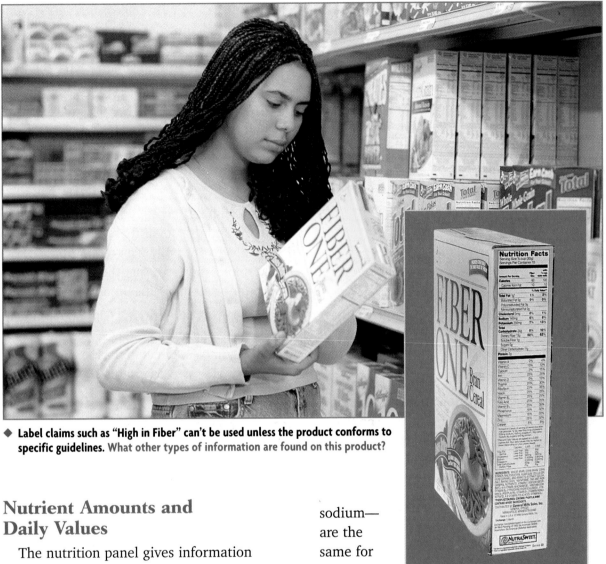

◆ **Label claims such as "High in Fiber" can't be used unless the product conforms to specific guidelines.** What other types of information are found on this product?

Nutrient Amounts and Daily Values

The nutrition panel gives information about some of the nutrients that are most important in a healthy eating plan. Amounts (in grams or milligrams) are given for total fat, cholesterol, sodium, total carbohydrate, dietary fiber, sugars, and protein.

For most of these nutrients, the label also lists "% Daily Value." Expressed as a percentage, **Daily Value (DV)** is a specific nutrition reference amount recommended by health experts. DVs are designed to help you put information about nutrient content into perspective. Two DVs—those for cholesterol and sodium—are the same for every adult. Others, including those for fat, saturated fat, total carbohydrate, and fiber, depend on how many calories you need daily.

For fat, saturated fat, cholesterol, and sodium, the DV listed is an upper limit. In other words, a person's goal is to consume no more than that amount each day. For total carbohydrate, fiber, vitamin A, vitamin C, calcium, and iron, the DV is a minimum. In this case, a person's goal is to take in at least that amount each day.

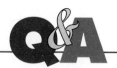

Q If I am supposed to eat no more than 30 percent fat per day in my eating plan, does that mean I should stay under 30 percent Daily Value for fat?

A No, because 100 percent Daily Value for fat represents 30 percent fat for a 2,000-calorie eating plan. So, if you need about 2,000 calories per day, you can have up to 100 percent Daily Value for fat; if you need about 1,500 calories, then allow 75 percent Daily Value for fat; for a 2,500-calorie diet, allow 125 percent Daily Value for fat.

Label Language

In these health-conscious times, many food labels promise "reduced calories," "good source of fiber," or some similar claim. What do these claims mean? Here are the legal definitions of some of the most common ones:

◆ **"Low- . . ."** The terms *low- . . .* and *low in . . .* can be used on food labels if the food could be eaten frequently without exceeding recommended amounts of the indicated nutrient. Generally, these terms are used in conjunction with *fat, saturated fat, cholesterol, sodium,* or *calories.*

◆ **"Reduced . . .," "Less . . .," or "Fewer . . ."** To display these terms, the product must have at least 25 percent less of something (such as fat or calories) than a comparable food. The term *reduced* is used when the product has been nutritionally altered. For example, reduced-fat cheddar cheese has at least 25 percent less fat than regular cheddar cheese. Look for a specific comparison on the label.

◆ **"High in . . ."** This means that one serving of the food provides at least 20 percent of the Daily Value for the specified nutrient. For instance, an orange juice label might state "High in vitamin C."

◆ **"Good source of . . ."** This means that one serving of the food contains 10 to 19 percent of the Daily Value for a particular nutrient.

◆ **". . . -Free."** A food package that uses this claim has an amount of the ingredient in question so small that it is not likely to affect your body. The term *fat-free,* for example, indicates that the product has no fat or an insignificant amount of fat.

◆ **"Organically grown."** This and a similar claim, "organically produced," both describe the manner in which a fresh or processed food was grown or produced—typically, without synthetic pesticides or fertilizers. To display this claim, a processed food must be at least 95 percent organically produced. The term *natural,* however, can mean whatever the food processor wants it to mean.

The purpose of these and other definitions is to ensure that food manufacturers do not use terms in ways that will mislead consumers. Remember, if you're not sure what a label term means, read the "Nutrition Facts" panel. It will give you the specific amounts of nutrients and calories.

Health Claims

If foods meet specific requirements, health claims might appear on their labels. Such claims are regulated by the FDA and must be supported by a significant portion of the scientific community. They are limited to relationships between the food or nutrient and a particular disease or health condition. For instance, a health claim might link calcium and osteoporosis or fats and cancer.

Product Dating

Product dating is a voluntary, industry-wide system. Except for infant formula and some baby food, the federal government does not require food manufacturers or processors to provide this information. Some food packagers use **open dating**, a practice in which a date is stamped directly on the product for the benefit of the consumer. The exact meaning of the date varies, depending on the product and the wording:

◆ **"Sell by" date.** This type of date indicates the last day the product should remain on the store shelf. It allows a reasonable amount of time for home storage and use after the date. Dairy products and cold cuts are among the foods that often carry "sell by" dates. The package may state "Sell by (date)" or "Best if purchased by (date)."

◆ **"Use by" date.** Some packages state "Best if used by (date)." The product may still be safe to eat after the date has passed. However, the quality will start to go down. If a date alone appears on baked goods, such as breads and rolls, it is usually a "use by" date.

Dates are helpful to ensure a product's freshness; however, a package date does not guarantee quality. That depends on the manufacturing and the handling of the product.

Code dating refers to a series of numbers or letters that indicates where and when the product was packaged. It is used by manufacturers for products with long shelf lives. If a recall is necessary, the products can be tracked quickly and removed from the marketplace. Federal law requires code dating on most canned food.

Other Information

You will find many other types of helpful information on food labels. For example, some products carry grades on their packaging, such as "U.S. Grade A." Grading is a voluntary program for identifying the quality of foods. You will learn more about food grades as you study specific foods in Unit Four.

Some label information is required only for certain products. For example, beverages that contain juice must list the percentages of juices.

The label often includes a picture of the product. If the product is not shown exactly as it appears in the package, the photo must be labeled "serving suggestion."

You may see directions on the label for using the product. If the product requires special handling, you will find instructions on the label, such as "Refrigerate after opening" or "Keep frozen."

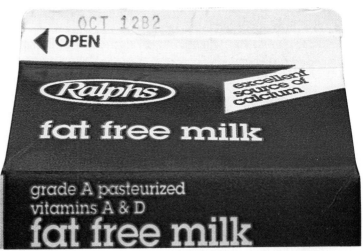

◆ The date stamped onto this milk carton provides critical information. What does it tell you?

UPC

You have probably noticed a pattern of black stripes similar to the one shown here on most products. This symbol, the **UPC**—or Universal Product Code—is a bar code that can be read by a scanner. Below the UPC is its numeric equivalent. The first five digits of this number identify the manufacturer; the second five, the product size and flavor (if relevant).

The UPC has specific uses. Many store checkout counters are equipped with electronic scanners that can read UPCs, thereby allowing the cashier to determine the correct price for a product automatically. It also enables the store to keep an automatic inventory of the product.

◆ **The UPC symbol on this package helps both the consumer and the merchant.** Explain how.

Section 12-2 Review & Activities

1. Identify three pieces of basic information found on all food labels.

2. Why is it important to consider serving size when reading a "Nutrition Facts" panel?

3. What is the purpose of the "% Daily Value" information on a "Nutrition Facts" panel?

4. What are the differences between "sell by" dates and "use by" dates? Why are such dates not a guarantee of quality?

5. Synthesizing. Why do you think it is difficult to define *natural* as a label term?

6. Evaluating. If an apple is organically grown, does it mean it's more nutritious than a nonorganic apple? Why or why not? Would you spend more money on organically grown produce? Why or why not?

7. Applying. Bring to class "Nutrition Facts" panels from two different foods. Use the panels to identify each food's nutritional pluses and minuses. Develop a rating system that can be applied to all foods—for example, a food with a DV for dietary fiber that is at least double that for fat and/or sodium rates a 10. Share your system with classmates.

In the Supermarket

When you walk into a supermarket, you are faced with hundreds of items displayed in an eye-catching fashion. Consumer skills can help you pinpoint foods that combine good nutritional value and quality at the best price. In this section, you will learn how to apply these skills.

Objectives

After studying this section, you should be able to:

- Describe ways of getting the most for your money when food shopping.
- Explain how to choose and handle food to preserve nutrition, quality, and safety.
- Give guidelines for courteous shopping.

Look for These Terms

bulk foods

comparison shop

unit price

store brands

generic

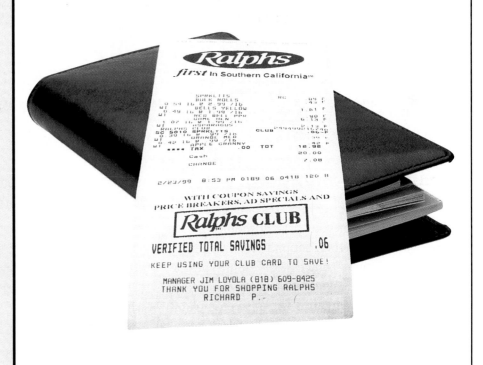

How Stores Are Organized

Some stores are so big they may seem like food mazes. Understanding how they are organized can help you navigate through them.

Most of the space in a supermarket is taken up by aisles lined with shelves stacked with shelf-stable foods in cans, jars, bottles, boxes, and packages. You might also find the following specific departments or sections:

- A produce department, where fresh fruits and vegetables are sold.
- A meat, poultry, and fish department.
- A refrigeration section. Often taking an entire aisle, this is where you will find dairy products, eggs, cured luncheon meats, and fresh pasta.
- A freezer section. Here you will find a variety of convenience foods and products meant to be consumed in their frozen state, such as ice cream.

Still other departments you might find include a meal center, delicatessen, salad bar, or bakery where you can buy fresh prepared foods. Some stores feature a department that specializes in **bulk foods**—shelf-stable foods that are sold loose in covered bins or barrels.

You place as much food as you want in a plastic bag, tie it, and attach a tag or sticker to the bag so that the checkout clerk can identify the contents. Foods that may be sold in bulk include grain products, nuts, dried fruits, dry beans and peas, snack foods, flour, sugar, herbs, and spices.

Departments with higher-profit items are usually located at the front of the store. These might include the floral department, bakery, deli, meal center, and produce department. The pleasant aromas and eye appeal of these departments are carefully designed to encourage the customer to spend money on these items.

◆ **Most stores provide the unit price on a shelf tab for the convenience of consumers.** How is this helpful to the consumers?

Comparison Shopping

No matter what size your food budget, getting the most for your money should be one of your goals when shopping. Yet, when faced with so many choices—different types of products, brands, and sizes—how can you spot the best bargain? The answer is to **comparison shop**, that is, to match prices and characteristics of similar or like items to determine which offers the best value. Among the methods used in comparison shopping are calculating unit price, computing cost per serving, and trying store brands or generic items.

Unit Prices

Which is a better buy, a 12-ounce jar of spaghetti sauce for $1.32 or a 16-ounce jar for $1.52? To find out, you need to know the **unit price**, an item's price per ounce, quart, pound, or other unit. In many stores, the unit price is shown on the shelf tab below the item, next to the total price. This gives you a quick and easy way to compare prices. If the unit

price is not shown, you can calculate it yourself by dividing the total price of the item by the number of units.

In the example given before, the smaller jar of spaghetti sauce costs 11 cents per ounce ($1.32 ÷ 12). The larger jar costs 9.5 cents per ounce ($1.52 ÷ 16), so it is a better value.

Cost Per Serving

Sometimes the unit price is not the best basis for comparison, particularly when you are shopping for fresh meat, poultry, or fish. These foods are best compared by the cost of a serving. Suppose you were trying to decide between fish fillets on sale at $1.80 per pound (500 g) and a whole broiling chicken at $1.06 per pound. At first, the chicken might seem like a better bargain. However, because the chicken includes bones, skin, and fat, there is less usable meat. Even though the fish has a higher unit price, you would need less fish to feed the same number of people served by the chicken.

A first step to finding the cost per serving is determining how many servings a given amount will provide. (See the chart below.) Divide the price for that amount by the number of servings it will provide. The result will be the cost per serving. In the example on page 348, the cost per serving of fish fillets would be 45 cents. ($1.80 ÷ 4 servings). The cost per serving of a pound of chicken with bones, meanwhile, is 53 cents. ($1.06 ÷ 2 servings).

You can use cost per serving to help you in meal planning and budgeting. For instance, you could find the cost per serving of a homemade recipe by adding the cost of the ingredients and dividing by the recipe yield. You could find the cost per serving of a packaged food by dividing the total price by the number of servings indicated on the label.

Store Brands and Generics

A third strategy for saving money is to buy and try items other than commercial name-brand items. **Store brands** (also called private labels) are brands specially produced for the store. They are generally equal in quality to name brands but less expensive. **Generic** items, items produced without a commercial or store brand name, are usually even less expensive. The labels of generic products aren't as eye-catching as those of name brands, but your taste buds may not know the difference. Finding out which store brands and generics are good quality may take some experimenting, but the savings can make the effort worthwhile.

Servings per Pound of Meat, Poultry, and Fish

Meat		
	Lean, boneless or ground	3 to 4 servings per pound
	Some bone or fat	2 to 3 servings per pound
	Large amount of bone or fat	1 to 2 servings per pound
Poultry		
	Boneless or ground	4 servings per pound
	With bones	2 servings per pound
Fish		
	Fillets or steaks	4 servings per pound
	Dressed	2 servings per pound
	Whole or drawn	1 serving per pound

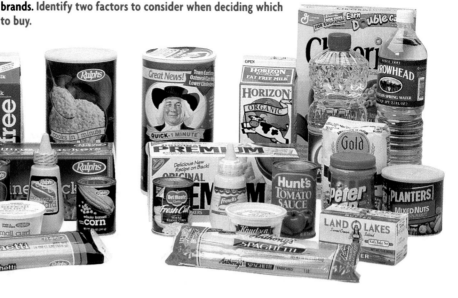

◆ **Many stores offer a choice between store brands and name brands.** Identify two factors to consider when deciding which to buy.

Other Money-Saving Ideas

Here are some additional suggestions for saving money at your food store:

◆ Use your shopping list, but be flexible. Look for sale items that you can substitute for the ones on your list.

◆ When using coupons, be sure you are really getting the best buy. Another brand may be less expensive even without a coupon.

◆ Join a shoppers' club if your store offers one. Customers are given an identification card that entitles them to reduced prices on certain items. Without the card, they would have to pay full price. Unadvertised specials are also available to club members.

◆ Periodically recheck the unit price of products you buy regularly. Manufacturers sometimes keep the same price but reduce the amount in the package.

◆ Consider bulk foods. They cost less because they are not prepackaged. In addition, you can buy just the amount you want.

◆ Don't buy more food than you can store properly, or more than can be used before spoiling.

◆ Be aware of strategies designed to encourage impulse buying. Don't be tempted by small, high-profit items, such as candy and magazines, placed next to the checkout lanes.

◆ Take advantage of the many customer services provided by the store. You may find a coupon rack, for example, or brochures with tips on meal planning, food budgeting, and shopping.

◆ Surf your supermarket's Web site, if one's available. Doing so enables customers with computers to communicate with the store. Customers can learn of future sales, send their suggestions through e-mail, print out coupons, and in some cases, order groceries.

Nutrition, Quality, and Food Safety

Shopping involves more than looking for low prices. To get the most value for your money, you must also pay attention to nutrition, quality, and food safety.

Remember to read labels carefully. Be sure you're getting the product and amount you want. Check the date on the package. Use the "Nutrition Facts" panel (explained in Section 12-2). Also look for additional nutrition information on shelf tags or signs.

Avoid packages that are dirty, rusty, leaking, or damaged in any other way. Harmful bacteria may have gotten into the food. If packages of meat, poultry, and fish leak, the juices can contaminate other foods with harmful micro-organisms. To be safe, put meat, poultry, or fish packages in plastic bags so that they won't drip onto other foods in your cart—and, later, in your shopping bag.

When buying frozen foods, avoid packages that are frosted with ice. The frost means the package may have thawed a little and was then refrozen. This can affect food quality and possibly contribute to food-borne illness.

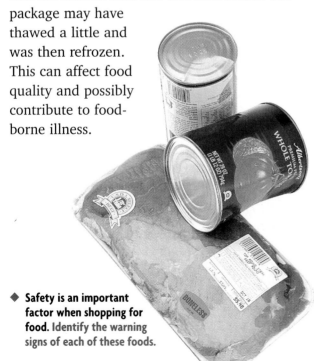

◆ **Safety is an important factor when shopping for food.** Identify the warning signs of each of these foods.

Keep fragile items in one part of your cart. As you add heavier items, move the fragile ones up so that they are always on top and won't be crushed.

Plan your route through the store. The freezer section and the meat, poultry, and seafood department should be your last stops. This plan ensures that your food stays at safe temperatures.

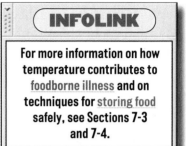

INFOLINK

For more information on how temperature contributes to foodborne illness and on techniques for storing food safely, see Sections 7-3 and 7-4.

Courtesy When Shopping

Be considerate of other shoppers. Although there are no "supermarket police" to give traffic tickets, obey the same rules you would when driving. Don't race your cart through the store (especially around corners), and keep to the right side of aisles. If you bump into someone or have to pass another shopper, excuse yourself. Avoid blocking the aisles or other busy areas.

Any food that is damaged by shoppers is wasted. Consumers pay for the damage in the long run—the cost is added to the price of food. Remember:

◆ Do not open containers to look at or sample contents.

◆ Return a product to its proper place if you decide not to buy it.

◆ Handle produce gently. Do not squeeze it or throw it back into a bin.

◆ When you buy bulk foods, use the scoop or tongs provided. Do not taste the food or touch it with your hands. Close the bin or barrel when you are through.

Finishing Your Shopping

When you've selected all your items, it's time to head for the checkout lane. If you choose an express lane, be sure you have the right number of items. Don't choose a cash-only line if you intend to pay by check.

Watch the display as the prices are rung up. The clerk could make a mistake. If the store has computerized checkouts, the incorrect price might have been entered into the computer. If you think you are being charged incorrectly, politely ask the clerk to check the price for you.

Food stores vary regarding what forms of payment they will accept. To pay by check, you may need a store check-cashing card. Some supermarkets also accept credit cards or automated banking cards. Don't let the ease of using a card tempt you to go over your food budget.

Take your purchases home right away, and store them properly. Put frozen foods away immediately so that they don't thaw. Store refrigerated foods next, and finally, shelf-stable ones. Remember to repackage bulk foods in airtight, durable containers.

If you come home and discover a food you selected is spoiled or of poor quality, return it to the store as soon as possible. Do the same if you have any other problems with your purchases. Take the store receipt with you. Stores are interested in keeping their customers and will do their best to satisfy you.

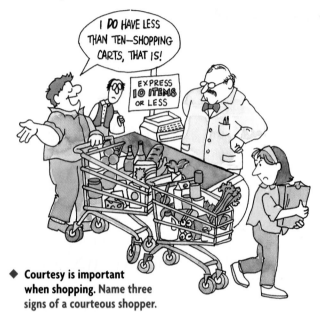

◆ **Courtesy is important when shopping. Name three signs of a courteous shopper.**

Section 12-3 Review & Activities

1. What is the formula for calculating unit price?

2. Give three examples of ways to save money when shopping.

3. Why is it important to avoid buying food in damaged containers?

4. Evaluating. Do you think it is fair of stores to pass the cost of carelessness and mishandling of food by shoppers along to other customers? What solutions can you recommend to prevent shoppers from mishandling food?

5. Synthesizing. Some people will not buy store brands or generic items. Why do you think this is so? What might you say to such people?

6. Applying. Working in pairs, write and perform a skit demonstrating at least three poor shopping strategies. Have the rest of the class identify them.

CAREER WANTED

Individuals who counsel others, communicate clearly, and are assertive without being aggressive.

REQUIRES:

- degree in government and/or law
- on-the-job training in legal issues and violations
- good management skills

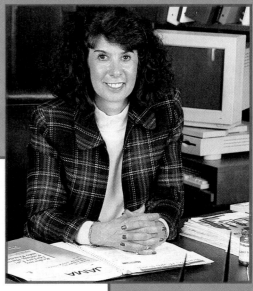

"I help people get a fair shake,"
says Consumer Advocate Alana Burch

Q: Alana, what is your background?

A: I started out as a private practice attorney. Then, I thought I wanted to go into politics so I could help more people in need. Finally, one Sunday, I happened to see a newspaper ad for a consumer advocate at a local family service agency. I have been happy ever since!

Q: What is the biggest consumer problem facing older citizens?

A: They're often treated as "second-class" citizens. I recently convinced an area supermarket to enlarge shelf signs so they could be read more easily by people with diminishing eyesight. They also added "Seniors" to the shopper's club so that their food would go even farther.

Q: What are some obstacles you experience in your line of work?

A: The toughest challenge is getting your message heard initially. Once "my foot's in the door" I can do my job.

Q: What advice do you have for young people interested in a career in consumer advocacy?

A: There's no time to start like the present. When I was in high school, I volunteered with the local Red Cross and at the local hospital. Understanding people's needs is the foundation of a good consumer advocate!

Career Research Activity

1. What is the difference between a paralegal specialist and a legislative assistant? Which career would you be most interested in? Why?

2. Research how the increasing government role in regulating food and food safety will increase the need for consumer advocates. Create an illustration that expresses your findings.

Related Career Opportunities

Entry Level
- Administrative Assistant
- Safety Patrol Officer

Technical Level
- Paralegal Specialist
- Social Services Assistant
- Magazine Writer

Professional Level
- Attorney
- Consumer Advocate
- Legislative Assistant

Chapter 12   Review & Activities

Summary

Section 12-1: Before You Shop

- A well-planned shopping trip begins with deciding where and when to shop.

- You can buy food from a number of types of stores. Which type you choose depends on your priorities.

- Preparing a shopping list helps prevent impulse buying.

- Collecting coupons is another money-saving strategy.

Section 12-2: Food Labels

- All food labels must include certain basic information.

- Nearly all food labels also include a "Nutrition Facts" panel to help you decide how well the product meets your nutritional needs.

- The use of certain terms and health claims on food labels is regulated by law.

- Open dating can help consumers judge how long products will remain safe.

Section 12-3: In the Supermarket

- Shopping skills can help you find nutritious, high-quality foods at the best price.

- Comparison shopping is easier if you know how to find the unit price and the price per serving.

- Choose quality foods and handle them carefully to help maintain nutritional value and safety.

- Food purchases should be taken home right away and stored properly.

Checking Your Knowledge

1. How do supermarkets and specialty stores compare in terms of foods sold, services offered, and price?

2. List four basic steps in making a shopping list.

3. What is the difference between a cents-off coupon and a rebate coupon?

4. What does *net weight* mean?

5. In what way is the Daily Value for sodium on a "Nutrition Facts" panel different from that for vitamin C?

6. What does "low-fat" on a food label tell you about the fat content of the food?

7. What kinds of health claims does the FDA allow on food products?

8. Describe the procedure for buying bulk foods.

9. Why is it helpful to calculate the cost per serving when buying fresh meat, poultry, or fish?

10. Name five signs that tell you a package of food may be unsafe.

Working IN THE Lab

1. *Foods Lab.* Make up a basic shopping list that could be stored on the computer. Explain how you would use the list.

2. *Taste Test.* Compare the taste, texture, and appearance of store brands or generic items with their name-brand equivalents. Compare a variety of types of foods, such as canned vegetables, breakfast cereals, and frozen juices. What conclusions can you draw?

Thinking Critically

1. Comparing and Contrasting. One of the items on Miguel's shopping list today is breakfast cereal. When he reaches the cereal aisle of his supermarket, he notices a large banner advertising double value on store coupons every Wednesday. Among the newspaper coupons he has clipped and brought with him is a rebate that returns one-third of the cost of any size package of this particular cereal as long as the coupon is mailed before December 31. What factors does Miguel need to take into account before he decides which coupon will give him the most value for his food dollar?

2. Recognizing Assumptions. Rhoda and her son Mark are shopping for a large turkey for a family gathering. All the bigger birds in the supermarket's meat case have ice crystals clinging to them. When Rhoda begins to reach for one of the birds, Mark reminds her that her shopping list specifies "fresh turkey." "This one is fresh," his mother replies. "See the sign?" She is pointing to a sign over the meat counter that states: "All our poultry is fresh, all the time." How might you respond if you were Mark?

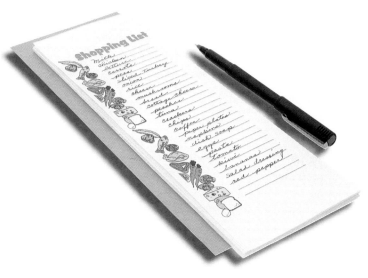

Reinforcing Key Skills

1. Directed Thinking. Compare the prices of at least four different foods with those of their nutritionally modified equivalents (for example, cheddar cheese with reduced-fat or fat-free cheddar cheese). What are some possible reasons for the price differences?

2. Leadership. Devise a plan for increasing consumer awareness of food safety issues in food stores in your community. Put your plan into effect. Include a suggestion box, and use any responses received to assess the usefulness of your campaign.

Making Decisions and Solving Problems

While buying milk, you notice some cartons marked "Reduced for quick sale." You see the "sell by" date is the day after tomorrow. You wonder whether you should buy one of the reduced-price cartons.

Making Connections

1. Social Studies. Using library or online resources, find information about how people in other cultures do their food shopping. How are their shopping practices similar to and different from those in your own culture?

2. Math. Suppose you need chicken for a party for eight people. Check the prices and selections of different forms of chicken at the supermarket. Use the "Servings per Pound of Meat, Poultry, and Fish" chart on page 349 to determine which form offers the most value. What other factors would affect your decision?

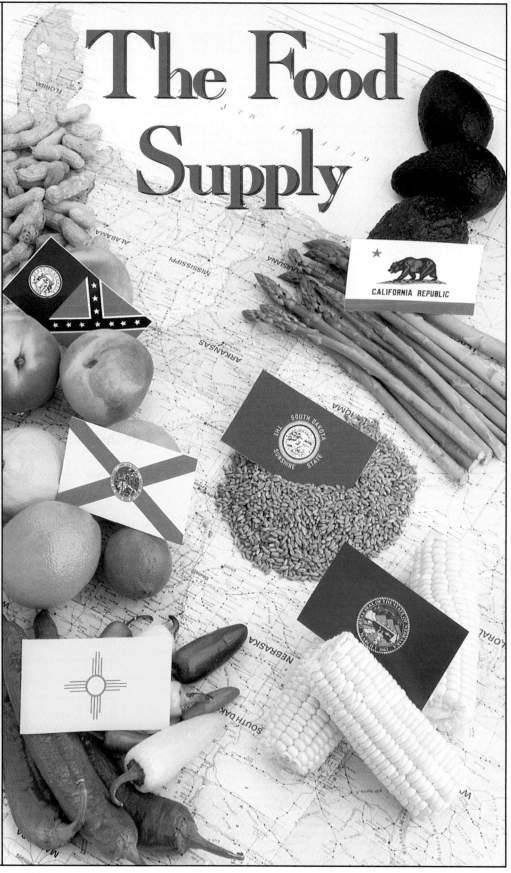

CHAPTER

13

The Food Supply

André leaned back from his homework. Looking out his window, he could see huge snowflakes falling. He reached across the kitchen table for a favorite snack, an orange. As he peeled it, he noticed a sticker indicating that the orange came from California. André chuckled: His food had traveled farther than he ever had in his entire life.

SECTION 13-1

Where Does Food Come From?

Like André's snack, most of the foods on your table at home have traveled hundreds or thousands of miles. In this section, you will learn about that journey and about the professionals through whose hands every food passes at various steps.

Objectives

After studying this section, you should be able to:

- Trace the route food takes from farm to marketplace.
- Describe innovative farming, processing, and packaging techniques.
- Identify factors that influence food prices.

Look for These Terms

sustainable farming

hydroponic farming

aquaculture

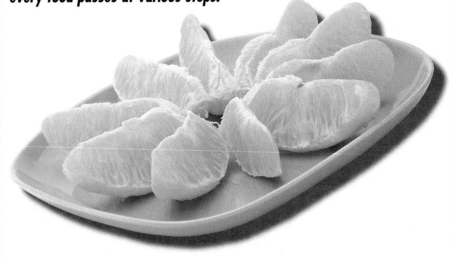

From Farm to Marketplace

Most food begins its journey on farms where it is grown. Farmers in the United States and Canada produce enough food not only for their own countries but also for sale elsewhere.

The Farmer

In recent years, several concerns have prompted a search for new farming technologies. One is the impact of traditional farming methods on the environment. Traditional methods rely on the use of potentially harmful chemicals in fertilizers and pesticides.

Among the alternative methods are the following:

- ◆ **Sustainable farming** is the cutting back on, or elimination of, chemicals in farming. In this method, animal manure replaces chemicals as a fertilizer. Nonchemical measures are also used to get rid of pests and weeds. One of these—integrated pest management—uses "good" bugs to destroy "bad" ones.

- ◆ **Hydroponic** (hy-druh-PAH-nik) **farming** is a method of growing plants without soil. Various materials, such as water, gravel, or sand, can be used to hold the plants.

Nutrient-enriched water provides food for the plants. Hydroponic lettuce, cucumbers, and tomatoes are currently available in many supermarkets.

◆ **Aquaculture** is a method of growing fish or seafood in enclosed areas of water. Fish farms may be areas located near the shore that are closed off with special nets, or they may be special ponds. Aquaculture is one of the fastest-growing industries in the world. The U.S. Department of Commerce predicts that by 2010, aquaculture will provide over a third of all fish eaten in this country.

The Processor

Once food is harvested, it is shipped to processors. The specific type of processing facility to which it travels depends on the type of food and the form in which it ultimately will be sold.

Processing ranges from very simple to complex. Fresh produce, for instance, needs minimum processing. It may just need to be cleaned, packaged, and shipped to the marketplace.

As part of the processing, many perishable foods are preserved to prevent spoilage and lengthen shelf life. Some commercial preservation methods include:

◆ **Canning.** Foods are sealed in airtight metal or glass containers and heated to destroy harmful microorganisms.

◆ **Freezing.** Foods are quickly frozen to slow down the growth of harmful bacteria.

◆ **Curing.** Ingredients such as salt, spices, sugar, sodium nitrate, and sodium nitrite are added to the food. This method is widely used in processing meats such as ham, bacon, and corned beef. It is also used to preserve fish, pickles, and some vegetables.

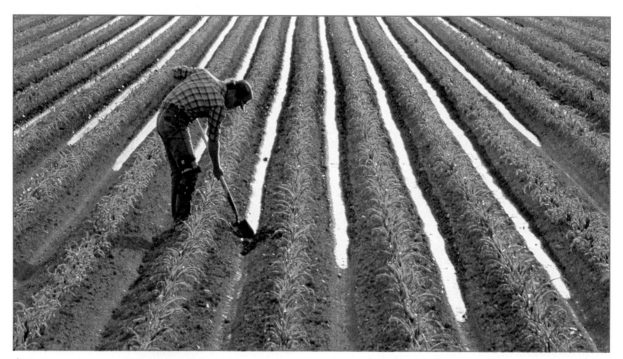

◆ Farmers are continually on the alert for ways to produce more and better quality food. Name some technological advances in farming during the past fifty years.

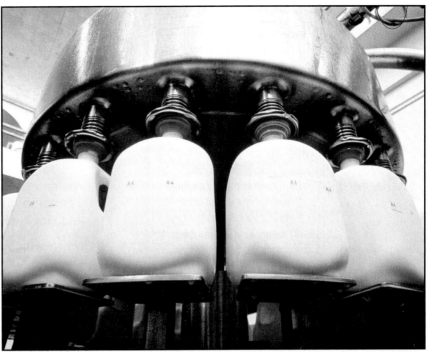

◆ **Milk goes through various amounts and types of processing before it is ready to be delivered to stores.** Research the processing of milk and outline the process.

◆ **Drying.** Moisture, needed by harmful microorganisms, is removed from the food. Drying is used for foods such as grains, dry beans, milk, and fruit.

◆ **Freeze-drying.** Food is first frozen and then dried. More flavor, texture, and nutrients are retained than with drying alone. Freeze-drying is used for foods such as instant coffee, dried soup mixes, strawberries, and mushrooms.

◆ **Controlled atmosphere storage.** Food is held in a cold area where the amounts of nitrogen, oxygen, and carbon dioxide in the atmosphere are controlled. This helps extend the shelf life of some foods, especially fruits.

Packing Technology

Several recent developments in packaging have enabled food manufacturers and processors to expand the kinds of products they offer. Here are some examples:

◆ **Aseptic** (ay-SEP-tick) **packages.** Also known as "juice boxes." Are made of layers of plastics, paperboard, and aluminum foil. The food and the package are sterilized separately, and the package is filled under sterile conditions.

◆ **Plastic cans and trays.** Are used for shelf-stable foods that can be heated in a microwave oven. Some trays also can be used in a conventional oven.

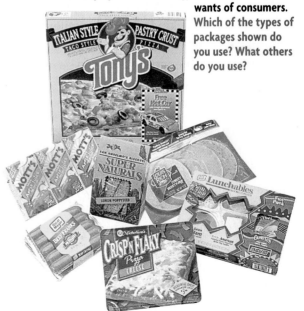

◆ **Packaging methods are continually being updated to keep up with technology and the needs and wants of consumers.** Which of the types of packages shown do you use? What others do you use?

◆ **Modified atmosphere packaging.**
A mixture of carbon dioxide, oxygen, and nitrogen is inserted into the package before it is sealed. The gas mixture slows down bacterial growth. With this method, foods such as fresh pasta, prepared salads, and cooked meats can be kept, refrigerated, up to four weeks.

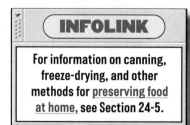

INFOLINK

For information on canning, freeze-drying, and other methods for <u>preserving food at home</u>, see Section 24-5.

The Distributor

Once food is processed and packaged, it is shipped to the distributor. Distributors are the link between food processors and retailers (the stores where you buy food). There are many different kinds of distributors, depending on the food involved. Generally, the food is shipped to large warehouses, where it is stored before being sent to the retailer.

The Retailer

From the distributor, food is shipped to the many different kinds of food retailers. Supermarkets, which offer a wide selection of products, are the most popular type of retail food outlet in this country. Others are described in Section 12-1.

A primary job of the retailer is to present food to the consumer. In an effort to satisfy consumers, food processors and manufacturers constantly develop new products. Some stores review as many as 100 new products a week. Because shelf space is limited, they cannot accept every new product. If new products are accepted but do not sell well, they are removed from the shelves.

Connecting Food and Health

Waste Not

Food processors have begun developing packages that are more "environment-friendly." As a consumer, you can also do your part for the environment.

- Use "convenience" packaging only when absolutely necessary. For meals eaten at home, avoid using juice boxes and single-serving packages.

- Learn which resources are recyclable and which are not. When you have a choice, buy food in packages that can be recycled.

- Be a leader and set a good example for friends and family members, especially younger brothers and sisters. Help them follow the motto "Waste not, want not."

Think About It

- Make an inventory of food packages in your home pantry and refrigerator. Note which foods come in recyclable packages and which do not. Share your inventory with your family, and discuss ways to make responsible shopping choices.

Food Prices

For every dollar a consumer spends on food, between 3 and 25 cents goes to the farmer. The rest of the money covers processing, packaging, advertising, and distribution. Generally, the more a food is processed, the more it will cost the consumer. Food prices tend to go up or down for other reasons as well.

- **Supply and demand.** If consumer demand for a food is greater than the supply, the price will go up. If supply is greater, as it is when crops reach their peak growing seasons, prices are low. Other foods, offered in limited supply, are high-priced.

- **Natural disasters.** Storms, earthquakes, floods, and droughts affect the price of food. For example, a severe freeze in California or Florida can damage orange trees, reducing the supply for the whole season. The reduced supply results in higher prices.

- **Consumer damage.** Careless consumers sometimes damage food when they shop. The damaged items may have to be thrown out by the store. Such losses are added to the prices consumers pay.

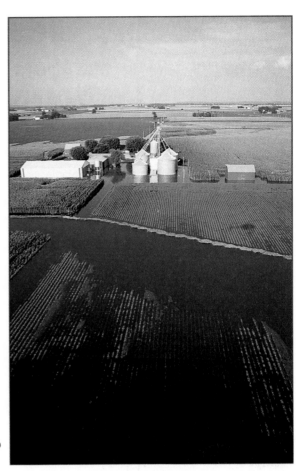

- **Floods and similar natural disasters can destroy crops and drive up the price of food. Identify two other factors that affect the prices of food.**

Section 13-1 Review & Activities

1. Name the four parts of the food supply network.

2. How and why is food preserved?

3. What factors affect food prices?

4. **Analyzing.** Why do you think there is a need for finding new farming technologies?

5. **Comparing and Contrasting.** What foods on your table at home or school might be grown or processed within 100 miles of your home? Which foods do you think travel the greatest distance to reach your local stores?

6. **Applying.** Interview a parent or another relative who shops for food regularly. Ask that person to think of any food or beverage products he or she used to buy at the supermarket but can no longer purchase there. Why might the product no longer be stocked? Has the person found a different brand of the product? Compile a class list of discontinued products.

A Safe Food Supply

When Brittany was shopping for cucumbers at the store, she noticed they were all shiny but felt a bit sticky. She asked the produce clerk why. He explained that they were coated with a wax to prevent loss of moisture and improve their appearance. He assured her that this process met government regulations for food safety.

Objectives

After studying this section, you should be able to:

- Explain how the government helps ensure the safety of the food supply.
- Identify and discuss food safety issues.

Look for These Terms

food additives

recall

irradiation

genetic engineering

tolerance levels

contaminants

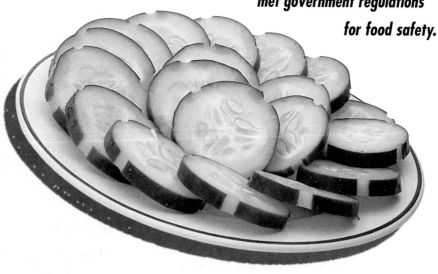

Safeguarding the Food Supply

Government and industry make every effort to provide a safe food supply. In doing so, they face a number of challenges. One is testing food additives to be sure they will cause no harm. **Food additives** are chemicals added to food to preserve freshness or enhance color or flavor.

Another challenge is seeing that foods are handled properly on their way to the marketplace so that harmful microorganisms do not reach dangerous levels. A third challenge is staying on top of new food technologies and taking steps to ensure that harmful chemicals do not get into food accidentally.

Government Agencies

In the United States, several federal agencies are responsible for monitoring the safety of the country's food supply:

◆ **Food Safety and Inspection Service (FSIS).** This section of the United States Department of Agriculture (USDA) is responsible for the inspection and safety of meat, poultry, and eggs.

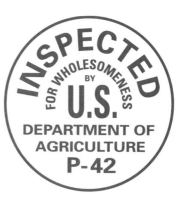

INSPECTED
FOR WHOLESOMENESS
BY
U.S.
DEPARTMENT OF
AGRICULTURE
P-42

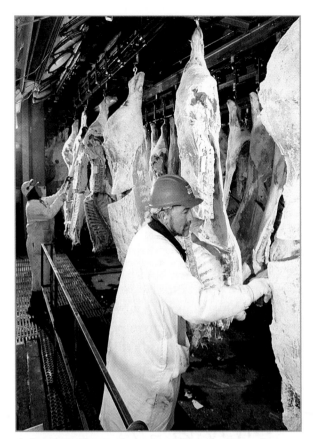

◆ **Inspectors from various government agencies work to protect the food supply.** Choose one agency and explain the work it does.

◆ **Food and Drug Administration (FDA).** The FDA is responsible for the general safety of food other than meat, poultry, and eggs. It enforces laws that regulate additives, food purity, packaging, labeling, and new foods and processing methods.

◆ **National Marine Fisheries Services.** This agency within the Department of Commerce offers a voluntary inspection program to fish processors.

◆ **Environmental Protection Agency (EPA).** The EPA registers pesticides and sets legal limits for pesticides in food. It also regulates disposal of hazardous wastes.

What happens if tests or consumer complaints show that a food is unsafe? The FDA may first ask the manufacturer to withdraw the product voluntarily. If the manufacturer refuses, or if the situation is a life-threatening one, the FDA will order a **recall**—the immediate removal of the product from store shelves and notification of the public through the media. The brand name and package code numbers are announced. Consumers who have purchased any of this food are asked to return it to the store.

Food Safety Issues

Many issues related to food safety are controversial. It is important to understand the facts as well as the opinions on both sides of each issue.

Food Additives

When you think of additives, you probably think of ingredients on food package labels with long, hard-to-pronounce names. Did you know, however, that spices are additives? Currently, some 3,000 additives are in use.

FDA approval for additives can be a lengthy process. An additive is first tested extensively. If it proves to be safe, the FDA approves it and sets regulations for its use. Additives with a long history of safe use are classified by the FDA as "Generally Recognized as Safe" (GRAS). Additives on the GRAS list can be used by food processors without further approval from the FDA. However, even these substances must be retested as standards change.

Even though additives are approved by the FDA, consumers sometimes raise questions about their safety. In some cases, the FDA undertakes a process of study and review.

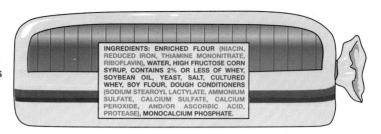

◆ Additives are used in many foods to improve the quality or lengthen the shelf life. **What is the meaning of the acronym "GRAS"?**

Consumers who are concerned about particular additives can avoid foods that contain them by reading ingredients lists carefully.

Sugar Substitutes

Sugar substitutes sweeten food while adding few or no calories. They can benefit people who must restrict the amount of sugar they eat, such as those with diabetes. Critics are not certain how helpful they may be for weight loss. Common artificial sweeteners include *aspartame* (ASS-pur-tame), *acesulfame-K* (ay-see-SULL-fame—KAY), and saccharin (SACK-uh-ruhn).

Some controversy has surrounded sugar substitutes. For example, saccharin was banned in 1977 after studies linked it with cancer in laboratory animals. By public demand, the ban was later lifted. The new rule allows products containing saccharin to be sold if a warning appears on the label and in the store.

Fat Substitutes

Fat substitutes are natural or artificial substances that replace fat in processed foods such as fried foods, baked goods, and ice cream. They are also used in reduced-fat foods, such as low-fat cheeses.

Some natural fat substitutes are based on proteins from ingredients such as nonfat milk or egg whites. Others are based on carbohydrates from sources such as cornstarch and oat bran. Natural substitutes are considered safe.

Artificial fat substitutes have also been developed. Since they do not break down during digestion, they add no fat or calories to the foods containing them. Specific FDA approval is required for artificial fat substitutes. One such substitute, *olestra* (oh-LESS-truh), was approved in 1996. However, some studies of this additive claim it removes some fat-soluble nutrients and phytochemicals from the body. The studies also indicate that olestra may cause mild digestive problems in some consumers. Because of these studies, the FDA requires that a warning label be on all packages of food that contain olestra, alerting consumers to these possible health risks.

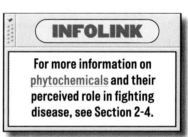

INFOLINK

For more information on phytochemicals and their perceived role in fighting disease, see Section 2-4.

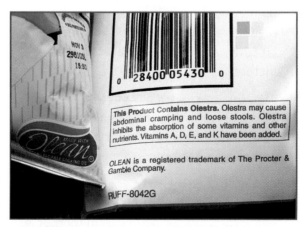

◆ Olestra, a synthetic fat, was first approved by the FDA for public consumption in 1996. **Compare and contrast the** advantages **and disadvantages of a product like olestra.**

Some experts are concerned that fat substitutes will not help people learn healthful eating habits. An eating plan heavily weighted toward fat-free treats may lack the proper balance of foods from the Food Guide Pyramid.

Irradiation

Irradiation is the process of exposing food to gamma rays to increase its shelf life and kill harmful microorganisms. Irradiation does not make foods radioactive. It can, however, cause minor changes in flavor and texture and slight vitamin loss.

Those in favor of irradiation mention its potential to improve food safety. It could reduce food-borne illness and eliminate the need for dangerous pesticides.

Critics of irradiation point to other concerns. They claim that irradiation produces harmful by-products that can lead to cancer and birth defects. They also fear that the radioactive chemicals used in irradiation plants pose a danger to workers and the community.

The FDA first approved the use of irradiation for spices. It has also been approved for fruits, vegetables, poultry, ground beef, and seafood. Irradiated foods must be identified with the symbol shown at the top of this page.

Genetic Engineering

Genetic engineering is a method of enhancing specific natural tendencies of plants and animals. This is done by altering genes, tiny

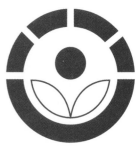

◆ **Irradiation plants use a conveyor system to move foods along.** Explain the purpose of irradiation.

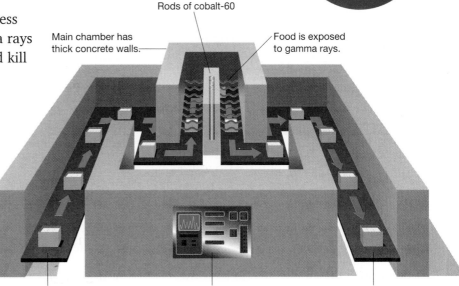

Rods of cobalt-60

Main chamber has thick concrete walls.

Food is exposed to gamma rays.

Packaged food is loaded on conveyor belt.

Computer controls conveyor speed and amount of radiation.

Food after irradiation

segments of matter that pass hereditary traits on from one generation to the next. Scientists have already used genetic engineering to produce new, hardier varieties of tomatoes, squash, and potatoes. They are working to develop other plants that are easier to grow and process, stay fresh longer, and have more nutrients.

Some critics have questioned the safety of foods that have been genetically altered. The FDA has developed guidelines for assessing the safety of such foods as they become available to consumers. It has also considered the question of product labeling. As with all foods, labeling is required if the product contains a substance that could trigger an allergic reaction or if the nutritional content has been altered.

Some people are concerned that genetic engineering could result in a food supply that is dependent on a few specifically designed plants. If so, unforeseen problems, such as a sudden change in climate, could endanger the entire food supply. Others, however, see genetic engineering as a way to increase the diversity of the world's crops.

This much is certain: Genetic engineering raises issues that have never had to be dealt with before. They will probably be debated for years to come.

Illegal Chemical Residues

In recent years, concern about chemical residues in food has increased. These residues are substances left behind in food after processing. Chemical residues have the potential to cause health problems, some of which can be serious.

Chemical residues can come from a variety of sources. In meat and poultry, they are usually from drugs used to improve animal health or from pesticides in animal feed. Residues gather in animal tissues. In plant foods, including grains, fruits, and vegetables, pesticides are usually the main residues.

Government agencies establish **tolerance levels**—maximum safe levels for certain chemicals in the human body. It is illegal for foods to contain more of a chemical than the tolerance level set for it. Government agencies test food samples regularly for illegal residue levels.

Safety Check

Never dump household chemicals down the drain or on the ground. The chemicals could contaminate the water and food supply. Follow package directions for proper disposal, or call your local sanitation department.

Contaminants

Contaminants are harmful substances that accidentally get into food as it moves from the farm to the table. One type of contaminant is chemical pollutants. Hazardous chemicals from industries, farms, or careless consumers can easily get into water supplies. Plants drawing on polluted water can become contaminated. Fish and other animals are also affected.

Microorganisms are another source of contamination. Salmonella bacteria, for example, can contaminate eggs and chickens, causing foodborne illness. *Aflatoxins* (AF-luh-TOCK-sunz) are poisonous substances produced by certain types of mold. They can sometimes be found in grains, milk, cheese, and peanuts.

As with illegal residues, various government agencies test food for contaminants to ensure the safety of the food supply.

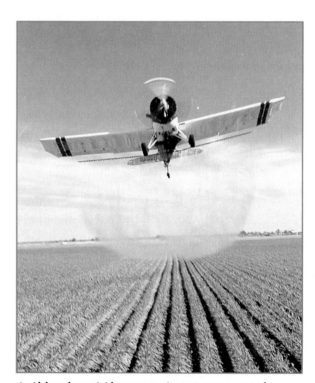

◆ **Although pesticides serve an important purpose, they also pose a health threat.** Explain the threat.

What Consumers Can Do

Contradictory reports regarding the safety of the food supply can be confusing to consumers. For reliable information, turn to a reputable consumer group concerned with food safety. Many such groups serve as watchdogs of both government and industry. Before you accept facts presented by a consumer group, however, be sure you know how it is funded. Some are merely agents for food and chemical industries.

Here are some additional suggestions for promoting a safe food supply:

◆ Support consumer groups that reflect your views.

◆ Avoid buying products from companies whose policies you do not support.

◆ Keep track of any laws that are being introduced relating to food. Write to your representatives. Tell them how you feel about any aspect of food safety.

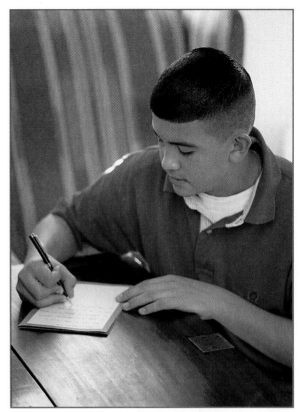

◆ **Writing to your representatives in government is constructive action you can take to ensure a safe food supply.** Name two other things you can do to ensure this.

Section 13-2 Review & Activities

1. Name four government agencies responsible for food safety.

2. What is a recall? Why are recalls important?

3. What is a food additive? Give two examples.

4. How might irradiation improve food safety?

5. Evaluating. How large a role do you think government should play in trying to make sure the country has a safe food supply? Explain your response.

6. Comparing and Contrasting. Form two groups to debate this statement as it applies to genetic engineering: "There are certain things humans should not meddle with."

7. Applying. Select a food safety issue you are concerned about. Write a letter to the appropriate government agency. Identify your concern, and ask for information on the government's role in this issue.

The Global Food Supply

In a perfect world, everyone would have plenty to eat. In the real world, many individuals and families go to bed hungry every night.

What accounts for the differences in the amounts and types of food available to different regions? This section will provide some answers.

Objectives

After studying this section, you should be able to:

- Explain why staple foods differ around the world.
- Identify the causes of food shortages.
- Discuss the possible ways to remedy global food problems.

Look for These Terms

industrialized nations

developing nations

staple foods

famine

subsistence farming

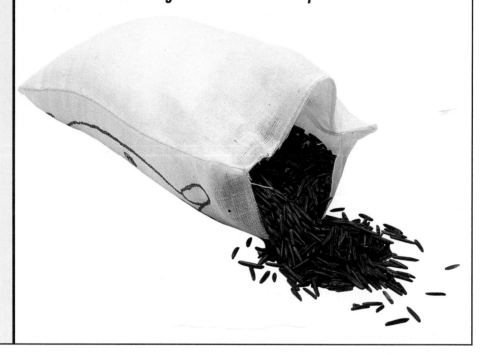

The Global View

One reason for differences in the food supply around the world is differing economic conditions. Countries are often categorized according to their economic progress. The **industrialized nations**, also called developed countries, are the richest. These are countries that rely on sophisticated, organized food industries to supply their citizens with food.

Developing nations are countries that are not yet industrialized or are just beginning to become so. People in such places cannot afford to buy food and must grow their own.

Some countries rank between industrialized and developing countries. As they progress economically, they are able to provide more food for their people.

Staple Foods

The food supply in any region also depends on what foods can be grown there. Only certain foods can be grown in each region. These **staple foods** are foods that make up the region's basic food supply. Several factors determine the staple foods for a given area:

- ◆ **Geography.** Food is most easily grown in areas where the soil is rich, such as valleys or plains. In mountainous areas, farming is more difficult. Animals that can live on rocky slopes, such as goats, may be raised.

- **Climate.** Moderate temperatures make it possible to grow a wide variety of food. In some climates, temperatures vary and food can be grown only during the warm months. Extreme temperatures, either high or low, limit the kinds of food that can be grown.

- **Rainfall.** Some crops thrive in areas that receive a lot of rainfall annually. Little, if any, food can be grown in dry areas such as deserts.

In many parts of the world, grains are the main staple foods. This is especially true in developing countries. Each type of grain, such as wheat, rice, corn, and rye, is best suited to a particular climate. For example, rice grows in warm, wet climates.

Grain is also fed to animals used for food. However, animals are inefficient in converting grain to meat. With cattle, for example, it takes about 8 to 10 pounds (3.6 to 4.5 kg) of grain to produce 1 pound (500 g) of meat.

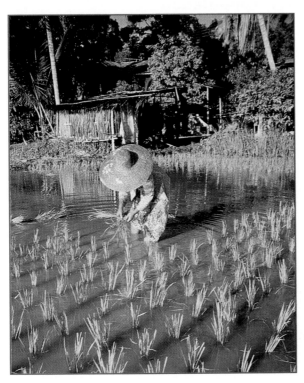

Food Shortages

It's estimated that about 700 million of the world's people don't have enough to eat. For some, that means going hungry for several days at a time. The most severe form of diminished food supply is **famine**—food shortages that continue for months or years. Many die of starvation during periods of famine.

The problem of world hunger is a complex one. Some of the basic causes are economics, inefficient farming methods, fuel shortages, overpopulation, wars and politics, and natural disasters. These factors may affect food production, or they may cause problems in distributing or using the food.

Economics

In many developing countries, most people are too poor to buy food and live instead on very meager meals consisting of home-grown foods. This practice of maintaining a small plot of land on which a family grows its own food is known as **subsistence farming**.

Some farmers have enough land to grow crops they can sell, or *cash crops*. However, when cash crops are exported, local food shortages often occur. Also, world food prices change so frequently that cash-crop farmers cannot depend on steady incomes.

In developing countries, good roads are rare. Villages are separated, with no modern transportation to connect them. As a result, it's difficult to distribute food. One area may have a surplus of food while a few miles away, people have nothing to eat. During famine, poor distribution keeps food aid from reaching starving people.

◆ Rice paddies like this one provide supplies of the staple grain throughout much of Southeast Asia. Investigate other foods that play a role in the diet of people in Cambodia or Vietnam.

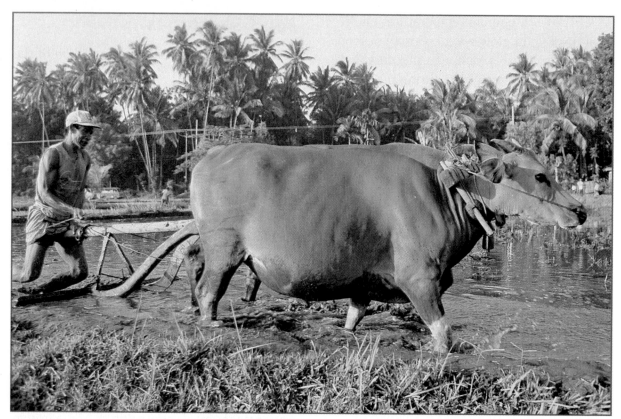

◆ **Subsistence farming relies on simple tools powered by people or animals.** Why is modern machinery not used for these tasks?

Inefficient Farming Methods

Subsistence farming makes use of ancient methods. Animals, instead of gas-powered machinery, supply the power. Farm tools are simple, having designs that date back hundreds of years. With such outdated tools and methods, food production is low. However, modern farming equipment and methods are costly and not always suited to the crops and conditions in developing countries.

Fuel Shortages

Most food must be cooked before being eaten, which means that fuel for cooking is essential. In developing countries, wood is the most common cooking fuel. Unfortunately, many areas are experiencing serious shortages of wood. Without fuel for cooking, people may go hungry.

Overpopulation

The world population, which has been growing steadily, could increase to 15 billion people by 2010. The most rapid increase has been in developing countries. As population grows, so does the demand for food. At the same time, more land is taken for housing, leaving less land for farming. When people clear forests to get more farmland, they destroy their source of fuel.

Will the food supply keep up with the increase in population? Some experts think not.

Wars and Politics

Wars can have a devastating effect on food supplies. Animals are killed and crops destroyed. People are forced to abandon their farms. Fighting disrupts food distribution systems.

Food is also used as a political weapon. Opposing parties may interfere with food distribution or manipulate supplies. Food aid may never reach the needy because it is stolen and sold on the black market.

During the 1900s, millions of people in Africa died of starvation because of civil wars in many countries.

Natural Disasters

Natural disasters such as floods and earthquakes can destroy a region's food supply. Crops may be damaged and animals killed. If soil erosion occurs or roads are destroyed, food supplies can be affected for many years. Prolonged drought, especially in developing countries, can result in famine and starvation.

What Can Be Done?

Many efforts are being made to increase the global food supply. The most common goal is to educate people in developing countries to help themselves. They are too poor to afford modern farming machinery and methods. Therefore, programs help people within the means available to them.

The United Nations, government agencies such as the Peace Corps, and private nonprofit organizations, such as the American Friends Service Committee and Oxfam International, are involved with the education process. They show farmers how to improve farming methods and equipment and how to increase water supplies. In Ethiopia, for instance, food production increased as a result of broadening the tiny steel blade on the crude wooden plows used by farmers.

The Role of Technology

Food technology also has an important role in increasing the world's food supply. Through genetic engineering, scientists hope to produce varieties of grains and other plant foods that are resistant to drought and other environmental problems.

Nutritious products are also being developed. Because people in some developing countries cannot easily digest milk or milk products, an alternative product is being introduced around the world. This new product is made by grinding leaves into a paste, which is then made into a highly nutritious crumbly cake.

Solar energy offers much hope as a solution to the problem of fuel shortages. It has great potential where the climate is sunny and dry most of the year. Several types of solar cookers are available, including one made inexpensively from cardboard, aluminum foil, and a plastic bag. These cookers can be used for most meal preparation tasks, such as simmering rice, baking potatoes, cooking casseroles and stews, and even pasteurizing milk. The solar cookers are being used in various areas, including India, China, Africa, Central America, and the southwestern United States.

Nutritionists from nonprofit organizations teach area residents how to use solar cookers. They also teach the basics of good nutrition.

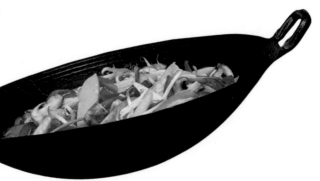

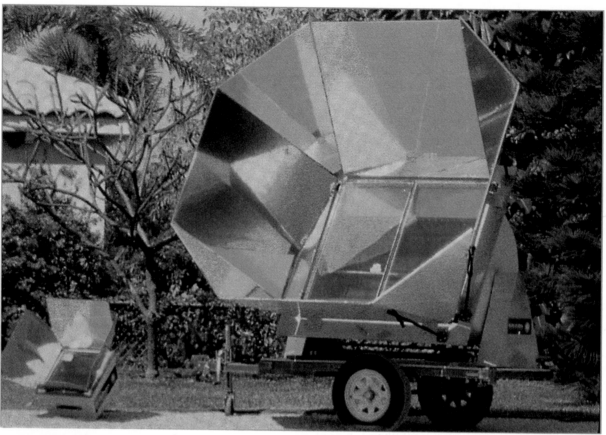

◆ **Solar-powered cookers like this one provide a means of cooking food in areas where fuel is scarce.** What current developments worldwide may increase the need for solar cookers in the future?

Section 13-3 Review & Activities

1. What is meant by the term *staple foods*? Name two factors that determine the staple foods found in a given place.

2. Identify five causes of food shortages.

3. Name two ways in which technology is being used to increase the global food supply.

4. **Analyzing.** Put the following statement in your own words: "To learn about hunger, you need look no farther than your own backyard." Explain what factors account for the problem alluded to in the statement.

5. **Extending.** What problems could result from trying to introduce modern farming machinery and methods in developing nations?

6. **Applying.** In magazines and newspapers, find articles about regions that are experiencing famine. Write a one-page report about one such locality, along with any recommendations you can make for curtailing the problem.

CAREER WANTED

Individuals with good communication and leadership skills; background and experience in the food industry.

REQUIRES:

- degree in food science or related field
- supervision of others
- passage of FDA exam

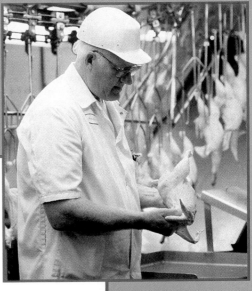

"Food safety is critical,"

says Louis Panopolous, FDA Inspector

Q: Louis, just what do you do as a food safety inspector?

A: I work for the U.S. Food and Drug Administration. I visit food production plants and check for violations such as inaccurate product labeling and possible contamination. I meet with plant managers, inspect their production lines, and collect product samples. My primary responsibility is public health and safety.

Q: What happens to the information you gather?

A: The samples are sent to an FDA lab to be analyzed. I write up my findings and present it to the FDA. If a problem is found, the firm must correct it and recall unsafe products.

Q: What is your work environment like?

A: I spend a lot of time traveling from one inspection site to another. My hours are often long and irregular. However, I enjoy meeting lots of people and seeing America. I also attend seminars to keep up with changes in FDA rules and regulations, as well as new developments in food science and technology.

Q: Is the need for food safety inspectors expected to grow in the coming decades?

A: Yes, very much so. Genetic engineering will continue to increase the need for inspectors. It is critical that we assure food safety as technology advances.

Career Research Activity

1. After researching one of the careers listed, create an informative brochure about it.

2. Visit the FDA or USDA web site and search for job openings. Compare the qualifications and salary ranges for three different positions. Write a one-page summary and explain why you would or would not be interested in pursuing each of the three different jobs.

Related Career Opportunities

Entry Level
- Food Service Worker
- Lab Assistant

Technical Level
- Laboratory Testing Technician
- Health Inspector
- Quality Control Technician

Professional Level
- FDA Food Safety Inspector
- Microbiologist
- Public Health Administrator

Chapter 13   Review & Activities

— Summary —

Section 13-1: Where Does Food Come From?

- Most food begins its journey to the consumer as a farm product.

- New farming technologies have been developed that do not use fertilizers or pesticides, which can harm the environment.

- From the farm, food is sent to a processor, where it is prepared for its final use.

- The processor sends food to the distributor, who sells it to the retailer. The retailer then sells the food to the consumer.

- The price consumers pay for the food depends on many factors.

Section 13-2: A Safe Food Supply

- In the United States, the federal government monitors the safety of the nation's food supply. Various government agencies inspect food for contamination and regulate food processing, packaging, and labeling.

- Food safety issues that are a source of concern include the use of food additives, food irradiation, genetic engineering, chemical residues from food processing, and contaminants that threaten the food supply.

Section 13-3: The Global Food Supply

- The basic food supply, or staple foods, of a region depends on geography, climate, and rainfall.

- Food shortages are caused by a number of factors that affect food production and distribution.

- International agencies and scientists are working to increase the food supply in developing countries.

Checking Your Knowledge

1. Give two examples of sustainable farming practices.

2. List four commercial preservation methods.

3. How does supply and demand affect food prices?

4. Identify what *FDA* and *FSIS* stand for. What types of food is each agency responsible for keeping safe?

5. What types of food additives are found on the GRAS list?

6. What are chemical residues? How do they get into food?

7. How does food production differ in industrialized nations and developing nations?

8. Explain the problems associated with growing cash crops in developing countries.

9. Explain the relationship between the growing population, food supplies, and fuel supplies.

10. How can genetic engineering be used to help increase the world's food supply?

Working IN THE Lab

1. *Taste Test.* Cook or heat equal amounts of two forms of the same vegetable. Compare for taste, texture, appearance, price per serving, and convenience.

2. *Food Science.* Conduct an experiment using two loaves of bread—one homemade and the other a store brand with preservatives. Place one slice of each on a plate, uncovered. Wrap another slice of each in plastic wrap. After two, five, and seven days, compare for mold and other signs of spoilage. What conclusions can you draw?

Review & Activities Chapter 13

Thinking Critically

1. Identifying Ambiguous Statements. Brad had just bought a package of crackers from the school vending machine. He was about to take a bite when Serena, a classmate, stopped him. "I'm doing you a huge favor," she said. "Those crackers are loaded with additives. If you want a safe snack, I have an extra apple in my backpack. I'll be happy to give it to you." On the basis of information provided in the chapter, how would you advise Brad to respond? Explain.

2. Determining Credibility. Imagine that a respected scientist testifies before the FDA that a certain pesticide is safe and effective. Later it is discovered that the university where the scientist teaches receives large donations from the company that makes the pesticide. How does this affect your opinion of the scientist's findings?

Reinforcing Key Skills

1. Communication. You are grocery shopping for the family dinner. When you reach the produce department, you find that most of the fruits and vegetables are bruised, wilted, or otherwise damaged. Knowing that this drives prices up, decide whom you would speak to and what you would say. Write out the text of your message.

2. Leadership. A friend tells you that, unless you are a scientist or politician, there is nothing you can do to increase the world's food supply. You want to prove him wrong by reducing food waste and helping the hungry in your community. Tell what action you would take.

Making Decisions and Solving Problems

Your friend wants to lose weight. She tells you that her weight-loss plan is based mainly on low-calorie foods and beverages made with artificial sweeteners and fat substitutes. She asks for your opinion. What do you say to her?

Making Connections

1. Language Arts. Using library or online sources, investigate the history of a food additive that has been in use for at least 100 years. Write a short autobiography, in which you take the point of view of the additive. Discuss the reason you were "born" (your original purpose), what kind of popularity you have enjoyed, and any controversies that might lead to your untimely demise. Your autobiography may be humorous, but keep it informative. Read your work aloud to classmates.

2. Social Studies. Using library sources, locate five farming regions on at least three different continents. For each region, identify the main crops, describe the geography and climate conditions that make the crops successful, and tell what products they are used in. Share your findings in a brief report.

Chapter 13 ◆ Review & Activities 375

Section 14-1
Consumer Skills

Section 14-2
Choosing Kitchen Equipment

Section 14-3
Designing a Kitchen

Shopping for a new refrigerator took Shasta's family to several different appliance stores. Using information she had learned in her family and consumer sciences class, Shasta helped her parents compare features on different models.

Some day you may be making a purchase like this for your own home. In this chapter, you will learn what you need to know.

Buying for the Kitchen

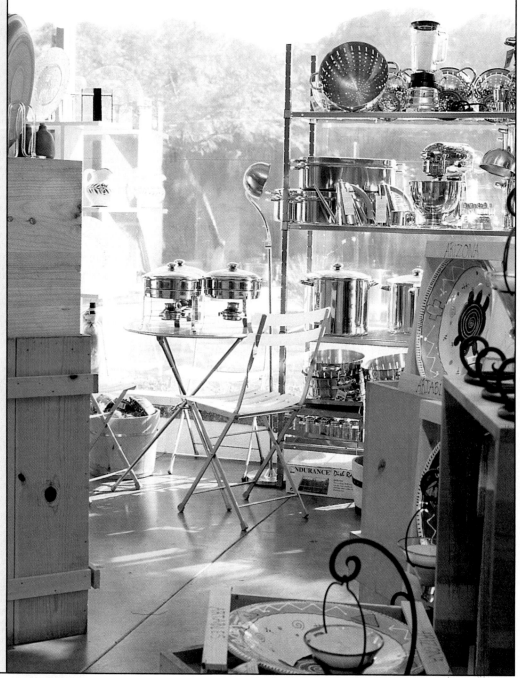

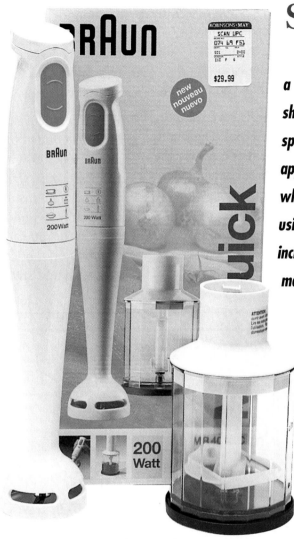

SECTION
14-1

Objectives

After studying this section, you should be able to:

- Describe the decisions that must be made before shopping for kitchen equipment.
- List four important shopping guidelines that can help you make wise kitchen purchases.

Look for These Terms

credit
principal
interest
annual percentage rate (APR)
finance charge
warranty
EnergyGuide label
service contract

Consumer Skills

Buying equipment for a kitchen can vary from shopping for a mixing spoon to buying a major appliance. No matter what you plan to buy, using consumer skills will increase your chances of making a smart purchase.

Before You Shop

Have you ever bought an article of clothing that ended up unworn in a drawer or closet? Before you buy anything, you need to think about your reasons for making that purchase. This step is particularly important when you are making a major purchase.

Begin by asking yourself these questions. If you are updating an item you already have, will the replacement be enough of an improvement to justify its cost? If you are buying a new item, will you use it? How much can you afford to spend? How will you pay for the item? Shasta's family asked themselves these questions. The refrigerator they ended up buying cost less than they initially planned to spend!

Paying for Your Purchase

Most people pay cash for small items. Some save so that they can pay cash for larger purchases, too. Many people, however, use credit for at least part of the cost of major purchases.

Buying on Credit

Credit is money you borrow from a lender. The lender may be a bank, as is the case with most credit cards, or it may be a different kind of financial institution. Buying on credit is more expensive than paying cash, but it allows you to use the item while you pay for it.

Credit has a vocabulary of its own. The money you borrow is the **principal**. The lender charges you interest. **Interest** is a fee for the loan, expressed as a percentage of the amount you borrow. Interest rates vary. By law, they must be stated in terms of **annual percentage rate (APR)**, which gives you the yearly cost of a loan.

When considering credit, look carefully at the **finance charge** —the total amount you will pay for borrowing. It includes interest and other costs, such as service charges and credit-related insurance premiums. Monthly payments are usually computed by dividing the total cost (principal + finance charge) by the number of months of the loan.

For major purchases, you may have several financing options. Many stores offer financing. Loans are available from institutions such as banks and finance companies. Credit cards can also be used.

Shop for credit as carefully as for your purchase. Ask each lender for the APR and finance charges so that you can compare the cost of borrowing. The differences in total cost may surprise you.

One problem with using credit is that you may be tempted to spend more than you can afford. Failure to make monthly payments on time can cause significant problems. The items you purchased can be taken away from you, and you may find it difficult to get credit in the future. You can avoid these problems by deciding on a price range you are comfortable with and sticking to it.

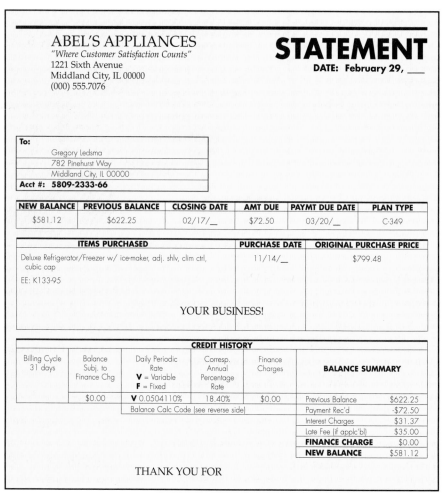

◆ People who buy on credit periodically receive bills that look something like this. What is the annual percentage rate on this loan?

◆ **Some consumer publications are run by not-for-profit organizations that permit them to conduct unbiased tests on goods and products.** How can you determine which publications rely on these types of tests?

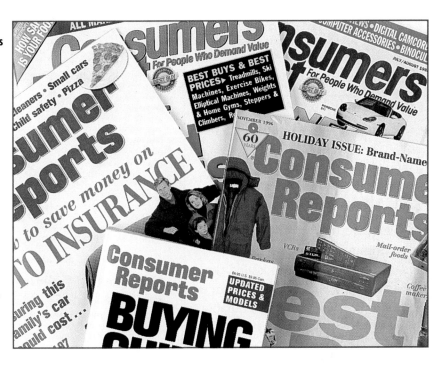

Buying Guidelines

Following a few simple shopping guidelines can help you make wise choices when buying for the kitchen. Any item you plan to keep a long time should be chosen with special care.

Consider Your Needs and Wants

Begin by identifying the characteristics and features most important in the item you plan to buy. For instance, if you're buying a new appliance, write down the measurements of the space where it must fit. If your new dishes must be microwave-safe, note that.

Also write down the features you would like the item to have. Rank your wants from most to least important. Setting priorities is helpful because you may not be able to find an item within your price range that has all the features you want.

Gather Information

Well-informed shoppers usually are happy with the items they purchase and often get a good price. Many sources of information are available. Look for advertisements and articles in magazines and newspapers. Some consumer magazines conduct unbiased tests to compare similar items from different manufacturers.

You can also contact manufacturers directly for up-to-date information.

The reliability of the store is also important, especially for major purchases. Check with the closest Better Business Bureau to see if the business has had complaints from consumers and if the complaints have been settled satisfactorily.

Look for Consumer Safeguards

As you shop, look for consumer safeguards. Government agencies, manufacturers, and dealers have provided means for ensuring the quality of products.

Seals of Approval

Seals of approval are given by nonprofit testing agencies to show that a product meets certain standards for safety and performance.

◆ On gas appliances, look for the *American Gas Association* seal. It indicates that a gas appliance's design, performance, and reliability have been tested and certified.

◆ **The EnergyGuide label gives the appliance's estimated energy cost. Why is this information important?**

◆ On electrical appliances, look for the *Underwriters Laboratories* seal. It indicates that an electrical appliance design is reasonably free from the risk of fire, electric shock, and other hazards.

Other seals of approval may be found on a product or a package. Find out more about who issued the seal and what it means. Don't assume that every seal comes from a reliable product-testing agency.

Warranties

A **warranty** is a manufacturer's guarantee that a product will perform as advertised. If you have problems with the product, the manufacturer promises to replace it or repair it. A warranty often has limits on the length of time it is in effect and what is covered.

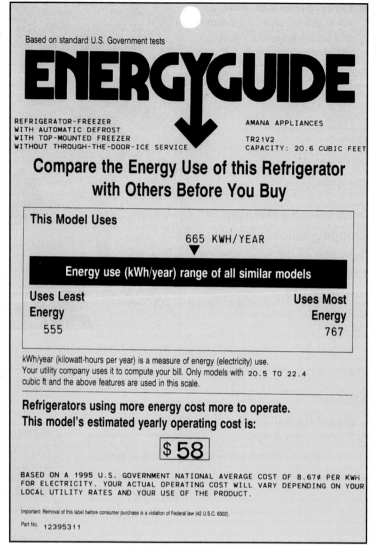

Based on standard U.S. Government tests

ENERGYGUIDE

REFRIGERATOR-FREEZER
WITH AUTOMATIC DEFROST
WITH TOP-MOUNTED FREEZER
WITHOUT THROUGH-THE-DOOR-ICE SERVICE

AMANA APPLIANCES

TR21V2
CAPACITY: 20.6 CUBIC FEET

Compare the Energy Use of this Refrigerator with Others Before You Buy

This Model Uses

665 KWH/YEAR
▼

Energy use (kWh/year) range of all similar models

Uses Least
Energy
555

Uses Most
Energy
767

kWh/year (kilowatt-hours per year) is a measure of energy (electricity) use. Your utility company uses it to compute your bill. Only models with 20.5 TO 22.4 cubic ft and the above features are used in this scale.

Refrigerators using more energy cost more to operate. This model's estimated yearly operating cost is:

$ 58

BASED ON A 1995 U.S. GOVERNMENT NATIONAL AVERAGE COST OF 8.67¢ PER KWH FOR ELECTRICITY. YOUR ACTUAL OPERATING COST WILL VARY DEPENDING ON YOUR LOCAL UTILITY RATES AND YOUR USE OF THE PRODUCT.

Important: Removal of this label before consumer purchase is a violation of Federal law (42 U.S.C. 6302).

Part No. 12395311

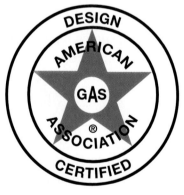

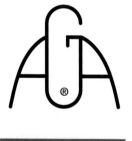

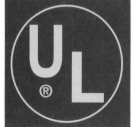

◆ **Looking for seals of approval is one consumer skill that can help you make an informed decision. Describe two other skills.**

EnergyGuide Labels

An **EnergyGuide label** gives information to help you estimate the energy costs of an appliance. Such labels are required for most major appliances. A dollar figure tells the average yearly cost for that model. You can compare the costs for different models. You can also project your own energy expenses based on the cost of gas or electricity in your area.

Service Contracts

A **service contract** is repair and maintenance insurance purchased to cover a product for a specific length of time. It is usually sold by the store that sells you the product. Service contracts often don't cover the total cost of repairs and parts. They may duplicate the protection received free with the warranty. Service contracts are often expensive and are only as good as the company that issues them.

Be an Active Shopper

While shopping, don't just look. Think about how the product will perform and last.

◆ Keep written notes. Making a list of your likes and dislikes as you shop can help you make a final decision.

◆ Consider accident prevention. Look for a seal of approval. Check carefully for potential hazards as well as features that protect against accidents.

◆ Handle tools, cookware, and appliances. Do they seem comfortable to use and durable?

◆ Look at the warranty and owner's manual. What exactly does the warranty cover? Will the item be easy to use and care for?

◆ Compare prices. More features and better quality usually mean a higher price. Some brands are generally more expensive than others. Sometimes, however, lower-priced items are a better buy.

◆ Ask the dealer about additional costs. Are there separate charges for delivery and installation?

Connecting Food and Health

Let the Seller Beware

Suppose you *do* buy something that doesn't work. What recourse do you have as a consumer? Here are some places you can turn for help:

• **Department of Consumer Affairs.** These offices exist at the municipal level. They are staffed by people trained to know local regulations and procedures. You can find the number in your local telephone directory.

• **Media action programs.** More than 100 newspapers and 50 radio and TV stations across the nation offer action or hot line services for consumers who need help.

• **Government agencies.** The Consumer Product Safety Commission (CPSC) and Federal Trade Commission (FTC) are just two of many federal agencies that protect your interests and rights.

Think About It

• Gather information at your local library, online, or from your local telephone directory about specific services in your community that aid consumers. Use a computer to make a guide to these services; explain the type of services each offers and how to contact each organization. Make copies of your guide available in your school and community.

When You Get Your Purchase Home

You will probably bring home some important documents with your purchase, especially if it's an appliance. You may have your receipt, a warranty, and an owner's manual. Keep these documents together in a safe place. If the warranty has a registration card, fill it out and send it in. Even if you don't have problems with the product, the manufacturer may need to notify you if a product poses a danger to the user.

Read the owner's manual before you use the product. Then test the product to make certain it works. If it doesn't, return it to the store or call the dealer.

Section 14-1 Review & Activities

1. What are two questions you should ask yourself before shopping for kitchen equipment?

2. What is credit? What is interest?

3. List the four guidelines to follow when shopping for the kitchen.

4. What should you do when you get your purchase home?

5. **Synthesizing.** What are some ways the choice of kitchen equipment affects how a family plans and prepares meals?

6. **Extending.** Review the definition of *impulse buying,* introduced in Chapter 12 (page 337). Discuss whether you would advise a friend who buys on impulse to apply for a credit card. Explain your reasons.

7. **Applying.** Collect magazine and newspaper advertisements for different brands of a major kitchen appliance. Make a chart that compares the various features that are available.

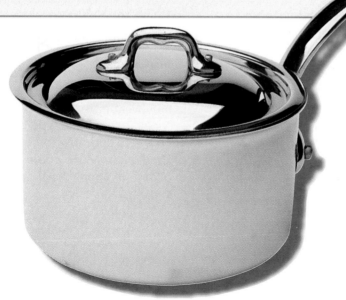

Choosing Kitchen Equipment

Just what kinds of equipment are included in a kitchen depends on budget, space, and personal preference. Equipping a kitchen can be an expensive process. Most people start with the basics and then add equipment over the years.

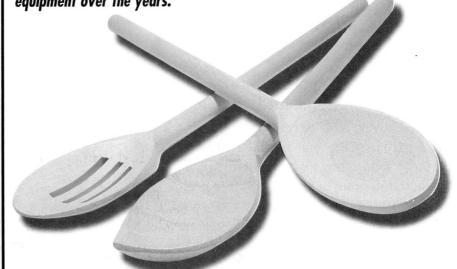

Objectives

After studying this section, you should be able to:

- Give examples of choices available in appliances, small equipment, and tableware.
- Discuss features to look for when buying items for the kitchen.

Look for These Terms

self-cleaning

continuous-cleaning

Buying Appliances

Appliances can take up a major portion of your kitchen equipment budget. So it pays to shop carefully.

Refrigerator-Freezers

Today there are more options than ever before in refrigerator-freezers. The freezer may be placed at the top, side, or bottom. Some models defrost the freezer automatically. Manual-defrost models must be emptied, thawed, and cleaned regularly.

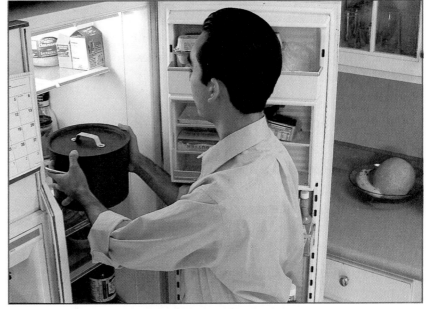

◆ **Some refrigerator-freezers have adjustable shelves for more flexibility.** Name two other special features. Identify their advantages and disadvantages.

Special features add not only to convenience but also to cost. Decide which features are most important and within your budget. In the refrigerator, choices include adjustable shelves, temperature- and humidity-controlled compartments for vegetables and meat, and special areas for tall or large items such as milk and soda. You will also find automatic ice makers and doors with ice and chilled water dispensers on the outside.

Ranges, Cooktops, and Ovens

When buying a major cooking appliance, you'll have to make some basic decisions first. Are you looking for an all-in-one range, a countertop oven, or separate built-in cooktop and oven units? Do you want a gas or an electric model? If you are replacing appliances in an existing kitchen, these decisions may already be determined. If you are remodeling or planning a new kitchen, your options are probably more open.

Cooktops

Although traditional gas burners or electric coils are still most typical, many new choices in cooktops are available. For example:

◆ **Sealed gas burners.** Have no visible flame and no pilot light. This feature adds safety and aids cleanup.

◆ **Smooth cooktops.** Are easy to clean. They include induction cooktops, which use electromagnetic energy. Heat is generated when a pan made of a magnetic metal is placed on the induction cooktop.

◆ **Modules.** Units that allow greater flexibility. A grill, griddle, or other accessory can be substituted for standard surface units.

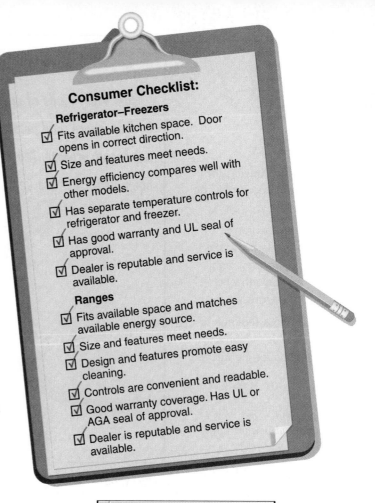

Consumer Checklist:

Refrigerator–Freezers

☑ Fits available kitchen space. Door opens in correct direction.

☑ Size and features meet needs.

☑ Energy efficiency compares well with other models.

☑ Has separate temperature controls for refrigerator and freezer.

☑ Has good warranty and UL seal of approval.

☑ Dealer is reputable and service is available.

Ranges

☑ Fits available space and matches available energy source.

☑ Size and features meet needs.

☑ Design and features promote easy cleaning.

☑ Controls are convenient and readable.

☑ Good warranty coverage. Has UL or AGA seal of approval.

☑ Dealer is reputable and service is available.

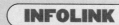

INFOLINK

For more on cooktops and the advantages and limitations of the different types, see Section 9-1.

Ovens

Shopping for an oven—as a separate unit or as part of a range—begins with the choice of conventional, convection, or microwave models. You may prefer a range with two ovens—one below the cooktop and a smaller one at eye level. Another option is an oven that combines two or more cooking methods in a single unit, such as a microwave-convection oven. As noted in Chapter 9, convection ovens use a fan to circulate the heated air and reduce cooking time.

Conventional and convection ovens are available with easy-clean options. A **self-cleaning** oven has a special cleaning cycle that uses high heat to burn off food stains. A **continuous-cleaning** oven has special rough interior walls that absorb spills and splatters. Soil residue can be easily wiped off.

Microwave ovens have many features. Some come equipped with a turntable. Others have a rack, which increases the capacity of the oven. Another feature is electronic programming, which can be used to cook food automatically. Browning units improve the appearance of microwaved foods. Temperature probes allow heating to a specific temperature.

Small Appliances

From sandwich makers to automatic bread machines, the list of small appliances available seems endless. Small electrical appliances can save time, money, and energy. However, having too many can cause storage problems. Before you buy, consider whether the appliance will be helpful enough to justify the cost and space required. Will you use it, or will you just store it in the back of a cabinet?

As with any other kitchen equipment, look for features that promote safety, comfort, ease of use, and ease of care. Doing research ahead of time will help you learn what to look for and which features you may want or need. For example, if you are shopping for a food processor, you will want to consider models that include a safety lock, a food pusher, and an overload switch—all these are important safety features.

Buying Other Equipment

Equipment needs don't end with major and small appliances. Kitchens also need cookware, bakeware, and tools.

Cookware and Bakeware

As discussed in Chapter 9, utensils used for cooking and baking can be made from a variety of materials, depending on their intended use. Each material has advantages and disadvantages.

Both cookware and bakeware are available as sets or by the individual piece. Keep in mind that both are major investments that should last for years. Consider these purchasing guidelines:

◆ Look for materials and finishes that are strong and durable enough to withstand daily use. Edges should be smooth. Handles should be heat-resistant.

◆ Choose high-quality items. Look for seamless construction. Metal should be heavy enough to resist warping.

◆ Check the balance of each piece. Look for flat bottoms and secure lids.

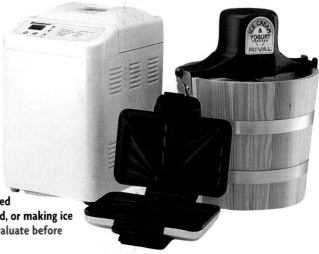

◆ Many small appliances serve just one specific function, such as making toasted sandwiches, automatically baking bread, or making ice cream. What factors do you need to evaluate before making such a purchase?

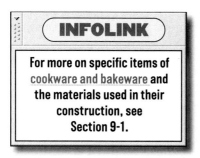

INFOLINK

For more on specific items of
cookware and bakeware and
the materials used in their
construction, see
Section 9-1.

Tools

As explained in Chapters 8 and 9, dozens of
hand tools are available to make the process
of preparing food faster and more convenient.
Many of these tools are designed for specific
tasks. Others can be used for several different
jobs. Follow these guidelines when selecting
kitchen tools:

◆ Choose tools that fit a real need. Avoid
buying ones you will seldom use.

◆ Well-designed, high-quality tools are easy
to use and will last for a long time. Knives,
for example, should have sturdy handles
that are firmly attached to the blades. Look
for at least two rivets (fasteners) through
the handle and the blade. Higher-quality
knives have three.

◆ Tools used for hot foods should be
heat-resistant.

◆ Keep storage in mind. If you can't store the
tool in a convenient place, you probably
won't use it very often.

Buying Tableware

The term *tableware* refers to any item
used for serving and eating food, including
dinnerware, flatware, glassware, and linens.
The amount, type, and formality of tableware
people choose vary. Some people have one
set; others have two or more.

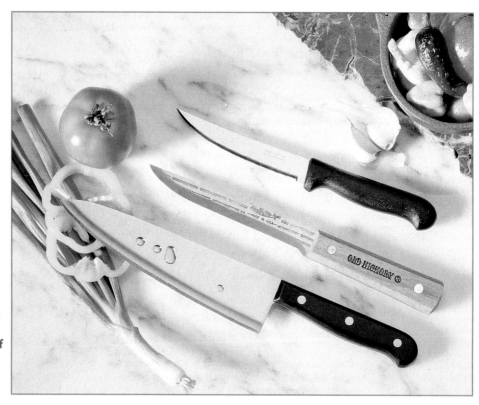

◆ **Look for quality kitchen
tools when stocking
essential items.** Which of
these knives would you
be most likely to buy?
Explain your answer.

Dinnerware, flatware, and glassware are available with many different designs, or patterns, on them. Remember, however, that patterns in tableware do not have to match. You can mix and match pieces that complement one another.

Most tableware is priced and sold by the place setting—the pieces used by one person to eat a meal. Sometimes you can buy sets for a number of people. Serving pieces may be sold individually or grouped as a set. Some tableware is also sold as open stock, meaning you can buy each piece separately.

Prices for tableware vary widely depending on quality and brand name. Fine china, crystal glassware, and silver flatware are the most formal and most expensive choices. Most people who have these items use them only for special occasions. For everyday use, there are many less costly, easy-to-care-for, yet attractive options. These include stainless steel flatware, informal glassware, and dishes made of stoneware, glass-ceramic, or plastic. Microwave-safe dinnerware and dishwasher-safe tableware are practical choices.

➕ Safety Check

Lead is a toxic metal that can travel from a container into food. It may be present in tableware and cookware made from pottery. Lead crystal glassware also contains lead. Do not use lead crystal regularly or store beverages in lead crystal for more than a few hours.

Section 14-2 Review & Activities

1. Give four examples of options available in range cooktops.

2. List three things to look for when buying cookware and bakeware.

3. What does buying tableware as open stock mean? What is another way tableware may be sold?

4. Extending. Suppose you and a friend decided to share an apartment while in college. What considerations might determine how you go about equipping a kitchen effectively?

5. Analyzing. Why should the observation "You get what you pay for" be the motto of anyone furnishing a home kitchen?

6. Applying. Choose a large or small kitchen appliance. Using magazines or other resources, make a list of the special features that are available.

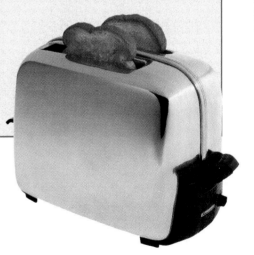

Designing a Kitchen

As Jenna approached Taylor, she noticed that her friend was reading a magazine on home improvements. "Why are you reading that?" Jenna asked.

"We're planning to remodel our home kitchen," Taylor replied. "I'm reading up on remodeling to help my mom make a checklist of things to think about."

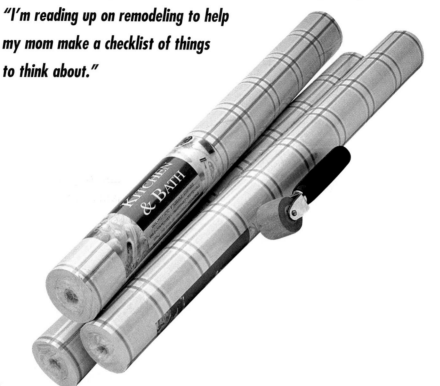

Objectives

After studying this section, you should be able to:

- Discuss considerations in kitchen design.

- Explain how the floor plan and other elements of a kitchen can affect safety and convenience.

- Give examples of barrier-free kitchen designs.

Look for These Terms

work flow

peninsula

island

grounding

task lighting

life-span design

Kitchen Design Basics

Taylor and her mom are smart! If you are remodeling a kitchen or moving to a new home, knowing something about kitchen design can help you evaluate how convenient and accident-free a kitchen is. This knowledge can also come in handy if you're ever in a position to plan a totally new kitchen. Even if you're not planning to remodel, you can use the information to find low-cost ways to improve your kitchen. Finally, knowing basics of kitchen design can open the door to some exciting career possibilities.

Planning a successful kitchen begins with recognizing the lifestyle of the people who will use it. Following well-researched principles of kitchen design helps ensure efficiency.

Considering Lifestyle

Taylor and her mother live alone. Their kitchen needs are different from those of a larger family. Some questions to think about when considering the design of a kitchen are:

◆ What activities, besides cooking, will take place in the kitchen? Will it be used, for example, for eating? For entertaining?

- How much kitchen equipment and food must be stored?

- Will more than one person at a time generally work in the kitchen?

- What are the needs and preferences of those who will use the space?

Designing for Efficiency

An efficient kitchen starts with a well-designed floor plan. It should provide enough space for working but also keep walking to a minimum. It should also optimize the **work flow**, that is, the recurring patterns of activity and repetitive tasks associated with any type of job routine. In a kitchen, these tasks revolve around food preparation—food is removed from storage, washed if necessary, prepared, and served—and involve moving from one place in the kitchen to another.

The Work Triangle

As noted in Section 7-1, the sink, cooking, and cold storage centers are the three major kitchen work centers. They make up the primary path of work called the "work triangle." In this common design, each work center is located at a point in the triangle. For an efficient work flow, the legs of the triangle should total between 12 and 22 feet (3.6 and 6.7 m).

When only one person works in the kitchen, the work triangle is an efficient arrangement. However, today's kitchens are often used by several people at once. Additional work space and duplicate work centers help avoid traffic jams. For example, a second sink or a separate microwave oven can give space for two cooks. The kitchen may then have adjacent or overlapping work triangles.

The kitchen should be arranged so that people going from one room to another do not pass through the work triangle. Such traffic can cut efficiency and may cause accidents.

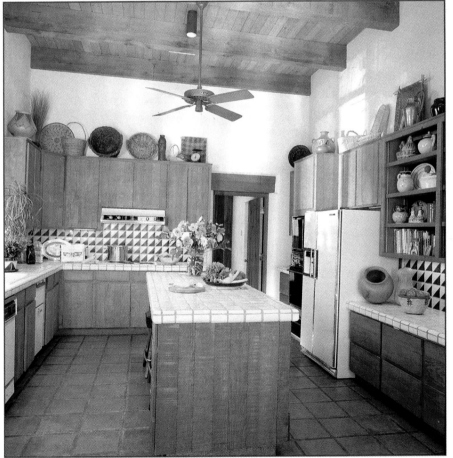

- Kitchen design should be based on how the space and appliances will be used. Identify two other factors that need to be considered.

Basic Kitchen Plans

Kitchens are often categorized by the location of the cabinets and major appliances. These common types have certain characteristics:

◆ **One-wall.** All three work centers are on one wall. One-wall kitchens tend to be small, with limited storage and counter space.

◆ **Corridor.** The work centers are located on two parallel walls. This pattern is efficient for one cook. However, efficiency is lessened if the corridor is a traffic lane through the kitchen.

◆ **L-shaped.** The work centers are on two connecting walls. No through traffic interrupts work.

◆ **U-shaped.** This efficient plan has work centers on three connecting walls, forming a U shape.

These basic kitchen plans may be modified by the addition of a peninsula or an island. A **peninsula** is an extension of a countertop. An **island** is a freestanding unit, often in the center of the kitchen. Both can include storage space below the countertop. They can be equipped with a sink or cooktop, or they may serve as an eating area.

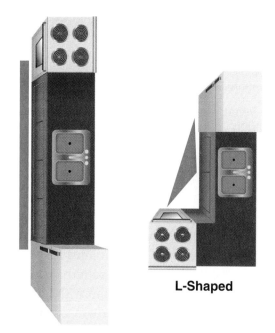

L-Shaped

One-Wall

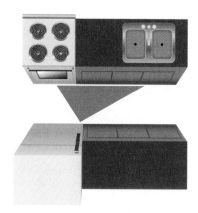

Corridor

◆ In basic kitchen designs, the sink, cooking, and cold storage centers are seen as forming three points of a "work triangle." What particular needs are served by each of the basic plans shown? What other considerations would affect which kitchen plan a family might choose?

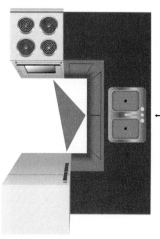

←**U-Shaped**→

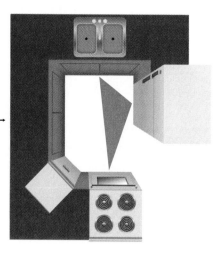

Storage and Work Space

The amount of storage and counter space in the kitchen also affects how pleasant and efficient it is to work in.

Storage

Many kitchens lack adequate storage space. As discussed in Section 7-1, items should be stored near the area where they will be used. For new or remodeled kitchens, the key is to identify storage needs and develop a plan to meet them. In existing kitchens, storage can often be improved inexpensively.

Kitchen cabinets include base cabinets, which rest on the floor, and wall cabinets. Base cabinets are generally 36 inches (91 cm) high and 24 inches (61 cm) deep. Wall cabinets, placed on the wall above the countertop, vary in size. Kitchens may also include some floor-to-ceiling cabinets for additional storage.

Many storage aids can be ordered as part of new cabinets. Some of these can also be added to existing cabinets. Here are a few such aids:

◆ Roll-out shelves.

◆ Cabinets with vertical dividers for baking sheets and trays.

◆ Pull-out, ventilated baskets for produce such as potatoes and onions.

◆ Pop-up shelves in base cabinets for appliances such as mixers.

Cabinets can be made of a variety of materials, including wood and plastic laminate. Look for well-made units with durable hardware. Cabinets receive more use than most furniture in a home, so durability is important.

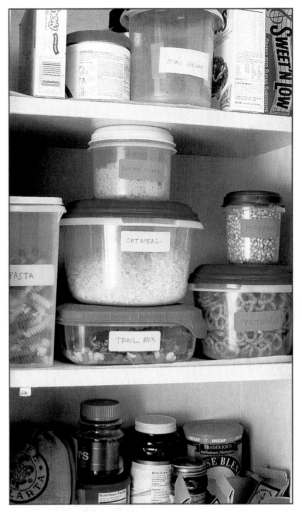

◆ **Different kitchen storage solutions exist.** Name three space-saving storage options for a small kitchen.

Counter Space

Each work center needs its own counter space. Additional counter areas are needed for preparing and mixing food.

Work space can be improved in an existing kitchen without remodeling. A cart, a table, or an island can provide additional work space. So can a flip-down shelf, a pull-out breadboard, or an adjustable cutting board that fits over the sink.

Countertops should be durable and easy to clean. Plastic laminates are the most common material. Solid surfacing is seamless and easier to clean than laminates. It is also more expensive. Ceramic tile is attractive but requires more care.

The Kitchen Environment

Cabinets and major appliances are the primary elements of a kitchen. Other components, however, also make up the kitchen environment. Some of these are essential but operate behind the scenes. Others make the kitchen comfortable and attractive.

The Electrical System

Much of the electrical usage in a home comes from the kitchen. Small appliances, many large appliances, and lighting all depend on electrical power.

If you are planning a new kitchen or remodeling an old one, providing adequate electricity should be a priority. This means having enough electric power coming into the kitchen, sufficient outlets, and a grounded electrical system. **Grounding** is a method of minimizing the risk of electrical shock by providing a path for current to travel back through the electrical system, rather than through your body. The National Electrical Code requires that new homes have grounding wires as part of their wiring systems. Outlets with three holes usually indicate the wiring is grounded. (Check with an electrician to be certain.) These outlets accept three-pronged plugs from grounded appliances. For a grounded system with two-hole outlets, you can use special adapters to plug in grounded appliances.

◆ Grounding appliance plugs is a safeguard against electrical shock. In older dwellings that have outlets with two holes, an adapter can be used to ground appliances. Inspect the appliances in your kitchen at home. Alert adults in the household to any appliances that lack proper grounding.

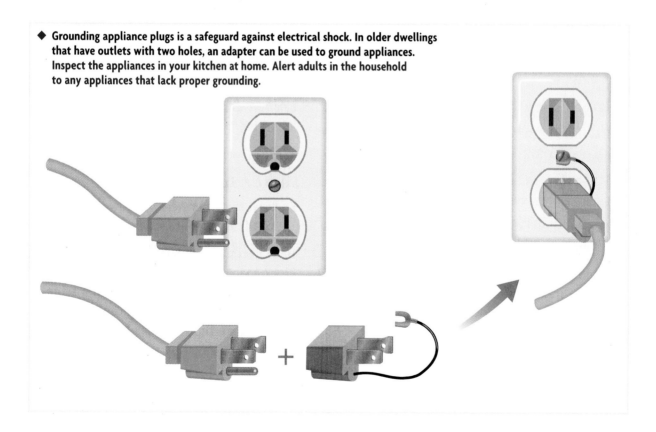

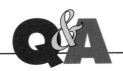

Q *The power in my kitchen often goes out when I am using several appliances. What can I do about this?*

A You may have an overloaded circuit or have tripped a breaker. Have a qualified electrician check out the electrical system. The condition you describe is one symptom of inadequate wiring, which can cause fires. Other telltale signs of a problem include lights dimming when an appliance goes on, appliances taking a long time to heat up, mixers and motors slowing down, and needing to use extension cords regularly with appliances.

Lighting

Good lighting is essential in a kitchen for both comfort and safety. General lighting, usually from lighted ceiling panels or a ceiling light fixture, provides overall light. During the day, natural light from windows may also help light the room. Modern kitchen design also frequently makes use of **task lighting**— bright, shadow-free light over specific work areas. Task lighting is usually used over the countertops, sink, and range. Spotlights or fluorescent fixtures are often mounted beneath overhead cabinets to light countertop areas. Recessed spotlights or track lights on the ceiling can also be positioned to light specific locations. Dimmer switches allow adjustment of the light to any level of brightness.

Ventilation

Cooking produces moisture, heat, grease, and odors. Good ventilation is needed to clear these from the kitchen. Windows, exhaust fans, and range hoods can all provide ventilation.

Some cooktops and grills have built-in ventilation systems called downdraft systems.

Plumbing

The plumbing system brings water to the kitchen and takes away waste water. With the addition of a garbage disposal, most food waste can also be carried away.

Sinks are the most visible parts of the system. Alternatives to traditional sinks include ones mounted without rims and ones that are part of the countertop itself. In addition, there are many bowl shapes, sizes, and combinations.

Walls and Floors

Wall coverings and flooring must look good and be durable and easy to clean. Options are available at varying price levels:

◆ **Wall covering.** May be paint or wallpaper. Look for "scrubbable" types. Kitchen walls have to be cleaned frequently, especially near the sink and range.

◆ **Flooring.** Should be durable and easy to clean, as well as comfortable to stand on. Ceramic tile has excellent durability but can be uncomfortable after long periods of standing. Vinyl or hardwood floors are resilient and easier on the feet. Choose flooring that does not have to be waxed or polished.

Barrier-Free Kitchens

Because food preparation is a basic activity, kitchen designers are working to make it easier for everyone. Their efforts are part of a movement known as **life-span design**. This is a design approach in which living space is adapted to the needs of people of various ages and degrees of physical ability. Life-span designs incorporate wider doorways and aisles in the kitchen to accommodate wheelchairs or walkers.

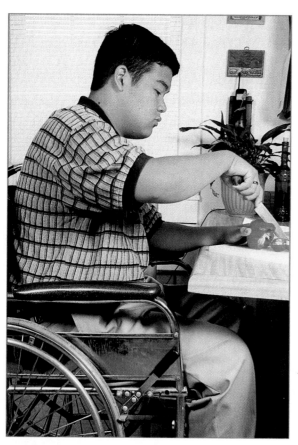

Work surfaces are placed at various heights so that preparation can be done sitting or standing. Open shelving and drawers, rather than closed cabinets, provide easier access.

Kitchens can also be designed, remodeled, or adapted to meet specific physical challenges. For example, cabinet knobs can be replaced with easy-to-grasp handles. Braille controls can be added to appliances. Kitchen designers, appliance manufacturers, and support organizations are good sources of information about special-needs designs.

◆ **Barrier-free kitchen design makes it easier for everyone to use the kitchen.** What specific features would make a kitchen convenient for the person shown?

Section 14-3 Review & Activities

1. List three questions to consider when planning the design of a kitchen.

2. Give two guidelines for evaluating the efficiency of a kitchen floor plan.

3. Identify three storage aids that can be ordered as part of new cabinets or added to existing cabinets.

4. What is meant by the term *life-span design?* Give an example.

5. Evaluating. David and Emily are a young couple just starting out. They enjoy entertaining and plan someday to raise a family, but right now their resources are limited. What type of kitchen would best suit their needs now and in the future? Explain your choices.

6. Extending. Imagine the kitchen in which you'll be preparing food 20 years from now. How will it be different from the kitchen of today? Explain your answer.

7. Applying. Describe how you could reorganize one work center in your kitchen at home. List tasks done at the center as well as food and tools located there. Tell what should be added and what should be moved to a different location.

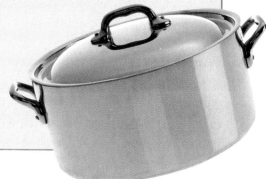

CAREER WANTED

Individuals who are creative, self-disciplined, can communicate with others, and follow directions.

REQUIRES:

- completion of an accredited art/design school or a degree in business
- knowledge of design trends and materials

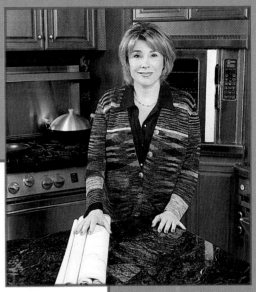

"Beauty + functionality is the key,"
says Kitchen Design Consultant Leigh Smith

Q: Leigh, what do you do as a kitchen design consultant?

A: I work as the link between the client, the architect, and the builders. I learn about my client's taste. Then, I sketch ideas for them to review. When one is chosen, I work to implement that design by interfacing with the architect and the builders.

Q: How do homeowners who want to build or remodel a kitchen contact you?

A: Mostly through ads that I run in home improvement magazines and the yellow pages. Word of mouth is also important. So, leaving your clients satisfied is essential!

Q: How do you keep your clients satisfied?

A: First, by listening. I take notes about what they do for fun and how they live. This can have an impact on the kind of kitchen that will suit them. Then, I sit down and talk over each stage with them. Communication is important.

Q: What problems do you encounter?

A: My biggest problem is with clients who want to "overdesign." They see an appliance or gadget and say "I want that." Before you know it, the design becomes so cluttered there is hardly any room left to walk! It is difficult talking a client out of making impulse additions.

Career Research Activity

1. Research "automated home system" and similar technological advances in home design. Make a list of ten ways these innovations are making a kitchen design consultant's job both easier and tougher.

2. Interview someone who has one of the jobs in each of the three levels on the right. Find out about the education and training needed for this exciting line of work. Share this information in a pictorial report that shows similarities and differences among the three careers.

Related Career Opportunities

Entry Level
- Cost Estimator
- Carpenter's Assistant
- Real Estate Agent

Technical Level
- Building Contractor
- CAD Specialist

Professional Level
- Architect
- Kitchen Design Consultant
- Multimedia Designer

Chapter 14   Review & Activities

Summary

Section 14-1: Consumer Skills

- Before you buy any kitchen equipment, be sure you need and will use it.

- People who decide to buy on credit need to investigate the costs of borrowing.

- When you shop for equipment, consider your needs and wants.

- Look for consumer safeguards, and consider your purchase carefully.

Section 14-2: Choosing Kitchen Equipment

- It is easier to shop for appliances, cookware, bakeware, tools, and tableware when you are familiar with some of the basic options you will find. A wide range of choices is available.

- Some features are essential for safety and quality, while others depend on personal needs and preferences.

Section 14-3: Designing a Kitchen

- A kitchen should be planned for efficient use by everyone.

- The floor plan should allow an uninterrupted work flow.

- Storage units and counter space should be adequate, accessible, and durable.

- Electricity, lighting, and plumbing should provide safety and convenience.

- Life-span design helps make the kitchen easier to use for people of various ages and degrees of physical ability.

Checking Your Knowledge

1. Name one advantage and one disadvantage of buying on credit.

2. What is an EnergyGuide label? How can it be helpful when you are shopping for appliances?

3. List four ways of being an active shopper.

4. Identify three special features that may be found in refrigerator-freezers.

5. List three things to consider when buying small appliances.

6. Describe two signs of quality construction in knives.

7. List four basic kitchen floor plans.

8. In kitchen design, how does a peninsula differ from an island? What is the purpose of both?

9. Why is good lighting important in a kitchen?

10. Identify three features of good flooring.

Working IN THE Lab

1. **Demonstration.** With one or two classmates, role-play an appliance shopping trip. One member of the group is to be a customer interested in buying one of the appliances in the foods lab. Another is to be the salesperson. Identify the points to consider when buying appliances.

2. **Foods Lab.** Design an efficient kitchen floor plan. Include the location of large appliances and the dimensions of the work triangle.

Review & Activities Chapter 14

Thinking Critically

1. Analyzing Decisions. One evening, you and your family go shopping for a microwave oven. At the first store you visit, the salesclerk shows you a model that has most of the features you want and is on sale. When you state that you would like to shop a little further, the clerk informs you that the sale ends that day. Would you advise your family to go ahead and make the purchase? Why or why not?

2. Comparing and Contrasting. James is helping his dad shop for appliances for the kitchen of their new apartment. They have been comparison shopping using newspaper ads from appliance stores. Some of the ads show appliances with features that James and his dad would not be likely to use that often. The remainder of ads for the same types of appliances are for models that lack needed features. Putting yourself in James's place, prepare a list of pros and cons for the two different categories that will help your father make an informed decision.

Reinforcing Key Skills

1. Communication. Sources of information about a product could include advertisements, reports in consumer magazines, and comments from salespeople. Which do you think would be the most accurate and reliable? Explain your answer.

2. Leadership. Conner and his family are planning to buy a new refrigerator. His sister likes the ice cube dispenser in one model; his father, the self-defrosting freezer; his mother, the adjustable shelves. The list of special features is so long that the only refrigerator that would suit the family is way beyond their budget. What action can Conner take to help his family decide which refrigerator to purchase?

Making Decisions and Solving Problems

A new student in your foods lab group uses a wheelchair. The appliances, storage areas, and work space are sometimes difficult for him to use. Your teacher has asked you to suggest long-range and short-range solutions to the problem. What recommendations would you make?

Making Connections

1. Math. Visit an appliance showroom in your community, and compare the EnergyGuide labels on three different models of the same appliance. Calculate the cost of using each for one week, one month, and one year. Determine the difference in energy costs, and rank the appliances from least to most expensive to use.

2. Art. Plan and sketch an attractive, efficient kitchen design for a small apartment. Point out the features that make the kitchen efficient (either on the drawing or in a separate written description). Use colored pencils, paint chips, or wallpaper samples to show the color scheme. Display your finished design in an in-class "gallery."

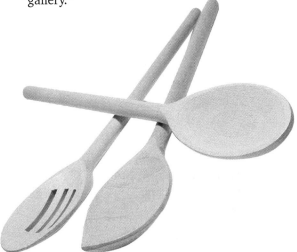

UNIT

4

Foods for

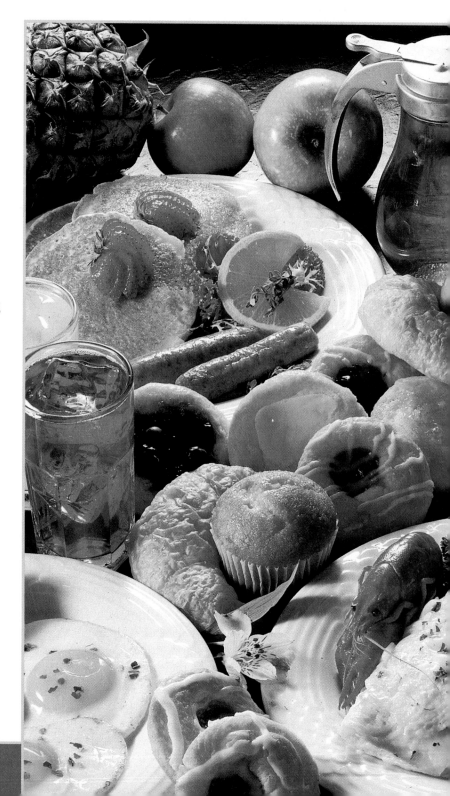

Meals and Snacks

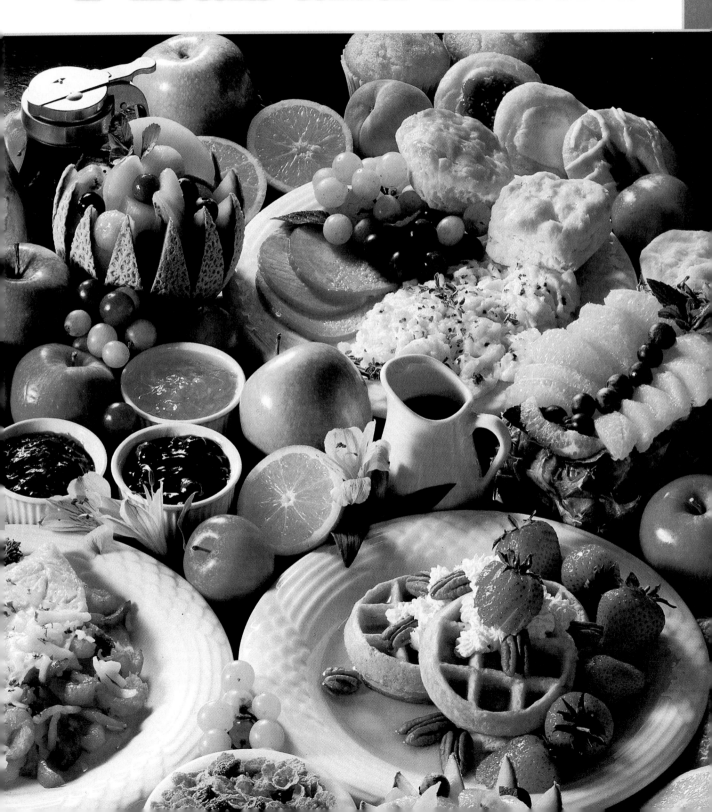

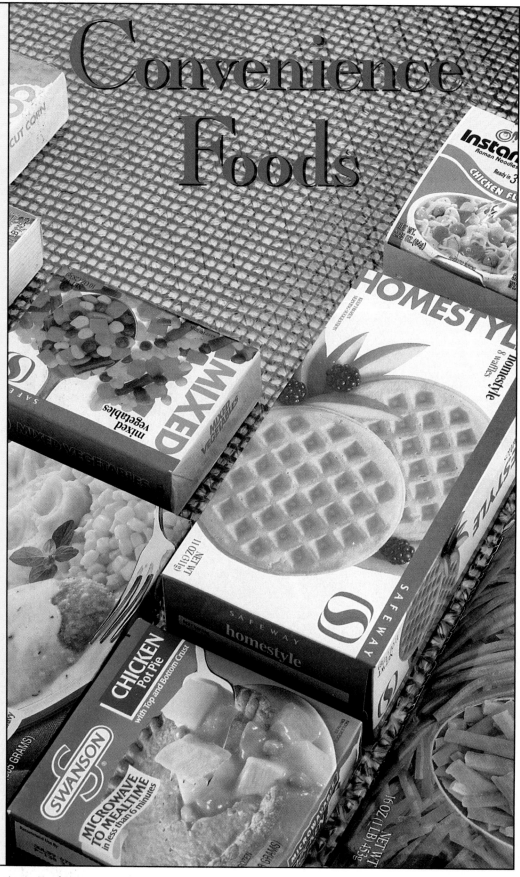

Convenience Foods

What does the term *convenience foods* mean to you? To Joanne, it means foods that are easy to cook and require little cleanup. Ricco thinks of packaged mixes that save time. Chantel uses the term to describe any ready-to-eat foods.

No matter how you define the term, convenience foods can be part of a healthful eating plan. In this chapter, you will find out how.

Choosing Convenience Foods

Through technology, we live in an age of instant communication. Is it any wonder that people want food the minute they feel hungry? The demand for on-the-spot meals has given rise to a new generation of convenience foods.

Objectives

After studying this section, you should be able to:

- Identify different types of convenience foods and their uses.
- Discuss the pros and cons of using convenience foods.

Look for These Terms

manufactured food

analogues

formed product

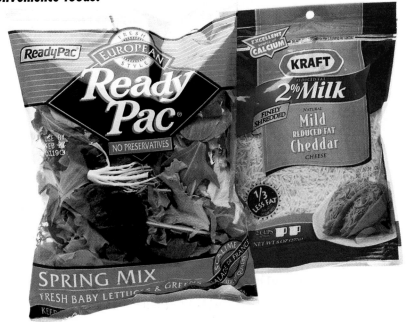

Convenience Foods

In general, a convenience food is one that has been commercially processed to make it more convenient to store or use. Some convenience foods have been around for such a long time that they have become staples in the American food supply. You might not think, for example, of packaged sliced bread or bottled salad dressing as convenience foods. When they first appeared, though, these products were viewed as time-saving innovations.

Convenience foods include items that have been processed for a longer shelf life. Nonfat dry milk can be stored without refrigeration and kept for a longer time than fluid milk.

Another purpose of convenience foods is to reduce meal preparation time. Food that is partially prepared when purchased—cheese that is already shredded or vegetables that are already washed and cut up—can save time in the kitchen. Some foods are combined and packaged for specific uses, such as a mixture of frozen stew vegetables. Dry mixtures are available for everything from macaroni and cheese to salad dressing to baked goods. Often you need only add one or two ingredients and complete a few simple steps to prepare the food.

Of course, convenience can go even further. You can buy snacks, main dishes, side dishes, desserts, and even complete meals that are already prepared. Some need only be thawed

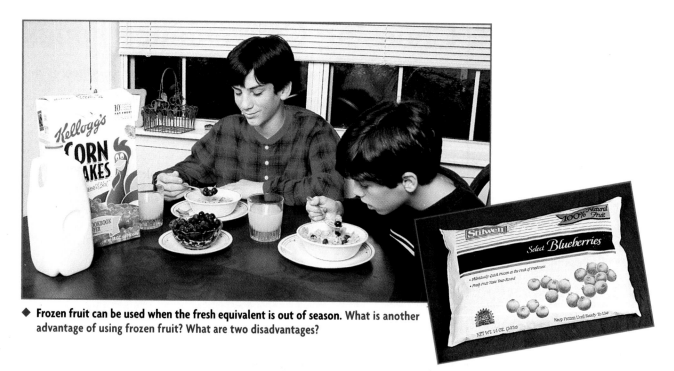

◆ **Frozen fruit can be used when the fresh equivalent is out of season.** What is another advantage of using frozen fruit? What are two disadvantages?

or heated. Others are ready to eat right out of the package.

Manufactured Foods

Have you sampled a meatless burger? Known by several different names, vegetable patties are one example of a **manufactured food** —a product developed to serve as a substitute for another food. Many manufactured foods have been developed to meet special nutritional needs or to provide low-cost alternatives. There are several types of manufactured foods:

◆ **Analogues. Analogues** (AN-uh-logs) are foods made from a vegetable protein and processed to resemble animal foods. They can be made from textured soy protein (TSP), tofu, vegetables, or grains. When flavored and processed, they are made into foods such as breakfast links, meatless burgers, pot pies, and hot dogs. These products are generally low in fat and cholesterol. TSP can also be purchased as granules so that you can make your own meatless dishes.

◆ **Egg substitutes.** These manufactured foods are usually made from egg whites with other ingredients added. Because they have no yolks, they have little or no saturated fat and cholesterol. They are usually sold in the freezer or refrigerator sections of the supermarkets. You can also buy ready-to-cook and ready-to-eat foods made with egg substitutes.

◆ **Formed products.** A **formed product** is a food made from an inexpensive food source processed to resemble a more expensive one. An example is *surimi* (soo-REE-mee)—white fish flavored and shaped to resemble lobster or crab. The prices of imitation foods are lower than the prices of the foods they replace. Such foods must be labeled "imitation" and can't be called by the name of the food they replace.

Sometimes manufactured foods are substituted for more expensive ingredients in convenience products. For example, "blueberry waffles" often do not contain real blueberries.

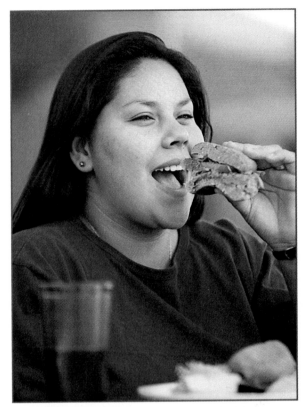

◆ Vegetable patties like this one are a manufactured substitute for red meat. Visit a local supermarket and examine the package label of a product like this one. In your Wellness Journal, note both advantages and disadvantages of using such products.

Instead, blueberry "buds"—a manufactured food consisting of sugar, oil, artificial flavor, salt, dyes, and other additives may be used.

Pros and Cons of Convenience Foods

Every day, about 30 new convenience foods appear in the marketplace to meet the growing demand. These foods can be a blessing to today's busy families. Yet, as a smart consumer, you need to be aware of the downside of using convenience foods.

◆ Formed foods, such as surimi products, can be a good value. Think of other ways in which formed foods might be used.

Cost

Convenience can be costly. Every additional step in processing adds to the price of a food. At the supermarket, for example, a ready-to-cook meat loaf costs more than twice as much as regular ground beef. Similarly, the cost per serving of cut-up chicken pieces is usually higher than that of a whole chicken.

Before buying any convenience food, evaluate the per-serving cost against other factors, such as time. Would you save money if you cut up the chicken yourself?

Nutrition

Processing usually destroys some nutrients. Heat, for example, destroys vitamin C. When grains are processed, much of the fiber and some of the nutrients are lost. Many convenience foods also tend to be high in added sodium, sugar, and fat.

What can you as a consumer do? Here are several suggestions:

◆ Look for convenience foods that are low in sodium, fat, and sugar. With the increasing awareness of good nutrition, such convenience foods are becoming more common. Instead of canned fruit packed in heavy sugar syrup, for example, look for fruit packed in water or its own natural juice.

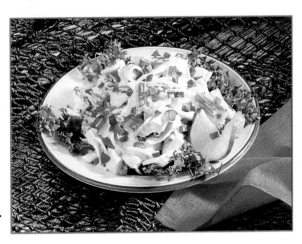

◆ Choose frozen plain vegetables over canned ones. The frozen type tend to lose the fewest nutrients during processing. Unlike their canned counterpart which usually have some salt added, frozen vegetables contain no added sodium, sugar, or fat.

◆ Use ready-to-cook and ready-to-eat foods sparingly. These often contain high amounts of sodium and fat. Ready-to-eat take-home food is the biggest culprit of all in terms of fat content.

Meal Appeal

Processing affects the flavor, color, and texture of food. Often, additives are used to make the final product resemble its fresh counterpart. The flavor and appearance of certain convenience foods may not compare with similar foods that are homemade.

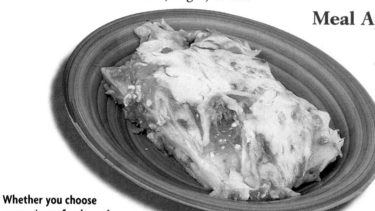

◆ **Whether you choose convenience foods or the homemade version, you may have to make some tradeoffs.** Using the skills for food choices you have learned, make a list of the pros and cons of convenience and homemade versions of lasagne or one of your favorite foods.

Section 15-1 Review & Activities

1. What is a manufactured food? What is an analogue?

2. In what three areas are there potential downsides to using convenience foods?

3. Identify two ways to make the most of convenience foods from a nutrition perspective.

4. Comparing and Contrasting. Form two groups and conduct a debate on the advantages and disadvantages of using convenience foods. Each group should present facts and views from this section.

5. Analyzing. With today's busy schedules, many people consider convenience foods essential and use them regularly in meals. What might be some effects of this trend?

6. Applying. Compare the cost and nutrition of at least three different convenience forms of a food. For example, you might want to compare different forms of spaghetti (canned prepared, boxed mix, frozen). Which form might be the best choice? Why?

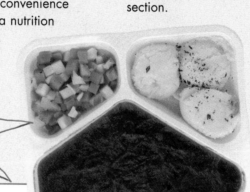

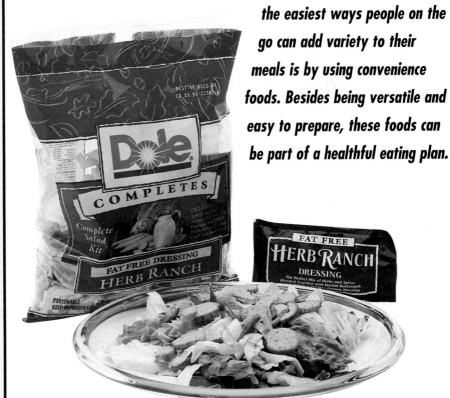

Cooking with Convenience

You may have heard the saying, "Variety is the spice of life." One of the easiest ways people on the go can add variety to their meals is by using convenience foods. Besides being versatile and easy to prepare, these foods can be part of a healthful eating plan.

Objectives

After studying this section, you should be able to:

- Give suggestions for planning healthful meals around convenience foods.
- Describe general methods for preparing basic convenience foods.
- Discuss the benefits of making your own convenience foods.

Look for This Term

reconstitute

Planning Meals with Convenience Foods

Meals that use convenience foods can be nutritious and help you meet your daily food needs. Here are some guidelines for making daily food choices when you use convenience foods:

- If you use convenience products for one part of the meal, plan the rest of your choices carefully. Make other parts of the meal from fresh or frozen foods that can be prepared quickly. These include fresh or frozen plain fruits and vegetables, whole-grain breads and cereals, and low-fat dairy

products. The FDA allows plain frozen fruits and vegetables to be labeled "healthy" if they meet certain requirements.

- When using dry mixes to make main dishes, side dishes, and sauces, reduce the amount of fat called for in the directions. Use fat-free milk or water instead of whole milk.

- Use quick-cooking grains as a side dish to add variety to meals. These include rice, bulgur, millet, kasha, and couscous.

- Keep shelf-stable or frozen main dishes and meals on hand for emergencies, but try to avoid using them regularly for meals.

◆ **Macaroni and cheese can be the center-piece of a meal that provides needed nutrients. What fresh foods would you serve to balance this main dish?**

INFOLINK

For more information on the steps in planning meals, see Section 11-1.
For more on the nutrients in grains of various kinds, see Section 17-1.

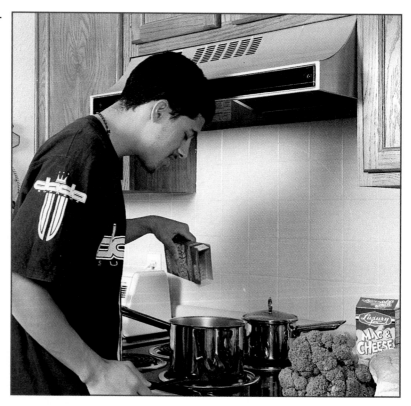

Preparing and Using Convenience Foods

Most convenience foods have directions for use on the package. Always read the directions carefully, even if you have used the product before. Manufacturers sometimes change the ingredients or the preparation methods.

If you want microwavable convenience foods, check the package directions before buying. Not all convenience foods can be successfully microwaved.

Here are some general guidelines for using common convenience foods. You'll also find information about specific convenience foods in later chapters.

◆ **Canned foods.** Many canned foods are ready to eat or need little preparation other than heating. Some canned soups must be mixed with water or milk. Once canned foods are opened, any leftovers must usually be refrigerated.

◆ **Frozen foods.** Some frozen foods may need only to be thawed. Others must be cooked without thawing. Check the package for special directions, such as "Do not heat in toaster oven."

◆ **Chilled foods.** Use the same care in handling chilled convenience foods—fresh pasta and sauces, for example—that you do when preparing the same foods from scratch. Keep them refrigerated until you are ready to use them. Use a chilled food product by the date shown on the package, or check to see if it can be frozen. As an alternative, consider using it in a recipe that can be frozen.

◆ **Dried foods.** Many dried foods, such as nonfat dry milk, need to be reconstituted. To **reconstitute** means to add back the liquid that was removed in processing.

◆ **Dry mixes.** Most mixes contain the dry ingredients needed to prepare the food. You add other ingredients, such as liquids. Along with the basic directions, the package may have suggestions for variations.

✚ Safety Check

Before opening canned goods, wipe the top of a can with a clean, wet dishcloth. Doing so will keep dirt and harmful microorganisms from getting into the food.

HEATING INSTRUCTIONS

MICROWAVE OVEN:
Microwave ovens vary. Heating time may require adjustment.
• Remove dinner from carton.
• Cut and remove film cover from fruit compartment only.
• Cut a slit in center of film cover over main entree.
• Heat on HIGH 6 to 7 minutes or until hot, rotating dinner once.
• Let stand in microwave oven 1 to 2 minutes.
• Stir main entree before serving.
When heating TWO dinners, follow instructions above, heating approximately 12 to 14 minutes or until hot, rotating once.

CONVENTIONAL OVEN:
Preheating oven is not necessary.
• Remove dinner from carton.
• Cut and remove film cover from fruit compartment only.
• Cut a slit in center of film cover over main entree.
• Heat at 350°F on COOKIE SHEET in center of oven 30 to 35 minutes or until hot.
• Remove dinner from oven on COOKIE SHEET.
• Let stand 1 to 2 minutes before serving.
Temperatures above 350°F AND/OR failure to use a COOKIE SHEET may cause damage to the plastic tray, food, and/or oven.

NOTE: When removing cover, be careful to avoid steam burns.
Do not prepare in toaster oven.

Ready-to-Eat Food

One category of convenience foods that needs special attention is ready-to-eat take-home foods. Although these foods are piping hot when you buy them, they may cool by the time you get them home, allowing harmful bacteria and microorganisms to grow. Before serving any such food, test the temperature with an instant-read thermometer. If it is not at least 160°F (72°C), reheat the food until it reaches the proper temperature. Remember to refrigerate or freeze any leftovers.

Making Your Own Convenience Foods

Even though people are busy, they may be concerned about the cost or nutritional quality of convenience foods. Some solve the problem by making their own convenience foods. Homemade convenience foods have several advantages:

◆ You decide on the kind and quality of ingredients to put into the product.

◆ You can control the amount of sodium, sugar, and fat used.

◆ Homemade convenience foods often cost less to prepare than commercial ones.

◆ They have few or no additives.

◆ You enjoy meals with a homemade appearance and flavor.

On the next three pages are some ideas for making your own convenience foods.

◆ Many convenience food packages today include two sets of heating instructions. Follow them exactly for best results. What cautions are given on the package directions shown here?

Pre-prepared Ingredients

Perhaps there are some basic ingredients that you often use in recipes. You can save time by preparing a quantity of these foods ahead of time and refrigerating or freezing them.

◆ **Sautéed chopped vegetables.** Many recipes call for sautéed chopped garlic, onions, celery, or green pepper. Chop and sauté the vegetables or combinations you use most often. Freeze them in recipe-size quantities, such as ¼ cup (50 mL). You can also freeze chopped vegetables without sautéing them, as long as you plan to cook them. Freezing softens crisp vegetables.

◆ **Dry beans and grain products.** Cook dry beans and grain products, such as rice and pasta, in quantity. Freeze them in 1-cup (250-mL) portions. Use them for salads, casseroles, soups, and side dishes.

◆ **Cubed or shredded cheese.** Cube or grate the kind of cheese you use frequently, such as cheddar or mozzarella. Store in a container with a tight-fitting cover, and keep refrigerated or frozen until used.

◆ **Bread crumbs or cubes.** Cut bread into cubes and dry them. For crumbs, grind dried bread slices in a blender or food processor. You can also crush them with a rolling pin between two pieces of waxed paper or in a large, sealed plastic bag. Store the crumbs or cubes in an air-tight container in the refrigerator or freezer. For added flavor and fiber, use whole wheat bread.

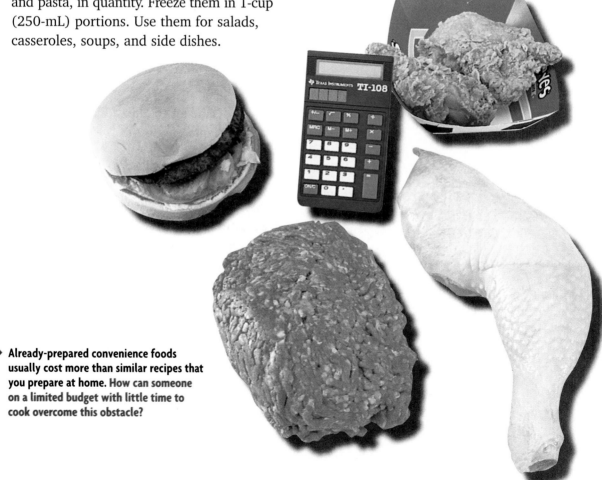

◆ **Already-prepared convenience foods usually cost more than similar recipes that you prepare at home.** How can someone on a limited budget with little time to cook overcome this obstacle?

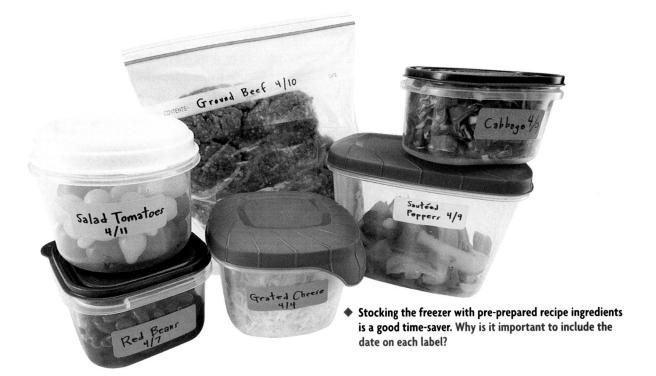

◆ Stocking the freezer with pre-prepared recipe ingredients is a good time-saver. Why is it important to include the date on each label?

Frozen Main Dishes

Although it may sound time-consuming to cook your own meals and freeze them, doing so can save you time and money in the long run. The advantages may be worth the extra time it takes.

Some busy people set aside one or two weekend days to cook for the freezer. They prepare as many of their favorite recipes as they can and then freeze them. Karen's mother gets the entire family involved in the "cooking weekend." They have a large freezer and can prepare and store enough main dishes to last about two months. Because everyone is involved, it has become a fun activity the family enjoys.

Others cook for the freezer regularly by preparing more than they need whenever they cook. The leftover food is frozen for future meals. One particularly handy tip is to freeze extra broth and other clear soups in ice cube trays. Once frozen, the cubes can be transferred to a plastic freezer bag for future microwaving to make a quick meal or to add to other recipes.

Storing Frozen Main Dishes

When packaging the food, consider how it will be used. If family members eat at different times, freeze the food in single-serving packages.

When labeling the packages, include any instructions needed to serve the food. For example, if the recipe is to be served over rice, write that on the package so that the rice can be thawed at the same time as the other foods.

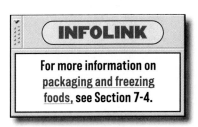

INFOLINK

For more information on packaging and freezing foods, see Section 7-4.

Homemade Mixes

You can make your own mixes for foods that you prepare regularly, such as quick breads or beverages. Seasoning mixes are great time-savers because you handle just one container instead of many different jars of herbs and spices.

The secret of making a successful mix is to be sure the ingredients are thoroughly combined and evenly distributed. Then, when you measure out the quantity you need, you will be sure to get the right amount of all the ingredients. Some ingredients may be heavier than others and may settle down in the container. Before measuring the amount you need, mix well to be sure the ingredients are evenly distributed.

You may not be able to store homemade mixes as long as commercial ones, which usually have preservatives added to extend the shelf life. Therefore, make only the quantity you think you will use before the mix has a chance to spoil.

Section 15-2 Review & Activities

1. List three tips for healthfully using convenience foods in meals.

2. Why is it important to read the directions on convenience foods even if you have used the product before?

3. Name two guidelines for using chilled convenience foods.

4. Synthesizing. Gloria's homemade pumpkin bread has long been a family favorite. Recently, Gloria discovered a mix that produces a result fairly close to her own, in addition to being less expensive. What reasons could you give Gloria for continuing to make her pumpkin bread from scratch?

5. Synthesizing. How might you and your family use homemade convenience foods? What types of foods would be most helpful?

6. Applying. Plan an entire dinner or lunch menu that combines a main dish convenience food with easy-to-prepare fresh foods as side dishes. Evaluate the meal for nutrition, cost, and appeal.

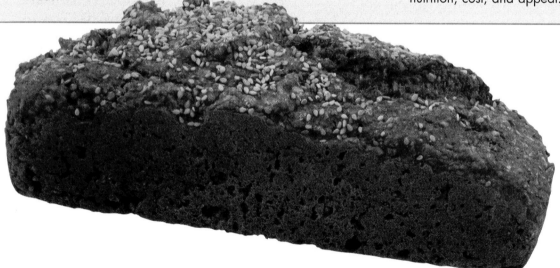

RECIPE FILE

Whole Wheat Quick Bread Mix

Homemade convenience mixes can save time and money in the kitchen.
Compare the "Favorite Wheat Pancakes" recipe on the next page to other
recipes you may have tried made with purchased convenience mixes.

Customary	Ingredient	Metric
6 cups	Whole wheat flour	1500 mL
3 cups	All-purpose flour	750 mL
1½ cups	Instant nonfat dry milk	375 mL
1 Tbsp.	Salt	15 mL
1 cup	Sugar	250 mL
½ cup	Wheat germ	125 mL
¼ cup	Baking powder	50 mL

Yield: About 12 cups (3 L) baking mix

Directions

1. Combine all ingredients in a large bowl.
2. Place the baking mix in a large container with a tight-fitting cover. Label with the
name of the mix and the date.
3. Store baking mix in the refrigerator. Use within 12 to 14 weeks.

Note: Mix well again before measuring
to use in recipes.

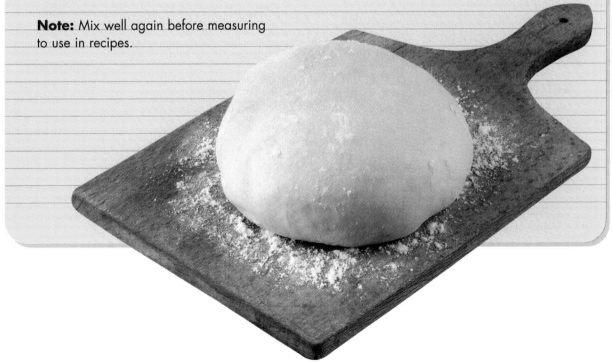

RECIPE FILE

Favorite Wheat Pancakes

Customary	Ingredient	Metric
	Vegetable oil cooking spray	
1	Egg, slightly beaten	1
1½ cups	Water	375 mL
2 Tbsp.	Vegetable oil	30 mL
2¼ cups	Whole Wheat Quick Bread Mix	550 mL

Yield: About 15 4-inch (10-cm) pancakes
Equipment: Non-stick skillet
Temperature: Medium-high

Directions

1. Spray skillet with vegetable oil cooking spray. Preheat.
2. Combine egg, water, and oil in medium bowl.
3. Stir in Whole Wheat Quick Bread Mix just until moistened.
4. For each pancake, ladle ⅓ cup batter into skillet. Tilt skillet slightly to spread batter into rounds.
5. Cook until top of pancake is speckled with bubbles. Turn and cook on the other side until golden brown, about 3 or 4 minutes.
6. Serve hot with syrup, sliced bananas or berries in season, if desired.

Nutrition Information

For each 3-pancake serving: 244 calories, 8 g protein, 39 g carbohydrate, 7 g fat, 43 mg cholesterol, 259 mg sodium
Good source of: potassium, iron, vitamin E, B vitamins, calcium, phosphorus

Food for Thought

• In what way were the pancakes different from others you have tasted that were prepared from a mix? Were they better? Explain.
• What other foods could be made from the Whole Wheat Quick Bread Mix? Where could you find recipes for these foods?

CAREER WANTED

Individuals who are safety conscious, have an eye for detail, and have a good work ethic.

REQUIRES:

- high school diploma
- on-the-job training

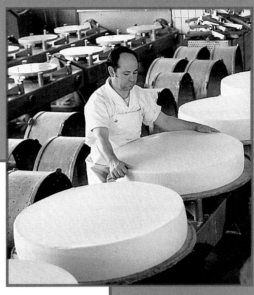

"Quality is our main concern,"

says Food Processing Plant Worker Carl Coran

Q: Carl, what does your job involve?

A: I work in a large food processing plant. My current job involves inspecting and sorting ears of corn before they are frozen and packaged. We pull the ears that are bruised or defective in any way off the conveyor system.

Q: What is it like working in a large plant?

A: It is hard to handle repetitive tasks quickly and accurately without making mistakes. You also need to work well as part of a team. The biggest thing to adjust to is the noise. In fact, everyone is required to wear special ear protection. Safety is another concern. We all must pay strict attention to safety rules every minute. The company makes us take breaks every 20 minutes to help ensure safety.

Q: What career moves are in your future?

A: I'm in line for a promotion to machine operator. My long-term goal is to become a supervisor or manager. As a first step toward that goal, I volunteered to lead the quality control team in my work unit.

Career Research Activity

1. Profile a processing plant in your own community. Create an information checklist that includes what the plant processes, what the work environment is like, and what advancement opportunities exist for processing plant workers.

2. Technology has replaced many assembly-line workers. Describe what you think a processing plant will be like in 50 years and what the job description would be for a food processing plant worker. How are things different? The same?

Related Career Opportunities

Entry Level
- Machine Operator
- Processing Plant Worker
- Counter Worker

Technical Level
- Quality Control Technician
- OSHA Inspector

Professional Level
- Food Processing Plant Manager
- Sanitarian
- Industrial Engineer

Chapter 15   Review & Activities

—— Summary ——

Section 15-1: Choosing Convenience Foods

- Convenience foods are items that have been processed for longer shelf life, ease of preparation, or both.

- Manufactured foods are developed to serve as substitutes for other foods.

- Although convenience foods can save time and energy, they may be more costly, less nutritious, and less appealing than home-prepared or fresh foods.

Section 15-2: Cooking with Convenience

- With careful planning, convenience foods can be part of a nutritious meal.

- Prepare convenience foods according to the package directions.

- You can make your own convenience foods by pre-preparing ingredients, freezing main dishes, and making homemade dry mixes.

Checking Your Knowledge

1. In what way is nonfat dry milk more convenient than fluid milk?

2. Name two reasons why manufactured foods have been developed.

3. What is TSP? How is it used?

4. Identify two nutritional disadvantages of some convenience foods.

5. What does the term *reconstitute* mean?

6. Identify three types of recipe ingredients that you can pre-prepare.

7. Describe two practices many people use to make and freeze main dishes.

8. Do homemade dry mixes last as long as commercial varieties? Explain.

Working IN THE Lab

1. *Food Preparation.* Prepare a ready-to-cook entrée or side dish and a similar recipe from scratch in the foods lab. Compare them for meal appeal and nutritional value.

2. *Food Science.* Using a recipe from this book or another source, prepare a dry mix. Store it and a similar commercial variety under identical conditions. Check both mixes regularly for texture and appearance. Prepare recipes using the mixes at regular intervals. How does time effect the quality of each mix?

3. *Foods Lab.* Prepare a commercial dry mix according to the basic package directions. Prepare another batch using a variation suggested on the package or one of your own creation. Compare the two recipes for taste, texture, appearance, and nutritional value.

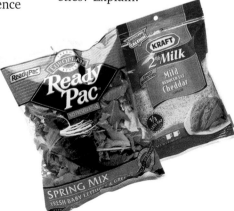

Thinking Critically

1. Identifying Ambiguous Statements. Peter comes from a family that enjoys preparing meals in the kitchen from scratch. His friend Simon comes from a family where everyone is so busy with activities outside the home that the term *home-cooked meal* has come to be synonymous with heating a convenience food in the microwave. How is each of the friends likely to react to an advertisement for a new food product that promises a "great home-made flavor"? Explain your answer.

2. Recognizing Stereotypes. Hattie and two friends were hungry after hockey practice and agreed to stop for a bite to eat. "I don't know exactly what I'm in the mood for," Hattie said. "Hey, how about the new pizza restaurant that opened on Maple Street?" Rita suggested. "Count me out!" Heather said pointedly. "I was walking by there yesterday and I saw a microwave oven on the counter. That's a sure sign that the food is awful!" What stereotype is reflected in this conversation? What logical flaw, if any, can you find in the argument?

Reinforcing Key Skills

1. Management. Emilia forgot to shop earlier in the week for the family dinner she was supposed to cook tonight. She had planned to make a shrimp and crab pasta entrée, salad, and fruit salad for dessert. Use information from the chapter to help Emilia organize her dinner plan—which includes sticking to a modest budget.

2. Directed Thinking. You are preparing your family's dinner when some old friends of the family drop by. You would like to invite them to stay for the meal, but you aren't sure you have enough food. Explain how to use convenience foods to stretch the recipes.

Making Decisions and Solving Problems

Your family uses convenience foods every day. You are worried about the effect on the family's health and on the budget. What would you do?

Making Connections

1. Social Studies. Trace the history of convenience foods. What were some of the first commercially sold convenience foods? What technologies make them possible? How has their use affected family life? Present your findings in an illustrated time line.

2. Math. Prepare a homemade convenience food. Calculate the cost per serving. Compare this with the per-serving cost of a similar commercial variety. Express the price difference in dollars and cents and as a percentage.

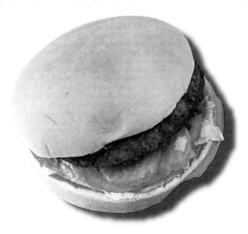

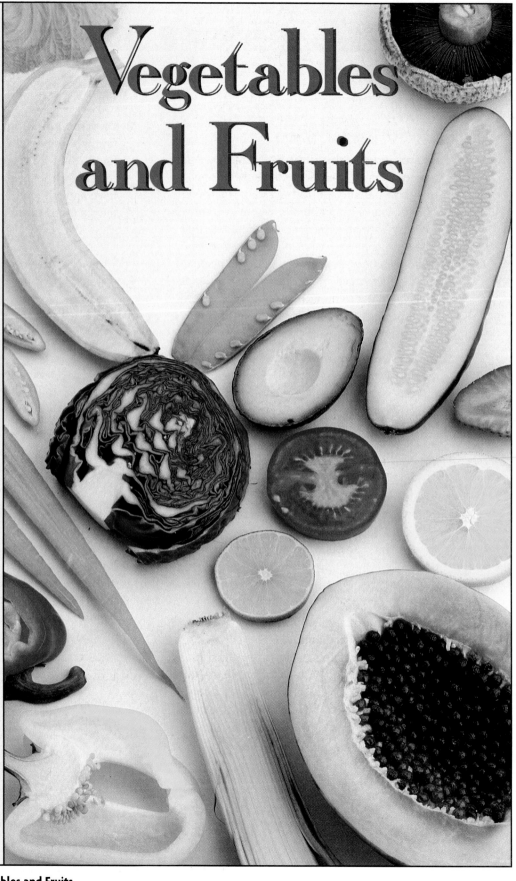

Vegetables and Fruits

Not only are vegetables and fruits some of nature's most delicious foods, they also are packed with important nutrients. In this chapter, you'll learn how to select fresh produce and other forms of vegetables and fruits. You'll also learn strategies for making the most of these foods once you get them home.

Choosing Vegetables and Fruits

Objectives

After studying this section, you should be able to:

- Identify the nutrients found in vegetables and fruits.
- Recognize qualities to look for when buying vegetables and fruits.
- Discuss guidelines for storing fresh produce.

Look for These Terms

cruciferous vegetables

tuber

mature fruits

ripe fruits

Picture yourself at a picnic, biting into an ear of tender, sweet corn. Imagine the crunch and tart, juicy goodness of a crisp, ripe apple. Vegetables and fruits appeal to all the senses. They are also an excellent source of many of the nutrients your body needs.

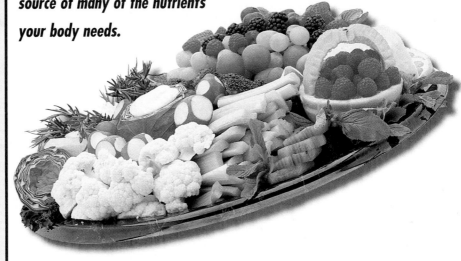

Nutrients in Vegetables and Fruits

Fresh vegetables and fruits are low in fat and sodium and have no cholesterol. At the same time, they are high in carbohydrates. They are also chock-full of important micronutrients, including antioxidants—substances that may lower the risk of some cancers and heart disease. Among the antioxidants that vegetables and fruits provide are

- **Vitamin C.** Many people, when they think of vitamin C sources, think of citrus fruits. However, many other vegetables and fruits are rich in this vitamin, including kiwifruit, strawberries, cantaloupe, cabbage, and potatoes.

- **Vitamin E.** Apples and warm-weather fruits such as apricots, nectarines, and peaches are good sources of vitamin E. So are **cruciferous** (kroo-SIH-fur-uhs) **vegetables**—vegetables in the cabbage family. These include bok choy, broccoli, brussels sprouts, cauliflower, collards, kale, kohlrabi, mustard greens, rutabagas, and turnips and their greens.

- **Beta carotene.** The body uses this phytochemical—a health-promoting substance found in foods from plants—to make vitamin A. It is found in yellow or orange vegetables and fruits, as well as in cruciferous vegetables.

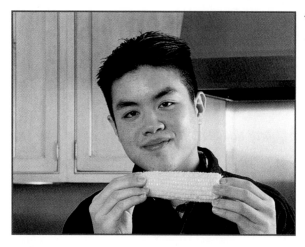

◆ **Fresh vegetables and fruits appeal not only to the sense of taste but to sight, smell, touch, and even sound.** Choose two fruits or vegetables. For each one, give a word describing its appeal to each of the five senses.

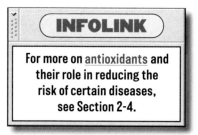

INFOLINK

For more on <u>antioxidants</u> and their role in reducing the risk of certain diseases, see Section 2-4.

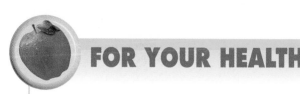

FOR YOUR HEALTH

Vegetable and Fruit Serving Equivalents

According to an old saying, you can't add apples and oranges. You *can*, however, substitute equivalent servings of fruits and vegetables depending on your tastes and preferences. Knowing this can help you get the daily servings of fruit and vegetables the Food Guide Pyramid recommends. If you don't like snacking on raw carrot sticks, try a glass of chilled tomato juice instead. Single-serving cans or packs of applesauce are an easy and tasty way to get a serving of fruit. The Food Guide Pyramid, on page 98, contains other suggestions.

Following Up

1. Which items might be best to take along on a weekend camping trip? Which might make a great appetizer at dinner? Explain your choices.

2. Think about specific foods you enjoy eating that equal one serving of fruits or vegetables. Maintain a list of these in your Wellness Journal. Refer to the list often.

Types of Vegetables

Do you know what tomatoes and cucumbers have in common? If you answered that both are often used as salad ingredients, you are right. Another and perhaps more surprising link is that both are really fruits, not vegetables. Strictly speaking, a fruit is any part of a plant that holds the seeds.

Types of Fruits

Most supermarkets carry a wide variety of fruits. Some may be from neighboring areas; others may come from across the country or halfway around the world. Here are some you might find in your supermarket:

◆ Many kinds of melons, from cantaloupe to casaba.

◆ Citrus fruits, including grapefruit, oranges, and tangerines.

◆ A bounty of berries—raspberries, strawberries, blueberries, and more—as well as grapes.

◆ Many kinds of apples and pears.

◆ Cherries, plums, peaches, apricots, and other drupes (fruits with a central pit enclosing a single seed).

◆ Tropical fruits, including bananas, pineapple, papayas, kiwifruit, carambola (star fruit), and mangoes—the list is endless!

What Is a Vegetable?

Vegetables can come from many different edible plant parts. They are all vegetables, but they may also be stems, fruits, or even flowers!

Look and Learn:

How might the nutrient content of a vegetable be related to the part of the plant that it comes from?

Seeds. Corn, beans, and peas are the seeds of the plants themselves. Seeds are high in carbohydrates and other nutrients because they are the part of the plant from which new plants grow.

Roots. Carrots, beets, and turnips are examples of root vegetables. Roots store a plant's food supplies and send nutrients and moisture to the rest of the plant.

Leaves. Spinach, lettuce, and cooking greens such as kale and collards are leafy vegetables. Leaves are the plant's manufacturing areas. Through the process of photosynthesis (foh-toh-SIN-thuh-suhs), they turn sunlight, carbon dioxide, and water into high-energy carbohydrates.

Stems. Celery is a common stem vegetable.

Fruits. In addition to tomatoes and cucumbers, eggplants are a fruit commonly considered a vegetable.

Tubers. A **tuber** is a large underground stem that stores nutrients. Potatoes are tubers.

Bulbs. Onions and garlic are examples of bulbs. A bulb is made up of layers of fleshy leaves surrounding part of the stem.

Flowers. Broccoli is an example of a vegetable that includes the flowers of the plant, along with the attached stems.

◆ There are several types of fruit in this photo. Choose different fruits for variety and good nutrition. Try a fruit you have never eaten before and give your reaction to it.

Buying Fresh Produce

Produce is sold many ways, including loose or in a bag or a plastic-covered tray. Some items, like broccoli, are sometimes sold in bunches held together with a rubber band or plastic tie. If you want less of a prepackaged item, ask a clerk to open it and repackage the amount you want. Here are some other guidelines for buying produce:

◆ Inspect produce carefully. Stains on the package or an unpleasant odor may be a telltale sign that the item is damaged or spoiled.

◆ Avoid produce that looks wilted, shriveled, bruised, or decayed. Some produce may have natural blemishes, which do not affect quality. Grapefruit and oranges, for instance, may have brownish surface areas.

◆ Buy by weight, when possible. Except for leafy vegetables, vegetables and fruits should feel heavy for their size. Buy top-quality vegetables and fruits. They will give you more nutrients for your money and will last longer.

◆ Buy only what you can store and use. Most high-quality vegetables and fruits last about a week in the refrigerator.

◆ Remember that some vegetables, such as greens, cook down from their original volume. For example, 1 pound (500 g) of raw mustard greens yields 1½ cups (350 mL) of the cooked vegetable.

Seasonal Produce

Some vegetables and fruits, such as spinach, broccoli, bananas, apples, and grapes, are available the year round. Others—asparagus, peaches, and plums, for example—have a specific growing season. During this season, when the vegetable or fruit is plentiful, prices drop and quality goes up. When shopping, look for year-round favorites and items that are in season. Seasonal produce is often available during the off-season months but tends to cost more then.

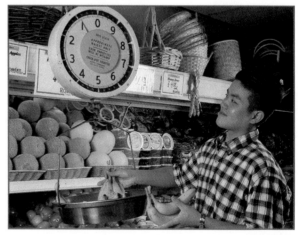

◆ When you can, buy produce by weight. The next time you are at the supermarket, weigh an average sized vegetable or fruit that is sold loose. Note this in your Wellness Journal for future reference.

◆ Washing produce before storing it speeds up decay.
Name two steps you *should* take when storing produce.

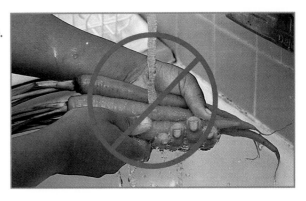

Ripeness

Vegetables and fruits are usually harvested when they are mature. **Mature fruits** are fruits that have reached their full size and color. However, fruits are not always ripe when harvested. **Ripe fruits** are fruits that are tender and have a pleasant aroma and fully developed flavor.

As shown in the chart below, some fruits continue to ripen after they are harvested. Buy these fruits at the stage of ripeness you want—ripe, if you plan to use them right away, or less ripe, if you plan to use them several days later. Some fruits are naturally green when they are ripe, such as many varieties of apples and pears. However, avoid other fruits that are green (except bananas), since they will not ripen well.

Test for Ripeness

To test for ripeness on most fruits, press very gently. Ripe fruit will give slightly under the pressure. Don't press so hard that you damage the fruit.

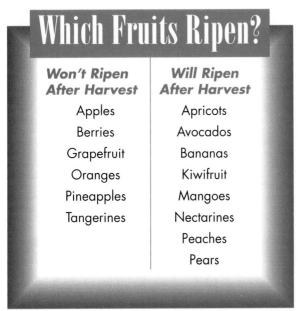

Which Fruits Ripen?

Won't Ripen After Harvest	Will Ripen After Harvest
Apples	Apricots
Berries	Avocados
Grapefruit	Bananas
Oranges	Kiwifruit
Pineapples	Mangoes
Tangerines	Nectarines
	Peaches
	Pears

Storing Fresh Produce

Unless produce is dirty, it should not be washed until you are ready to use it. Added moisture will speed up the action of bacteria, causing spoilage. Moisture remaining on produce can also cause mold to grow. If you need to wash produce before storing it, be sure it is thoroughly dry.

◆ **Storing unripe fruits.** For faster ripening, place them in a brown paper bag at room temperature. For slower ripening, refrigerate. As you need ripe fruit, take it out of the refrigerator and let it ripen at room temperature.

◆ **Storing potatoes, sweet potatoes, and onions.** Store in a cool, dark, dry place. They will keep longest at a temperature of about 45°-50°F (7°-10°C). If you must store potatoes and onions at room temperature, buy only what you can use in a short time. If refrigerated, onions and sweet potatoes will mold and decay, and the flavor of potatoes will change as their starch turns to sugar.

◆ **Storing other vegetables and fruits.** Refrigerate in the crisper section or in brown paper bags. If you use plastic bags, punch holes in them so that some of the moisture can escape. Don't line the bottom of the crisper with paper towels; they get soggy and cause the produce to decay or turn moldy.

Potatoes that are exposed to light sometimes develop a greenish color. This color indicates that the potato may contain a harmful, bitter-tasting compound called solanine. Solanine may also be found in potato sprouts. Cut away green portions and sprouts before using potatoes. Discard potatoes that have a bitter taste.

Convenience Vegetables and Fruits

Convenience forms of vegetables and fruits can be a real help in today's busy families. Canned and frozen vegetables and fruits can be stored longer than fresh produce and can be prepared quickly. They often cost less than fresh produce, yet provide similar amounts of vitamins and minerals.

Juices are also convenient and refreshing. You can buy vegetable and fruit juices in bottles, cartons, cans, or as frozen concentrate. Read the label carefully when you shop. If the label says "juice," the product is 100 percent juice. Products that are not pure juice must be called by another name, such as "fruit drink."

Quick and Easy Convenience Fruits

Canned, frozen, and dried fruits offer convenient choices. Here are tips for using them:

◆ For a quick, low-fat dessert, purée canned fruit in a blender and serve over angel food cake.

◆ To serve frozen fruits, thaw only partially. The ice crystals that remain will help the fruit stay firm.

◆ Dried fruits are sweet and chewy—a concentrated form of energy. They can be eaten as snacks, cooked, or used in recipes.

Buying Convenience Vegetables and Fruits

Challenges	Solutions
Canned fruits are often high in added sugar.	Look for fruits packed in natural juice instead of sugar syrup.
Canned vegetables are often high in sodium.	Look for low-sodium varieties. Drain the liquid from high-sodium vegetables before heating.
Some frozen vegetables are relatively expensive.	Buy frozen vegetables in bags. They cost less than those in boxes. Buy plain vegetables without sauces and other extras. Add your own special touches, such as a sprinkling of herbs.

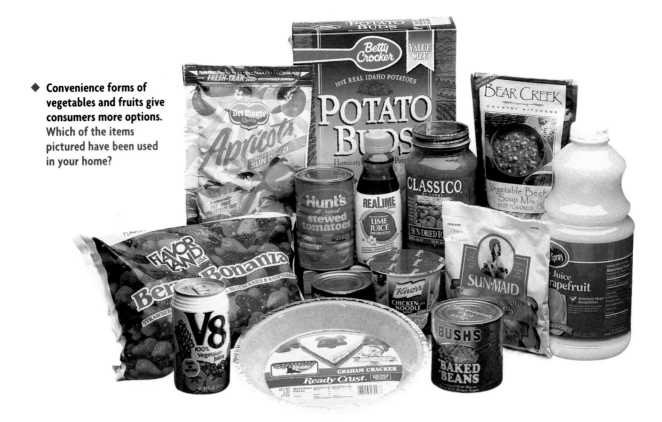

◆ **Convenience forms of vegetables and fruits give consumers more options.** Which of the items pictured have been used in your home?

Section 16-1 Review & Activities

1. Name three nutrients found in fresh vegetables and fruits. Identify specific vegetables and fruits that contain these nutrients.

2. What are three qualities to look for when buying fresh produce?

3. Identify similarities and differences between mature and ripe fruit. Under what circumstances would you buy one or the other?

4. Why should produce be stored unwashed?

5. Analyzing. Twenty-five years ago, supermarkets and produce stands did not offer as great a variety of vegetables and fruits as many do today. What are the reasons for this change? From a nutritional standpoint, how does this change benefit consumers?

6. Synthesizing. The supermarket where Chet shops is having a sale on bananas. Most of the bananas are green. What information would you need to know before you could advise Chet on how much of the fruit to buy?

7. Applying. Use the information from this section to create a Produce Storage Checklist. Armed with your checklist, inspect the state of produce storage in your home. Discuss any problems you encounter with adults in the family, and clarify any myths or misinformation that may exist.

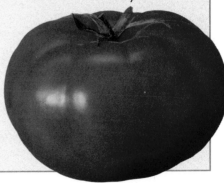

SECTION 16-2

Preparing Raw Vegetables and Fruits

Objectives

After studying this section, you should be able to:

- Describe how to wash fresh produce.
- Give suggestions for healthful and attractive ways to prepare and serve raw vegetables and fruits.

Look for This Term

enzymatic browning

Fresh raw vegetables and fruits are one of nature's convenience foods. They take almost no time to prepare. In minutes, you can have slices of sweet pepper to scoop up your favorite dip. Even when time is short, you can add zip to your morning cereal—and important nutrients to your eating plan—with fresh strawberry or peach slices.

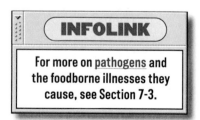

Washing Fresh Produce

Before you eat or cook any fresh vegetable or fruit, you need to wash it. Washing removes pesticide residues, dirt, and pathogens. Even vegetables that are going to be peeled need to be washed first to prevent transferring pesticides and dirt to the edible parts. For tender vegetables and fruits, wash thoroughly in cool, clear water. Be sure to remove all visible dirt. For thicker-skinned produce, such as winter squash, scrub with a stiff brush. Also scrub potatoes and other vegetables that tend to have a lot of dirt. To minimize nutrient loss, do not soak produce in water.

INFOLINK

For more on pathogens and the foodborne illnesses they cause, see Section 7-3.

✚ Safety Check

Never use detergent when washing produce. The produce can absorb the detergent, which can make people ill if it's swallowed. Detergent sometimes reacts with pesticides and waxes found on the produce. The chemicals that result from such reactions can be harmful to humans.

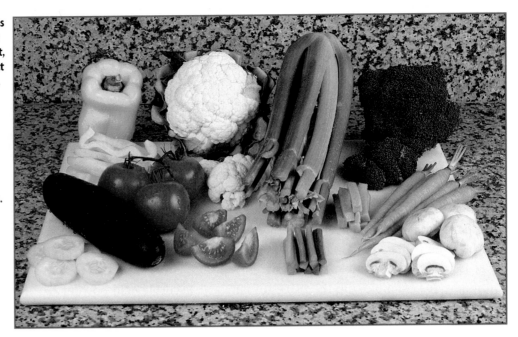

◆ The raw vegetables pictured are easy to chew and digest, making them great snacking options. In your Wellness Journal, record two interesting ways of making these or other raw vegetables a part of your meals and snacks.

Cutting Fresh Produce

After it is washed, some produce needs to be peeled—for example, potatoes and oranges. Other produce, such as jicama, may need to be pared. Inedible parts, including the seeds of sweet peppers, the stems of fruit, and any soft spots or damaged areas, also need to be removed.

For more nutrients and fiber, eat edible skins rather than paring them away. However, if you're concerned about removing wax and residues, pare the produce. Even though some nutrients will be lost in paring, most will remain.

Cutting vegetables and fruits into pieces makes them easier to eat and adds eye appeal. Keep the chunks fairly large when cutting, and serve them as soon as possible. That way, you retain the nutrients. Vegetables and fruits can be cut into dozens of interesting shapes. Sweet peppers, carrots, and zucchini can be presented as strips. Carrots can be sliced crosswise; so can kiwifruit and bananas.

Tomatoes and peaches can be cut into wedges. One eye-catching way to present fresh fruits is to cut them into bite-size shapes and serve them with wooden picks. You can also use a melon baller or small scoop to make balls of soft-fleshed fruits, such as cantaloupe.

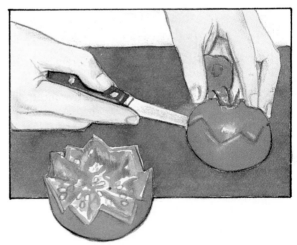

◆ Some raw produce, such as a tomato, can be cut in a decorative shape to make it more visually appealing. Name two other types of raw produce that might be cut into creative shapes.

Preventing Cut Fruits from Darkening

Some fruits turn dark after they are cut. This discoloration, which results from the exposure of a fruit's flesh to the air, is called **enzymatic** (EN-zih-mat-ik) **browning**. Although oxygen in the air will eventually cause any fruit to turn brown, the reaction occurs more quickly in fruits that contain a certain enzyme.

An easy way to avoid enzymatic browning is to coat the fruits with some form of ascorbic acid (vitamin C) as soon as they are cut. You might, for example, dip the pieces of cut fruit in lemon juice. Another option is to buy

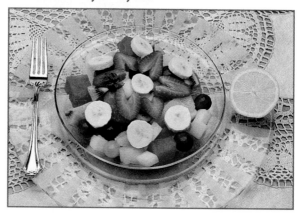

◆ Lemon juice can keep banana slices from turning dark. Would you need to use lemon juice on any other fruits in this salad? Why or why not?

ascorbic acid powder to mix with water and sprinkle on cut fruit.

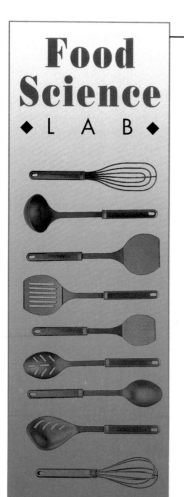

Food Science
◆ L A B ◆

How Quickly Do Different Fruits Darken?

If you were preparing a fruit salad, how would you keep one fruit from darkening while you prepared the others? To answer, you need to know which fruits undergo enzymatic browning and at what rate of speed.

Procedure
1. Working with four classmates, simultaneously cut an apple, a pear, a banana, an orange, and a cantaloupe into small cubes. Place the cubes on a glass plate.
2. Carefully inspect each fruit for discoloration at 2-minute intervals. At the first sign of browning, note how long it took for enzymatic browning to begin.

Conclusions
◆ Which fruits underwent enzymatic browning? Which didn't?
◆ How can this information help you when preparing an entire meal?
◆ Repeat the experiment, this time coating the pieces of fruit with lemon juice after they are cut. Then taste the fruit. How does the juice affect the fruit's flavor?

Unlike fruits, the majority of vegetables do not turn brown when cut. If they are allowed to stand for several days, however, they may begin to darken.

Serving and Storing Cut Produce

An assortment of cut-up raw fruits and vegetables can be a healthful touch when entertaining. Instead of just heaping the fruits and vegetables on a plate or in a bowl, use your imagination. You'll have more fun preparing the food, and the people you are serving will appreciate the extra effort. You might arrange different kinds of produce in ever-widening rings or in wedges like a pie. Keep in mind that color contrast makes a pleasing display.

If you don't plan to serve the produce immediately, cover your arrangement tightly with plastic wrap. Squeeze out as much air as possible, and refrigerate until serving time. You might want to serve the produce with a tasty low-fat dip, possibly one made with yogurt.

Try keeping cut-up vegetables in the refrigerator as handy snacks. Store them in a tightly sealed plastic bag or on a plate covered with plastic. Again, squeeze out as much air as possible to keep nutrients from being destroyed by oxygen.

Section 16-2 Review & Activities

1. Why is it important to wash produce before eating it?

2. Explain enzymatic browning in your own words. Explain how it can be prevented.

3. Analyzing. Why is keeping cut-up fruits and vegetables on hand as snacks a good idea from a nutritional standpoint?

4. Extending. Identify ways in which the presentation of cut vegetables and fruits might be used to increase young children's interest in these foods. Sketch possible fun shapes that would be easy to prepare. If possible, try presenting these foods to a toddler and record his or her reactions.

5. Applying. With a small group of classmates, discuss ways of communicating to teachers and students in your school that vegetables and fruits are the ultimate convenience food. For example, you might create a public service announcement or series of original posters. Assess the effectiveness of your campaign by randomly interviewing members of the school community in the days and weeks following.

Cooking Vegetables and Fruits

If given a choice, would you rather eat vegetables that look bright and colorful, or ones that look tired and washed out? It probably isn't a difficult choice to make.

This visible difference relates to how the vegetables were cooked. Paying close attention to cooking methods can affect not only the look but also the flavor and even the feel of a vegetable or fruit.

Objectives

After studying this section, you should be able to:

- Identify the effects of heat and cooking on vegetables and fruits.
- Describe methods for cooking vegetables and fruits.

Look for This Term

chlorophyll

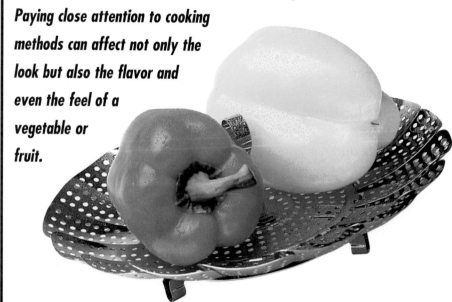

Effects of Cooking on Vegetables and Fruits

Cooking causes changes in vegetables and fruits. One of the most important changes is not observable to the human eye. It is a loss of vitamin C and other nutrients. You can minimize these losses when cooking by:

- Keeping vegetables and fruits whole or in large pieces.
- Cooking them quickly using methods that require only a small amount of water—for example, steaming, simmering in a tightly covered pan, or microwaving.
- Serving cooked vegetables and fruits with the cooking liquid whenever possible.

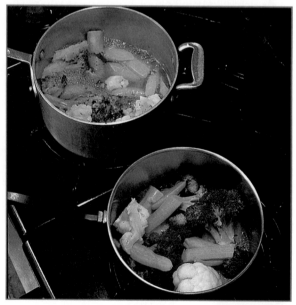

◆ **The difference in cooking time affects the appeal of fresh vegetables.** Give three adjectives to describe the vegetables in each pot.

Sensory Changes in Cooked Vegetables and Fruits

In addition to nutrient loss, cooking results in changes to the texture, color, and flavor of vegetables and fruits.

◆ **Texture.** Heat softens the cell walls, making vegetables and fruits more tender. Many vegetables, such as green beans and winter squash, must be cooked to be edible. Starchy vegetables are easier to digest when cooked. If overcooked, vegetables and fruits become mushy.

◆ **Color.** When properly cooked, vegetables and fruits retain pleasing colors. Green vegetables get their color from **chlorophyll** (KLOR-uh-fil), the chemical compound that plants use to turn the sun's energy into food. If overcooked, green vegetables can turn an unpleasant olive green.

◆ **Flavor.** The heat of cooking releases flavors, making them more noticeable. Fruit flavors mellow somewhat and taste less acid. Herbs, spices, or other foods can be added during cooking, allowing their flavors to mingle with the natural flavor of the vegetable or fruit. When overcooked, vegetables and fruits lose their flavor or may develop an unpleasant flavor.

Cooking Fresh Vegetables

Fresh vegetables can be cooked by several different methods. The timing and method depend on the tenderness of the vegetable and the size of the pieces into which it has been cut.

Steaming Vegetables

Steaming is one of the most healthful ways to cook vegetables. Fewer precious nutrients are lost because the vegetables are not cooked

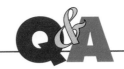

Q How can you prevent discoloration when cooking vegetables?

A Adding a small amount of an acid food, such as vinegar or lemon juice to the cooking water, will stop red cabbage and beets from discoloring. To retain the color of green vegetables, steam them. If you boil them, don't add baking soda, as some people recommend. The chemical reaction that takes place destroys phytochemicals and other nutrients, and creates a mushy texture.

in water. Because steaming takes a little longer than some other methods, be sure to build ample time into your meal preparation plan.

To steam vegetables, place a steamer basket in a saucepan with a tight-fitting lid. Add water to a depth just below the bottom of the steamer. Cover the pan and bring the water to a boil. Add the vegetables to the steamer basket and cover. Reduce the heat slightly, but not so much that the water stops boiling and producing steam. Steam the vegetables until tender.

Simmering Vegetables

Vegetables can be simmered in a covered pan in a small amount of water. Be sure to use a pan made of stainless steel, enamel, or glass. Do not use aluminum or copper. These minerals react with sulfur compounds in vegetables, resulting in a loss of vitamin C, folic acid, and vitamin E. They can also create unpleasant odors and flavors in foods.

Allow about ½ cup (125 mL) of water for four servings of vegetables. Pour the water into a medium-size saucepan, cover, and bring to a boil. Add the vegetables, cover, and bring to a boil again. Then lower the heat until the water just simmers. Cook, covered, until vegetables are tender.

FOR YOUR HEALTH

Low-Fat Flavor Alternatives

Vegetables are naturally low in fat. Yet when butter, mayonnaise, cheese, or rich sauces are added, the fat content soars. Is it possible to add zip to vegetables without adding the fat grams? Here are some ways:

Instead of . . .	Try . . .
• Sour cream	• Plain, nonfat yogurt
• Mayonnaise or salad dressing	• Low-fat or fat-free dressing
• Butter or margarine	• Butter flavoring

You might also like to flavor vegetables with herbs or lemon juice. Try a flavored vinegar—ordinary vinegar that has been allowed to steep with fresh herbs or even fruit added to it.

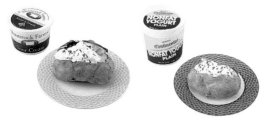

Following Up

1. Examine the nutrition labels of sauces or toppings that you or people you know put on vegetables. How many grams of fat per serving does each contain? What percentage of your Daily Value for fat does this amount represent?

2. Experiment with flavored mustards and other lower-fat alternatives to dressing up vegetables. Write about your findings in your Wellness Journal.

Microwaving Vegetables

Microwaving cooks vegetables quickly using only a small amount of water. As a result, the vegetables lose few nutrients and keep their color, texture, and flavor.

Remember, larger pieces will take longer to cook than smaller ones. Keep in mind, too, that pieces the same size will cook more evenly. If parts of a vegetable are less tender than others—for example, the stems of broccoli and asparagus—arrange the tender parts toward the center and the less tender ones toward the edge of the baking dish.

When cooking whole vegetables that have a skin, such as potatoes or squash, pierce the skin with a fork. This will keep the vegetables from bursting. Always be sure to cover the container to keep in moisture. Follow the directions in the owner's manual or cooking guide for cooking times, power settings, and any special instructions.

Baking Vegetables

Vegetables with a high moisture content can bake in the dry heat of an oven. Vegetables of this type include winter squash, potatoes, and sweet potatoes.

Winter squash is usually cut in half, the seeds removed, and the halves placed on a baking sheet. Squash usually bakes at 350°F (180°C) for 30 minutes or longer, until it is tender. The time depends on the variety and size of the squash.

Potatoes baked in the skins are usually placed right on the oven rack. They can bake at any temperature between 300°F (150°C) and 450°F (230°C). The baking time will depend on the temperature. This flexibility in temperatures makes it possible to bake potatoes with other foods that need more exact temperatures. For example, you can bake muffins at 375°F (190°C) and still bake potatoes at the same time.

Sweet potatoes can also be baked with the skin on. Put them in a shallow pan in case juices begin to run out. They bake best at 400°F (200°C).

Pared whole vegetables such as carrots, onions, and potatoes can be baked in the same pan with a roast. This method adds fat to the vegetables, but it also browns them nicely and gives them a tasty crust.

Frying Vegetables

Some vegetables, including onion, garlic, celery, and sweet pepper, are sometimes chopped and sautéed before they are used in recipes. Sautéing brings out the flavor of the vegetables. Stir-frying and deep-frying are other popular methods of cooking. Except for potatoes, deep-fried vegetables are usually covered with a batter before frying.

Keep in mind that frying in even a small amount of oil adds fat and calories to vegetables. This is especially true when the vegetables are deep-fried.

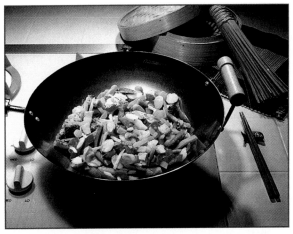

◆ **Vegetables stir-fried with other foods use just a small amount of added fat.** In a print or online source, learn about one different culture that makes use of stir-frying. Share your findings with the class.

Connecting Food and Social Studies

Vegetables: A Bird's-Eye View

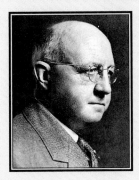

If the frozen food section of your supermarket sometimes feels as cold as the Arctic, perhaps that is no accident. Clarence Birdseye—the scientist without whose pioneering work there might be no frozen food—wouldn't have it any other way!

Birdseye was born in 1886 in Brooklyn, New York. Before graduating from college, he was offered a job as a biologist for the

United States government. While on assignment to the Arctic, he discovered that the extreme cold temperatures would flash-freeze fish placed on the ice. When cooked later, the fish tasted almost the same as if it had been caught fresh. Birdseye went on to conduct further experiments. By 1930, he had perfected the freezing of vegetables, fruits, fish, and meats. Thus, the frozen food industry was born.

Think About It

• Using print or online resources, learn more about Birdseye's contributions to a related industry—the refrigerated shipping of foods. In a brief report, explain how refrigerated shipping has allowed us to enjoy fruits and vegetables once unknown to this part of the world.

Cooking Fresh Fruits

Cooking fruits is a nice alternative for adding variety to your food choices. Cooked fruits can be served hot or chilled. They may be eaten as part of the main course, as dessert, or as a snack.

Like vegetables, fruits can be cooked by several different methods. These include poaching, turning them into a fruit sauce, baking, and microwaving.

Poaching Fruits

Poaching, or stewing, is the cooking of fruit in enough simmering liquid to cover it. The goal is to retain the shape of the fruit as it cooks.

Fruits that can be poached include plums, berries, apples, and pears. Small fruits, such as berries, are left whole. Apples and pears may be cooked whole or cut into large pieces.

Add sugar at the beginning of the process. The sugar is not just for sweetness but to help the fruit keep its shape during cooking

by strengthening the cell walls. For more flavor, you can also add lemon or orange rind, a cinnamon stick, or vanilla. Simmer, uncovered, just until the fruit is tender.

Fruit Sauces

You have almost certainly eaten applesauce, but have you ever tried peach sauce, plum sauce, or pear sauce? All these fruits can be made into sauce. Different fruits can even be combined in a sauce to create tasty, new flavors.

Fruit sauces are made by cooking the fruit in a liquid. Unlike poaching, however, the goal when making a fruit sauce is to break down the texture. Sugar, therefore, is not added until after cooking.

To make a fruit sauce, pare the fruit and cut it into small pieces for faster cooking. Add water to a saucepan to a depth of about ¼ inch (0.6 cm), and place the fruit in the pan. Bring to a boil, lower the heat to simmer, and cover. Cook, stirring occasionally, until the fruit has broken down. The time will vary, depending on the kind of fruit and the size of the pieces. Sweeten as desired with sugar, honey, or syrup. Spices or other flavorings may also be added.

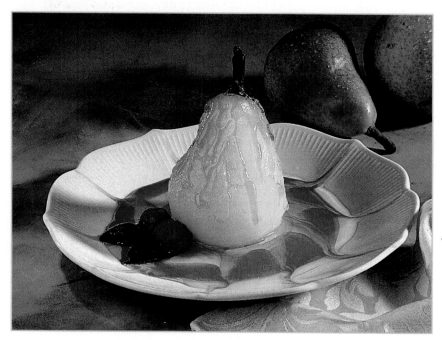

◆ **Poaching adds flavor to fruit while retaining the shape for an attractive presentation. Some contemporary chefs flavor fruits with pepper. Identify two other spices that might give fruits an interesting taste.**

Baking Fruits

When you bake fruits, you need to take care to avoid overcooking them. Best results are obtained with firm fruits—such as apples, pears, and bananas—that are whole or in large pieces.

Apples are probably the most popular baked fruit. They are easy to prepare and make a delicious ending to any meal. Use a variety of apples suited to cooking, such as Rome Beauty. Before cooking, core the apples, and cut a thin strip of skin from around the middle. This will allow the apples to expand as they cook, so that they won't burst. You can fill the cavity with raisins and sweet spices such as cinnamon and nutmeg. Place the apples in a baking dish and pour hot water around them to a depth of ¼ inch (0.6 cm). Bake at 350°F (180°C) until tender, about 45 to 60 minutes.

Microwaving Fruits

Fruits are easy to prepare in the microwave oven. They cook quickly and keep their fresh flavor and their shape. Because they are so tender, however, they can easily overcook. Watch the timing carefully.

Cover fruits when microwaving them, but leave a small opening for excess steam to escape. If you are cooking whole fruits, such as plums, pierce them with a fork in several places to keep them from bursting.

The basic steps in poaching, making a fruit sauce, and baking fruit are similar for microwave and conventional cooking. Power level and cooking time will vary, so check the owner's manual or a microwave cookbook.

Section 16-3 Review & Activities

1. Name three undesirable changes that can occur if vegetables or fruits are overcooked.

2. Explain in a step-by-step fashion two methods for cooking vegetables.

3. Choose one cooking method that is used for both vegetables and fruits. Identify similarities and differences in the method's application to the two types of produce.

4. What are some of the ways in which cooked fruits can be used?

5. **Analyzing.** How can a knowledge of the nutritional impact of cooking on vegetables and fruits benefit an individual shopping for produce?

6. **Synthesizing.** A saying popular in professional kitchens is that people "eat with their eyes." How does this saying apply to the cooking of fruits and vegetables?

7. **Applying.** Write an article for the food page of a newspaper. In your article, provide ideas for cooking vegetables that help retain nutrients, appearance, texture, and flavor. If your local newspaper has a food page, send the article to the paper.

RECIPE FILE

Herbed Vegetable Combo

This quick and easy dish combines several colorful, nutritious vegetables of summer. If you like, experiment with other seasonings, such as basil or lemon juice.

Customary	Ingredient	Metric
2 Tbsp.	Water	30 mL
1 cup	Thinly sliced zucchini	250 mL
1 cup	Thinly sliced yellow summer squash	250 mL
½ cup	Green pepper strips	125 mL
¼ cup	Diced celery	50 mL
¼ cup	Chopped onion	50 mL
½ tsp.	Caraway seed	3 mL
⅛ tsp.	Garlic powder	0.5 mL
1 medium	Tomato, cut into wedges	1 medium

Yield: 4 servings
Equipment: Large nonstick skillet with cover

Directions

1. Heat water in skillet over medium heat.
2. Add vegetables. Cover and cook until vegetables are tender-crisp, about 4 minutes.
3. Sprinkle seasonings over vegetables. Top with tomato wedges.
4. Reduce heat to low. Cover and cook about 2 minutes, or just until tomato wedges are heated.
5. Serve hot.

Nutrition Information

Per serving (approximate): 24 calories, 1 g protein, 5 g carbohydrate, trace of fat, 0 mg cholesterol, 12 mg sodium
Good source of: vitamin C

Food for Thought

• How much time would you allow for pre-preparation tasks for this recipe?
• Why is this a healthful method for cooking vegetables?

CAREER WANTED

Individuals who enjoy facilitating business linkages among various enterprises and people.

REQUIRES:
- flexibility and organizational skills
- computer skills

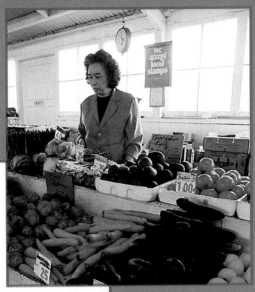

"I put fruit on the nation's table,"

says Produce Wholesaler Lian Yang

Q: Lian, what exactly do you do as a produce wholesaler?

A: I am the link between retail produce buyers—such as supermarkets, school cafeterias, and restaurants—and farmers and food processing firms. I strive to get my clients the best possible prices.

Q: How did you get started in this line of work?

A: I got a part-time job on the loading dock of a produce distributor to help pay my way through college. I enjoyed the wholesaling process and soon I began to work full-time. By the time I finished college, the challenge of running my own produce wholesaling business was hard to resist.

Q: What sorts of skills do you need in your line of work?

A: You have to be able to use computer databases. That's how we keep track of inventory. You also need basic accounting and marketing skills to set appropriate prices and guarantee product availability.

Q: What's the biggest challenge facing someone who wants to pursue a career as a produce wholesaler?

A: My challenge is constantly managing so many different tasks and people all at one time. There are the vendors, store executives, loading dock employees, and the people who handle advertising—just to name a few. I feel like a juggler keeping four balls in the air at once.

Career Research Activity

1. The expression "wearing many hats" is used to refer to people like Lian Yang. Choose three careers from the chart on the right and make a list of the "hats" they wear. Discuss why they must be flexible and organized.

2. Investigate the role technology plays in the availability of fresh produce—from harvesting to transportation. Write a "forecast" of how technological developments will change produce wholesaling in the next 50 years.

Related Career Opportunities

Entry Level
- Salesperson
- Produce Wholesaler
- Summer Camp Counselor

Technical Level
- Game Warden
- Grain Broker

Professional Level
- Food Marketing Representative
- Personnel Administrator
- Purchasing Agent

Chapter 16 Review & Activities

— Summary —

Section 16-1: Choosing Vegetables and Fruits

- Vegetables and fruits are sources of nutrients vital to the body.

- Shop carefully for the best quality and value on in-season and year-round produce.

- Some fruits can be ripened after purchase.

Section 16-2: Preparing Raw Vegetables and Fruits

- Fresh produce should be washed just before use.

- To retain the most nutrients, keep paring and cutting to a minimum.

- Adding ascorbic acid (vitamin C) will prevent cut fruits from turning dark.

Section 16-3: Cooking Vegetables and Fruits

- Cooking affects the nutrient value, texture, color, and flavor of produce.

- Overcooking can result in discoloration and loss of texture, flavor, and nutrients.

- Fresh vegetables and fruits can be cooked in a variety of ways.

- Deep-frying vegetables adds fat and should be done sparingly.

Checking Your Knowledge

1. Give three examples of cruciferous vegetables. What is a possible health benefit of eating them?

2. Why are the roots in vegetables an excellent source of phytochemicals?

3. Why is it best to buy fresh produce in season?

4. Why is it important to wash produce, even if you are going to peel it before eating?

5. Under what circumstances might you buy ascorbic acid powder, mix it with water, and sprinkle it on fruit?

6. How should cut produce be stored?

7. How can you minimize vitamin C loss when cooking vegetables and fruits?

8. Explain the process of simmering vegetables.

9. Give three suggestions for microwaving vegetables.

10. What characteristic makes some fruits better for baking than others?

Working IN THE Lab

1. **Food Science.** Select two similar potatoes. Store one in a cool, dry, dark place. Store the other in the refrigerator. After at least one week, bake the potatoes. Compare their taste and texture. What caused the difference?

2. **Food Science.** Based on what you know about the effects of lemon juice on cut fruit, make a prediction about the action of other juices on cut fruits. Test it by conducting a brief experiment. Was your prediction correct? Why or why not?

3. **Food Preparation.** Select any vegetable or fruit, and prepare it using three of the methods detailed in the chapter. Compare the results for appearance, taste, texture, and convenience. Identify when you might want to use each method.

Thinking Critically

1. Distinguishing Between Fact and Opinion. While out with three friends, Nadine revealed her plan to eat only fruit from now on. Each friend had a different response, as follows: (a) "Eating that much fruit would be boring." (b) "Fruits have a lot of nutrients, but they don't have all the nutrients you need." (c) "Out-of-season fruits taste awful." Evaluate each response. For any that are opinion, restate the same or a similar idea in a way that gives factual information.

2. Determining Credibility. While standing in the supermarket checkout line, Margot notices a tabloid headline that states, "New Scientific Study Shows Eating Fried Vegetables Reduces Disease Risks." Next to this article is a story about a woman who claims she is married to a Martian. What would you advise Margot about the reliability of the article on fried vegetables? Why? How could she find out more about the study mentioned in the headline?

Reinforcing Key Skills

1. Directed Thinking. Rae's supermarket has just expanded its produce section. Before Rae fills her shopping cart with exotic produce, what questions should she ask the produce clerk? What questions should she ask herself about the storage capabilities of her home pantry?

2. Management. Elio is preparing the family meal tonight. He plans to include a tossed salad along with the main course, and assorted fresh fruit for dessert. Before you could advise Elio about meal preparation plans, what other information about the fruit would you need to have? About the meal as a whole?

Making Decisions and Solving Problems

Adam understands the health benefits of eating two to four servings of fruits each day, but he has a small appetite. By the time he has finished his sandwich at lunch or main course at dinner, he is often too full to eat fruit. What could Adam do?

Making Connections

1. Math. By using newspaper ads or visiting a local supermarket, compare the per-serving costs of fresh, frozen, and canned versions of a specific fruit or vegetable. Use package labels or cookbooks to compare the preparation time for each form. Show your findings with two bar graphs: one for price and one for preparation time.

2. Social Studies. Using cookbooks, food magazines, or online sources, learn about a vegetable or fruit widely used in another culture. In that culture, how is the vegetable or fruit purchased and stored? Is it eaten raw or cooked? What methods are used in its preparation? Share your findings with the class in the form of an illustrated report.

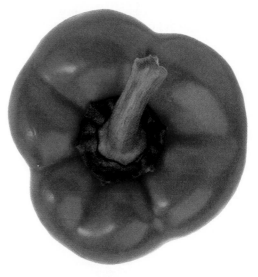

CHAPTER

17

Grains, Legumes, Nuts, and Seeds

Among the earliest
crops raised by humans
for food, grains remain
a staple in many cultures
around the world. In this
chapter, you will learn
about choosing and
using grains in a health-
ful eating plan.

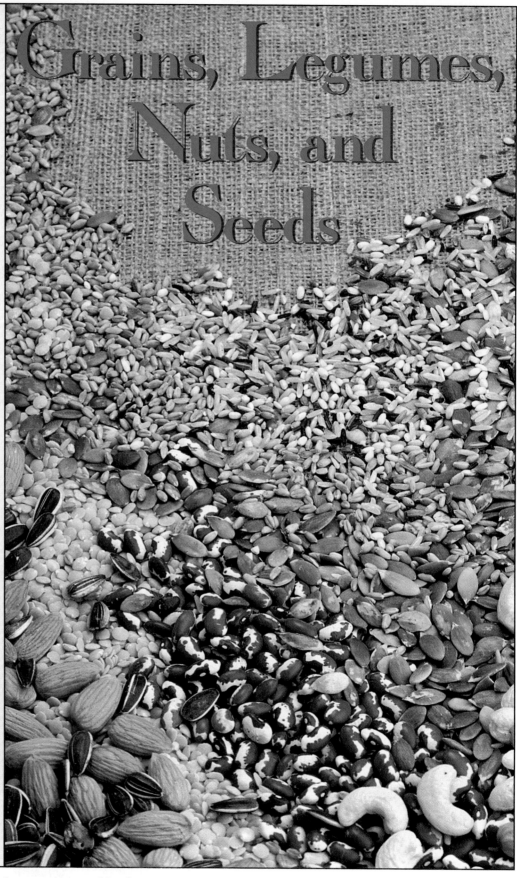

Choosing Grains and Grain Products

Objectives

After studying this section, you should be able to:

- Describe the nutrients in grains and grain products.
- Identify different grain products and their uses.
- Give guidelines for buying and storing grain products.

Look for These Terms

germ
endosperm
bran
whole grain
enrichment
fortification

Grains have been the most important staple in the world's food supply for thousands of years. How many grains and grain products do you eat? How many can you name? After reading this section, you may become familiar with some different grains and grain products.

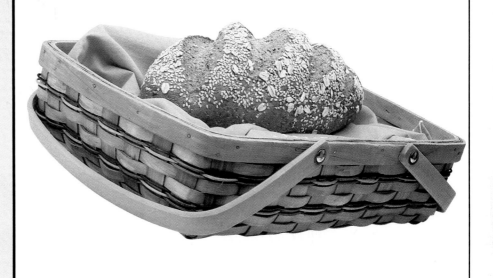

What Are Grains?

Grains are the seeds of plants in the grass family. Common grains in North America include wheat, rice, corn, buckwheat, oats, rye, triticale (trih-tih-KAY-lee), barley, and millet.

Every seed, or kernel, of grain is composed of three main parts:

◆ **The germ.** The **germ** is a tiny embryo in a seed that will grow into a new plant.

◆ **The endosperm.** The **endosperm** is the food supply for a seed's embryo, made up of proteins, starches, and other nutrients. It takes up most of the inner part of the grain.

◆ All three parts of the grain kernel are nutritious. What is the function of each part?

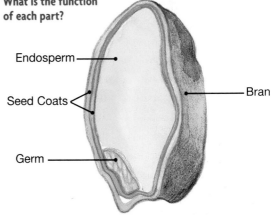

Endosperm

Seed Coats

Germ

Bran

◆ **The bran.** The **bran** is the edible, outer protective layers of a seed.

Nutrients in Grains

Grains get a lot of attention in health news because they are naturally packed with nutrients. The endosperm is high in complex carbohydrates and proteins, with just a small amount of vitamins and minerals. The bran is rich in fiber, B vitamins, and some trace minerals. The germ provides B vitamins, vitamin E, iron, zinc, and other trace minerals; some protein; and a small amount of saturated fat.

Grain Processing

Before consumers can use them, all grains must be processed. This begins with the removal of the outer husk, a natural fibrous material, which exposes the kernel. What happens from that point on will affect the nutrient value of the grain or grain product.

When the **whole grain**—the entire edible grain kernel—is used, the resulting product contains most of the kernel's original nutrients. Examples of whole-grain products are whole wheat flour and whole-grain breakfast cereals.

Very often, the bran and germ are removed during processing—along with the grain's fiber and many of its nutrients. White flour and many breakfast cereals are products made in this fashion. Usually, these products undergo **enrichment**, a process in which some nutrients lost as a result of processing are added back to the product to near original levels. Some products may also undergo **fortification**, a process of adding 10 percent or more of the Daily Value for a specific nutrient to a product by the manufacturer. Most fortified foods supply about 25 percent of the Daily Value for one or more nutrients. Some have 100 percent of many nutrients.

The Food Guide Pyramid recommends eating 6 to 11 daily servings of enriched or whole grains and grain products. Typical servings include one slice of bread; ½ cup (125 mL) cooked cereal, rice, or pasta; or 1 ounce (30 g) of ready-to-eat cereal.

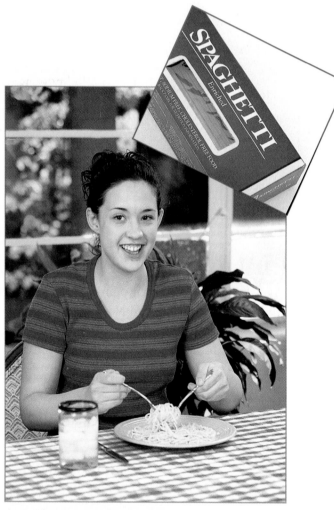

INFOLINK

For more about the benefits of including <u>fiber</u> in your eating plan, see Section 2-2. For more on <u>Daily Value (DV)</u> and how to use this important information to improve your eating habits, see Section 12-2.

◆ Enriching grain products restores some of the nutrients lost in processing. **Explain fortification.**

Buying Grains and Grain Products

When you buy grains and grain products, keep nutrition in mind. Choose whole-grain products as much as possible. Aim for at least three of your grain servings from whole grains each day. If a product you choose does not provide whole grains, be sure it is enriched. Look for products low in fat, added sugar, and sodium, too. Try different grains for variety.

When buying, read the labels to make certain you get the product you want. If the grain is visible in the package, inspect it carefully to be sure you are getting good quality. Pasta, for example, should not appear to be cracked or broken.

Which grains should you buy? That's a matter of personal taste, as well as knowing what's available.

◆ The type of rice you choose may depend on how you plan to use it. What else would you consider when buying rice?

Rice

Several different varieties of rice are grown. You can choose rice with short, medium, or long grains.

◆ **Short grains.** The grains are almost round. When cooked, the rice is moist and the grains stick together. Short-grain rice is a good choice for creamy dishes and for molded rice rings, or if you plan to eat with chopsticks.

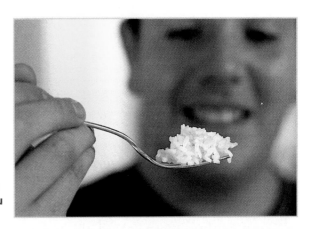

Connecting Food and Social Studies

Graham for Graham

The ideas that we should eat a variety of foods and that different foods provide different nutrients may seem new. However, these ideas can be traced back at least 150 years —to an American religious leader by the name of Sylvester Graham.

Graham was an early supporter of whole wheat bread. However, he felt that the whole wheat flour sold commercially at the time was not "pure" enough. Graham came up with his own recipe for a coarsely ground wheat flour, which he called "Graham flour." Graham used his flour in a special flat bread, which he served to the guests of Graham boarding houses. These were health clinics located throughout the country in the early 1800s. Whether the bread relieved stomach pains, as Graham claimed, most people who tasted it fell in love with it. Today, we know Graham's invention better as the graham cracker.

Think About It

• Using library or online resources, research two other nineteenth-century "health food" pioneers—Dr. John Henry Kellogg and Dr. Charles Post. In a brief report, identify how the two men (who knew each other) were connected and what food innovations each was responsible for.

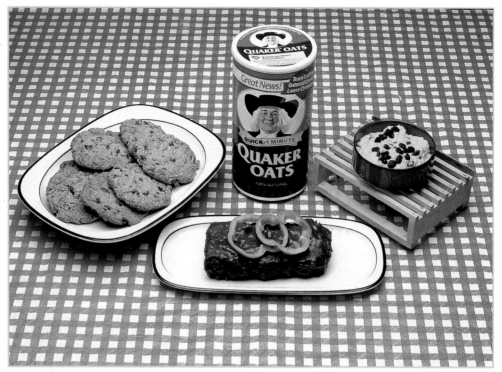

◆ Oats are a versatile grain. Rolled oats, the basis of oatmeal, can also be used in baked goods, meat loaf, and other recipes. In what other forms are oats sold?

◆ **Medium grains.** The grains are plump, tender, and moist. They stick together, but not as much as short-grain rice.

◆ **Long grains.** When cooked, the grains are fluffy and stay separated.

Rice can vary in the way it is processed. *Brown rice* is the whole-grain form of rice. Only the outer, inedible hull has been removed; the bran, endosperm, and germ still remain. *White rice* has had the bran and germ removed. *Converted rice* has been parboiled (briefly boiled) to save nutrients before the hull is removed. *Instant rice* has been precooked and dehydrated. It takes only a few minutes to prepare.

The fiber content of rice also varies—mostly as a result of the removal of the bran for white rice. The fiber content of brown rice is about three times higher than that of white rice.

How does wild rice fit in with the other types of rice? It's actually the seed of water grass, not a grain at all.

Other Grains

In addition to rice, many other types of grains can be creatively cooked and served as side dishes. Cooked grains are also popular as hot breakfast cereals. Some can be used in baking or other recipes. Here are some types of grains you may have eaten or may want to try:

◆ **Barley.** Mild-flavored, hardy grain. Usually used in soups and stews.

◆ **Brans.** The ground bran of oat, rice, or wheat can be purchased to use as a hot cereal or in baking. All are high in fiber. For instance, 1 ounce (30 g) of wheat bran has about 13 grams of fiber.

◆ **Bulgur.** Wheat kernels that have been steamed, dried, and crushed. Tender with a chewy texture. Used in main dishes, salads, and as a side dish. A popular use for bulgur is in tabbouleh, a Middle Eastern salad flavored with mint and parsley.

- **Cornmeal.** Coarsely ground dried corn. Available in yellow or white types. Used as a breakfast cereal and in baked goods.

- **Couscous** (KOOS-koos). Steamed, cracked endosperm of wheat kernel. Has a nutty flavor. Used as a cereal, in salads and main dishes, or sweetened for dessert.

- **Cracked wheat.** Crushed wheat berries with a very tough and chewy texture. Often added to bread.

- **Grits.** Coarsely ground endosperm of corn. Used as a breakfast cereal or side dish.

- **Kasha** (KAH-shuh). Roasted buckwheat that is hulled and crushed. Has a pleasant, nutty flavor. Used as a breakfast cereal or side dish.

- **Millet.** Small, yellow grains with a mild flavor. A staple in Europe, Asia, and northern Africa. Used in breads and as a breakfast cereal or side dish.

- **Oats.** Often eaten as a hot cereal or used in baked goods. Quick-cooking types are available.

- **Quinoa** (KEEN-wah). A small, ivory-colored, ricelike grain, quinoa cooks much faster than rice and is an excellent source of protein—higher than any other grain. Its neutral flavor makes it a perfect addition to side dishes, soups, meat loafs, and more.

- **Triticale** (trih-tuh-KAY-lee). A cross between wheat and rye, with more protein than wheat. Can be used in cereals and main dishes and combined with other cooked grains.

- **Wheat berries.** Whole, unprocessed wheat kernels. Can be cooked as a cereal or used in grain-based dishes.

Ready-to-Eat and Instant Cereals

Breakfast cereals are among the largest-selling foods in the United States. Each year Americans spend close to $1 billion on these products.

Besides tasting good, dry breakfast cereals can fit into a healthful eating plan. Just read the "Nutrition Facts" label on the box or bag to make sure you know what you're buying. Look for a product that is high in complex carbohydrates and fiber. It's not necessary for a cereal to provide 100 percent of the nutrients you need in a day. In fact, you can get a nutritious product often at a lower cost by buying cereals that are not highly fortified.

When eating a breakfast cereal in milk, keep in mind that some vitamins and minerals were added in the form of sprays and thus will dissolve in the milk. These nutrients are not lost as long as you finish the milk in the bowl along with the cereal.

Another ready-to-eat grain product is wheat germ. It has a pleasant, nutty flavor and is an excellent source of protein, vitamins, and minerals, along with a small amount of unsaturated fat. It also is a good source of fiber—more than 4 grams of fiber per ounce. Wheat germ can be added to yogurt, cereals, and other foods for a nutritional boost, and for extra crunch.

Some of the hot cereals already described, such as oats and grits, are also available in instant forms. Cooking time is shorter. Often sugar and other flavorings have been added.

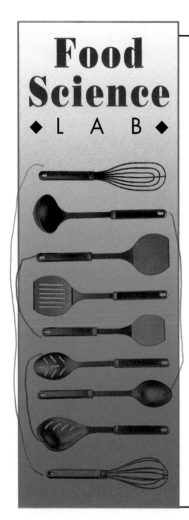

Food Science ◆ L A B ◆

Connecting Fiber and Flavor in Cereals

Some people believe that high-fiber, whole-grain cereals may not be as tasty as low-fiber cereals made from processed grains. Is this always the case?

Procedure

1. Blindfold a classmate for a blind taste test.

2. Pour out ¼-cup (50-mL) portions of three cereals that are high in fiber (at least 5 grams of fiber per serving) and three that are not (2 grams of fiber or less per serving).

3. Have your subject taste each sample and record his or her reactions. Products are to be assigned a rating of 1 or 2, where 2 is high-fiber and 1 is low-fiber.

4. Compare the ratings for each cereal with the actual fiber content on the Nutrition Facts panel for the product.

Conclusions

◆ How did your subject's rankings compare with the actual fiber content of each cereal?

◆ How can this information help in your future purchases of cereal?

◆ How does cost correlate with flavor or fiber content?

Pasta

Did you know that *pasta* is the Italian word for "paste"? Like paste, pasta dough is made from flour and water. After it is rolled thin, pasta dough can be formed into hundreds of different shapes. Examples include spaghetti, corkscrews, bow ties, and macaroni.

Both enriched and whole wheat pastas are available. Whole wheat pasta has almost three times as much fiber as traditional, enriched pasta. Some pastas are flavored and colored with carrots, spinach, tomatoes, or other foods. Noodles are pasta made with eggs. Noodles can also be made without egg yolks, which makes them lower in fat and cholesterol than regular noodles.

Packages of dried pasta are found in the grocery section with other shelf-stable foods. You may find fresh pasta in the refrigerated section.

Choosing pasta can be fun. Selecting a variety of pasta shapes and sizes can add appeal to many meals.

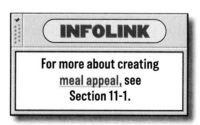

INFOLINK

For more about creating meal appeal, see Section 11-1.

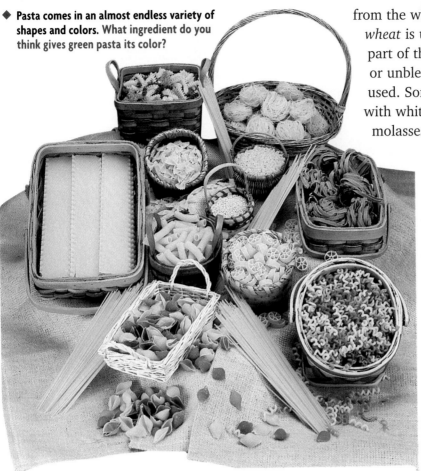

◆ **Pasta comes in an almost endless variety of shapes and colors.** What ingredient do you think gives green pasta its color?

from the whole grain. If only the word *wheat* is used, it usually means some part of the grain has been removed, or unbleached white flour has been used. Some dark breads are made with white flour with caramel or molasses added for color.

Storing Grains and Grain Products

To maintain the quality of grains and grain products, follow these storage guidelines:

◆ Store whole grains and whole-grain products in the refrigerator if you plan to store them for a couple of weeks or more. Because they contain oil, they can spoil at room temperature if not used quickly.

◆ Refrigerate fresh pasta.

◆ Store other uncooked grains and grain products, such as white rice and dried pasta, in a cool, dry place in tightly covered containers.

◆ Store breads at room temperature for short-term storage. Otherwise, freeze them. Hard-crusted bread gets stale faster when refrigerated. However, in humid weather, refrigerate bread to prevent mold from growing.

◆ Store cooked grains in the refrigerator if they will be used within a few days. For longer storage, freeze.

Breads

Breads range from enriched white bread to whole wheat and mixed whole grains. They come in assorted flavors, shapes, and sizes, including individual rolls.

Leavened (LEV-uhnd) breads are made with a leavening ingredient, such as yeast or baking powder, which causes the bread to rise. Unleavened, or flat, breads, like tortillas, are made without leavenings. Pita bread is a flat bread that can be split horizontally to make a pocket and then filled with a variety of foods.

When buying bread, read the label carefully. *Whole wheat* means the product is made

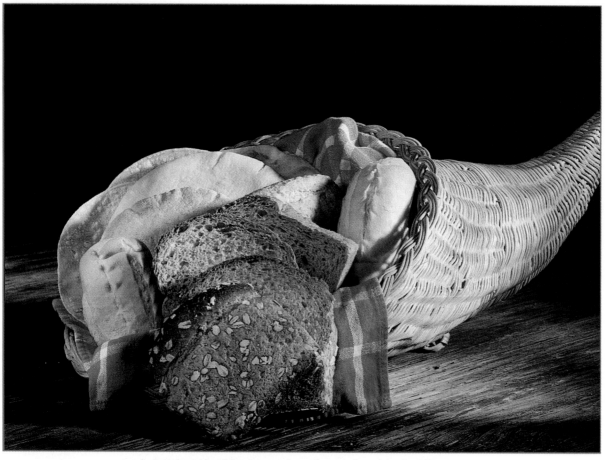

◆ **Breads can be either leavened or unleavened. Explain the difference.**

Section 17-1 Review & Activities

1. Identify the three parts of a grain kernel and the nutrients found in each.

2. Name four grains that can be cooked and eaten as side dishes.

3. What should you look for when choosing a nutritious ready-to-eat cereal?

4. Synthesizing. For years, Suki's grain selections were limited to white bread, white rice, and pasta made with white flour. What health consequences may she be at risk for later in life as a result of her choice of grains?

5. Analyzing. What qualities have made grain products so popular around the world?

6. Applying. Find three recipes, each of which uses a different grain or grain product. Make a chart in which you identify the type of grain or grain product, and describe its nutritional value.

Preparing Grains and Grain Products

Properly prepared, grains can be a nutritious, flavorful part of any meal, from breakfast to dinner. You can serve them plain or top them with vegetables, seasonings, and sauces. You can even serve some as desserts by adding sweeteners or fruits.

Objectives

After studying this section, you should be able to:

- Explain the general principles of cooking grains.
- Describe how to prepare rice and other grains, pasta, and breakfast cereals.

Look for This Term

al dente

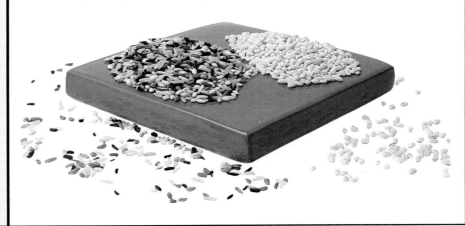

Principles of Cooking Grains

Because they are dry, grains need to be prepared in liquid—usually plain or salted water. Many grains can also be simmered in broth or stock. Even though most grains are cooked in a similar way, cooking methods and times vary. Always follow package or recipe directions.

Unless package directions state otherwise, do not rinse enriched grains prior to cooking. Rinsing can cause a loss of added B vitamins.

Microwaving grains is not always practical. Because grains need time to absorb liquid to soften, microwaving does not usually save time. Pasta, for instance, takes just as long in the microwave as it does to cook conventionally.

Nevertheless, go ahead and check the package for microwave directions.

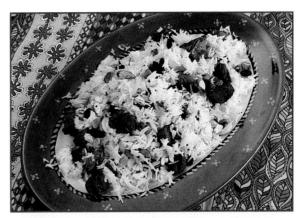

◆ Biryani—a delicious blend from India of basmati rice, meats, raisins, nuts—is a healthful way of satisfying several nutrient requirements. Consult cookbooks or online resources for other rice-based one-dish meals. Share your findings with the class.

Preparing Rice and Other Grains

Rice is usually simmered, using just the amount of liquid that the grain can absorb. Bring the liquid to a boil, add the rice, cover, and bring to a boil again. Then reduce the heat so the rice simmers gently.

Package directions may tell you to stir the rice at intervals as it cooks. Do not stir long-grain rice unless necessary. Stirring can scrape off starch, making the grains stick together.

Near the end of cooking time, check the rice for doneness. It should be moist and tender but firm. There should be no liquid left in the pot. If any liquid remains, continue cooking without the cover until the excess liquid is absorbed or evaporates. Instant rice requires a slightly different cooking method. Follow package directions.

Barley, grits, kasha, and many other grains are cooked in much the same way. One that is not is bulgur, which is "cooked" by pouring boiling water over the dry grain and letting it stand 30 minutes.

Preparing Pasta

Unlike rice and some other grains, pasta is cooked uncovered in a large amount of boiling water. Pasta is one of very few foods that must be boiled. The boiling helps circulate the pasta so that it cooks evenly.

Check the package for the amount of water to use. With dry spaghetti, for example, use about 1 quart (1 L) of water for every 4 ounces (120 g) of spaghetti. Be sure the pot is large enough for the amount of water used and the boiling action of the water.

Grain Measurements and Cooking Times

Grain (1 cup, or 250 mL, dry)	Amount of Liquid	Cooking Time	Cooked Yield (approximate)
Barley (pearl)	2½ cups (625 mL)	40 minutes	3 cups (750 mL)
Cornmeal	4 cups (1 L)	25 minutes	3 cups (750 mL)
Grits (regular)	4 cups (1 L)	25 minutes	3 cups (750 mL)
Kasha	2 cups (500 mL)	20 minutes	2½ cups (625 mL)
Millet	2½ to 3 cups (625 to 750 mL)	35-40 minutes	3½ cups (875 mL)
Rice (long- or medium-grain)	2 cups (500 mL)	45 minutes (brown) 15 minutes (white)	3 cups (750 mL)
Bulgur	2 cups (500 mL)	None	2½ cups (625 mL)

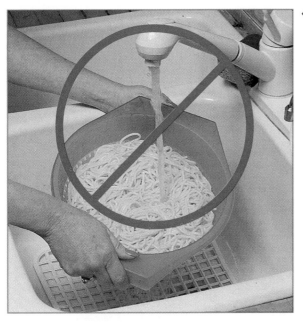

◆ Never rinse pasta after cooking. Doing so washes away valuable nutrients. **Give two tips for preserving the flavor and nutrient value of pasta.**

After cooking, drain the pasta in a colander or strainer. Never rinse pasta after cooking it—this removes nutrients. To keep cooked pasta hot, set the colander or strainer over a pan of hot water and cover.

If you have leftover cooked pasta, freeze it. First, stir 1 teaspoon (5 mL) cooking oil into the drained pasta to keep it from sticking. Freeze in serving-size portions.

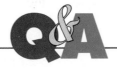

Dry pasta is generally cooked to a doneness stage known as **al dente** (ahl DEN-tay), firm to the bite. Cooking time varies from 5 to 20 minutes, depending on the thickness of the pasta. If the pasta is to be further cooked in a recipe (such as lasagne), cook it for a shorter time so that it is slightly more firm. Unless directions state otherwise, fresh pasta will cook in a fraction of the time needed by dry pasta.

Q How can I keep pasta from sticking together during or after cooking?

A Start by using plenty of water. Bring the water to a rapid boil, then add pasta slowly so that the water continues boiling. Stir frequently. After cooking, if the pasta still seems to be sticking together, toss it with 1 teaspoon (5 mL) of cooking oil per portion.

Dry Pasta Quantities

Type of Pasta	Dry Weight	Dry Volume	Cooked Yield (approximate)
Small pasta shapes—macaroni, shells, spirals, twists	4 ounces (120 g)	1 cup (250 mL)	2½ cups (675 mL)
Long, slender pasta strands—spaghetti, angel hair, vermicelli	4 ounces (120 g)	1-inch (2.5-cm) diameter bunch	2 cups (500 mL)

Preparing Cereals

A bowl of steaming hot cereal can really jump-start your body on a cold morning. Even if you live in a region that has mild temperatures year-round, a bowl of oatmeal or other hot cereal makes a tasty breakfast.

Some hot cereals can be prepared with either water or milk. Check the package directions. Instant hot cereals usually require only that you add boiling water. Some ready-to-eat cereals can be microwaved to serve hot.

Whether hot or cold, have your cereal with milk, especially if you don't drink much milk otherwise. It will help you get one of the servings from the Food Guide Pyramid you need as a growing teen. For natural sweetness and added nutrients, try adding fresh or dried fruit, such as strawberries, raisins, dried apricots, or sliced bananas.

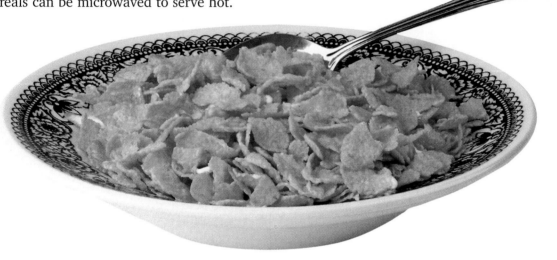

Section 17-2 Review & Activities

1. Why shouldn't you rinse grains before cooking them?

2. Does microwaving grains save time? Explain.

3. How can you tell when rice is properly cooked?

4. Extending. Are there advantages to using fresh pasta instead of dry pasta? If yes, what are possible advantages?

5. Synthesizing. When preparing grains at home, what are some creative ways you can use them with your meals?

6. Applying. Find recipes for a variety of pasta sauces. Which appear to be low in fat and high in fiber? How might you reduce the fat in the other recipes? How might you increase the fiber?

Legumes, Nuts, and Seeds

Legumes have been eaten all over the world for more than 10,000 years. Legumes include dry beans, peas, and lentils. All these foods come in different shapes, sizes, and colors. No matter what form or shape, they are packed with flavor, nutrition, and meal appeal.

Objectives

After studying this section, you should be able to:

- Identify the nutrients in legumes, nuts, and seeds.

- Give guidelines for buying, storing, and preparing legumes, nuts, and seeds.

Look for This Term

legumes

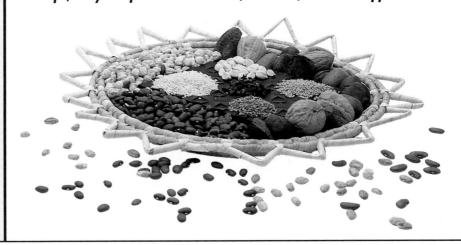

Nutrients in Legumes

Technically, **legumes** are plants whose seeds grow in pods that split along both sides when ripe. They are excellent sources of complex carbohydrates (especially fiber), proteins, B vitamins (including folate), iron, calcium, potassium, and some trace minerals. Nearly all are low in fat. In addition, their use has been linked to reduced risk of heart disease, some cancers, and other lifestyle diseases.

Because of their rich concentration of plant proteins, legumes are grouped along with other protein sources—including meat, poultry, and fish—in the Food Guide Pyramid. Health experts urge eating dry beans, peas, or lentils instead of meat at least twice a week. When totaling your servings, count ½ cup (125 mL) of cooked dry beans as 1 ounce (28 g) of lean meat. Legumes can also do double duty as a vegetable serving.

Legumes and Grains

Legumes and grains work perfectly as a team. Each has the amino acids (building blocks of proteins) the other lacks. By eating both any time during a day, you can get all the essential amino acids needed for good health. The soybean is the only legume that naturally contains all the building blocks of proteins necessary for health. Grains and legumes make up about two-thirds of the proteins eaten by people all around the world.

INFOLINK

For more on specific illnesses grouped under the label "lifestyle diseases", see Section 3-1.
For more on the essential amino acids and how to obtain them, see Section 2-2.

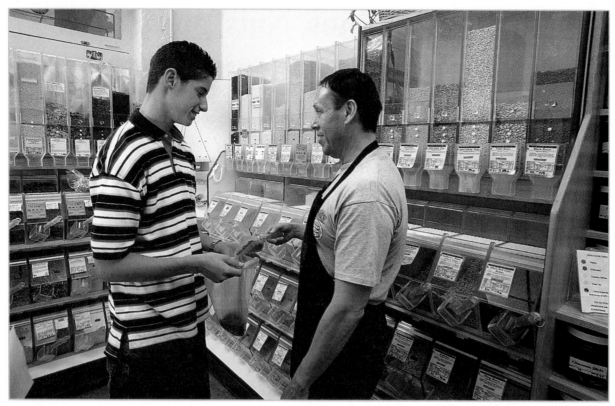

◆ Legumes are considered "crossover" foods. They can be grouped with meats, poultry, and fish in the Food Guide Pyramid, but they can also be grouped with vegetables. How would you classify red beans served as a main-dish casserole?

Buying and Storing Legumes

Because legumes continue to dry out when stored, a good rule of thumb is to buy only as much as you will use within six months. The drier they are, the longer they will take to cook.

If legumes are visible in the package, inspect them carefully. Look for bright color, no visible damage, and uniform size. Mixed sizes result in uneven cooking, since smaller ones cook faster than larger ones.

Store dry legumes in a cool and dry place. Once the package has been opened, transfer the remainder to a tightly covered container.

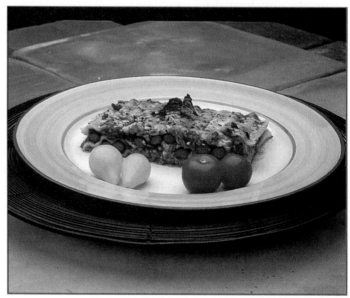

◆ This lasagne combines pasta sheets with cooked dry beans. What are the advantages of using legumes as a protein source?

Types and Uses of Legumes

Type of Legumes	Uses	Popular Recipes
Black beans (turtle beans) Black skin, cream-colored inside, sweet flavor.	Soups, stews, Latin American and Asian dishes	Cuban rice and beans
Black-eyed peas Actually beans, not peas. Small, oval, with black "eye" on one side.	Main dishes with ham or rice, curries	"Hoppin' John," a Southern recipe
Dry peas Available whole or split, green or yellow.	Soups	Split-pea soup
Garbanzo beans (chickpeas) Round, roughly shaped, nutlike flavor, firm texture. Hold their shape when cooked.	Dips, main dishes, salads, roasted as a snack	Hummus, a Middle Eastern dip
Lentils Thin, tiny, disc-shaped. Come in colors ranging from grayish brown to green to reddish orange.	Soups, stews, salads, curries, side dishes	Main ingredient in East Indian dish, dal
Lima beans White, flat beans in assorted sizes. Baby limas are smallest with mild flavor. Butter beans are largest with a rich, buttery flavor.	Soups, casseroles, salads, side dishes	Succotash
Pink and red beans Vary in size, flavor, and intensity of color. Kidney beans are largest, with a hearty flavor.	Stew, mixed bean salads, Latin American main dishes	Chili con carne
Pinto beans Pink and white, speckled. Similar in flavor and texture to pink and red beans.	Chili, stew, Mexican rice and beans	Refried beans
Soybeans Distinct flavor. High in protein and fat. Difficult to digest.	Soy products—tofu and soy milk	Some meatless burgers, tofu
White beans Vary in size and flavor, but all have a firm texture. Great Northern are largest. Navy beans are medium in size.	Soups, casseroles, mixed dishes	Boston baked beans

Cooked legumes can be stored in the refrigerator if you plan to use them within three days. For longer storage, freeze them. When putting the beans in freezer containers, add enough cooking liquid to cover them so that they will not dry out. Frozen cooked beans can be thawed in a microwave oven or in the refrigerator.

Preparing Legumes

Like grains, legumes are versatile and easy to prepare. They tend to pick up the flavor of bay leaf, onion, or other seasonings you add to the cooking water. Just be sure to give them time to absorb water until they are soft enough to eat.

Once cooked, beans and other legumes can be served whole, mashed, or puréed, as a side dish, or as a main ingredient in casseroles, soups, stews, chilis, burritos, and salads. Dry peas and lentils are tasty in soups and stews. To be really creative, try a lasagne made with beans or a lentil loaf instead of a meat loaf.

Sorting and Rinsing

Before cooking, sort legumes carefully. Pick out foreign material such as pebbles and stems. Also discard any legumes that are damaged, are smaller than others, or have a greenish tint.

Rinse the legumes carefully by placing them in cool water. Drain, then rinse again. Repeat, if necessary, until the water is clear.

Soaking Beans

Dry beans normally take from one to two hours to cook. Soaking before cooking can cut down on cooking time by 15 to 30 minutes. Dry peas and lentils do not have to be soaked.

To soak dry beans, use a large pot. For every pound (500 g) of any kind of beans, sorted and washed, add about 10 cups (2.5 L) hot water. Simmer for two to three minutes; then turn off the heat and cover the beans. Let them soak for at least an hour. The longer beans soak, the less cooking time they need. If beans have been soaked, drain and rinse them before proceeding with the recipe.

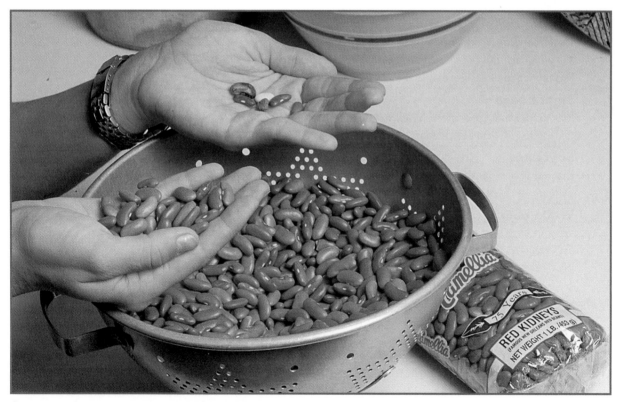

◆ Sorting legumes is an important step in the cooking process. Describe the next two steps.

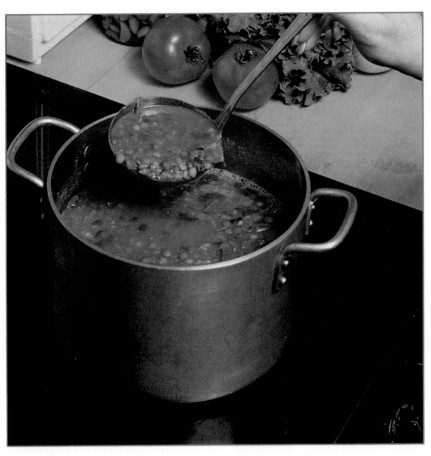

◆ **Soups based on legumes make for hearty, cold-weather fare.** What would you serve with this lentil soup to help balance your daily nutrient intake?

are a bit firmer. If you plan to mash them, cook longer so that they are a little softer.

When done, the beans should have a little cooking liquid left. Although beans retain most of their important nutrients, serve the cooking liquid with the beans—it contains small traces of B vitamins. If you plan to use only the beans, save the liquid for soups, sauces, or broth.

Simmering Beans

Place the beans in a large pot—they double in volume as they cook. Add water, using the amount specified on package directions. More water may be needed if the legumes are old and dry. If you like, you can spice up the cooking water by adding chopped onions, garlic, or dried herbs.

Cover the pot and bring the water to a boil. Then lower the heat to a simmer. Follow package directions for cooking time. For best results, start checking at the minimum cooking time specified. If the beans are not tender enough, continue cooking. If the beans are used in a salad or for further cooking in a recipe, cook them a shorter time so that they

Other Methods

A convenient way to cook beans is with a slow cooker. Do not presoak them. Check the slow cooker owner's manual for exact directions. In general, the beans are combined with boiling water in the cooker. Mix well, cover, and cook on the high setting. This method generally takes three to eight hours, depending on the kind of beans.

Beans also can be cooked in a pressure cooker. Again, follow the directions in the owner's manual.

Legumes can be cooked in the microwave, too. It takes about the same amount of time as conventional cooking.

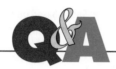

A Tough beans sometimes get that way when the recipe calls for salt or an acid food, such as vinegar or tomatoes. If your recipe does, add these ingredients near the end of the cooking time. To prevent beans from getting mushy or having the skins break, cook them gently, leaving the lid slightly ajar. One more tip: If you don't have time to cook dry beans, don't let that stop you from using them in meals. Use canned beans—they're a time-saver.

Nuts and Seeds

Like legumes, nuts and seeds are included in the Meat Group of the Food Guide Pyramid. Nuts and seeds are high in protein and B vitamins. They're also high in fat, though not the saturated kind. When eaten in moderation, they can be a beneficial part of a heart-healthy eating plan.

Among the wide assortment of nuts available are almonds, filberts, cashews, and Brazil nuts. Even though peanuts are legumes, people use them as they do other nuts. The same is true of walnuts, which are actually seeds. Other popular edible seeds include sunflower, pumpkin, squash, and sesame seeds.

◆ Nuts and seeds, such as sunflower seeds, can be used to add flavor, texture, and nutrients to many recipes. What is the best advice for storing nuts and seeds?

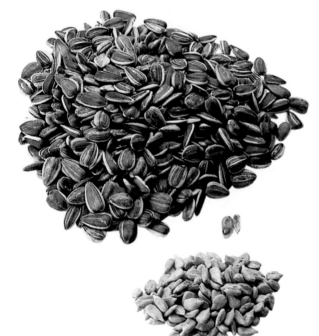

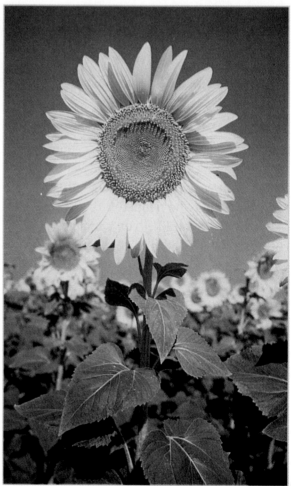

Buying and Storing Nuts and Seeds

Nuts and seeds are sold both with and without the shell. Many varieties are available raw or roasted—either in oil or dry roasted, a special process in which no oil is added.

Nuts and seeds can be ground into a thick, spreadable paste. The most common example is peanut butter. Tahini (tuh-HEE-nee), a spread made from ground sesame seeds, is popular in Middle Eastern cooking.

When buying nuts and seeds, avoid those in shells that are cracked or broken. Harmful pathogens may be present in the edible parts.

If you're not planning on using them quickly, store nuts and seeds in the refrigerator. Because they contain oil, even in their raw state, they can spoil at room temperature over time.

Using Nuts and Seeds

You can enjoy nuts and seeds in a variety of ways. Chopped or ground nuts and seeds add flavor and texture to baked goods, salads, cereal, and yogurt. They can also be used in meatless baked dishes for added protein. Nut butters and spreads can be used in sandwiches or recipes.

When using nuts and seeds in low-fat cooking, first toast them in the oven or on the range. Toasting enhances flavors, so you can use less and still get the same full flavors.

Section 17-3 Review & Activities

1. Name five nutrients supplied by legumes.

2. Within how many months should dry legumes be used? Why?

3. What are the three basic steps in preparing dry beans?

4. **Evaluating.** Since nuts and seeds are high in fat, how can you include them in a healthful eating plan? List at least three examples.

5. **Analyzing.** What characteristics of legumes do you think explain their long history as staples in the world food supply?

6. **Applying.** Look through cookbooks to find recipes that use legumes in each of the following: a vegetarian main dish, a main dish with meat or poultry, a soup, and a salad. Be prepared to discuss how the recipe directions relate to the preparation principles you have learned in this section.

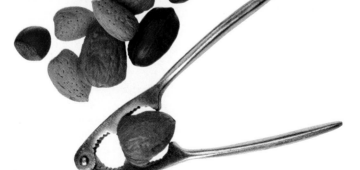

RECIPE FILE

Western Beans and Rice

This recipe combines legumes and rice to provide complete proteins. It also combines conventional and microwave cooking techniques with convenience forms of rice and legumes. Serve this dish with a tossed salad, fruit, and milk for a complete meal.

Customary	Ingredient	Metric
(See package directions)	Brown rice	(See package directions)
(See package directions)	Water	(See package directions)
1 Tbsp.	Vegetable oil	15 mL
1 cup	Chopped onion	250 mL
1 cup	Diced celery	250 mL
3 cups	Canned pinto beans, drained and rinsed	750 mL
1 8-oz. can	Reduced-sodium tomato sauce	224-g can
½ cup	Water	125 mL
¼ tsp. (or to taste)	Hot pepper sauce	1 mL (or to taste)

Yield: 6 1-cup servings
Equipment: Saucepan; 1-qt. (1-L) microwave-safe dish with cover
Power level: 100%

Directions

1. Prepare instant brown rice in saucepan according to package directions, using amount of rice and water to make 3 cups cooked rice.
2. While rice is cooking, combine onion, celery, and oil in microwave-safe dish. Cover.
3. Cook onion and celery at 100% power for 2 minutes, stirring after 1 minute.
4. Stir in beans, tomato sauce, ½ cup water, and hot pepper sauce. Cover.
5. Cook mixture at 100% power for 5 to 8 minutes, stirring after 4 minutes.
6. Let stand 1 minute.
7. Serve over hot, cooked rice.

Nutrition Information

Per serving (approximate): 250 calories, 9 g protein, 46 g carbohydrate, 4 g fat, 0 mg cholesterol, 531 mg sodium
Good source of: potassium, iron, vitamin E, B vitamins, phosphorus

Food for Thought

• What foods provide the most protein in this recipe?
• If you were preparing this recipe to serve as a side dish, what foods could you serve it with?

CAREER WANTED

Individuals interested in specialty or health foods, who like meeting people and like change.

REQUIRES:

- degree in food science or retailing
- some on-the-job training

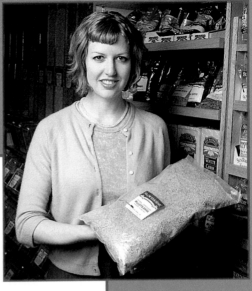

"Eating well is key to good health,"

says Health Food Store Nutritionist Margery Kleinerman

Q: When did you open your store?

A: It actually began as a family business over 75 years ago. My grandfather, who came here from Greece, settled in this neighborhood. To make a living, he began importing olive oil, nuts, cheeses, and spices.

Q: When did it become a health food store?

A: The transition was recent. With the trend toward healthier eating, more and more people have turned to ethnic recipes, which are often meatless. We offer Greek specialties, including a dozen varieties of olive oil, which are all low in saturated fat. We also sell organically grown fruits and vegetables.

Q: You refer to yourself as a "nutritionist." Do you have special credentials in that area?

A: As a matter of fact, I do. I have a degree in food science. I also keep up with health trends.

Q: What makes your specialty food store successful?

A: Our dedication to quality. Plus, we are now online. I get orders from all over the world. I'm even writing a specialty foods organic cookbook.

Career Research Activity

1. Visit a specialty or health food store or restaurant in your community. Try to find out how the store or restaurant was established. Ask how technology has impacted their business and what trends they see among customers.

2. Choose two of the careers listed on the right and investigate the ways in which technology has changed the way people work in that field. For example, do importer/exporters travel as much as they used to? Why or why not?

Related Career Opportunities

Entry Level
- Sales Clerk
- Canteen Operator
- Dietetic Aide

Technical Level
- Importer/Exporter
- Health Food Nutritionist
- Dietetic Technician

Professional Level
- Epidemiologist
- Health-Science Librarian

Summary

Section 17-1: Choosing Grains and Grain Products

• Grain kernels are made up of the germ, endosperm, and bran.

• Grains are generally high in complex carbohydrates, proteins, fiber, vitamins, and minerals. However, the nutritional value of grains depends on how they are processed.

• Cooked grains are popular as side dishes and breakfast cereals; grain products include instant and ready-to-eat cereals, pasta, and breads.

• Look for nutrition and quality when buying.

• Store grains and grain products properly to maintain their quality.

Section 17-2: Preparing Grains and Grain Products

• Grains must be cooked before eating.

• Although cooking methods for many grains are similar, always check the package directions.

• Rice and many other grains are simmered in only as much water as they can absorb.

• Pasta is boiled in a large amount of water and then drained.

• Breakfast cereals are served hot or cold, often with milk and fruit.

Section 17-3: Legumes, Nuts, and Seeds

• Legumes are high in protein, fiber, and other nutrients. Most are low in fat.

• The many types of legumes can be used in main dishes, side dishes, and salads.

• Dry beans require long cooking in water. Soaking them first decreases the cooking time.

• Nuts and seeds are high in protein and unsaturated fat. In moderation, they may be eaten plain or added to baked goods and other dishes.

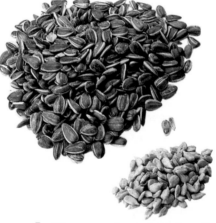

Checking Your Knowledge

1. What is the difference between whole-grain and enriched products?

2. Describe the following grain products and tell how they are used: couscous, kasha, and triticale.

3. Name three specific instances when grains or grain products should be refrigerated.

4. Why must grains be cooked before they are eaten?

5. What type of rice should not be stirred during cooking? Why?

6. What term is used to describe properly cooked pasta? What does it mean?

7. Describe the following legumes and tell how they are used: chickpeas, lentils, soybeans.

8. Give three guidelines for buying legumes.

9. Briefly describe how to cook beans.

10. What nutrients are found in nuts and seeds?

Review & Activities Chapter 17

Thinking Critically

1. Drawing Conclusions. Hallie, an aging adult with gastric problems, has been advised by her health professional to avoid using whole-grain products. What might be the reason for this advice? Why might the advice be sound, even though non-whole-grain products often lack the bran and germ, and hence, are less nutritious?

2. Recognizing Assumptions. A friend of yours who wants to lose weight tells you she plans to avoid pasta because it is fattening. Do you agree? Explain your answer.

3. Identifying Cause and Effect. Saril has found a recipe for a stew that includes lentils, tomatoes, and onions. He says, though, that the last time he cooked lentils, they came out tough and chewy. What are some possible explanations for this result? What precautions should Saril take when preparing the recipe?

Working IN THE Lab

1. Food Preparation. Prepare a variety of different grains, such as couscous, bulgur, and millet. Compare them for taste, texture, and appearance. Decide what types of dishes or recipes each grain might be used in. Give reasons for your answers.

2. Food Preparation. Prepare a dessert dish using rice or pasta. What nutritional value does rice or pasta add to the dessert?

Reinforcing Key Skills

1. Communication. Imagine that you work as a media consultant. A company that manufactures and sells pasta has come to you, asking you to develop a campaign to increase public awareness about the goodness and nutritive values of their product. Make a list of the facts to include in your campaign.

2. Management. Sean cooked too much rice for his family's dinner. He wonders what to do with all the extra rice. Help Sean find a solution.

Making Decisions and Solving Problems

Your family relies mostly on processed grain products and eats very few whole grains. You would like to introduce more whole grains to make your family's meals more nutritious. You have had limited success introducing new foods in the past.

Making Connections

1. Social Studies. Using library sources, write a report on a grain product that is popular in a specific culture. How was the grain introduced in that country? Why is it popular? How is it used? What percentage of the population is employed in growing and processing the grain?

2. Math. Draw a graph comparing the cooking times of various grains and legumes. If available, use a computer to develop the graph. Post your graph in a high-visibility location near the classroom foods lab for quick reference.

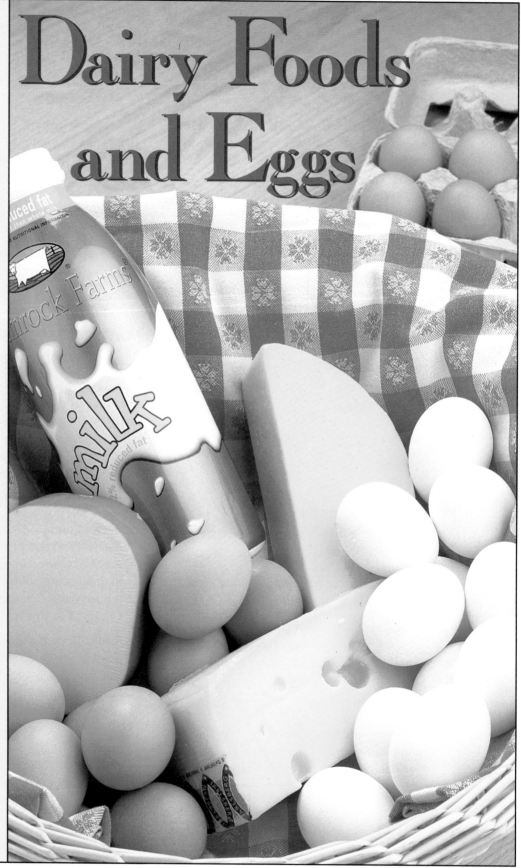

18

Dairy Foods and Eggs

Section 18-1
Choosing Dairy Foods

Section 18-2
Preparing Dairy Foods

Section 18-3
Egg Basics

Section 18-4
Using Eggs in Recipes

Todd had worked up a big thirst during football practice. He went straight to the refrigerator and poured himself a tall, cold glass of milk. Like many teens, Todd knows milk tastes great. In this chapter, you will learn about the many benefits of milk, other dairy foods, and eggs.

462   **Chapter 18 ◆ Dairy Foods and Eggs**

Objectives

After studying this
section, you should be
able to:

- Identify nutrients in
  milk and other dairy
  foods.

- Describe the types of
  dairy foods available.

- Give guidelines for
  buying and storing
  dairy foods.

Look for These Terms

pasteurized

homogenization

cultured

ripened cheese

unripened cheese

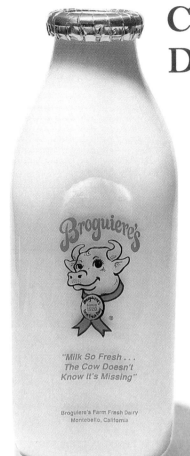

Choosing Dairy Foods

Dairy foods include milk and the many products made from milk, such as yogurt and different kinds of cheeses. Daily servings of milk and other dairy foods provide many nutrients that promote good health.

Nutrients in Milk

Milk has been called an almost perfect food. It is especially high in proteins, vitamin A, riboflavin, vitamin B_{12}, calcium, phosphorus, magnesium, and zinc. When fortified, it is an excellent source of vitamin D. The Food Guide Pyramid recommends two to three servings a day of milk or other dairy foods.

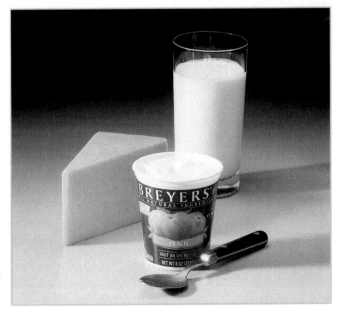

◆ Milk and milk products are loaded with important vitamins and minerals. Name three micronutrients found in milk.

Types of Milk

Although whole milk contains some saturated fat and cholesterol, lower-fat and fat-free forms are available. These products, which appear in the chart on the right, also have less cholesterol than whole milk.

Fresh whole milk contains about 87 percent water and 13 percent solids, some of which are milk fat. The other solids, which are fat-free, contain most of the protein, vitamins, minerals, and lactose (milk sugar) found in milk. These fat-free milk solids are also found in reduced-fat, low-fat, and fat-free milk.

Processing of Fluid Milk

When shopping, look for milk that has been **pasteurized**. To help ensure food safety, milk is heat-treated to kill enzymes and harmful bacteria. Enzymes in milk can make it spoil quickly. Sometimes milk is

Fat in Milk

Type of Milk	Amount of Fat
Whole milk	8 g fat per 8-oz. (250-mL) serving
Reduced-fat milk	5 g fat per 8-oz. (250-mL) serving
Low-fat milk	2.5 g fat per 8-oz. (250-mL) serving
Fat-free milk	Trace of fat

ultra-pasteurized, heated to a higher temperature than in pasteurization. This permits it to be kept longer in the refrigerator. When exposed to even higher temperatures—as in the case of UHT (ultra-high temperature) processing—milk becomes a shelf-stable product that can be packaged in aseptic containers.

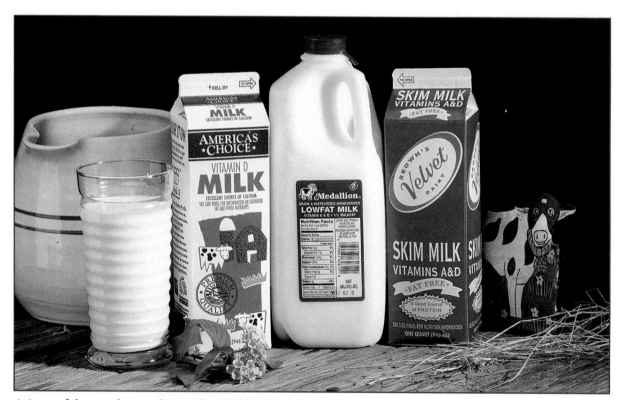

◆ Is one of these products used in your household? Identify the fat content of each product by percent.

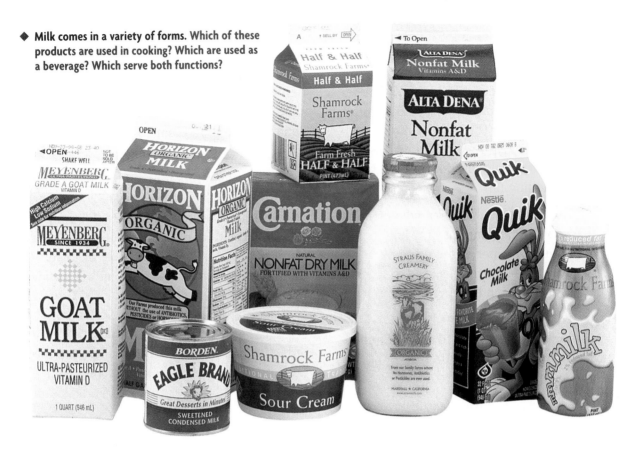

◆ Milk comes in a variety of forms. Which of these products are used in cooking? Which are used as a beverage? Which serve both functions?

Milk fat is lighter than other milk fluids and easily separates, rising to the top of the milk. **Homogenization**, the process whereby fat is broken down and evenly distributed in the milk, prevents this from happening. When fat is removed from milk, most of the vitamin A is removed along with it. By law, any vitamin A removed during the process must be replaced. In addition, most manufacturers voluntarily fortify milk with vitamin D. You can also buy milk with added calcium.

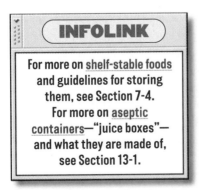

INFOLINK

For more on shelf-stable foods and guidelines for storing them, see Section 7-4. For more on aseptic containers—"juice boxes"— and what they are made of, see Section 13-1.

Other Types of Milk

Besides plain fluid milk, various flavored milks and convenience milk products are available:

◆ **Buttermilk.** Has a tart, buttery flavor and smooth, thick texture. These properties are a result of its having been **cultured**— fermented by a harmless bacteria added after pasteurization. Other familiar cultured dairy products are yogurt and sour cream.

◆ **Kefir** (kuh-FEER). A cultured beverage similar in flavor to yogurt. The authentic Middle Eastern product is made of fermented camel's milk. In the United States, kefir is made from cultured cow's milk.

◆ **Chocolate milk.** Has chocolate or cocoa and sweetener added.

- **Fat-free dry milk.** A powdered form of fat-free milk. When reconstituted, fat-free dry milk needs to be handled like liquid milk, which includes refrigeration. The instant variety of fat-free dry milk mixes easily with water. The powder may also be added directly to recipes to increase nutrients, especially protein and calcium, without adding fat.

- **Evaporated milk.** Canned whole or fat-free milk that contains only half the amount of water as regular milk. Evaporated fat-free milk is used as a cream substitute in beverages.

- **Sweetened condensed milk.** A concentrated, sweetened form of milk, used to make candy and desserts.

- **Lactose-free or reduced-lactose milk.** Available for people with lactose intolerance.

Other Dairy Foods

Many dairy products that start off as milk reach the market in other forms. Among these are yogurt, cheeses, cream, butter, and frozen dairy desserts.

Yogurt

Yogurt is made by adding a harmless bacteria culture to milk. The result is a thick, creamy, custardlike product with a tangy flavor. Yogurt is available plain or with added flavorings, such as vanilla and fruits. For an added nutrition boost, as well as a tasty and refreshing snack, try adding fresh sliced fruit, such as a banana or kiwi, to plain yogurt.

A concentrated form of milk, yogurt is higher in calcium than liquid milk. One cup (250 mL) of fat-free yogurt has 452 milligrams of calcium, compared with 302 milligrams in the same quantity of fat-free milk. Yogurt can also have a fat content as low as, or lower than, that of comparable fluid milk. Consider that a serving of nonfat yogurt has 1.5 grams or less of fat per serving and a serving of low-fat yogurt has between 1.5 and 5.7 grams of fat. To get the least fat, carefully read the label on the container before making your purchase.

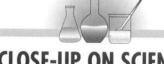

CLOSE-UP ON SCIENCE:
C H E M I S T R Y

Coagulating Milk Protein

Milk contains many different proteins, but two major ones are involved in making milk products such as yogurt and cheeses. The two proteins are casein (KAY-seen) and whey. When an acidic food or milk-clotting enzymes such as rennin (REH-nuhn) are added to milk, the two proteins separate. Casein clumps together into solid groups called curds, as in cottage cheese. The whey is a thin, bluish liquid that remains after the curds clump. Many different dairy products are made by turning proteins into curds.

🚑 Safety Check

After pouring milk, return the container to the refrigerator immediately. Do not pour milk that has been sitting out in a serving pitcher back into the original container. Instead, if the milk has been at room temperature less than two hours, refrigerate it in a separate container and use it soon. Discard milk that has been left at room temperature more than two hours.

Cheeses

When you want to add zip to a sandwich or a tangy touch to pasta, say "Cheese!" Cheese is a natural food made from milk curds with the whey drained off. There are two basic categories of cheeses:

◆ **Ripened cheese.** Also called aged cheese. Made from curds to which ripening agents —bacteria, mold, yeast, or a combination of these—have been added. The cheese is then aged under carefully controlled conditions. Aging time depends on the kind of cheese. The result is a cheese that can be stored for a relatively long time. The texture of ripened cheeses ranges from soft to very hard. In between is a wide range of textures, including semisoft, semihard, and hard.

◆ **Unripened cheese.** Made from curds that have not been aged. Most unripened cheeses will keep only a few days in the refrigerator.

Specialty cheeses are created by combining several ripened cheeses by either cold or hot processing methods. *Cold pack cheese* is a blend of ripened cheeses processed without heat. Flavorings and seasoning are often added. *Pasteurized process cheese* is a blend of ripened cheeses processed with heat. Examples are process American cheese, cheese spread, and cheese food.

Types of Cheese

		Appearance	*Texture and Flavor*
Ripened Cheeses	Blue Cheese	White cheese with a blue vein.	*Semisoft.* Tangy flavor.
	Brick	Light yellow color.	*Semisoft.* Sweet, mild but pungent flavor.
	Brie (BREE)	White, edible crust with a creamy, yellow interior.	*Soft.* Mild to pungent flavor.
	Camembert (KAM-ehm-behr)	White, edible crust with a creamy, yellow interior. Similar to Brie.	*Soft.* Mild to pungent flavor.
	Cheddar	White to orange color.	*Hard.* Mild to sharp flavor.
	Colby	Similar to cheddar, but moister.	*Hard.* Mild to sharp flavor.
	Edam (EE-duhm)	Creamy, yellow Dutch cheese with red wax coating.	*Semihard.* Mild, nutlike flavor.
	Feta (FAY-tuh)	White, crumbly cheese.	*Semihard.* Salty, pickled flavor.

		Appearance	Texture and Flavor
Ripened Cheeses (cont'd)	Gouda (GOO-duh)	Creamy, yellow cheese with red wax coating. Similar to edam, but higher in fat.	*Semihard.* Mild nutlike flavor.
	Monterey Jack	Creamy, white cheese with tiny cracks.	*Semisoft.* Mild flavor.
	Muenster (MUHN-stir)	Orange exterior and white interior.	*Semisoft.* Mild flavor.
	Parmesan (PAHR-muh-zahn)	Creamy, white, granular cheese.	*Very hard.* Tangy, robust flavor.
	Provolone (proh-vuh-LOH-nee)	Creamy, golden yellow, plastic-like cheese.	*Hard.* Bland to sharp, smoked flavor.
	Romano (roh-MAH-noh)	Creamy, white cheese. Similar to parmesan.	*Very hard.* Rich, tangy flavor.
	Swiss	Creamy, white cheese with holes in it.	*Hard.* Nutlike flavor.
Unripened Cheeses	Cottage Cheese	Moist, soft cheese with large or small curds.	Bland flavor, but flavorings such as chives may be added. May be creamed.
	Cream Cheese	Smooth, spreadable, white cheese.	Mild, slightly acid flavor. Flavorings such as straw-berry may be added.
	Farmer's Cheese	Firm and dry. Similar to cottage cheese.	Bland flavor.
	Mozzarella	Creamy, white, plastic-like cheese.	*Semisoft.* Mild flavor.
	Ricotta	Moist, white cheese.	Mild, sweet flavor.

Cream

Cream is a liquid separated from milk. Several types, which vary as to fat content, are available. Heavy cream, the highest in fat, whips easily. Light cream, which is not as high in fat, is often used in coffee. Half-and-half is a mixture of milk and cream. Sour cream, made by adding lactic acid bacteria to cream, is thick and rich with a tangy flavor. It's also relatively high in fat and calories. Add it sparingly to your baked potato, or select a reduced-fat or fat-free sour cream product. Another alternative is using thickened yogurt. You'll learn how to make thickened yogurt in Section 18-2.

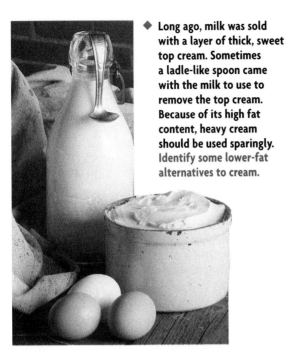

◆ Long ago, milk was sold with a layer of thick, sweet top cream. Sometimes a ladle-like spoon came with the milk to use to remove the top cream. Because of its high fat content, heavy cream should be used sparingly. **Identify some lower-fat alternatives to cream.**

Butter

Butter is made from milk, cream, or a combination of the two. Because it's high in saturated fat and also contains cholesterol, the most healthful choice is to use it in moderation.

Butter is graded for quality by the USDA. *Grade AA* is superior in quality. It has a delicate, sweet flavor and a smooth, creamy texture, and it spreads well. It may be purchased salted or unsalted. *Grade A* butter is very good in quality and has a pleasing flavor with a smooth texture. *Grade B* butter is made from sour cream and has a pleasing flavor.

Frozen Dairy Desserts

Several different types of frozen desserts are available. They differ in fat content and ingredients. All come in a variety of flavors. Here are some examples:

◆ **Ice cream.** A whipped, frozen mixture of milk, cream, sweeteners, flavorings, and other additives. In addition to regular ice cream, you can buy reduced-fat, low-fat, fat-free, and no-sugar-added versions.

◆ **Frozen yogurt.** Similar to ice cream, but with yogurt cultures added. Low-fat and fat-free varieties are the most popular.

◆ **Sherbet.** Made from milk fat, sugar, water, flavoring, and other additives. It generally has less fat and more sugar than regular ice cream.

As an occasional treat on a hot summer's day, a frozen dairy treat can be just the thing. Just be cautious in choosing a product. As an alert consumer, you need to go beyond the

FOR YOUR HEALTH

The Scoop on Frozen Dairy Desserts

What's in a name? When it comes to frozen dairy desserts, the answer is "a whole lot!" All of the products in the list below vary in terms of fat, sugar, and calorie content. None, however, could be described as a low-calorie treat. Use the following information when choosing a frozen dairy dessert. Numbers of calories and fat grams are based on a ½-cup (125-mL) serving.

	Calories	Fat (grams)
Premium ice cream	175	12
Regular ice cream	135	7
Low-fat ice cream	92	3
Sherbet	135	2
Low-fat frozen yogurt	125	3

Following Up

• Think about some of the ways frozen dairy treats are served—for example, in sundaes. Investigate how various toppings and other additions affect the total fat and calorie content. What strategies can you think of for increasing the nutrient value of frozen treats?

name and descriptions on the label. Above all else, pay attention to portion size. Remember, even fat-free ice cream can have up to 300 calories per cup!

Buying and Storing Dairy Foods

When buying dairy products, look for the date on the package. Most milk products can safely be used for up to five days beyond the "sell by" date if they have been stored properly. Yogurt and some ripened cheeses may be stored for longer periods of time. Be sure containers are sealed tightly and have not been opened before you buy them.

Dairy foods are highly perishable. Store them immediately when you get home from shopping. Refrigerate all dairy foods in their original containers, if possible.

Here are some additional tips for storing dairy foods:

◆ Tightly close milk and cream containers. These products can pick up aromas from other foods and develop off-flavors.

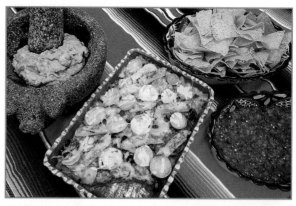

◆ Cheese can be frozen for later use in cooked dishes, such as this Mexican casserole of tortillas layered with chicken and tomatillos (green tomatoes). What other dishes do you like that have cheese in them?

◆ Store milk away from light. Light destroys the riboflavin (a B vitamin) in milk.

◆ Keep cheeses tightly wrapped.

◆ Hard cheeses can be frozen, but the texture will change. Freeze in ½-pound (250-g) portions. Use crumbled, shredded, or in cooked dishes.

◆ Refrigerate butter up to several weeks. For longer storage, freeze up to nine months.

◆ Store ice cream tightly covered in the freezer.

Section 18-1 Review & Activities

1. Identify four nutrients in milk and milk products.

2. Why is milk pasteurized?

3. What is the difference between ripened and unripened cheese?

4. Give three tips for storing milk and milk products.

5. Analyzing. Make a chart of the shelf-stable dairy products detailed in the chapter. For each product, identify common uses as well as other situations in which it might be used.

6. Evaluating. Discuss the benefits of using fat-free yogurt over other dairy foods in cooking.

7. Applying. Use the chart "Nutritive Value in Foods," in Appendix B, to compare the nutrients in various dairy products. Which are highest in calcium? Which are lowest in fat?

Preparing Dairy Foods

Ted was heating milk to make cocoa when the phone rang. He knew that if he left the milk to get the phone, the milk might boil over. So he let the answering machine take the call.

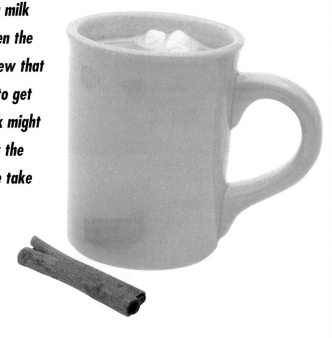

Objectives

After studying this section, you should be able to:

- Identify ways to prevent problems when cooking with milk.
- Discuss ways to use yogurt in recipes.
- Identify guidelines for preparing cheese.

Look for This Term

scalded milk

Cooking with Milk

Ted was aware that dairy foods are delicate proteins. They must be cooked carefully at moderate temperatures and for a limited amount of time.

Milk can be the base for preparing delicious cooked foods, including cocoa and soups. However, several problems can arise when you're cooking milk:

- **Forming a skin.** As milk cooks, protein solids clump together, forming a skin on the surface. The skin can make the milk bubble up and boil over. To keep a skin from forming, cover the pan or stir the mixture regularly. If a skin forms, use a wire whisk to beat it back into the mixture. Removing it removes nutrients.

- **Scorching.** When milk solids fall to the bottom of a pan, they stick and burn. To prevent milk from scorching, use low heat. Stir the mixture to keep the solids circulating. Cooking milk in a double boiler can help prevent scorching.

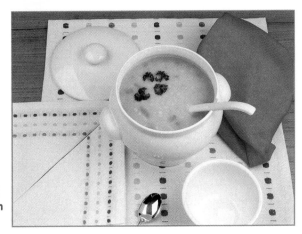

◆ When milk-based recipes such as this corn chowder are cooked carefully, the result is smooth and flavorful. How did the person who cooked this chowder avoid scorching the milk?

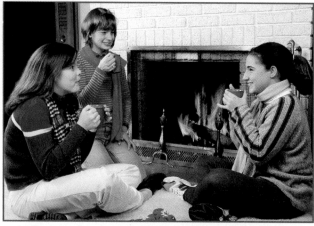

♦ **Cocoa is a favorite cold-weather beverage made with milk.** Name two ways of preparing cocoa.

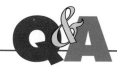

Q When making cocoa, how can I cut down on fat and prevent problems—such as lumping and scorching—from occurring?

A Use fat-free milk to reduce fat. To prevent lumping, mix the cocoa powder and sugar thoroughly. Gradually add a little liquid, stirring well to make a smooth paste. Then continue adding the rest of the liquid, stirring constantly. Use low heat to prevent scorching, or cook the cocoa in the microwave.

♦ **Curdling.** When milk curdles, it has separated into curds and whey. Curdling may occur when milk is heated with acidic foods, such as vegetables and fruits. It can also be caused by salt or high heat. To prevent curdling, use low temperatures, stir the mixture, and combine milk with acidic foods gradually.

Some recipes call for **scalded milk**, milk that is heated to just below the boiling point. Use low heat and cook only until bubbles appear around the sides of the pan.

Milk and milk-based recipes can be prepared easily in the microwave oven. Be sure to use a large enough container in case the milk foams up.

Using Yogurt in Recipes

Yogurt can be a nutrient-dense substitute for sour cream, cream cheese, milk, and mayonnaise. You can use it in many recipes, from soups to main dishes to salads.

Here are some basic guidelines to remember when cooking with yogurt:

♦ Yogurt can be cooked, baked, or frozen. The active bacteria cultures may not survive, but the nutrients will still be the same.

♦ Whey may separate from the curd in yogurt when it is stored. Stir the whey back into the yogurt before you use it.

♦ Cook yogurt at moderate temperatures for only the time needed. Yogurt is just as delicate as other dairy foods. If overcooked, it will curdle.

♦ To keep yogurt from separating during cooking, blend 1 tablespoon (15 mL) cornstarch with a small amount of yogurt. Combine with the remaining yogurt, and use according to recipe directions.

♦ You can thicken yogurt by letting the whey drain off. Line a strainer with a double thickness of cheesecloth. Empty the yogurt into the strainer and set the strainer over a bowl. (The bowl should be a size and shape that prevent the strainer from touching the bottom.) Refrigerate up to 12 hours or until enough whey has drained off to give the desired thickness. If the yogurt is thick enough, you can use it as a cheese. Use the nutrient-rich whey in soups and casseroles, or substitute it for water, buttermilk, or milk in baking.

You can also use yogurt as a salad dressing, dip, sauce, or dessert topping. For example, top cooked vegetables such as asparagus with plain yogurt; then sprinkle with chopped nuts and minced chives.

Preparing Cheese

Serve unripened cheeses, such as cottage cheese and cream cheese, chilled. Add seasonings and chopped vegetables to them to make zesty dips.

Ripened cheese tastes best when served at room temperature. Remove it from the refrigerator at least 30 minutes before serving. You can also bring it to room temperature by microwaving it. Follow the directions in the owner's manual.

Follow these guidelines when cooking cheese:

◆ Heat cheese just long enough to melt it. If overcooked, cheese gets stringy and tough.

◆ To speed up cooking time, shred, grate, or cut cheese into small pieces.

◆ Be careful when microwaving cheese—the fat in it attracts microwaves. The cheese may be hotter than the rest of the microwaved food.

◆ To lower the fat in recipes with cheese, choose sharp-flavored varieties. Since they have more flavor, you can use less cheese.

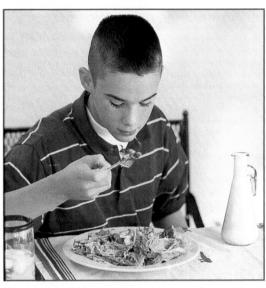

◆ **This zesty salad dressing was made by blending fresh herbs and plain, nonfat yogurt.** What other ways can yogurt be used in cooking?

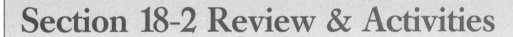

Section 18-2 Review & Activities

1. List two ways to prevent milk from curdling.

2. How can yogurt be used as a substitute for cheese?

3. What happens to cheese if it is overcooked?

4. Extending. Ronit's six-year-old daughter doesn't like milk or cheese. What recommendations can you make for using milk and/or other dairy products in cooking that can help Ronit meet her daughter's nutritional needs?

5. Synthesizing. Would you try to dovetail other food preparation tasks with the cooking of dairy products? Why or why not?

6. Applying. Locate a recipe for homemade cream of tomato soup. Read through the directions carefully. What does the recipe recommend to prevent curdling? How might you improve upon the directions?

RECIPE FILE

Easy Macaroni and Cheese

Just about every home cook—and many professional ones, too—have a recipe for macaroni and cheese. Here's a version that's easy *and* good!

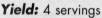

Customary	Ingredients	Metric
½ lb.	Elbow or corkscrew macaroni	250 g
4 oz.	Process cheese spread (sold in loaves)	125 g
½ cup	Green pepper, chopped	125 mL
¼ cup	Finely chopped onion	50 mL
1 tsp.	Butter or margarine	5 mL
1 cup	Evaporated fat-free milk	250 mL
¼ tsp.	Ground pepper	1 mL
½ cup	Dry breadcrumbs	125 mL
1 tsp.	Butter or margarine, melted	5 mL

Yield: 4 servings
Equipment: Saucepan; 1½ qt. (1.5 L) casserole
Oven Temperature: 350°F (180°C)

Directions

1. Cook macaroni according to package directions. Drain and set aside.
2. Preheat oven.
3. Cut cheese into cubes and set aside.
4. In a saucepan, sauté green pepper and onion over medium-low heat in 1 teaspoon (5 mL) butter or margarine, about 1 to 2 minutes, stirring constantly.
5. Stir in evaporated fat-free milk and cheese cubes.
6. Cook over medium-low heat, stirring constantly, until cheese is melted and mixture is well blended. Stir in pepper.
7. Combine milk and cheese mixture with macaroni in casserole. Mix gently.
8. Combine breadcrumbs and 1 teaspoon (5 mL) melted butter or margarine.
9. Sprinkle breadcrumb mixture over macaroni and cheese mixture.
10. Bake 20 to 30 minutes until hot and bubbly.

Nutrition Information

Per serving (approximate): 387 calories, 18 g protein, 57 g carbohydrate, 10 g fat, 19 mg cholesterol, 570 mg sodium

Good source of: potassium, iron, vitamin A, vitamin D, vitamin C, B vitamins, calcium, phosphorus

Food for Thought

- Why is the cheese cut into cubes before it is cooked?
- What are some low-fat foods you could serve with this dish to make a nutritionally-balanced menu?

SECTION 18-3

Objectives

After studying this section, you should be able to:

- Describe the structure of an egg.
- Identify the nutrients provided by eggs.
- Give guidelines for buying and storing eggs.
- Explain how to cook eggs by conventional and microwave methods.

Look for These Terms

albumen

chalazae

coagulate

shirred eggs

Egg Basics

Trudy watched in puzzlement as her father cracked eggs into a bowl and began to beat them. "Hey, Dad," she said. "Did you forget that it's dinnertime, not breakfast?" Trudy's dad knows that while many people enjoy eggs for breakfast, they can be featured in other meals as well. Eggs are an economical food source and can be prepared in a variety of ways.

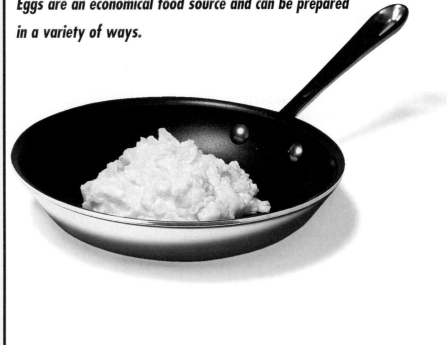

Structure of an Egg

An egg's shell is lined with several membranes. A pocket of air lies between these membranes and the shell at the wide end. As the egg ages, the air pocket grows.

Inside the egg is the **albumen** (al-BYOO-muhn), a thick, clear fluid commonly known as the egg white. The yolk—the round, yellow portion—floats within the albumen. Anchoring the yolk in the center of the egg are **chalazae** (kuh-LAH-zuh), twisted, cordlike strands of albumen.

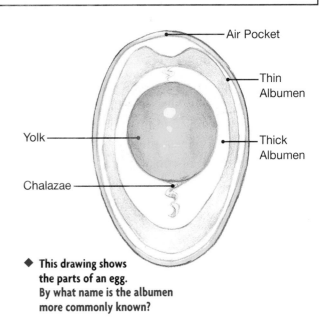

◆ This drawing shows the parts of an egg. By what name is the albumen more commonly known?

Nutrients in Eggs

Eggs are an excellent source of protein, riboflavin (a B vitamin), and iodine. In addition, they are good sources of vitamin A, some other B vitamins, vitamin D, iron, and trace minerals. However, egg yolks also contain saturated fats and cholesterol.

On the Food Guide Pyramid, eggs are part of the Meat, Poultry, Fish, Dry Beans, Eggs, and Nuts Group. When counting servings, remember that a single egg counts as 1 ounce (30 g) of meat. However, because whole eggs are so high in cholesterol, health experts recommend eating no more than four egg yolks a week. There is no limit on the number of egg whites because they are cholesterol-free.

Buying Eggs

Eggs are sold according to grade and size standards set by the USDA. Both grade and size are clearly marked on the package.

Grade

The USDA grade shield on the package means that the eggs have been federally inspected for wholesomeness. The grade is determined by the inner and outer quality of the egg at the time it was packaged. It has nothing to do with the freshness of the egg or its size.

The three egg grades are AA, A, and B. There is no difference in nutritive value among them. However, there is a difference in appearance when cooked. Grade AA and A eggs have a thicker white and are used when appearance is important, such as with fried or poached eggs. Grade B eggs are used when appearance is not important, as in baked products or scrambled eggs. As a rule, grades AA and A are the grades most commonly found in supermarkets.

Size

The size of an egg is determined by the minimum weight for a dozen. The sizes most commonly sold are large and extra large. As a general rule, recipes assume that large eggs will be used.

Eggs are usually priced according to size and supply. Check the unit price to determine which size is the best buy. Be sure to open the carton and inspect the eggs. They should be clean and whole, without any cracks.

Storing Eggs

Eggs are highly perishable. Store them immediately when you get home from shopping. Refrigerate eggs in the original carton. Do not put them in the egg tray commonly found in the refrigerator door—the drop in temperature each time the door is opened may cause the eggs to lose quality. In addition, egg shells are porous and pick up aromas from other foods if stored uncovered. Do not wash eggs before storing—washing destroys the egg's natural protective covering.

⊕ Safety Check

Harmful bacteria in raw or undercooked eggs have caused foodborne illness. To be sure that eggs are safe to eat:

- Do not use eggs that are cracked or broken. They may contain harmful bacteria.

- Always cook eggs thoroughly—until the whites and yolks are firm.

- Serve cooked eggs and egg-rich foods right after cooking.

- Never eat raw eggs or any foods containing raw eggs, such as homemade eggnog, homemade ice cream, or raw cookie dough. Raw eggs in commercial products are usually pasteurized, which destroys harmful bacteria.

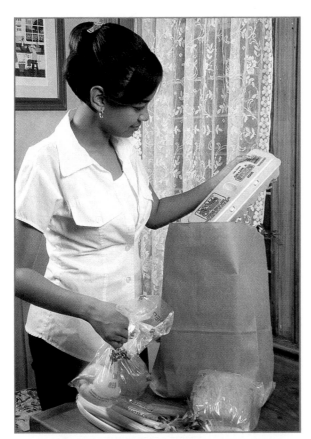

◆ **Knowing how to store eggs properly can make a difference when it comes to their quality and nutrient values. Name two things you should do and two things you shouldn't.**

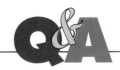

Q What's the best way to freeze eggs?

A To freeze whole raw eggs, beat the eggs until well-blended and pour them into freezer containers. Three tablespoons (45 mL) of beaten whole egg equals one large egg. To freeze raw whites, place the white of one egg in each compartment of an ice cube tray. After freezing, put frozen cubes in a tightly sealed freezer container and use as needed. Two egg whites equal one large egg. Use frozen eggs only in dishes that will be thoroughly cooked.

Refrigerate leftover raw yolks or whites in a covered container if you plan to use them within two to four days. For longer storage, freeze them. Refrigerate cooked egg dishes immediately and use them within three days.

Preparing Eggs

Like dairy foods, eggs are delicate proteins. They must be cooked at moderate temperatures for a limited amount of time. When overcooked, egg whites shrink and become tough and rubbery. When egg yolks are overcooked, they toughen and turn gray-green on the surface.

Eggs can be cooked on top of the range, in the oven, or in the microwave oven. Depending on which method you use, there are a few differences in basic cooking principles. In conventional cooking, use medium to low heat. Time the eggs carefully to be sure they are thoroughly cooked. The whites will **coagulate**, or become firm, before the yolks do.

When eggs are cooked in a microwave oven, the yolks cook faster than the whites. That is because the fat in the yolks attracts more microwaves than the whites do. Remove eggs from the microwave oven while they're still moist and soft. Standing time will complete the cooking.

Eggs can be prepared in several basic ways: cooked in the shell, fried, baked, poached, or scrambled.

Safety Check

Never microwave an egg in the shell. Steam builds up in the egg. When it can no longer be held in by the shell, the egg can burst and cause a serious injury.

Eggs Cooked in the Shell

When cooking eggs in the shell, place a single layer of them in a saucepan. Add water to a level at least 1 inch (2.5 cm) above the eggs. Cover the saucepan, and bring the water just to boiling. Turn off the heat. If using an electric range, remove the pan from the heating element. Let the eggs stand in the hot water, covered. If you want soft-cooked eggs, let them stand about 4 to 5 minutes for a safe doneness. For hard-cooked eggs, let stand about 15 minutes if you're using large eggs (about 18 minutes for extra-large eggs).

After cooking, immediately run cold water over the eggs to stop the cooking process. To serve soft-cooked eggs, break the shell with a knife and scoop the egg out of the shell into a serving dish. To remove the shell from a hard-cooked egg, gently tap the egg all over to crack the shell. Roll the egg between your hands to loosen the shell. Peel the shell away starting at the large end.

Fried Eggs

Eggs can be fried in a very small amount of unsaturated fat or in a nonstick skillet that has been coated with a vegetable-oil cooking spray. With this method, the excess fat is held to a minimum. To fry eggs healthfully:

1. Heat a skillet over medium-high heat until it is hot enough to sizzle a drop of water.

2. Gently break one egg at a time into a small bowl or custard cup. If the yolk breaks, save the egg for another use. Otherwise, gently slip the egg from the bowl into the heated pan.

3. Immediately reduce the heat to low. Cover the pan, and cook the eggs slowly until done.

4. Turn the eggs over to cook the other side.

Baked Eggs

Baked eggs, also known as **shirred eggs**, are easy to prepare and low in added fat. Begin by breaking the eggs into a small bowl, then slipping them into a greased, shallow baking dish or custard cup. You can use individual dishes or place several eggs in one dish. Top the eggs with a small amount of milk, if you like.

To bake conventionally, place in an oven preheated to 325°F (160°C). Bake until done—about 12 minutes for two eggs. To microwave, first pierce the yolks with the tip of a knife or a wooden pick so that steam can escape. Cover the baking dish with either waxed paper or cooking parchment, and vent it to allow steam to escape. Follow the power level and timing instructions in the owner's manual or in a recipe book.

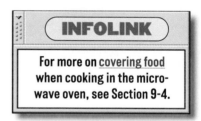

INFOLINK

For more on covering food when cooking in the microwave oven, see Section 9-4.

Poached Eggs

Poaching is a method of cooking eggs, out of the shell, in simmering water. To poach eggs conventionally, bring the water to a boil in a saucepan or deep skillet; then reduce the heat to a gentle simmer. Break one egg at a time into a small dish. Hold the dish close to the surface of the water and slip in the egg. Simmer about 5 minutes or until done.

You can also poach eggs in a microwave oven. Follow the directions in the owner's manual or in a recipe book. Be sure to pierce the yolks first to let steam escape.

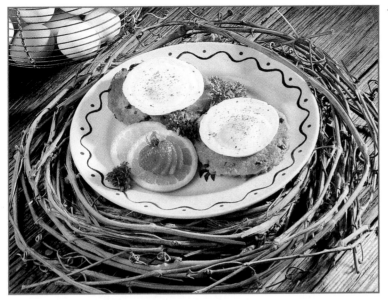

◆ Poached eggs are a healthful alternative to other forms of cooked eggs since they require no added fat. Here they are served over salmon patties. **What are three points to remember when poaching eggs?**

After cooking, use a slotted spoon to lift the eggs out of the water and drain them. Serve the eggs in a dish or over toast.

Scrambled Eggs

When making scrambled eggs, beat the eggs together with water or milk. Use 1 tablespoon (15 mL) liquid for each egg.

To cook conventionally, melt a small amount of butter or margarine in a skillet, or use a vegetable-oil cooking spray. Pour the egg mixture into the hot skillet. As the mixture starts to thicken, gently draw a spatula across the bottom and sides of the pan. This forms large curds and allows the uncooked egg to flow to the bottom of the skillet. Continue this procedure until the eggs are thickened and no visible liquid remains. Don't stir the eggs constantly. They will get mushy.

To make scrambled eggs in the microwave oven, cook the egg mixture in a custard cup or other microwave-safe container. Follow the power level and timing instructions in the owner's manual or in a recipe book. Stir once or twice during cooking and again at the end of the cooking time. Let stand to complete the cooking.

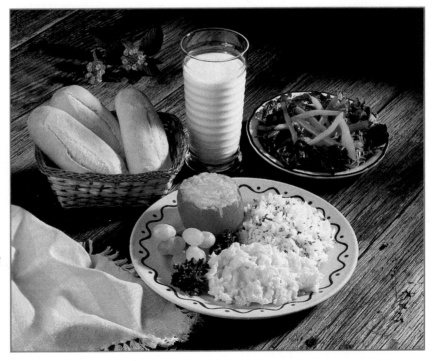

◆ Eggs are not just for breakfast. The centerpiece of this dinner is fluffy scrambled eggs accompanied by a broiled tomato, rice, grapes, and a green salad. **How many food groups in the Food Guide Pyramid are represented in this meal?**

Basic Omelet

A basic omelet, also called a French omelet, is made with beaten eggs, just as scrambled eggs are. However, you cook an omelet in a skillet without stirring the eggs. The result is shaped somewhat like a large pancake. During cooking, occasionally lift the edge of the omelet to allow uncooked egg to flow to the bottom. When the omelet is almost done, you may add a filling, such as sautéed vegetables. Fold the omelet in half to serve.

There are many variations on omelets. In the next section, you'll learn how to make a puffy omelet using beaten egg whites.

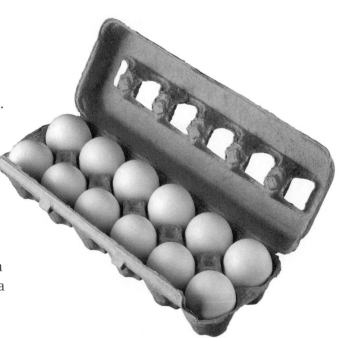

Section 18-3 Review & Activities

1. Describe the structure of an egg.

2. Name four nutrients found in eggs.

3. In what ways are eggs similar to and different from dairy foods?

4. Describe how eggs should be stored.

5. Extending. Imagine that it is 2090. Identify two synthetic, or human-made, products that have replaced dairy products mentioned in this chapter. Describe nutritive and other properties that led to the creation of these products.

6. Analyzing. Eggs have been called the most versatile food in the kitchen. Give reasons why this statement may have been made.

7. Applying. Design an advertisement to promote the use of eggs. You may want to focus on their versatility or nutritional value.

Italian Frittata

A *frittata* (fruh-TAH-tuh) is an Italian omelet. This open-faced omelet is full of flavorful ingredients. It can be served hot, warm, or cold as a lunch dish or a first course.

Customary	Ingredients	Metric
¼ lb.	Fresh mushrooms, thinly sliced	125 g
2	Green onions, minced	2
1½ Tbsp.	Butter or margarine	20 mL
6	Eggs	6
3 Tbsp.	Fresh parsley, chopped	45 mL
½ tsp.	Dried basil, crumbled	2 to 3 mL
¼ cup	Grated Parmesan cheese	30 mL
	Salt and pepper to taste	

Yield: 4 servings

Conventional Directions

Equipment: Large non-stick skillet with oven-safe handle
Oven Temperature: Broil

1. Sauté mushrooms and green onions in margarine or butter over medium heat until tender-crisp.
2. Preheat broiler.
3. Beat eggs in medium bowl.
4. Add parsley, basil, 2 tablespoons cheese, and salt and pepper to the eggs. Mix well.
5. Pour egg mixture over vegetables in skillet. Cook over medium heat, without stirring, until edges are lightly browned.
6. Sprinkle with remaining cheese.
7. Broil until top is golden brown.
8. Cut into wedges and serve hot.

Nutrition Information

Per serving (approximate): 227 calories, 13 g protein, 14 g carbohydrate, 17 g fat, 327 mg cholesterol, 424 mg sodium
Good source of: iron, vitamin A, vitamin D, vitamin E, B vitamins, calcium, phosphorus

Food for Thought

• How does the preparation method for this recipe differ from that for scrambled eggs?
• Name two ways you might reduce the amount of fat in the frittata.

Using Eggs in Recipes

Have you ever heard the expression "wearing many hats"? It means performing many different functions—which is just what eggs do in recipes. They add richness and nutrients. They bind ingredients together. They thicken foods such as sauces. When beaten, they incorporate air and can help baked products rise.

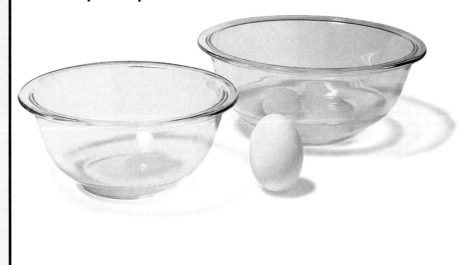

Objectives

After studying this section, you should be able to:

- Describe the difference between stirred custard and baked custard.
- Explain how to separate and beat egg whites.
- Identify uses of beaten egg whites.

Look for These Terms

quiche

soufflé

meringue

Custards

One example of a recipe made with eggs is custard. Custard is a tender blend of milk thickened with eggs. It serves as a base for main dishes, such as **quiche** (KEESH)—a pie with a custard filling that contains foods such as chopped vegetables, cheese, and chopped cooked meat. Sweetened, flavored custard is a popular dessert.

There are two types of custard, stirred and baked:

◆ **Stirred custard.** Is cooked on top of the range and stirred constantly until it thickens enough to coat a spoon. It is also known as soft custard. Stirred custard is pourable and creamy. You can serve it as a pudding or as a sauce over cake or fruit.

◆ **Baked custard.** Is baked in the oven. It has a firm, delicate consistency. If you are preparing it in individual custard cups, set the cups in a pan of hot water to keep the mixture from overcooking. Bake the custard until a knife inserted in or near the center comes out clean. Baking time varies, depending on the size of the pans. If overbaked, the custard will curdle. If not baked long enough, it won't set.

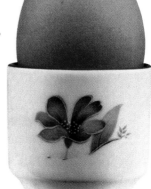

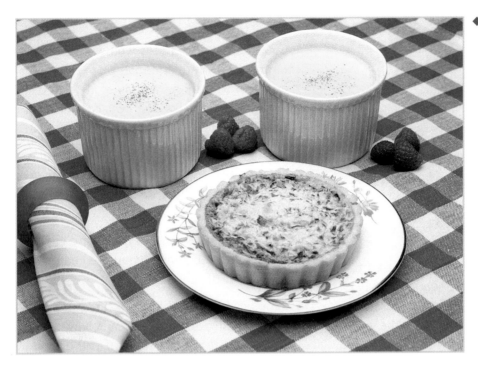

◆ Custard is a versatile combination of milk and eggs. It serves as a base for main dishes, such as quiche. **Describe the difference between stirred and baked custard.**

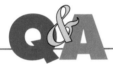

Q Is there anything I can do to rescue a stirred custard that curdles and looks lumpy?

A Pour the custard gradually into a blender or food processor and beat it. The sauce will be frothy instead of velvety. However, it will be usable unless it is very badly curdled.

Separating Eggs

Sometimes recipe directions call for only the yolk or white of the egg. In that case, you need to separate the egg. Eggs separate more easily when they are cold.

An easy, sanitary way to separate whites from yolks is to use an inexpensive egg separator. Simply break the egg carefully into the separator. The white will flow through, leaving the yolk in the separator.

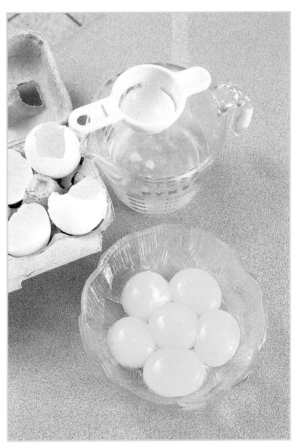

◆ Egg separators make it easy to separate whites from yolks. **What is another benefit of these devices?**

The traditional method for separating whites calls for passing the yolk back and forth from shell half to shell half. This method is no longer recommended. Bacteria may be present in the pores of the shell and could be picked up by the yolks and whites.

Beating Egg Whites

When egg whites are beaten, air is incorporated into them. Beaten egg whites can be used to add volume and lightness to baked products. For example, they can be used to prepare soufflés. A **soufflé** (soo-FLAY) is a dish made by folding stiffly beaten whites into a sauce or batter, then baking the mixture in a deep casserole until it puffs up.

Here are some guidelines for beating egg whites:

◆ When separating the yolks from the whites, be careful that no yolk mixes with the whites. Yolks contain fat, and even a drop of fat can keep whites from reaching full volume.

◆ Before beating, let egg whites stand at room temperature for 20 minutes. This will allow them to reach the fullest volume when beaten.

◆ Use beaters and bowls that are clean and completely free of fat. Plastic bowls tend to absorb fat, so use only glass or metal bowls.

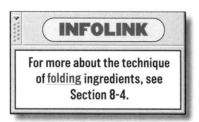

INFOLINK

For more about the technique of folding ingredients, see Section 8-4.

Forming Peaks

As you beat egg whites, you will notice them turning white and foamy. Eventually, they begin to form peaks. There are two different stages of peaks that eggs can reach. The terms for these stages frequently appear in recipes involving beaten eggs.

◆ **Soft-peak stage.** The peaks bend over slightly when the beaters are lifted out of the whites.

◆ **Stiff-peak stage.** The peaks are glossy and hold their shape when the beaters are lifted out of the mixture.

Stop beating egg whites as soon as they reach the stage called for in the recipe. Never try to beat past the stiff-peak stage. If you overbeat the whites, they will turn dry and dull and begin to fall apart. Since they have lost air and moisture, they can no longer be used.

When using beaten egg whites in mixtures, fold them in. If stirred or beaten, the whites lose air and volume. To fold beaten whites into a mixture, add them to the bowl containing the mixture. Use a flat tool, such as a rubber spatula, for folding.

Puffy Omelet

You can use beaten egg whites to make a puffy omelet. A puffy omelet is made by separating the eggs and beating the whites and yolks separately. Fold the stiffly beaten whites into the yolks. Pour the mixture into a skillet with an ovenproof handle. Cook it first on top of the range until it is puffed and lightly browned on the bottom, about 5 minutes. Then bake it at 350°F (180°C) for 10 to 12 minutes or until a knife inserted in the center comes out clean.

◆ Besides lending themselves to a variety of fillings, puffy omelets are light in texture. Create a recipe for a puffy omelet that includes a nutrient-dense filling. Try preparing the dish and write about your experiences in your Wellness Journal.

You can serve the omelet open-faced or folded. To serve the omelet folded, cut partially through the center of the omelet for ease in folding. Then fill the omelet with foods such as cheese, vegetables, or meats.

Meringues

A **meringue** (muhr-ANG), a foam made of beaten egg white and sugar, is used for desserts. There are two types of meringue, soft and hard. Soft meringue is used to top precooked pies and puddings. Hard meringue is used in the form of baked meringue shells that can be filled like a pie.

To make a meringue, beat the whites until they are foamy. Cream of tartar is sometimes added to the whites before beating to make the meringue more stable. When the whites are foamy, gradually beat in the sugar, one tablespoon at a time. Most soft meringue recipes call for 1 to 2 tablespoons (15 to 30 mL) sugar per egg white. A hard meringue may use 4 tablespoons (50 mL) sugar per egg white. Continue beating until the sugar is dissolved. To find out if the sugar is dissolved, rub a little meringue between the thumb and forefinger. If it feels gritty, not all the sugar is dissolved.

Soft Meringue

A soft meringue is made by beating egg whites to the soft-peak stage. Spread soft

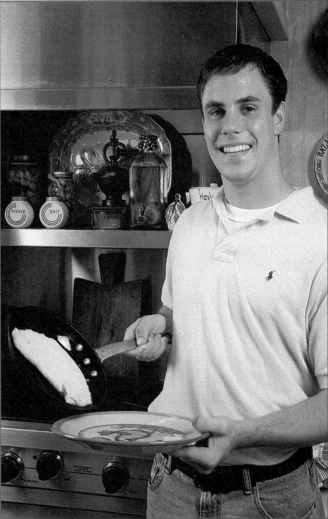

meringue over hot, precooked pie filling or pudding. On a pie, the meringue should touch the crust all around the edge. Otherwise, it may shrink during baking. Bake it in a preheated oven according to recipe directions until the peaks are lightly browned.

Sometimes a liquid accumulates between the meringue and pie filling, a condition known as weeping. This happens when the sugar is not completely dissolved or the meringue is not beaten to the soft-peak stage. Meringue weeps less when put on a hot filling.

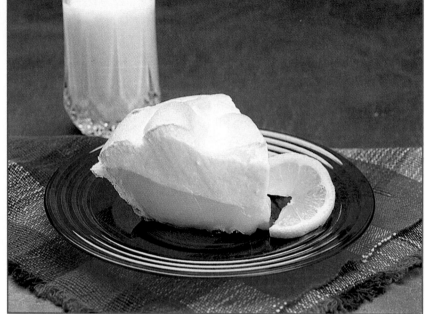

◆ Lemon meringue pie is a classic dessert. Identify the type of meringue used to make the delicate fluffy topping.

Hard Meringue

A hard meringue is made by beating egg whites to the stiff-peak stage. You can bake hard meringue on a baking sheet. Line the sheet with cooking parchment, waxed paper, or foil. Shape the meringue into individual or large shells using a spoon, spatula, or pastry tube.

A baked hard meringue is crispy. It must bake at a low enough temperature to dry out thoroughly but not overcook. Unless it dries well, the meringue may be sticky and chewy. Bake according to the time and temperature in the recipe directions. Turn off the oven and leave the meringue in it for at least another hour to dry out.

Section 18-4 Review & Activities

1. What is the difference between a baked custard and a stirred custard?

2. What is the safest way to separate egg whites from the yolks?

3. Name two dishes that use beaten egg whites.

4. Evaluating. Karl prefers to separate egg whites by breaking the egg into his bare hand and gently cradling the yolk, while the white slips between his fingers into a bowl. What problems, if any, can you see in this approach?

5. Extending. What might you fill baked meringue shells with?

6. Applying. Beat one egg white using ⅛ teaspoon (0.5 mL) cream of tartar. Beat another egg white without cream of tartar. Compare the results.

CAREER WANTED

Individuals concerned about the environment who are good at inductive, deductive, and mathematical reasoning.

REQUIRES:

- degree in agribusiness or related area
- acute visualization skills
- compassion for natural resources

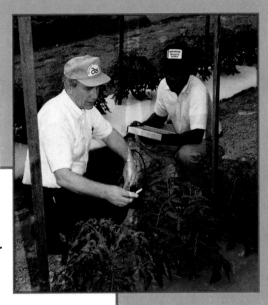

"Producing excellent crop yields is my goal,"

says Theo Hughes, Agronomic Engineer

Q: What is life like on a farm?

A: I grew up on a dairy farm. I love being out next to the soil. Farming is not just a career but a way of life.

Q: What kinds of responsibilities do you face in your line of work?

A: Farms like this one provide food for thousands of people each year. It takes long-range planning, knowledge of the land, weather, seeds, fertilizers, yield projections, and market fluctuations.

Q: It sounds like your work is very complex.

A: It is. Most people think farming is driving tractors and harvesting crops or feeding animals. However, it also requires a lot of planning, financial forecasting, accounting, and data analysis. The farm can only bear "fruit" when it is taken care of properly. Land is just like people—you need to address both internal and external factors in order to maintain wellness.

Q: What kind of preparation does someone need to become an agronomic engineer?

A: Education is vital. I have a Master's degree in agribusiness and a Ph.D. in agronomy. Growing up on a farm helped me understand the responsibilities and rewards of this career choice.

Career Research Activity

1. Investigate the career path of someone that starts out as a farm equipment dealer, then moves into the position of agricultural engineering technician, and ends up as a geologist. Make a poster noting the educational preparation, skills needed, and salary ranges for all three careers.

2. Think about what you believe to be the main tasks of a farm hand, a farm mechanic, and a farm manager. Then find out what each of these jobs entail. Write an essay explaining how these careers are similar and yet different.

Related Career Opportunities

Entry Level
- Farm Hand
- Farm Mechanic
- Farm Equipment Dealer

Technical Level
- Farm Manager
- Agricultural Engineering Technician

Professional Level
- Geologist
- Agronomic Engineer
- Dairy Technologist

Chapter 18 Review & Activities

—— Summary ——

Section 18-1: Choosing Dairy Foods

- Milk is high in protein, vitamin A, and B vitamins. A variety of milk products are available.

- Dairy products also include yogurt, cheese, cream, butter, and frozen dairy desserts.

- Dairy foods must be refrigerated or frozen.

Section 18-3: Egg Basics

- Eggs are good sources of protein, several vitamins, and iron. The yolks are high in fat and cholesterol.

- Eggs are sold by size and grade.

- Eggs should be refrigerated in their original cartons.

- Eggs may be cooked in the shell, fried, baked, poached, scrambled, or made into a basic omelet.

Section 18-2: Preparing Dairy Foods

- When heating milk, avoid scorching, curdling, and skin formation.

- Yogurt is a healthy substitute for higher-fat dairy products.

- Unripened cheese should be served chilled; ripened cheese tastes best at room temperature.

- Avoid overcooking cheese.

Section 18-4: Using Eggs in Recipes

- Eggs perform different functions in recipes.

- Custard serves as the base for both main dishes and desserts.

- Some recipes call for only egg yolk or white, requiring eggs to be separated.

- Egg whites can be beaten to add volume and lightness to recipes.

Working IN THE Lab

1. **Food Science.** Add 1 tablespoon (15 mL) lemon juice to 1 cup (250 mL) room-temperature milk. Let the milk stand for 10 minutes. Describe the results. What do you think is happening to the milk? What is this process called?

2. **Food Preparation.** Develop your own recipes for scrambled eggs. Experiment by adding seasonings and other ingredients. Evaluate the results for taste, appearance, nutritional value, and cost per serving.

Checking Your Knowledge

1. Identify the percentage of calories from fat in whole, low-fat, and fat-free milk.

2. Give two examples of cultured milk products.

3. How is pasteurized process cheese made?

4. What causes skin formation when milk is cooked? How can you prevent it?

5. Why should you save the whey from thickened yogurt? How can it be used?

6. Give two reasons why you should not store eggs in the egg tray on the refrigerator door.

7. Describe how to freeze leftover raw egg whites.

8. Briefly describe the procedure for making hard-cooked eggs.

9. Describe the characteristics of egg whites beaten to the soft-peak stage and the stiff-peak stage.

10. Identify two ways to keep meringue from weeping.

Review & Activities Chapter 18

Thinking Critically

1. Determining Accuracy. While standing in the checkout line at the supermarket, Delia is thumbing through a popular magazine and comes upon an article that explains how you can enjoy eggs, while still reducing the amount of cholesterol in your overall eating plan. She notices that the author of the article has the initials M.D. after her name in the byline, but the name itself is not one that Delia recognizes. Would you advise her to read the article or skip on to the next feature? Explain the factors that affect your recommendation.

2. Distinguishing Between Fact and Opinion. Chet receives an advertisement and a cents-off coupon in the mail for a new dairy dessert product. The ad claims that the product contains one-fifth the fat of regular full-fat ice cream and adds that a panel of qualified judges all agreed that the product was as rich and creamy as the leading brand of premium ice cream. How many of the claims made in the ad are fact and how many are opinion?

Reinforcing Key Skills

1. Communication. In the past, milk, other dairy foods, and eggs have been given a bad reputation by health care professionals. What information could you include in a press release aimed at reeducating the public about the advantages of including dairy foods and eggs in their eating plans?

2. Directed Thinking. Milk and other dairy foods are traditionally a part of the eating habits of cultures that raise herd animals, such as milk cows or goats. In other cultures, dairy foods are not a part of traditional eating styles. Use this and other information to answer this question: What impact do social influences have on food choices?

Making Decisions and Solving Problems

You offer to make a dip for a friend's party. You want to make it attractive and tasty but low in fat and cholesterol as well.

Making Connections

1. Math. Compare the per-serving price and nutritional value of sour cream and its lower-fat substitutes, including yogurt and reduced-fat sour cream products. Record your findings on a chart or bar graph. Also tell how each product's nutritional value affects your decision about which is the best buy.

2. Social Studies. Using print or online resources, write a report on the international origins of dishes mentioned in this chapter. Where and when did soufflés and meringues originate? What other international dishes use beaten egg whites?

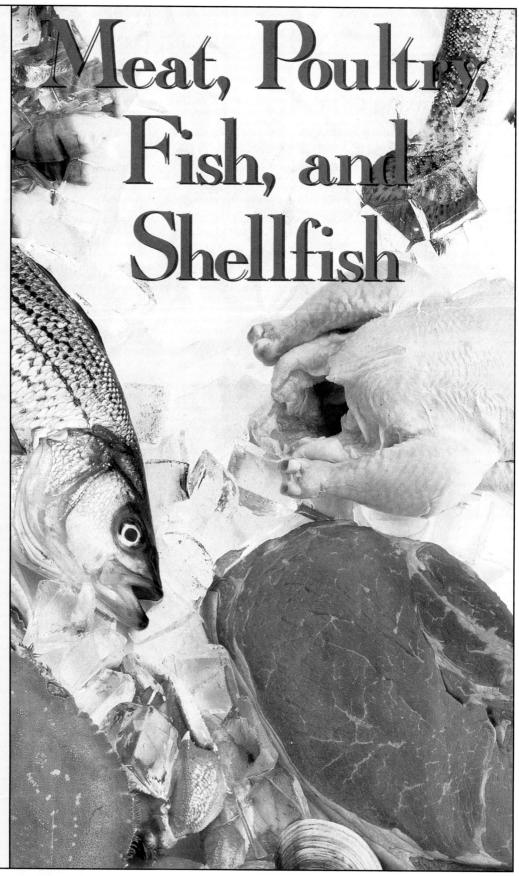

CHAPTER 19

Meat, Poultry, Fish, and Shellfish

Section 19-1
Looking at Meat, Poultry, Fish, and Shellfish

Section 19-2
Meat Selection and Storage

Section 19-3
Poultry Selection and Storage

Section 19-4
Fish and Shellfish Selection and Storage

Section 19-5
Preparing Meat, Poultry, Fish, and Shellfish

After reading this chapter, you will know how to make wise choices when buying or preparing meat, poultry, fish, or shellfish.

Looking at Meat, Poultry, Fish, and Shellfish

Objectives

After studying this section, you should be able to:

- Identify nutrients in meat, poultry, fish, and shellfish.
- Discuss factors that affect tenderness.
- Give guidelines for comparing costs of meat, poultry, fish, and shellfish.

Look for These Terms

cut

marbling

Most American meals are built around a main dish, often one containing meat. The meat might be a form of beef or pork. Families who favor poultry might sometimes choose turkey, duck, or goose instead of chicken. Fish and shellfish, lamb, and veal are other possibilities.

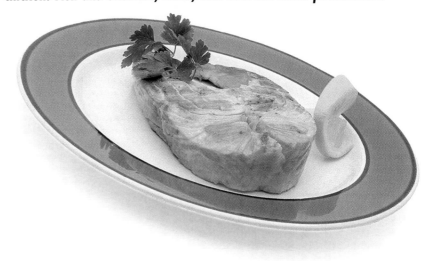

Cuts

A starting point when shopping for meat, poultry, fish, and shellfish is to recognize that each of these foods is sold in the form of fresh or frozen cuts. A **cut** is a particular edible part of meat, poultry, or fish. Cuts of meat, for instance, include steaks, chops, and roasts.

In addition to these raw cuts are numerous cured meat and poultry products, such as ham, bacon, cold cuts, and sausages. Many convenience forms are available as well.

How can you make wise decisions when shopping for meat, poultry, fish, and shellfish? Start by taking a look at how the different choices vary with regard to nutrition, tenderness, and cost.

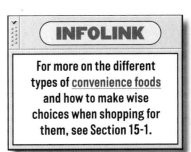

INFOLINK

For more on the different types of <u>convenience foods</u> and how to make wise choices when shopping for them, see Section 15-1.

Nutrition

Meat, poultry, fish, and shellfish are all nutritious foods. They are excellent sources of complete protein. All provide B vitamins, phosphorus, and certain trace minerals. Meat and poultry are good sources of iron and zinc. Fish, especially fatty fish such as salmon and tuna, are good sources of omega-3 essential fatty acids.

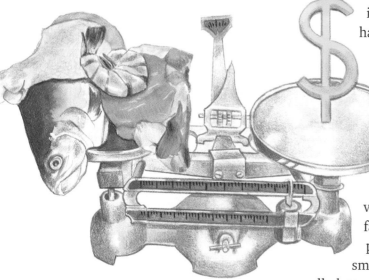

The Food Guide Pyramid recommends two to three servings daily from the Meat, Poultry, Fish, Dry Beans, Eggs, and Nuts Group. A typical serving can be 2 to 3 ounces (56 to 84 g) of cooked lean meat, poultry, or fish.

Many Americans eat servings of meat, poultry, and fish that are larger than the recommended portions. That means they eat more protein than needed. The larger servings may also add more fat and cholesterol to daily food choices.

Fat and Cholesterol

Because they are animal foods, meat, poultry, fish, and shellfish all contain cholesterol. All animal muscle contains about the same amount of cholesterol per ounce, except for organ meats (such as liver), which have more.

Fat content varies. Most fish is low in fat. So is turkey breast meat. Other poultry and meat cuts generally have more fat, but the amount varies depending on the cut and the preparation method. Meat, poultry, fish, or

shellfish that has less than 10 grams of fat in a 3½-ounce (98-g) serving is considered lean. It must also have less than 4 grams of saturated fat and less than 95 milligrams cholesterol.

Types of Fat

Meat and poultry contain both invisible fat—which is part of the chemical composition of the food—and visible fat. In meat, a layer of visible fat may surround the lean muscle portion of the cut. In addition, small white flecks of internal fat, called **marbling**, may appear within the muscle tissue of the meat. In poultry, most of the visible fat is located in the skin and in layers under the skin.

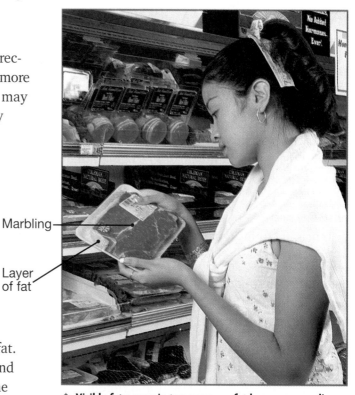

Marbling

Layer of fat

◆ Visible fat occurs in two ways—as fat layers surrounding muscle sections and as marbling within muscle sections. **Which type of fat contributes to a cut's tenderness?**

Comparing Fat and Cholesterol Content

Type of Food (3-oz. [84-g] serving)	Total Fat (g)	Saturated Fat (g)	Cholesterol (mg)
Fish and Shellfish			
Cod, cooked	1	0	45
Tuna, canned in water	1	0	35
Red salmon, canned	6	2	45
Mackerel, cooked	13	2	60
Shrimp, cooked	1	0	166
Poultry			
Chicken, light meat, without skin, roasted	2	1	70
Chicken, dark meat, without skin, roasted	7	2	80
Turkey, breast meat, without skin, roasted	1	0	55
Meat			
Beef, top round steak, trimmed, broiled	4	1	70
Beef, ground, regular, broiled	18	7	76
Beef liver, pan-fried	7	2	410
Pork loin, trimmed, roasted	6	2	65

◆ The fat and cholesterol content of different meats, poultry, fish, and shellfish vary. Which item has the most saturated fat? Which has the least total fat? How many milligrams of cholesterol is contained in a 3-oz. serving of waterpack canned tuna?

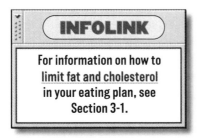

INFOLINK

For information on how to limit fat and cholesterol in your eating plan, see Section 3-1.

Tenderness

You've probably heard meat called "so tender it melts in your mouth" or "as tough as shoe leather." You can increase your chances of selecting a tender cut if you know a little about the makeup of meat, poultry, or fish. As you will see later on, the choice of cooking method can also be a factor in tenderness.

FOR YOUR HEALTH

Have Your Cut and Enjoy It, Too

There's no way to avoid fat and cholesterol completely when your eating style includes meat, poultry, fish, and shellfish. You can still enjoy these foods, however, while limiting fat and cholesterol.

- Keep serving sizes sensible. Follow recommendations in the Food Guide Pyramid.
- Cut down on amounts of meat, poultry, or fish, and increase intake of grains and vegetables.
- Substitute legumes for meats several times a week.
- Choose cuts with less fat.

- Trim fat layers from meat. Remove poultry skin before eating.
- Use low-fat cooking methods, such as broiling or roasting. Avoid frying and other cooking methods that add fat.

Following Up

- In your Wellness Journal, record everything you eat during the course of one day. Then make up a one-day menu that is low in fat and cholesterol. Compare the two menus. Then, if necessary, devise a strategy you could use to cut down on the amount of fat and cholesterol in your current eating plan.

Makeup of Meat and Poultry

Meat and poultry have very long, thin muscle cells (sometimes called muscle fibers). Some are as long as 12 inches (30 cm). They are thinnest in young animals and in parts of the animal that get little exercise, such as the back. As animals get older, the fibers thicken. They are thickest in those parts that get the most exercise—the legs, for example. As a rule, the thicker the muscle fibers, the tougher and coarser the cut.

Meat and poultry also have several kinds of connective tissue—protein material that surrounds cells. These, too, can affect tenderness.

- ◆ **Collagen** (KAHL-uh-juhn). A thin, white or transparent connective tissue. When meat or poultry is cooked using moist-heat methods, such as simmering in liquid, the collagen softens and turns into gelatin.

- ◆ **Elastin** (ee-LAS-tuhn). A very tough, yellowish connective tissue. It cannot be softened by heat. Other tenderizing methods

—pounding, cutting, or grinding—must be used to break down elastin.

Fat content can also have an effect on tenderness. Meat that has more marbling is more tender. In addition, fat gives meat and poultry flavor and helps keep it juicy as it cooks.

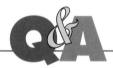

 What is one way to make a less tender cut of meat easier to eat?

 The lengthwise direction of the muscle cells is known as the grain. One solution for less tender cuts of meat is to cut across the grain. By doing this, you cut the long fibers into pieces, and the meat may be easier to chew. Most meats are generally cut this way for retail sale. It's also a good way to cut cooked meat and poultry for serving.

Makeup of Fish

The muscles in fish are arranged differently from those in meat and poultry. Instead of the long fibers found in meat and poultry, fish have very short fibers that are arranged in layers. The layers are separated by sheets of very thin, fragile connective tissue. When heated, this connective tissue turns into gelatin. As a result, all fish and shellfish are very tender. When cooked, the flesh flakes, or breaks up into small pieces, because the muscle fibers are short.

Comparing Costs

When shopping, cost is an important point of comparison. Meats, poultry, fish, and shellfish are generally the most expensive part of the food budget. However, cuts can vary widely in cost.

Remember to compare the cost per serving of different cuts of meat, poultry, and fish. If you find a bargain that is not on your shopping list, consider changing your plans. You may save a considerable amount.

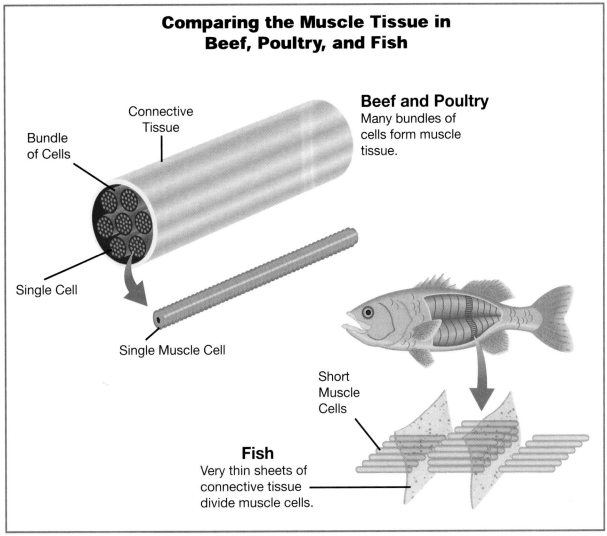

Comparing the Muscle Tissue in Beef, Poultry, and Fish

Connective Tissue

Bundle of Cells

Single Cell

Single Muscle Cell

Beef and Poultry
Many bundles of cells form muscle tissue.

Short Muscle Cells

Fish
Very thin sheets of connective tissue divide muscle cells.

◆ In beef and poultry, muscle tissue is held together in bundles by connective tissue. The thicker the fibers, the less tender the meat. Fish, by contrast, is made up of short muscle fibers and fragile connective tissue. Explain the connection between the size of muscle tissue and cost of a product.

Here are two general guidelines:

◆ Tender cuts are often more expensive than less tender cuts. Knowing how to cook less tender cuts can help you save money.

◆ Boneless meat and poultry are generally more expensive than cuts sold with the bone. You may be able to save money by removing the bones yourself. Remember, however, that boneless cuts yield more servings per pound. Be sure to check the cost per serving.

✚ Safety Check

When shopping for meat, poultry, or fish, be sure the market or department smells fresh. Foul odors could indicate leaking packages or temperatures that may be too high for safety. The fish department may have a characteristic fishy aroma but should have no foul odors.

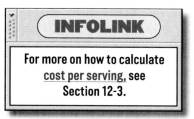

INFOLINK

For more on how to calculate cost per serving, see Section 12-3.

Section 19-1 Review & Activities

1. List three nutrients found in meat, poultry, and fish.

2. Identify two factors that affect the tenderness of meat and poultry.

3. What is the most accurate way to compare the cost of different cuts of meat, poultry, or fish?

4. Analyzing. What factors might affect the price of meat, poultry, and fish?

5. Evaluating. Lonette is shopping for a cut of meat she can broil. Having heard that fat can add flavor and tenderness, she is considering buying a cut that has a broad band of fat around it. Tell whether you would advise Lonette to buy this cut. State your reasons.

6. Applying. In magazines and cookbooks, find at least six recipes for meat, poultry, or fish. Identify the cut and preparation method for each recipe. Why do you think some preparation methods are preferred for certain cuts?

Meat Selection and Storage

Lee's family is on a tight budget. They shop carefully, check sale items, and try to get the most value for their money. Like Lee's family, the more you know about meat, the easier it will be for you to find the best buys. Even though there are many different cuts, an understanding of just a few basic guidelines can help you become a smart meat shopper.

Objectives

After studying this section, you should be able to:

- Describe the four basic types of meat.
- Identify tender and less tender cuts of meat.
- Identify processed meat products.
- Give guidelines for storing meat.

Look for These Terms

wholesale cuts

retail cuts

variety meats

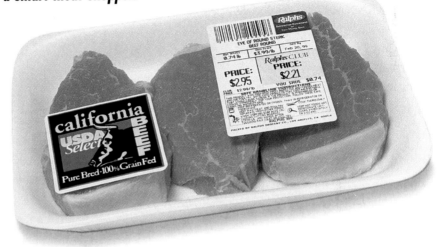

Types of Meat

Each of the four basic types of meat has a distinct flavor and appearance. When shopping, look for color typical of the meat.

- **Beef.** Meat from cattle more than one year old. It has a hearty flavor. The cuts have bright red flesh. The fat is firm, with a white, creamy white, or yellowish color.

- **Veal.** Meat from very young calves, one to three months old. It has a mild flavor and light pink color with very little fat. "Special fed veal" has been fed a special milk-based diet. The flesh is more tender, with a grayish-pink color and white fat.

- **Lamb.** Meat from young sheep. It has a mild but unique flavor. Cuts are a bright pink-red color with white, brittle fat. The fat is sometimes covered with a *fell*, a colorless connective tissue.

- **Pork.** Meat from hogs. It has a mild flavor. Fresh meat is a grayish-pink color with white, soft fat.

Cuts of Meat

Meat is first divided into **wholesale cuts**. Also called primal cuts, these are large cuts for marketing. These wholesale cuts are further divided into **retail cuts**—the smaller cuts that you can find in the supermarket. As an illustration, note that one of the wholesale cuts of beef is the chuck, from the shoulder area. Retail cuts from the chuck include blade roast and chuck short ribs.

◆ **Because of changes in breeding and feeding practices, the pork produced today is much leaner than in the past.** In a print or online resource learn about trichina (a microbe found in pork products in the past), the disease it caused, and measures that were taken to reduce this problem.

The price label on the meat package identifies the cut. The type of meat is listed first (beef, veal, pork, lamb). The wholesale cut is listed second. This tells you what part of the animal the meat comes from, such as chuck, rib, or round. The retail cut—for example, spareribs, chops, or steak—is listed third.

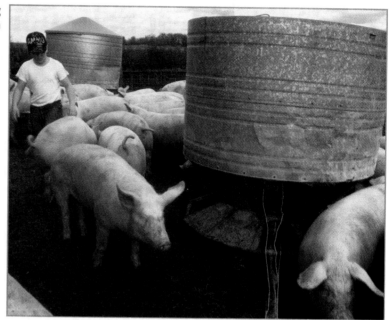

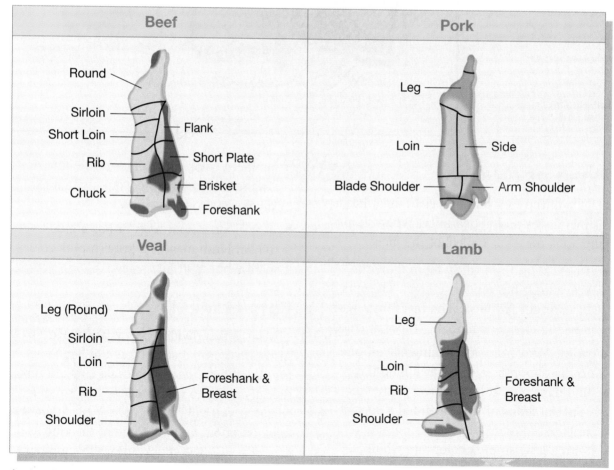

◆ **The wholesale cuts for the four types of meat animals are shown here.** Compare and give similarities and differences among the four types.

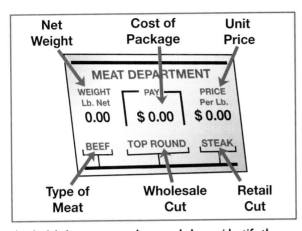

Net Weight	Cost of Package	Unit Price

MEAT DEPARTMENT

WEIGHT Lb. Net	PAY	PRICE Per Lb.
0.00	$ 0.00	$ 0.00

BEEF	TOP ROUND	STEAK

Type of Meat	Wholesale Cut	Retail Cut

◆ The label on a meat package can help you identify the retail cut. Identify four other pieces of information provided on the label shown.

Bone Shape

Each wholesale cut has a distinctive bone shape that can be used to identify the meat cut. These shapes—which are nearly identical in beef, pork, lamb, and veal—are also clues to the tenderness of the cut. For example, the rib and T-shaped bones, both of which are part of the backbone, indicate meat that is tender. Knowing this can help you decide what cooking method to use.

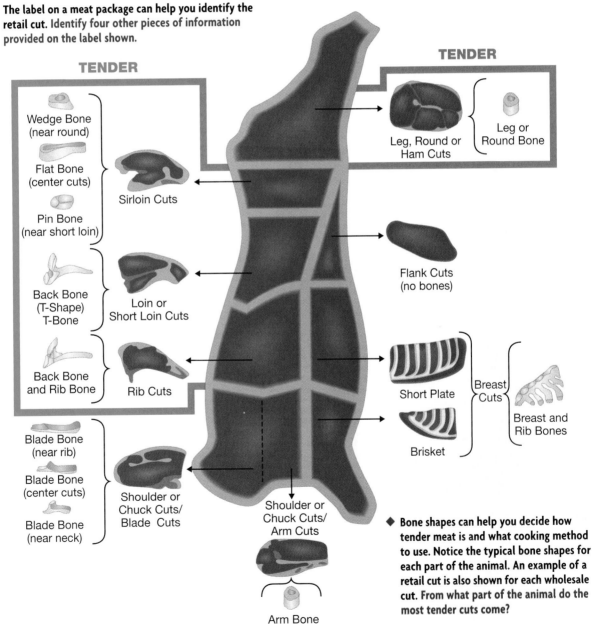

TENDER

Wedge Bone (near round)

Flat Bone (center cuts)

Pin Bone (near short loin)

Sirloin Cuts

Back Bone (T-Shape) T-Bone

Loin or Short Loin Cuts

Back Bone and Rib Bone

Rib Cuts

Blade Bone (near rib)

Blade Bone (center cuts)

Blade Bone (near neck)

Shoulder or Chuck Cuts/ Blade Cuts

Shoulder or Chuck Cuts/ Arm Cuts

Arm Bone

TENDER

Leg, Round or Ham Cuts

Leg or Round Bone

Flank Cuts (no bones)

Short Plate

Brisket

Breast Cuts

Breast and Rib Bones

◆ Bone shapes can help you decide how tender meat is and what cooking method to use. Notice the typical bone shapes for each part of the animal. An example of a retail cut is also shown for each wholesale cut. From what part of the animal do the most tender cuts come?

Which Cuts Are Lean?

When shopping for meat, look for these lean choices (less than 10 grams of fat, less than 4 grams of saturated fat, and less than 95 milligrams of cholesterol in a 3½-ounce [98-g] serving):

- **Beef roasts and steaks:** round, loin, sirloin, chuck arm.

- **Pork roasts and chops:** tenderloin, center loin, ham.

- **Veal cuts:** all except ground veal.

- **Lamb roasts and chops:** leg, loin, foreshank.

Appearance is the best indicator of leanness. It is important, therefore, to inspect the package carefully. The fat that surrounds the cut should be trimmed to less than ¼ inch (0.6 cm). If there is more than that, you are wasting money by paying for excess fat.

Ground Meat

Ground beef is made from beef trimmings. By law, ground beef cannot have more than 30 percent fat by weight. Lean ground beef is available, although it may cost more.

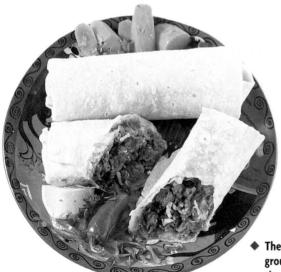

You may also find packages of ground lamb, pork, and veal. If not, you can ask to have meat ground for you.

Organ Meats

Edible animal organs are usually called **variety meats**. Here are some examples.

- Liver is highly nutritious and tender, with a pronounced flavor.

- Lamb and veal kidneys are tender, with a mild flavor. Beef and pork kidneys are strong-flavored and less tender.

- *Chitterlings* usually refers to the intestines of pigs, but they may also come from calves. They are thoroughly cleaned and sold whole in containers.

Other organ meats are brains, heart, tongue, tripe (the stomach lining of cattle), and sweetbreads (thymus gland).

Inspection and Grading

Before it can be sold, meat has to be inspected by the USDA for wholesomeness. A round inspection mark is stamped on the meat with a harmless vegetable dye. The inspection mark is stamped in only a few places on the animal, so you will probably not see it on retail cuts.

Meat may also be graded. Grading is a voluntary program available to the meat industry, which pays for the service. Meat is graded according to standards that include amount of marbling, age of the animal, and texture and appearance of the meat.

◆ These beef and bean burritos are just one example of the many uses for ground meat. When shopping, look for fat content on the label. Compute the fat content of a package of ground veal with the label "89 percent lean."

Following are the most common grades for beef:

◆ **Prime.** The highest and most expensive grade. The meat is well marbled with fat. It is very tender and flavorful.

◆ **Choice.** The most common grade sold in supermarkets. It has less marbling than prime but is still tender and flavorful.

◆ **Select.** Contains the least amount of marbling and is the least expensive. It is sometimes sold as a store brand.

Lamb and veal are also graded. The same grades are used as for beef, except that "Good" replaces "Select." Pork is not graded because the meat is more uniform in quality.

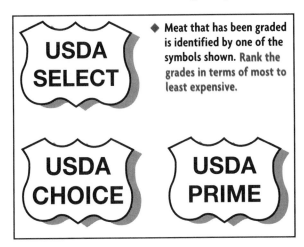

◆ Meat that has been graded is identified by one of the symbols shown. Rank the grades in terms of most to least expensive.

Processed Meats

About 35 percent of the meat produced in the United States is processed. Unlike other foods, which are processed mainly to extend shelf life, meats and other animal foods are processed to impart distinctive flavors. Typical processed meats include ham, bacon, sausage, and cold cuts.

The most common processing method is curing, placing the meat in a mixture of salt, sugar, sodium nitrate, potassium nitrate, ascorbic acid, and water. In addition to their function as preservatives, the nitrates also prevent the growth of botulin bacteria, a common cause of foodborne illness. The meat may be soaked in the solution, or the solution may be pumped into the meat.

Other processing methods include drying and salting, which help preserve meat, and smoking. Originally, smoking meant exposing the meat to wood smoke to preserve and flavor it. Today, only liquid smoke may be used for flavoring.

Often, more than one processing method is used. For example, bacon is cured and smoked. Chipped beef has been dried, salted, and smoked.

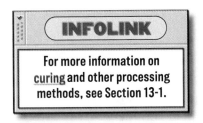

INFOLINK

For more information on curing and other processing methods, see Section 13-1.

Using Processed Meats

Ham is meat from the thigh of a hog that has been cured and either smoked or canned. Check the label carefully for instructions. Some hams are precooked, but others must be cooked before eating. If the label does not specify, cook the ham.

Sausages are made from ground meat, often mixed with fat, salt, sugar, preservatives, seasonings, and other additives. Many different types of sausages are available. Some, such as fresh pork sausage, must be cooked before eating. Others are ready to eat, although they may be heated. Again, check the label carefully.

Cold cuts are processed meats that have been sliced and packaged. They are ready to eat. So are deli meats—processed meats sold fresh and sliced to order at deli counters in supermarkets and other food stores.

FOR YOUR HEALTH

Go Easy on the Processed Meats

Cured meats are popular because of their wonderful smoky flavor. Unfortunately, the chemicals responsible for that flavor—nitrites and nitrates—have been linked with certain types of cancer. In addition, these meats are high in sodium, fat, or both. So enjoy an occasional hot dog or deli sandwich. Just remember to use these foods in moderation.

Following Up

• Approximately 35 percent of the nitrites and 13 percent of the nitrates in food are added during the manufacturing process. The rest occur naturally in certain vegetables—such as spinach, lettuce, and beets—and in baked goods. Discuss how this information might affect your eating style in the future.

Storing Meat

Meat requires cold storage. Use ground meat and variety meats within one to two days after storing them in the refrigerator. Other fresh meat will keep in the refrigerator for three to five days. For longer storage, freeze the meat.

INFOLINK

For more on cold storage temperatures of meats, see Section 7-4.

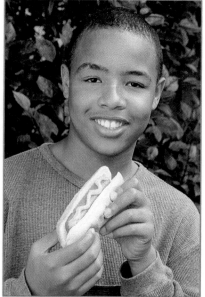

◆ Because of the high fat and sodium content in conventional hot dogs, many people are switching to chicken and turkey franks, which are generally lower in both. Still, health experts advise eating such cured meat products only occasionally. Discuss possible reasons for the view health experts take toward cured meat products.

Section 19-2 Review & Activities

1. Name three wholesale cuts of beef that are considered tender.

2. Give four examples of processed meat products.

3. How long can fresh meat be stored safely in the refrigerator?

4. Comparing and Contrasting. How do beef, pork, veal, and lamb differ in color and flavor?

5. Synthesizing. Identify three specific ways of including processed meats in a healthful eating plan.

6. Applying. Bring to class several clean price labels from packages of meat. Use the information on the labels, identify the animal, the wholesale cut, the retail cut, the unit price, and the total price for the package. Calculate the cost per serving of each package. Which cuts are the most economical? The least?

Poultry Selection and Storage

The term poultry refers to any bird raised for food. Some poultry is relatively low in fat, which makes it a good choice for health-conscious consumers. Its mild flavor lends itself to many different recipes.

Objectives

After studying this section, you should be able to:

- Describe types and market forms of poultry.
- Give guidelines for buying and storing poultry.

Look for This Term

giblets

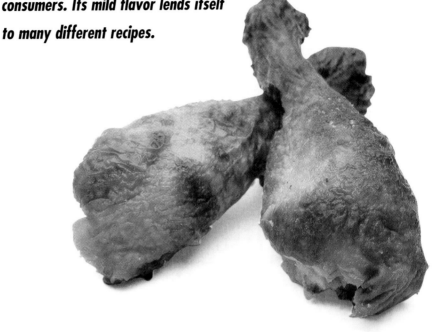

Types of Poultry

How do you want your poultry—whole, cut up, drumsticks only, boneless? Whether you want chicken, turkey, duck, or goose, you can buy different types of poultry in a wide variety of forms.

Chicken

Chicken has light and dark meat. The light meat is leaner and has a milder flavor than the dark meat.

The bird's age determines the tenderness of its meat and the cooking method to use. The terms used on the package label also give an indication.

- **Broiler-fryer chickens.** The most tender and most common. They can be cooked using almost any method.

- **Roaster chickens.** Raised to be roasted whole. They are slightly larger and older than broiler-fryers and yield more meat per pound.

- **Stewing chickens.** Older, mature birds. Since they are less tender than younger birds, they must be cooked in moist heat.

- **Rock Cornish game hens.** Young, small chickens of a special breed. They have less meat in relation to size than other chickens. One hen usually makes one serving. They can be broiled or roasted.

How to Cut Up a Whole Chicken

To cut up a whole chicken, follow the six steps shown below.

Look and Learn:

What are two advantages to buying a whole chicken and cutting it up yourself?

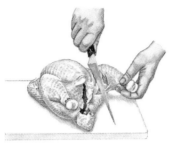

1. Slice the skin between one leg and the body.

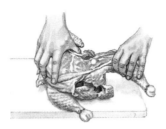

2. Bend the leg to crack the joint. Then cut through the joint and remove the leg. Repeat for the other leg and the wings.

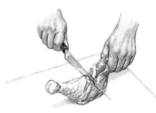

3. If desired, separate the drumstick from the thigh by cracking the joint and cutting through it.

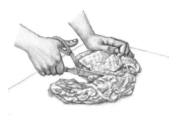

4. Use kitchen shears to cut along the backbone on both sides, separating the breast from the back.

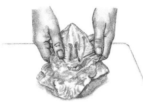

5. Hold the breast skin side down and snap it in two.

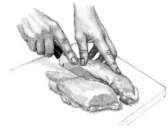

6. Cut the breast in half, leaving the breastbone on one of the halves.

◆ **Capons.** Desexed roosters under ten months old. Tender and flavorful, they are best roasted.

Poultry may be labeled in one of two ways, either fresh or frozen. *Fresh* poultry has never been chilled below 26°F (–4°C). *Frozen* means that the poultry has been chilled to below 0°F (–18°C).

Turkey

Turkeys are larger than chickens and have a stronger flavor. The light meat is leaner and more tender and has a milder flavor than the dark meat.

When buying a whole turkey, you have a choice of several types. They differ mainly in size. All are suitable for roasting, the most common method for cooking turkey.

504 **Chapter 19** ◆ **Meat, Poultry, Fish, and Shellfish**

- **Beltsville or fryer-roaster turkeys.** The smallest, with an average weight of 5 to 9 pounds (2.3 to 4.5 kg). They are not always available.
- **Hen turkeys.** Female. Weigh about 8 to 16 pounds (4 to 8 kg).
- **Tom turkeys.** Male. Can weigh up to 24 pounds (12 kg).

Whole turkeys are sold fresh or frozen. You can also buy turkey parts, such as drumsticks, thighs, and wings. Turkey breast is sold bone-in, boneless, or cut into tenderloins and cutlets.

Ducks and Geese

Ducks and geese have all dark meat, which is very flavorful but relatively high in fat. Usually, only whole, frozen ducks and geese are sold.

Ground Poultry

With the growing emphasis on healthful eating, ground chicken and turkey are found in many supermarket meat departments. When buying either product, read the label carefully. If it states "ground turkey breast" or "ground chicken," both the flesh and skin were used. As you may recall, most of the fat is in the skin. If the word *meat* is part of the description, such as "ground turkey breast meat" or "ground chicken meat," the poultry was ground without the skin. Poultry ground without skin is leaner.

You can use ground poultry in place of ground beef, but it results in a drier, blander product. Usually, you need to add a little more liquid and more seasonings to the recipe.

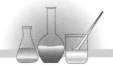

CLOSE-UP ON SCIENCE: BIOCHEMISTRY

Light and Dark Meat

Why does poultry have light and dark meat? The difference in color is due partly to the amount of exercise that different parts of the bird get. Muscles that get frequent, strenuous exercise need more oxygen than others. The oxygen is stored in a red-colored protein pigment called *myoglobin* (MY-uh-GLOW-bin). The amount of myoglobin in the muscle tissue determines the color. Dark meat is found in those parts of chickens and turkeys that get the most exercise, such as the legs. Because domesticated breeds of chickens and turkeys do not fly, their breast and wing muscles do not need as much oxygen to function. The tissue does not contain as much myoglobin, which makes breast meat lighter in color.

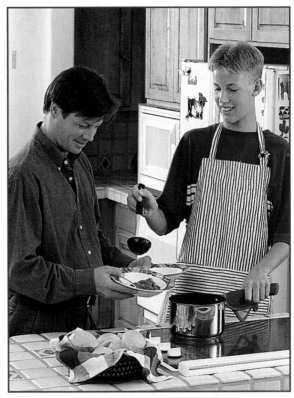

- Chili made with lean ground turkey has a flavor and texture strikingly similar to chili made with red meat. Think of two other dishes made with ground red meat in which ground turkey or chicken might be substituted.

Giblets

Edible poultry organs are called **giblets** (JIB-luhts). Giblets are usually included in a package stuffed inside the whole, cleaned poultry. They include the liver, gizzard (stomach), and heart. Chicken livers and gizzards are also sold separately.

Processed Poultry

Turkey is also processed into products such as ham and bacon. Turkey and chicken are also processed into frankfurters and other types of sausage.

Inspection and Grading

Poultry is inspected and graded by the USDA. Grading is a voluntary program, just as it is with meat. The inspection and grade marks can appear on the label or on a wing tag attached to the bird.

Grade A is the grade of poultry most commonly found in supermarkets. It indicates the poultry is practically free of defects, has a good shape and appearance, and is meaty.

Buying and Storing Poultry

When buying poultry, look for plump, meaty birds. The skin should be smooth and soft. Color of the skin may vary from a creamy white to yellow, depending on the food eaten by the bird. Avoid poultry with tiny feathers or bruised or torn skin.

Use poultry that has been stored in the refrigerator within one to two days. For longer storage, freeze.

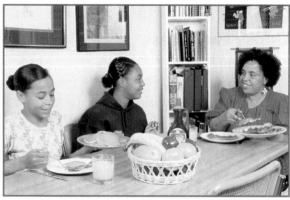

◆ **Processed chicken or turkey products, like this turkey bacon, may be lower in fat and sodium than processed meats.** What precautions should be taken if turkey bacon is to become a part of every breakfast?

Section 19-3 Review & Activities

1. What is the main difference among types of turkeys?

2. Why might ground chicken breast meat cost more than a product labeled "ground chicken breast"?

3. List three characteristics of good quality poultry.

4. Analyzing. Review the different forms of poultry. When might you prefer to buy each one?

5. Evaluating. Tell which cooking method is best for each of the following types of chicken: broiler-fryer, stewing chicken, capon. Explain your responses.

6. Applying. Make a list of as many different ways of using poultry in recipes as you can. Identify the type or form of poultry that might be used in each.

Fish and Shellfish Selection and Storage

Fish and shellfish have long been favorite foods of people living in coastal regions. Today, people almost everywhere can enjoy the nutrition and flavor of the many varieties of fish and shellfish that are available.

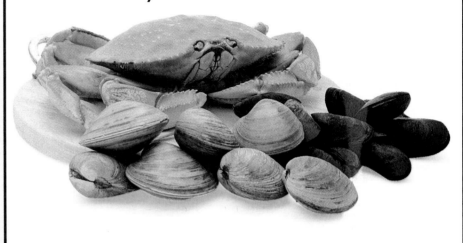

Objectives

After studying this section, you should be able to:

- Describe different types and market forms of fish.
- Identify different types and market forms of shellfish.
- Give guidelines for buying and storing fish and shellfish.

Look for These Terms

crustaceans

mollusks

Types of Fish and Shellfish

What is the difference between fish and shellfish? Most fish have fins and a bony skeleton with a backbone. Shellfish have neither fins nor bones, but have a shell instead.

Some fish and shellfish come from freshwater lakes, rivers, streams, and ponds. They are known as freshwater varieties. Saltwater varieties, also known as seafood, come from oceans and seas. Today, some types of freshwater and saltwater fish and some shellfish are raised on fish farms.

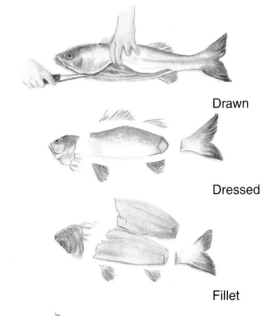

Drawn

Dressed

Fillet

Steaks

◆ **You can purchase drawn or dressed fish, fillets, or steaks.** Which would you choose if you wanted boneless fish?

Types of Fish

There are dozens of varieties of fish. For cooking purposes, many are similar. If a specific fish isn't available, you can substitute a fish similar in flavor, color, and/or texture. The chart on the right gives some examples.

As you have learned, most fish are very low in fat. A few of the darker fish have a higher fat content.

Market Forms of Fish

You can purchase fish in several market forms. See the drawings on page 507. The most common are

- **Drawn.** Whole fish with scales, gills, and internal organs removed.

- **Dressed or pan-dressed.** Drawn fish with head, tail, and fins removed.

- **Fillets.** Sides of fish cut lengthwise away from bones and backbone. Usually boneless. Large fillets may be cut into smaller ones.

- **Steaks.** Cross sections cut from large, dressed fish. May contain bones from ribs and backbone.

Shellfish

Shellfish generally have a mild, sweet flavor. Almost all shellfish come from oceans and seas, but a few come from fresh water. There are two types of shellfish: crustaceans (krus-TAY-shuhns) and mollusks.

Crustaceans

Crustaceans are shellfish that have long bodies with jointed limbs, covered with a shell. They include crabs, crayfish, lobsters, and shrimp.

- **Crabs.** Have an oval shell, four pairs of walking legs, and two claws. Different

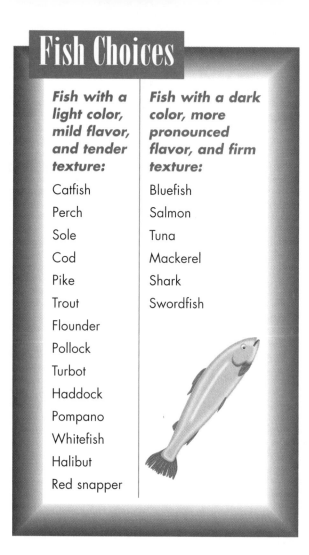

Fish Choices

Fish with a light color, mild flavor, and tender texture:	Fish with a dark color, more pronounced flavor, and firm texture:
Catfish	Bluefish
Perch	Salmon
Sole	Tuna
Cod	Mackerel
Pike	Shark
Trout	Swordfish
Flounder	
Pollock	
Turbot	
Haddock	
Pompano	
Whitefish	
Halibut	
Red snapper	

varieties and sizes are available. Whole crabs are sold live, cooked, or frozen. Crab legs and claws are sold cooked and frozen. Cooked crabmeat is available refrigerated, frozen, and canned.

- **Crayfish.** Freshwater crustaceans. They are also called crawfish or crawdads. They look like small lobsters. Crayfish are sold whole, live, or cooked.

- **Lobsters.** Have a long, jointed body with four pairs of walking legs and two large claws, all covered with a hard shell. Average weight is from 1¼ pounds (625 g) to 2¼ pounds (1125 g). Maine lobster is the most popular. Fresh lobster is sold live.

◆ **Shrimp.** Vary in size and color. They are usually sold frozen or previously frozen and thawed. You can buy raw shrimp, with or without the shell, as well as shelled, cooked shrimp.

Mollusks

Mollusks are shellfish with soft bodies that are covered by at least one shell. They include clams, mussels, oysters, scallops, and squid.

◆ **Clams.** Have two shells hinged at the back with edible flesh inside. Many varieties are available, from small to large. They are sold live (still in the shell) or shucked (removed from the shell).

◆ **Mussels.** Have a thin, oblong shell. Length varies from 1½ inches (3.8 cm) to 6 inches (15 cm). Shell colors also vary.

The flesh is creamy tan and not as tender as that of oysters or clams. Mussels are sold live in the shell.

◆ **Oysters.** Have a rough, hard, gray shell. They come in various sizes. The flesh varies in color, flavor, and texture. Oysters are sold live or shucked.

◆ **Scallops.** Grow in beautiful, fan-shaped shells. Only the muscle that hinges the two shells is sold. Bay scallops are very tiny— about ½ inch (1.3 cm) in diameter—sweet, and tender. Sea scallops are larger—about 1½ inches (3.8 cm) in diameter—and not as tender as bay scallops.

◆ **Squid.** Also known as calamari (kah-luh-MAH-ree). It is sold fresh. Squid is popular in Asia and the Mediterranean area and has become popular in the United States.

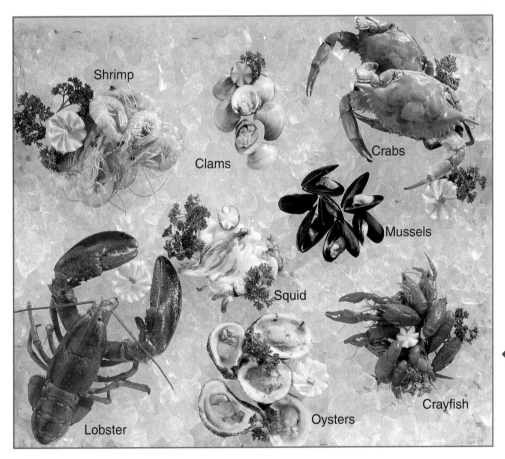

Shrimp

Clams

Crabs

Mussels

Squid

Lobster

Oysters

Crayfish

◆ Remember to look for signs of quality when buying fish and shellfish. How would you store the varieties shown here?

People with certain types of health problems—including liver disease, diabetes, and immune disorders—should be careful never to eat raw or undercooked fish or shellfish. If they do, they risk serious illness or even death. The cause is harmful bacteria that may be present in the fish or shellfish. Thorough cooking kills the bacteria.

Processed Fish

Fish may be dried, pickled, smoked, or cured. Sometimes more than one method is used. For example, lox is a type of cured, smoked salmon. Cod is often salted and dried. Herring may be cut into chunks, pickled in vinegar and spices, and then packed in jars.

Canned fish and shellfish are ready to eat as is, heat, or use in recipes. To cut down on fat, look for fish packed in water instead of oil. If the fish is packed in oil, drain it well

and rinse off the oil before using. Many other convenience forms of fish, such as frozen breaded fish fillets, are available.

Inspection and Grading

The Food and Drug Administration (FDA) has a modern food safety system for fish, known as Hazard Analysis and Critical Control Point, or HACCP (pronounced HAS-sip). All seafood processors, repackers, and warehouses—both domestic and foreign exporters to this country—must use it. The system focuses on identifying and preventing hazards that could cause foodborne illness.

A voluntary inspection and grading program is also carried on jointly by the FDA and the National Marine Fisheries Service of the U.S. Department of Commerce. The program attempts to focus on those parts of fish processing that may be risks to consumer

---

Connecting Food and Social Studies

Let's Potlatch!

In coastal regions today, the cost of fish and shellfish is much lower than elsewhere. At one time, these items were there for the asking. To the Native American people who inhabited the Pacific Northwest—the Tlingit, Kwakiutl, Haida, Tsimshian, and others—the clear, swift-flowing streams and rivers teemed with salmon and trout. The ocean offered an abundance of saltwater fish, and there were plenty of clams, oysters, and crabs.

With so many natural resources, there was much cause for celebration. The people became famous for their large gatherings, called *potlatches,* a word that in the Chinook language means "to give." Potlatch ceremonies were marked by the lavish distribution

of gifts and food to guests from other clans, villages, and tribes.

Potlatches often lasted as long as two weeks. Wearing ceremonial dress and masks, each family performed its songs and dances. Then they feasted on the gifts the waters gave them.

Think About It

- In 1885, the Canadian government enacted a law making the potlatch ceremony illegal. Why do you think the government interfered in this way? How do you think this affected the lives of the people of the Northwest Coast? Investigate government regulations on fishing in the United States and what effect these laws have had on the supply of fish and shellfish.

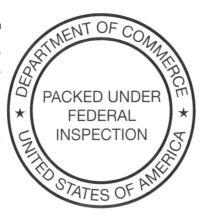

◆ **Fish that has been inspected carries this seal. Look for it on the package. What other safeguards can help you select fish that is at its peak of flavor and safe to eat?**

safety. Some state and local fish inspection services are also available.

Buying Fish and Shellfish

When you are buying fish, a fishy odor should make you suspicious. Fresh fish and shellfish that have gone bad will smell "fishy" or have an unpleasant ammonia odor. Here are some tips for buying fish and shellfish:

◆ Buy from a reliable source. Pay attention to the way fresh fish is displayed. If layers are piled on ice, the top layer may be too warm for safekeeping. Don't buy ready-to-eat fish that is piled next to fresh fish. Harmful bacteria from the fresh fish may have transferred to the ready-to-eat product.

◆ Use appearance, aroma, and touch to judge quality. Fresh fish should have shiny skin and a glistening color. Whole fish should have clear, full eyes and bright red or pink gills. Any fish should have a mild, fresh aroma, similar to that of cucumbers or seaweed. The skin should spring back when pressed.

◆ Some shellfish must be alive if bought fresh. Look for signs that they are alive, such as movement in lobsters. Mollusk shells should close when they are tapped.

Storing Fish and Shellfish

After you bring fish home, store it in the refrigerator or freezer immediately. Refrigerate live shellfish in containers covered with a clean, damp cloth. They need breathing space to stay alive. Do not put live saltwater shellfish in fresh water—they won't live.

Use fish stored in the refrigerator within one to two days. For longer storage, freeze.

Section 19-4 Review & Activities

1. Define the terms *crustacean* and *mollusk*. Give three examples of each.

2. List four signs to look for when buying fresh fish and shellfish.

3. How should live shellfish be stored?

4. **Comparing and Contrasting.** How are drawn fish and dressed fish alike? How are they different?

5. **Evaluating.** Do you think it would be safe to eat fish that you and your friends caught on a fishing trip? Why or why not?

6. **Applying.** Find recipes for fish and shellfish in magazines or cookbooks. Note whether each recipe calls for a light-colored fish, dark-colored fish, crustacean, or mollusk. Decide whether it would affect the finished product if you chose fresh, frozen, or canned fish. Which recipe would be most economical to serve to a group of six people?

Preparing Meat, Poultry, Fish, and Shellfish

Objectives

After studying this section, you should be able to:

- Explain how to select a cooking method for different cuts of meat, poultry, fish, and shellfish.
- Identify ways of preparing cuts for cooking.
- Tell how to test cuts for doneness.
- Give guidelines for cooking cuts by different methods.

Look for These Terms

marinating

marinades

doneness

Torey looked down at the supermarket's meat and poultry cases. "What should we have at the cookout?" he wondered. He pictured chicken breasts sizzling on the grill. Maybe thick swordfish steaks would be even better.

When it comes to cooking, meat, poultry, and fish have many similarities. Many of the same basic cooking methods can be used for each.

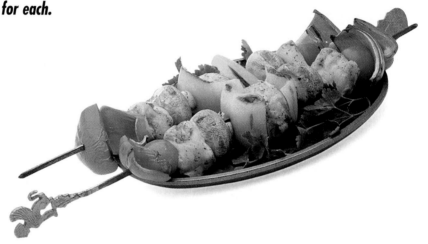

Cooking Meat, Poultry, Fish, and Shellfish

When cuts from animal foods cook, several changes occur in color, flavor, and texture.

- ◆ **Color.** The red color changes to brown. Beef, which is dark red, turns dark brown. Pork and the white meat of poultry, which are light pink, turn almost white.

- ◆ **Flavor.** Heat develops the flavor by creating chemical reactions within the cut.

- ◆ **Texture.** When heated, a cut loses fat and moisture. As a result, it shrinks. In addition,

muscle fibers get firmer and connecting tissue becomes more tender.

When cooked in dry heat, animal foods lose some juices, carrying off some B vitamins. Some thiamin is destroyed by high temperatures. In general, however, few nutrients are lost unless the food is overcooked.

When a cut is overcooked in dry heat, it dries out and gets tough, stringy, and chewy. In moist heat, an overcooked cut gets mushy and loses its flavor. When overcooked in a microwave oven, the cut can get so hard that you can't chew it.

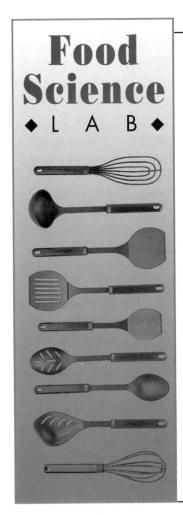

Food Science
◆ L A B ◆

More than "Meats" the Eye

Is there more to cooking a cut of meat than just applying heat? You are about to find out by comparing several methods.

Procedure

1. Divide a piece of shoulder or chuck steak into three pieces. Place one piece in a mixture of lemon and ¼ teaspoon (1 mL) ground black pepper for 1 hour. Pound a second piece on both sides with a mallet to break down the muscle fibers.

2. Broil the two prepared pieces along with the untreated third piece for the same length of time. Be sure you know which piece was prepared by which method.

3. Taste all three pieces, noting the relative tenderness of the meat.

Conclusions

◆ Which piece was the most tender? The least tender?

◆ What generalizations can you make about the relative tenderizing effects of heat, acid, and pounding on a cut of meat?

◆ Which piece had the most flavor? What explanation can you offer?

Choosing a Cooking Method

The cooking method you choose depends on the tenderness of the cut. You can cook tender cuts—for example, some steaks, chops, and rib and loin roasts—using dry-heat methods such as broiling and roasting. Broiling, the faster of the two methods, cooks tender cuts in a matter of minutes. Other foods that take well to dry-heat cooking methods include ground meat, poultry, fish, and some shellfish.

Less tender cuts—such as blade roasts, arm steaks, stewing hens, and some shellfish—need to be tenderized. This can take place either during cooking, by using a moist-heat cooking method, or before, by marinating.

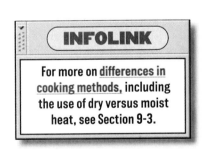

INFOLINK

For more on <u>differences in cooking methods</u>, including the use of dry versus moist heat, see Section 9-3.

Using Moist Heat

Applying moist heat to less tender cuts breaks down the collagen in them, making the meat tender. Moist-heat methods—simmering, stewing, and braising—all involve long, slow cooking that helps develop the meat's flavor.

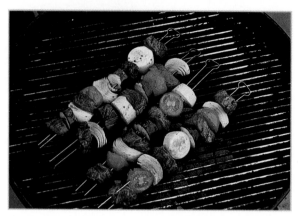

◆ When properly cooked, meat is tender and flavorful and retains most of its nutrients. The cubes of lean meat on these skewers have been marinated for extra tenderness. What simple starch would you serve with these kebabs to add a serving from the grains group?

Moist-heat methods also give you an opportunity to add seasonings, sauces, and other foods to the dish. You can create many different flavor combinations in this way. For this reason, you may sometimes choose to cook tender cuts in moist heat. If you do so, you should generally shorten the cooking time. Otherwise, the cut can easily be overcooked and fall apart.

Marinades

Marinating, or steeping in a liquid, is a method of tenderizing and adding flavor to foods before you cook them. **Marinades** (MAR-uh-nayds)—the flavorful liquids in which food is steeped—can turn less expensive cuts into tender, flavorful meals.

Most marinades contain three basic ingredients—oil, an acid, and seasonings. You can use any mild oil. The oil coats the outside of the food and keeps it from drying out as it broils or grills. The acid ingredient helps tenderize the food. Options include flavored vinegars, citrus juices, plain fat-free yogurt, and buttermilk. Seasonings add flavor. Try using herbs and spices or aromatic vegetables such as onions, peppers, garlic, and celery.

Pour the marinade ingredients into a large container, such as a reusable glass jar, and shake well. Place the food in a glass or plastic container, pour the marinade over the food, cover the container, and refrigerate. Occasionally turn or stir the food so that it marinates evenly. Do not marinate food in metal pans—the acid may react with the metal and give the food an unpleasant flavor.

Using Marinades

Marinating time depends on the food. Tender foods, such as fish, can marinate for an hour or less. Meat and poultry can marinate up to six or eight hours. Be careful not to over-marinate foods because they will get mushy. If you are marinating foods just for flavor, 30 minutes is usually long enough.

Before cooking, drain the food well. Discard marinade used for meat, poultry, fish, and shellfish, since it may contain harmful bacteria. If you want to baste with the marinade, make an extra batch to use for this purpose.

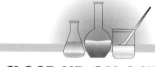

CLOSE-UP ON SCIENCE:
CHEMISTRY

Meat Tenderizers

Enzymes are proteins that control chemical activity in living organisms. One use of enzymes is in meat tenderizers. Three enzymes that come from a fruit called the papaya are diluted with salt to form a dry powder called *papain* (puh-PAY-in). The enzymes in papain attack the connective tissue in muscle fiber. By breaking down the muscle fiber, they make the meat more tender to eat.

Preparing to Cook

For best results, thaw frozen raw meat, poultry, and fish before cooking. If you don't thaw the cut, you will have to increase the cooking time. In general, increase the cooking time by about 50 percent. For example, if the normal cooking time is 40 minutes, the cooking time for frozen cuts would be about 60 minutes. However, the extra time needed depends on the size of the food and whether or not it was partially thawed.

Before cooking meat, poultry, or fish, be sure the cut is clean. Rinse it under cold water and pat dry with a paper towel. If you are cooking whole poultry, first remove the giblets and neck from the body and neck cavities. Rinse the cavities of whole poultry and drawn fish several times. Remove any foreign matter that may be present in the cavities.

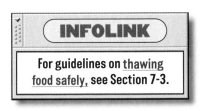

For guidelines on <u>thawing food safely</u>, see Section 7-3.

Trimming Fat

Before cooking meat and poultry, remove as much fat as possible. Trim visible fat from meat.

As you have learned, much of the fat in poultry is in or just under the skin. When cooking poultry in moist heat, remove the skin. However, when using dry-heat methods, leave the skin on to keep the poultry from drying out. Most of the fat will melt and drip away during cooking. Remove the skin before eating.

Judging Doneness

Doneness means having cooked a cut long enough for the necessary changes to take place so that a cut tastes good and is safe to eat. If any part is not cooked, there is a risk of foodborne illness.

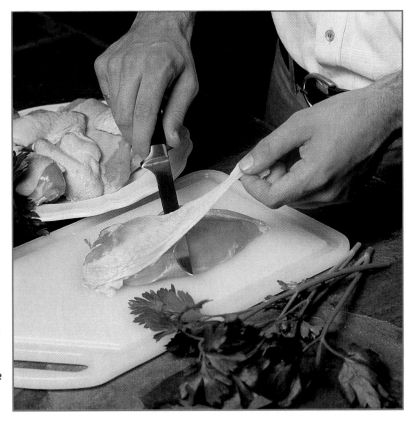

◆ Remove the skin from poultry that will be cooked in moist heat to reduce the amount of fat in the finished dish. Explain why you should not remove the skin from poultry that is broiled until just before eating.

Internal Temperatures for Meat and Poultry

Food	Internal Temperature	
	°F	°C
Beef		
Medium-rare (some bacterial risk)	145	63
Medium	160	71
Well-done	170	77
Pork, Lamb, Veal (Roasts, Steaks, Chops)		
Medium	160	71
Well-done	170	77
Poultry		
Whole chicken, turkey	180	82
Turkey breasts or roasts	170	77
Stuffing (cooked alongside bird)	165	74
Ham		
Fresh (raw) or shoulder	160	71
Precooked (to reheat)	140	60
Ground Meat and Poultry		
Turkey, chicken	170	77
Beef, veal, lamb, pork	160	71
Leftovers		
Meat in soups and stews (Bring soup and any grains to a rolling boil.)	165	74
Casseroles	160	71

Both meat and poultry are tested for doneness in the same general way. To be safe to eat, either should reach an internal temperature of at least 160°F (71°C).

Meat and poultry cooking times vary, depending on the method and the cut used. The cooking time given in the recipe is just a guide. Begin testing meat and poultry for doneness about 10 minutes before the end of the cooking time.

Testing Meat for Doneness

When roasting cuts more than 2 inches (5 cm) thick, don't rely on appearance alone as a test for doneness. Use a meat thermometer. This type of thermometer, usually made of metal, is inserted into the thickest part of the cut and left in place for the entire cooking period. Taking a reading in two or three different places yields an even more accurate sense of when a roast is done.

With other cooking methods or thinner cuts, use an instant-read thermometer. Do not use an instant-read thermometer in the oven while food is roasting. This type of thermometer is designed to be inserted into depths no greater than ½ inch (1 cm) and furnishes a reading within about ten seconds.

Testing Poultry for Doneness

When testing chicken, you may find the meat has turned dark around the bones. This is common in young broiler-fryers. Their bones have not hardened completely. During cooking, color pigment from the inside of the bone seeps out. The meat is safe to eat.

When testing cubes of poultry, pierce with a fork. If the fork slides easily to the bottom, the food is done.

How to Use a Meat Thermometer

A meat thermometer is an indispensable tool when cooking meat or poultry.

Look and Learn:

Explain the importance of inserting the thermometer into the thickest area of a cut or as close to the center as possible.

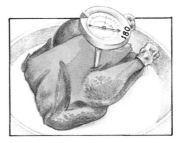

Whole Poultry

◆ Whole poultry: Insert the thermometer into the inner thigh, near the breast. It should not touch the bone. If the bird is stuffed, take a reading of the stuffing at the end of the cooking time.

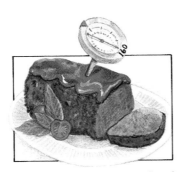

Ground Meat—Meat loaf

◆ Ground meat or poultry: Place the thermometer in the thickest part of the food.

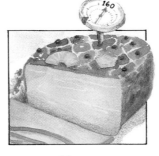

Ham

◆ Roast: Insert the thermometer into the center of the thickest part, away from gristle, fat, and bone.

◆ Casseroles: Insert the thermometer into the thickest portion. If the dish is shallow, check the temperature at the end of the cooking time with an instant-read thermometer. Insert it about ½ inch (1 cm) into the mixture.

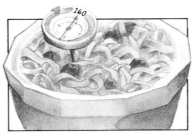

Casserole

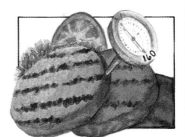

Ground Meat—Burgers

◆ Thin pieces: Insert the instant-read thermometer sideways until the tip is in the center of the burger.

Once you start to cook a cut, regardless of the method, finish cooking it. Don't cook food partially and then complete the cooking later. Partial or interrupted cooking often produces conditions that encourage the growth of harmful bacteria.

Testing Fish for Doneness

Fish is very tender and cooks in a short time. When using conventional cooking methods, remember the "10-minute rule." Cook fish 10 minutes for every inch (2.5 cm) of thickness, as measured at the thickest part. However, there are a few exceptions. If fish is being baked in a sauce, add about 5 minutes to the total cooking time. Some moist-heat recipes may call for longer cooking times to allow flavors to blend. Remember to increase the cooking time if the fish is frozen.

Begin to check for doneness about 2 or 3 minutes before the cooking time is up. Fish is done when its flesh turns opaque. When gently lifted with a fork, the flesh flakes easily.

Basic Cooking Methods

You can use a number of different cooking methods for meat, poultry, fish, and shellfish. These include roasting, broiling, poaching, and microwaving.

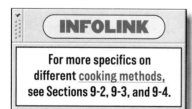

INFOLINK

For more specifics on different cooking methods, see Sections 9-2, 9-3, and 9-4.

Roasting or Baking

When you are roasting or baking meat, poultry, or fish, it is usually not necessary to preheat the oven. However, follow recipe directions. The roasting temperatures in a conventional oven should be at least 325°F (160°C) to keep harmful bacteria from growing. Fish can bake at higher temperatures, such as 450°F (230°C).

The way you prepare meat, poultry, and fish for roasting or baking varies.

◆ **Large meat roasts.** Put the roast, fat side up, on a rack in a pan to hold the cut out of the drippings. Some rib cuts of meat form a natural rack. Insert the meat thermometer so that the tip is in the center of the roast. The thermometer should not touch bone, fat, or thick connective tissues.

◆ **Whole poultry.** Make the bird as compact as possible so that it cooks evenly. Tie the legs together. Tuck tips of wings under the back. Insert a meat thermometer deep into the thickest part of the thigh next to the body. Be sure it is not touching bone or fat. Do not stuff the bird, which can lead to cross-contamination. Instead, cook the stuffing in a separate pan.

◆ **Poultry pieces.** Place in a shallow pan, skin side up.

◆ **Fish.** Place the fish in a lightly oiled, shallow baking dish. If baking fillets, place them skin side down so that you can test for doneness. To keep the fish moist, brush with seasoned melted fat or sauce. You can also bread the fish. If so, dot the fish with a teaspoon (5 mL) of butter or margarine after breading.

Follow recipe directions for turning the food. Generally, large roasts, whole poultry, and fish do not have to be turned. Poultry pieces may need to be turned after half the cooking time. To reduce fat, use broth or juice for basting instead of drippings. Roast or bake for the time specified in the recipe.

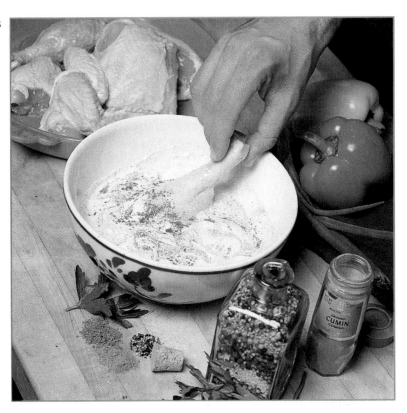

◆ Tandoori chicken, a favorite in India, is marinated in a savory blend of yogurt and spices before grilling or broiling. In addition to adding an interesting flavor, what function does the yogurt serve in this dish?

Broiling

Broiling is one of the quickest cooking methods. It is an ideal choice for families who are on the go but want to sit down together to a home-cooked meal.

To prepare meat for broiling, slash the fat around the edges. This will help keep the cut from curling. When broiling chicken, begin with the skin side down. Halfway through the broiling time, turn the skin side up. When broiling fish, which is lean, brush it lightly with melted butter or margarine to keep it from charring.

To add flavor to any broiled food, brush it with a sauce, such as barbecue sauce or salsa. For even greater variety, make kabobs. Thread cubes of meat, poultry, or firm fish onto skewers, alternating with tomato quarters, mushrooms, green pepper chunks, or other vegetables. Brush with melted butter or margarine, or a sauce, to keep the vegetables from drying out. Broil or grill, turning so that all sides are done.

Poaching

As noted in Chapter 9, poaching involves simmering whole foods in a small amount of liquid. Fish is one of the foods most commonly poached. Many people consider poached fish to be a delicacy, and it is often served in fine restaurants.

You may poach whole drawn fish, fillets, or steaks. The cooking liquid may be plain water, water with lemon or grapefruit juice, fish or vegetable stock, or milk. Usually, the liquid is seasoned to add more flavor to the fish. Try using herbs or spices—dill or grated fresh ginger, for example—and sautéed vegetables, such as onions and green peppers.

Poaching Fish Fillets

To poach fish fillets:

1. Pour the cooking liquid (seasoned as desired) into a large, deep skillet. Bring to a boil; then immediately reduce the heat to a simmer.

2. Place the fillets in a single layer in the pan. Add enough liquid, if necessary, to cover the fish by at least 1 inch (2.5 cm).

3. Cover the pan and simmer gently until the fish is just opaque throughout. Do not turn the fish while poaching.

Poaching Whole Fish

To poach whole drawn fish or fish steaks, first wrap the fish in cheesecloth. Allow enough length at the ends so that you can twist and knot them. Use the ends as handles to lower and raise the fish to prevent it from falling apart. Otherwise, follow the same procedure as for fillets.

If you like, you can serve hot poached fish with a sauce made from the cooking liquid. After removing the fish from the pan, boil the cooking liquid to reduce the amount of liquid and reach the desired flavor.

Poached fish may also be eaten chilled. You might serve cold poached fish with dill or cucumber sauce or use it in a salad.

Microwave Cooking

All types of meat, poultry, fish, and shellfish can be microwaved. When buying for microwaving, choose cuts that are uniform in size. Thaw frozen raw meat, poultry, fish, and shellfish completely before cooking in the microwave.

For best results, follow the directions in the microwave recipes exactly. Following are some general guidelines.

Microwaving Meat and Poultry

Remember that microwave ovens do not always cook evenly, even with a turntable. This is especially important to keep in mind when microwaving large cuts, such as meat roasts or whole poultry. Follow recipe directions exactly to be sure the meat or poultry cooks completely throughout.

When microwaving pork roasts, take special care to cook the meat thoroughly. Place the meat in a covered dish or in a loosely sealed, microwave-safe cooking bag. This will hold in moist heat to help ensure even cooking and tender, juicy meat. If you like, add a small amount of liquid, such as water, broth, fruit juice, or a sauce. You can also use a cooking bag for whole poultry.

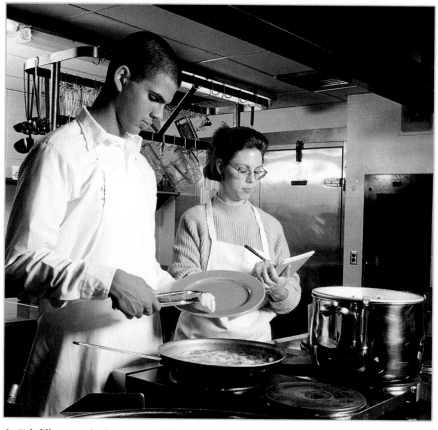

◆ Fish fillets poached in seasoned liquid emerge moist, tender, and flavored by the broth. Create your own recipe for poaching. Identify each step involved.

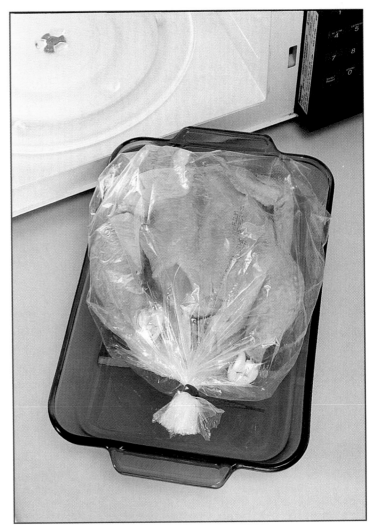

◆ A cooking bag can be used when microwaving roasts and whole poultry. Name two advantages of this method.

When microwaved, roasts and whole poultry are cooked at a lower internal temperature than with conventional cooking. This is because the internal temperature continues to rise during standing time. If the microwave oven has a temperature probe, you can program the oven to shut off when the food reaches the desired temperature.

During standing time, cover roasts loosely with foil to hold heat in. After standing time, check the meat or poultry in several spots with a meat thermometer to be sure it has reached the proper internal temperature throughout.

Light-colored cuts cooked in a microwave oven may look unappetizing because they have not yet browned. You may want to use one of the following methods to create a browned effect:

◆ Before cooking, brush or rub with a dark-colored sauce, such as barbecue, tamari, or Worcestershire.

◆ Use a browning dish or grill. These are specially made so that they become extremely hot. Press small cuts down against the bottom to brown them.

◆ After microwaving, put the cut in the broiler for a few minutes to brown it.

Microwaving Fish

When microwaving fish, allow about 3 to 6 minutes per pound (500 g) at 100 percent power. Thick fillets and whole fish take a little more time than thin ones.

Take care to avoid overcooking—fish is tender, and the microwave cooks quickly. Remove the fish from the microwave when it is still slightly underdone in the center. Let it stand for 5 minutes to complete the cooking; then test for doneness.

Shellfish cooks quickly, so be careful not to overcook it. If you do, it will get tough and rubbery.

Other Cooking Methods

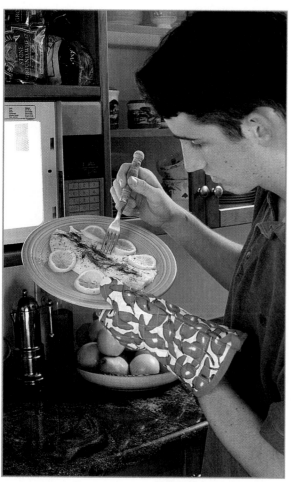

You may pan-fry meat, poultry, and shellfish. Often the food is breaded or dipped in batter first. Remember that food absorbs fat as it fries. If you do choose to fry, use as little fat as possible—no more than 1 teaspoon (5 mL) of oil. You may use a vegetable-oil spray for sautéing small pieces of meat, poultry, fish, or shellfish.

Most meat (except veal) is marbled with fat and can be pan-broiled—cooked in a skillet without added fat—instead of fried. Just be sure to remove the fat that accumulates during cooking.

Some cooking methods—such as stewing, braising, and stir-frying—usually involve cooking several different foods together, such as meat and vegetables.

◆ **When microwaving fish, remove the fish before it has completely finished cooking. The fish should feel slightly firm when lightly pressed with a fork. Check the manufacturer's instructions on a microwave oven in the foods lab or at home for any special tips on cooking fish. Record these in your Wellness Journal for future reference.**

Section 19-5 Review & Activities

1. Name two specific cooking methods you might use for tender cuts and two you might use for less tender cuts.

2. Name three steps that might be involved in preparing raw meat or poultry for cooking.

3. Name two signs that fish is done cooking.

4. Extending. What would you do if you came home and found that the meat for the evening meal was still in the freezer?

5. Evaluating. What is the advantage of knowing basic guidelines for a number of different methods of cooking meat, poultry, and fish?

6. Applying. Choose one of the cooking methods discussed in this chapter. Write the name of the method vertically down the left-hand side of a sheet of paper. Next to each letter, write a sentence that begins with that letter and gives a fact about the cooking method.

RECIPE FILE

Pan-Asian Microwave Chicken Deluxe

The soy sauce gives this tangy main course a Chinese touch; the yogurt gives it a taste of India. The recipe is also great as kabobs—cut into chunks and skewered.

Customary	Ingredient	Metric
4	Boneless, skinless chicken breast halves	4
2 Tbsp.	Reduced-sodium soy sauce	30 mL
½ cup	Plain fat-free yogurt	125 mL
½ tsp.	Grated onion	3 mL
½ tsp.	Prepared mustard	3 mL
½ tsp.	Seasoned salt	3 mL
Dash	Ground pepper	Dash

Yield: 4 servings, ½ breast each
Equipment: Round microwave-safe dish with removable rack
Power level: 100% power

Directions
1. Brush chicken pieces with soy sauce.
2. Arrange chicken on rack close to edges of dish. Cover loosely with waxed paper.
3. Microwave at 100% power for 6 minutes.
4. Mix together yogurt, onion, and mustard in small bowl. Set aside.
5. Remove chicken pieces from rack. Turn pieces over and place in bottom of dish, arranging them in a circle around the edge.
6. Spoon yogurt mixture over each piece. Cover loosely with waxed paper.
7. Microwave at 100% power for about 6 minutes, or until fork can be inserted in chicken with ease.
8. Sprinkle with seasoned salt and pepper. Let stand, covered, 2 minutes before serving.

Nutrition Information
Per serving (approximate): 215 calories, 31 g protein, 3 g carbohydrate, 8 g fat, 84 mg cholesterol, 593 mg sodium
Good source of: B vitamins, phosphorus

Food for Thought
- Why is it important to arrange and turn the chicken pieces as specified in the recipe?
- What is the purpose of the soy sauce?

RECIPE FILE

Beef Patties with Herbs

Building a better burger is a priority for many home and professional cooks. Here is a recipe that is more healthful and just as tasty as a pan-fried burger.

Customary	Ingredients	Metric
1 lb.	Extra-lean ground beef	500 g
½ tsp.	Ground pepper	3 mL
½ tsp.	Dried rosemary	3 mL
½ tsp.	Dried thyme	3 mL
4	Slices tomato	4
4	Thin slices onion	4
4	Crusty rolls, split	4

Yield: 4 servings, 1 sandwich each
Oven Temperature: Broil

Directions

1. Combine ground beef, pepper, and herbs until well blended.
2. Shape the ground beef mixture into four patties about ½ inch (1 cm) thick.
3. Place beef patties about 2 inches (5 cm) under the heat source. Broil 10 minutes, turning once after 6 minutes.
4. Serve patties with tomato and onion slices on crusty rolls.

Nutrition Information

Per serving (approximate): 351 calories, 28 g protein, 23 g carbohydrate, 16 g fat, 84 mg cholesterol, 313 mg sodium
Good source of: iron, B vitamins, phosphorus

Food for Thought

- If you substituted ground turkey meat for ground beef, what other changes might you need to make in the recipe? Why?
- What other serving suggestions could you make for these ground beef patties?

CAREER WANTED

Individuals who like fish, and are able to follow instructions and perform repetitive tasks.

REQUIRES:

- courses in biology, math, agriculture, and environmental studies
- on-the-job training

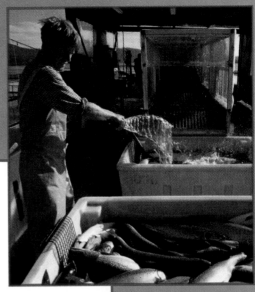

"We are helping preserve natural balance,"

says Fish Production Technician Troy Richter

Q: Troy, what does a fish production technician do?

A: I work for a privately owned fish hatchery that raises fish for food. My responsibilities include caring for the fish on a daily basis and keeping records of their activities.

Q: When you say "care for the fish," do you mean "feed them"?

A: That's part of it, but there's much more. Because we artificially breed fish, we need to regulate things like water depth, flow, temperature, oxygen level, and velocity. We also need to watch fish for possible disease and, when needed, administer medication.

Q: Your work sounds interesting.

A: It is. It can also be challenging when you have to attach small "tags" to individual fish so each one can be monitored. It's pretty slippery work, but it helps biologists study ways to increase the production of healthy fish.

Q: What does the future hold for fish production technology?

A: The industry is still in its infancy and is expected to keep growing. People are eating more fish nowadays. As for me, I plan to get another degree and eventually open my own fish hatchery.

Career Research Activity

1. Contact the USDA or the Environmental Protection Service about career possibilities in fish production technology. Determine ways in which the job descriptions they furnish are similar to and different from that of Troy Richter. Write a report summarizing your findings.

2. The U.S. Fish & Wildlife Service, the National Park Service, or the U.S. Forest Service jointly run a summer program for teens interested in this career area. How could you find out about this program? Would you be interested in this program? Why or why not?

Related Career Opportunities

Entry Level
- Deck Hand
- Fisher

Technical Level
- Fish Production Technician
- Environmental Health Technician
- Oceanographic Technician

Professional Level
- Marine Biologist
- Forest Ranger
- Fish Hatchery Manager

Chapter 19 Review & Activities

Summary

Section 19-1: Looking at Meat, Poultry, Fish, and Shellfish

- Meat, poultry, fish, and shellfish are sources of complete protein, B vitamins, and minerals. They also contain cholesterol and fat.

- Some cuts of meat and poultry are less tender than others.

- These foods are usually the most costly part of the food budget.

Section 19-4: Fish and Shellfish Selection and Storage

- Fish may be bought fresh or frozen in several market forms.

- Shellfish include crustaceans and mollusks. Many are sold live.

- Judge the quality of fish and shellfish by looks and aroma.

- Fish should be refrigerated or frozen.

Section 19-2: Meat Selection and Storage

- You can identify cuts by the package label or by bone shape.

- The USDA inspects meat for wholesomeness.

- Some meats are processed by curing and other methods.

- Store meat properly to retain its quality.

Section 19-5: Preparing Meat, Poultry, Fish, and Shellfish

- Tender cuts can be cooked with dry-heat methods. Less tender cuts need moist-heat methods.

- Thaw, clean, and trim fat before cooking.

- You can test for doneness by using a meat thermometer.

- Basic cooking methods include roasting or baking, broiling, poaching, and microwaving.

Section 19-3: Poultry Selection and Storage

- Chicken and turkey may be purchased fresh or frozen, whole or in parts. Ducks and geese are usually available whole and frozen.

- Poultry is inspected and may be graded by the USDA.

- Poultry requires cold storage.

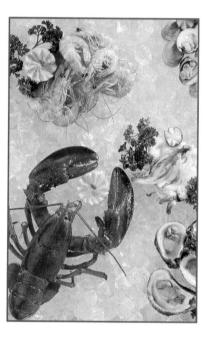

Checking Your Knowledge

1. Of beef, pork, chicken, and fish, which generally has the most saturated fat? The least?

2. What is elastin? Why is it a factor in meat and poultry preparation?

3. Give two examples of lean cuts of each of the following: beef, pork, lamb.

4. List and describe three grades of meat.

5. Name three types of chicken suitable for roasting.

6. What is the difference between ground turkey and ground turkey meat?

7. What does the term *seafood* refer to?

8. What is the difference between fish fillets and fish steaks?

9. Describe how cuts from animal foods change in color, flavor, and texture when cooked.

10. Give three tips for broiling meat, poultry, or fish.

Thinking Critically

1. **Identifying Cause and Effect.** Besides cost and tenderness, what other factors might affect your choice when buying meat, poultry, and fish?

2. **Making Generalizations.** Rona wants to try out a new recipe for pork roast that she glanced at in a magazine while waiting to get her hair cut. She has never cooked a roast. What specific information and techniques should she know about before attempting this recipe?

Working IN THE Lab

1. *Taste Test.* Compare the taste of different types of processed meat, poultry, or fish. Identify the processing method used, and tell what characteristics it gives the food.

2. *Foods Lab.* Choose a recipe calling for ground meat. Prepare it once using meat, and then using ground poultry instead. Compare the results.

3. *Foods Lab.* Poach a fillet of a firm-fleshed fish, such as salmon. Check the fish for doneness 2 or 3 minutes before the cooking time is due to end. When the fish is opaque and the flesh flakes easily, it is done.

Reinforcing Key Skills

1. **Management.** You would like to reduce the amount of money you spend on meat, poultry, and fish, while still providing your family with good-tasting, high-quality protein foods. What steps do you need to take before you can achieve this goal?

2. **Communication.** Elena refuses to try organ meats, giblets, or shellfish. She is sure she won't like them. Why might she feel this way? What might be some benefits of trying these foods? What arguments might you use to persuade Elena to give them a try?

Making Decisions and Solving Problems

You have just moved to a new town and would like to prepare dinner for some new friends. You choose a favorite recipe that calls for loin of lamb, but discover that none of the stores in your area carry it.

Making Connections

1. **Science.** Find information about meat processing methods. How were meats treated for preservation and flavoring in the past? How is this done today? What chemicals and chemical processes are involved? If possible, conduct an experiment or demonstration showing these principles at work.

2. **Math.** Compare the prices of similar forms of chicken and turkey in your area. Figure the cost per serving for each. Show the findings on a bar graph. List the possible reasons for any price differences.

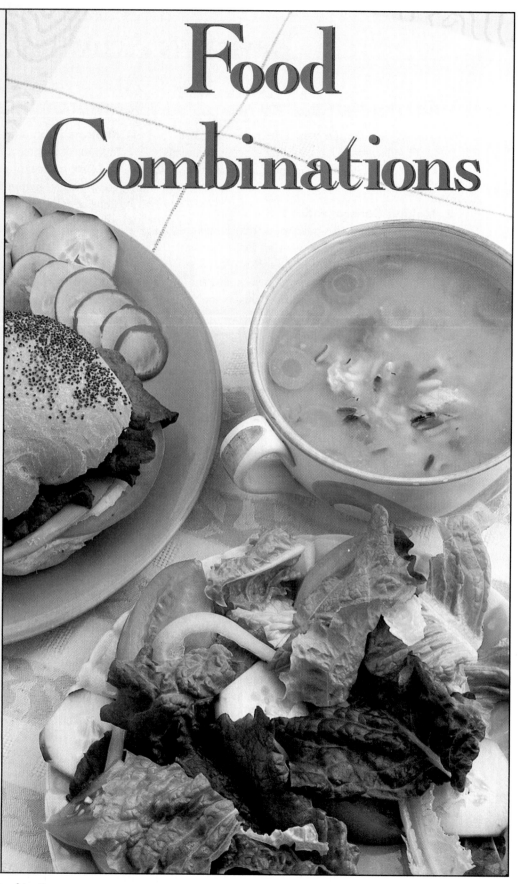

CHAPTER

20

Section 20-1
Sandwiches, Snacks, and Packed Lunches

Section 20-2
Salads and Dressings

Section 20-3
Soups and Sauces

Section 20-4
Casseroles and Other Combinations

Do you know people who have the same thing for lunch every day? Maybe you're one of those people. In this chapter, you'll learn some new, tasty twists on lunch and other interesting food combinations.

Food Combinations

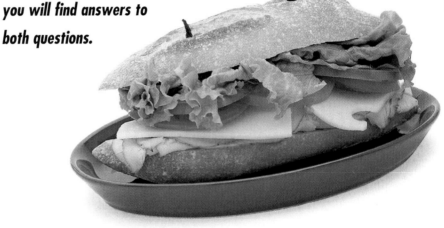

Sandwiches, Snacks, and Packed Lunches

You may think of the sandwich as an invention of Western culture. The truth is that people of many cultures, East and West, have been enjoying foods on bread for over 2,000 years.

What accounts for our fascination with sandwiches? How do they fit in with a healthful eating plan? In this section, you will find answers to both questions.

Objectives

After studying this section, you should be able to:

- Describe how to make sandwiches using a variety of breads and fillings.
- Give suggestions for nutritious snacks.
- Explain how to pack an interesting, nutritious lunch and keep it safe to eat.

Look for These Terms

club sandwich

vacuum bottle

Sandwiches

No matter how you slice it, the sandwich is undoubtedly America's favorite lunchtime food. Different types of foods can be put together to make an endless variety of sandwiches.

Making Sandwiches

The foundation of any sandwich is bread. When constructing a healthful sandwich, start with a whole-grain product. As a change from sliced bread, make sandwiches with rolls, pita bread, taco shells, bagels, or tortillas. Toast the bread for added texture.

The variety of fillings is limited only by your imagination. Choose cooked lean meat, poultry, or fish; deli meats; mashed, cooked dry beans; egg, chicken, or fish salad; or low-fat cheeses.

Top the fillings with other foods. Try tomatoes, lettuce, pickles, onions, shredded carrots, sliced apples, cucumbers, and other fruits and vegetables. Add mustard or salsa for extra flavor.

Sandwiches can be heated easily in a microwave oven. Prepare the sandwich, omitting fresh vegetables and fruit, which will wilt during heating. Add those later. Wrap the sandwich in a paper towel and microwave it on 100 percent power for 30 seconds or until heated.

◆ By using different breads, fillings, and flavorings, you can create an endless variety of sandwiches. Create a recipe for a favorite sandwich and bring a sample to class.

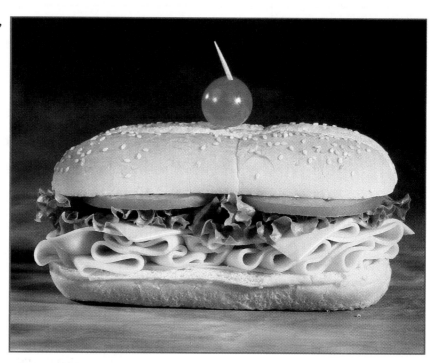

Specialty Sandwiches

Just as there is no end to the list of ingredients you can use to build a sandwich, so there are no constraints on the "architecture." Sandwiches can be flat, tall, round, or square. Here are some basic ways to make sandwiches:

◆ **Club sandwich.** A **club sandwich** is usually made with three slices of toasted bread and filled with chicken or turkey breast, bacon, tomato, lettuce, and mayonnaise. To make one, follow the same basic instructions as for a traditional sandwich, except that you use two layers of filling instead of one. To add eye appeal to the preparation, cut the sandwich into quarters, securing the quarters with decorative toothpicks.

◆ **Fancy sandwich.** Cut the bread into fun or fancy shapes with cookie cutters before or after you add the filling. Serve these sandwiches at formal events, on special occasions, or just for fun.

◆ **Filled pocket sandwich.** Make a pocket sandwich with pita bread, a hard roll, or a taco shell. To make a pocket from a pita, first warm the pita briefly in the microwave oven for easier handling.

Then cut the pita in half with a sharp knife. Gently slit or pull the two sides apart. To make a pocket from a hard roll, slice off the top and scoop out the bread to form a hollow for the filling. (Dry the leftover bread and crust for breadcrumbs.) To keep pockets from absorbing the filling, line them first with shredded lettuce or cucumber slices.

Healthful Snacks

As noted earlier, snacks are as much a part of your daily eating pattern as meals, especially during the teen years when your nutrient needs are particularly high. There are many simple, nutritious ways to satisfy between-meal hunger. Enjoy fresh fruits and vegetables as quick snacks. You could also have a glass of fat-free milk, a small sandwich, or a cup of soup with whole-grain crackers. A creamy fruit smoothie could also fill the bill.

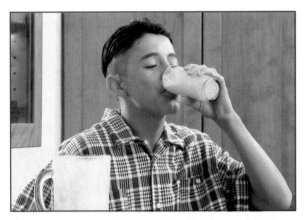

◆ Delicious refreshing fruit smoothies like the one shown here, made with fresh orange juice, can be made by blending fruit juice or fresh fruit with nonfat yogurt and ice cubes. What other combinations would make a great smoothie?

Here are more ideas for healthful, tasty snacks:

◆ **Yogurt pops.** Pour flavored yogurt into a paper cup. Put a wooden ice pop stick or a plastic spoon in the center. Freeze the yogurt pop for at least an hour. The stick or spoon serves as a handle.

◆ **Frozen fruit bites.** Freeze whole berries or grapes to make frozen candy-like snacks.

◆ **"Un-chips."** Cut tortillas or pita bread into six or eight wedge-shaped pieces. Spread a single layer in a baking pan. Bake them in a preheated oven at 450°F (230°C) for about 5 minutes or until crisp. Serve with salsa or bean dip.

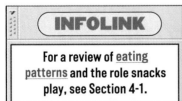

INFOLINK

For a review of <u>eating patterns</u> and the role snacks play, see Section 4-1.

FOR YOUR HEALTH

"Vegging" at Lunchtime

Many Americans fail to meet the minimum Food Guide Pyramid recommendation of three vegetable servings per day. One way to meet this requirement is to build a sandwich around vegetables. Here are some nutrition-packed vegetarian sandwich ideas:

• For a fresh and crunchy choice, top whole wheat bread with thinly sliced cucumber, diced green onions, fat-free cream cheese, and pepper.

• Instead of the usual grilled cheese, slip some sliced tomatoes in with low-fat cheese. You might also microwave cheese and tomato, open-face, on a bagel half.

• Place a mixed green salad or a grain salad, such as tabouleh, in a whole wheat pita pocket.

• Go Italian with mozzarella cheese, tomato, and fresh basil on Italian bread with a splash of flavored vinegar for a burst of flavor.

• Spread vegetarian refried beans, diced tomatoes, salsa, and shredded cheese on a tortilla. Roll up. Then heat and eat.

• Grill or roast your favorite vegetables. Then layer them on whole-grain bread and enjoy the natural taste of the veggies.

Following Up

• In the foods lab, create one of the sandwich ideas above, or invent one of your own. Cut the sandwich into bite-size pieces, insert a toothpick in each, and share the pieces with class members. Use their criticism as the basis for a campaign to educate people in your home on how to make healthful sandwich eating a part of the family's eating pattern.

Packing a Lunch

It is estimated that about 30 percent of American workers carry a packed lunch. Their reasons vary from saving money to having better food choices. As you know, packed lunches can be taken to school, too.

With a little organization, packed lunches can be easy to assemble. Follow these simple guidelines:

◆ Remember that safety comes first. Keep hot foods hot and cold foods cold.

◆ To pack hot soup, chili, stew, or similar hot foods, use a wide-mouth **vacuum bottle** —a glass or metal bottle with a vacuum space between the outer container and the inner liner. Vacuum bottles do a better job of keeping foods hot than less expensive foam-insulated bottles. Before packing the vacuum bottle, preheat it— fill it with hot tap water and let it stand a minute or two. Empty the water, fill the bottle with piping hot food, and close tightly.

◆ Pack foods that are easy to handle. Avoid foods that are drippy or oily. If foods must be cut up, cut them before packing the lunch.

◆ To speed up lunch packing, set aside an area in the freezer, refrigerator, and a nearby cabinet for lunch foods and equipment.

◆ Make packing lunches a family affair. Take turns being the family's "designated lunch packer" for the day.

◆ Remember these three "R's"—reduce, reuse, and recycle. For example, plastic containers from yogurt, sour cream, and cottage cheese can be washed out and used to pack foods. Reuse plastic bags from the grocery store as lunch sacks. Save used aluminum foil if it can be recycled in your area. Try to avoid one-use containers and wraps. Use cloth napkins instead of paper ones. These tips will help you save time and money and cut down on waste.

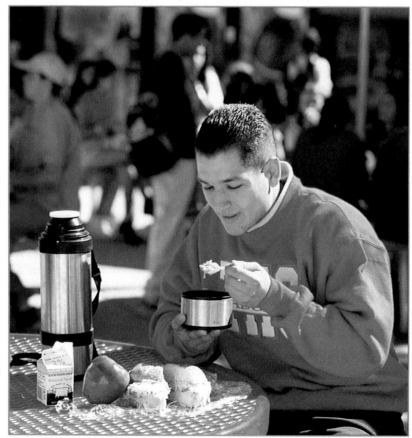

◆ Nutritious packed lunches should contain servings from several different groups on the Food Guide Pyramid. What food groups are represented by this lunch? How would you rate the lunch from a nutritional standpoint?

Safety Check

Is brown-bagging the safest way to carry lunch to school? If you pack perishable food that's left at room temperature more than two hours, the risk of foodborne illness increases. It's especially important to remember this if you typically store your lunch in a stuffy locker.

For the safest bet, use an insulated lunch bag. You can also freeze sandwiches and juice boxes to help keep cold foods cold. The foods will be thawed by lunchtime. Use ice packs or chilled, insulated vacuum bottles to help keep foods cool. Pack nonperishable foods such as dried fruit, boxed juice, and peanut butter with crackers.

Assembling the Lunch

To prepare an interesting and nutrient-rich lunch, use a variety of foods, following the guidelines in the Food Guide Pyramid. Use your imagination. Think of leftover foods you enjoy eating cold—baked chicken, meat loaf, roast turkey, or pizza. Heat up leftover chili, stew, or soup to pack in a vacuum bottle.

If you take salads with greens, mix fruits and vegetables, but pack dressing separately. Drizzle on the dressing just before eating.

Bean dips and spreads make tasty sandwich fillings. Try using them as dips for fresh fruits and vegetables, too.

For a healthful lunch, be sure your food choices include whole grains as well as fresh fruits and vegetables.

What will you choose for a beverage? Milk and fruit juice are both flavorful and nutritious choices. Fruit juice can be frozen ahead of time. In addition to helping keep food cool, it will be a cool, refreshing drink.

Don't forget to include such nonfood items as forks, spoons, and napkins. Tuck in a wipe or a wet washcloth in a plastic bag to clean your hands and wipe up spills.

Section 20-1 Review & Activities

1. Name four kinds of bread that might be used to make a sandwich.

2. Identify two healthful snacks made with fruit.

3. Describe how to preheat a vacuum bottle.

4. Comparing and Contrasting. How do the snack suggestions in this section compare with those you choose at home in terms of nutrition, expense, and ease of preparation?

5. Synthesizing. A club sandwich is not traditionally a low-fat choice. How would you prepare a low-fat version of a club sandwich?

6. Applying. Draw a diagram showing how you would set up an ideal lunch-packing area in your kitchen at home. Explain the advantages of your plan. Share it with other family members who pack lunches for themselves.

RECIPE FILE

Apple-Tuna Sandwiches

This sandwich combines a variety of foods for a complex blend of flavors and textures. For variety, try serving this sandwich in whole-wheat pita halves or rolled in a tortilla.

Customary	Ingredients	Metric
7-oz. can	Water-pack tuna, drained and flaked	198-g can
½ cup	Chopped celery	125 mL
2 Tbsp.	Chopped onion	30 mL
½ cup	Plain, nonfat yogurt	125 mL
4	Lettuce leaves	4
4 slices	American cheese (optional)	4 slices
1	Apple, cored and thinly sliced (about 12 slices)	1
4	Whole wheat buns, split	4

Yield: 4 servings, one sandwich each

Directions

1. Combine tuna, celery, onion, and yogurt.
2. Cover the bottom of each bun with a lettuce leaf. Be sure leaves are dry.
3. Place a cheese slice (if desired) on top of the lettuce leaf.
4. Spread tuna mixture on top of lettuce or cheese on each bun.
5. Place 3 apple slices on top of tuna mixture.
6. Cover with top half of bun.

Nutrition Information

Per serving (approximate–sandwich with cheese): 277 calories, 22 g protein, 29 g carbohydrate, 8 g fat, 35 mg cholesterol, 675 mg sodium
Good source of: iron, B vitamins, calcium, phosphorus

Food for Thought

• Which food groups are represented in this sandwich?
• What ingredients might you add or subtract for a flavor variation?

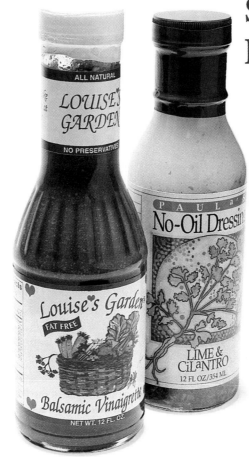

Salads and Dressings

Salads can be as simple as assortments of greens or fruits, or they can be hearty main dishes. Fresh fruit salads can be refreshing desserts or snacks. Depending on the ingredients, salads can provide servings from each of the five food groups.

Objectives

After studying this section, you should be able to:

- Describe how to select, wash, store, and serve several kinds of salad greens.
- Plan and assemble a salad using a variety of methods and ingredients.
- Identify ways to serve salads.

Look for These Terms

emulsion

base

body

Ingredients for Salads

Almost any ready-to-eat food from the five food groups can be used in a salad. Some of the basic foods include:

◆ **Salad greens.** To most people *salad* is synonymous with *lettuce*—which, in turn, translates to "iceberg lettuce." Yet, a wide variety of types of lettuce exist, from romaine, bibb, and Boston, to red leaf and curly leaf. Besides waking up a salad, these other lettuces, especially the darker greens, are higher in nutrients, such as vitamin C and iron. Beyond lettuce, the world of salad greens also includes spinach, arugula (uh-ROO-gyah-luh), escarole, chicory, watercress, and radicchio (rah-DEE-kee-oh). To add interest and nutrition, try a blend of greens in a salad. You can also buy pre-washed greens, packaged and ready to use.

◆ **Other vegetables and fruits.** You can toss any fruits and vegetables, fresh, canned, or cooked, in salads. They can be sliced, dried, shredded, quartered, or cubed. Use red or green cabbage for coleslaw or mixed with other greens.

◆ **Cooked and chilled pasta, grains, legumes, meat, poultry, fish, or eggs.** Prepare hearty main dish salads by mixing these foods with fruits and vegetables. Try this salad: Combine leftover chilled rice

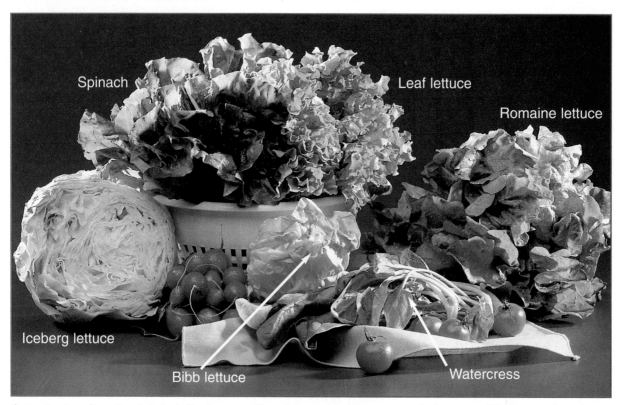

Spinach

Leaf lettuce

Romaine lettuce

Iceberg lettuce

Bibb lettuce

Watercress

◆ Varying ingredients in salads, including lettuce, adds variety to your eating patterns. Find as many of the lettuces shown here as you can in your local supermarket and note the price of each. Which type(s) would you eat on a daily basis?

and cooked dry beans, chopped onions, chopped tomatoes, seasonings, and greens. Sprinkle grated cheese as a topping. Serve with salsa or a splash of balsamic or cider vinegar.

Salad Dressings

Salad dressings not only add richness and flavor but also act as binding agents to hold salads together. There are several basic types of dressings:

◆ **Oil-based dressings.** Sometimes known as Italian or vinaigrette (vihn-uh-GREHT) dressings. Are a mixture of oil, vinegar, and seasonings. Typical vinaigrettes are made with 3 parts oil to 1 part vinegar. Oil-based dressings separate easily and must be mixed each time you use them.

◆ **Mayonnaise.** Made with oil, vinegar or lemon juice, seasonings, and eggs. Eggs create an **emulsion**—an evenly blended mixture of two liquids that do not normally stay mixed—which keeps the oil and acid from separating.

◆ **Cooked dressings.** Similar to mayonnaise, but use white sauce to replace some of the eggs and oil.

◆ **Dairy dressings.** Include ranch-type dressings. They usually have buttermilk, yogurt, sour cream, or cottage cheese as a main ingredient. Seasonings are added.

Low-Fat Dressings

Salad dressings are traditionally high in fat and calories—because of the oil used in making them. Today, however, many low-fat and

Some salad dressings and mayonnaise preparations contain raw eggs, placing you at risk for foodborne illness. When making dressings that call for raw eggs, cook the eggs in their shells to the soft-cooked stage, as described in Chapter 18. Beat the eggs together with the liquid in the dressing until the dressing achieves the proper consistency. Commercially manufactured mayonnaise and other egg-based dressings are made with pasteurized eggs, which makes them safe to eat.

fat-free dressings are available. Check the fat content on the label when you are selecting bottled or packaged salad dressings. Remember, the nutrients listed on the label are for one serving of 2 tablespoons (30 mL). Many people use far more than that. To counter this habit, think in teaspoons, not tablespoons, when dressing your salad.

When making salad dressing at home, try using nonfat yogurt to make a flavorful, low-calorie dressing. Add your favorite herbs and spices, prepared mustard and honey, or a dry prepared mix to vary the flavor. You can also experiment with fruit juices and flavored vinegars for some or all of the oil in recipes.

Making a Salad

What kind of salad should you put your dressing on? First, you need to decide how you plan to serve it. *Appetizer salads* are small, tasty salads served at the beginning of a meal to stimulate your appetite—for example, a shrimp cocktail or small garden salad. An *accompaniment salad* is a small salad served with a meal. Coleslaw, fruit salads, and mixed green salads are examples. *Main dish salads* make up the main course of a meal. They've become very popular on lunch menus.

They usually contain a protein-based food along with grains, fruits, and vegetables. For instance, a chef's salad is made with cooked meat, poultry, eggs, and cheese on a thick bed of assorted lettuce. A main dish salad is a great way to use leftovers. *Dessert salads* are usually made with fruit. Select a dessert salad for a sweet way to meet your daily requirement of at least two servings of fruit.

Preparing Salad Greens

If your salad has greens, you need to refrigerate them as soon as you get home from the supermarket. Greens grow close to the ground and thus may contain soil. Clean them before storing so that they will be ready to use.

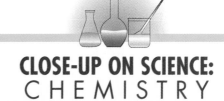

CLOSE-UP ON SCIENCE: CHEMISTRY

Emulsification

There is much truth to the saying that oil and water don't mix. You can shake the two liquids together to combine them temporarily. As soon as you stop shaking, however, the tiny oil droplets produced by the agitation begin to combine with one another. Soon the oil and water are separate again.

The egg yolks in mayonnaise contain a natural substance that acts as an *emulsifying* agent. This agent coats the oil droplets and causes them to repel one another. It also reduces the ability of the vinegar (which is mainly water) to repel the oil. Therefore, the oil stays in small droplets that remain evenly mixed throughout the dressing.

◆ **Iceberg lettuce.** Hold the head in your hands, core side down, as shown below. Hit the core on the counter once or twice to loosen it. Remove the core from the head. Let cold water run into the cavity for a minute or two until it pours out between the leaves. Place the head, core side down, in a colander and let it drain. Store the drained lettuce in a covered plastic container or in a plastic bag in the refrigerator.

◆ **Leafy greens.** Pull the leaves away from the core and wash them under cold running water. Place each leaf, stem side down, in a colander so that the water can drain off easily. You may also need to pat the greens dry before storage, but leave a little moisture to keep them crisp. Put the washed greens in a plastic container or in a large plastic bag, and refrigerate.

◆ **Premixed salad greens.** If you are using packaged premixed salad greens, don't assume they have been washed. Look for the words *washed* or *ready to eat* on the label. If they don't appear or if you're in doubt, wash the greens. Some mixed salad greens are sold in bulk in the produce section, where you use tongs to make your own selection. Always wash bulk mixed salad greens before using them.

Assembling the Salad

Salads are fun and easy to put together. Be creative: Choose a variety of textures and colors of greens, fruits, vegetables, or other foods for an attractive, healthful dish. The combinations are endless. So are the ways of presenting them. For an attractive touch, place a foundation of greens on the bottom of the salad bowl or plate—creating a **base** for

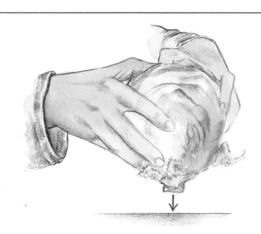

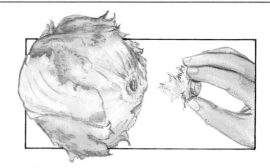

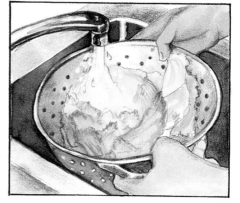

◆ Before washing iceberg lettuce, remove the core. Striking the head against a flat surface loosens the core so that it can be removed easily with the fingers. Drain leafy greens by standing them in a colander. Explain why it is important to wash lettuce even if you intend to use only the inner leaves.

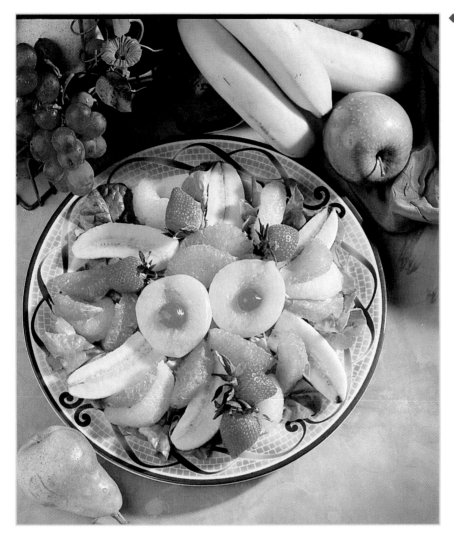

◆ **Making an arranged salad is an opportunity to develop your artistic skills. This refreshing fruit salad has been designed creatively.** Make a design for an arranged salad. Try to include items from at least three different groups in the Food Guide Pyramid.

your salad. Top with other salad ingredients to make up the **body**, or main part of the salad.

Here are a few hints, both plain and fancy, for presenting your salad creations:

◆ **Tossed or mixed salads.** This form of presentation includes the garden salad, a simple blend of greens and vegetables gently tossed with a dressing. For an attention-getting variation, present tossed salads in layers—for example, a layer of shredded greens, one of mashed cooked beans, and another of chopped tomatoes, all dressed with yogurt.

◆ **Arranged salads.** Salad ingredients can be arranged in one of a number of striking patterns, usually on a base of greens. One possibility is to fan fresh fruit slices around a mound of cottage cheese.

◆ **Molded salads.** Any salad mixture that holds its shape can be molded in a decorative container. Many molded salads are made with gelatin. Salads that contain a grain product, such as rice, and a binding agent, such as yogurt, also make attractive molded salads.

Serving Salads

Dress up your salads. Green salads often need the most help with their appearance. Arrange red pepper rings, grated carrots, sprouts, or other decorative vegetables on the greens. Then sprinkle with seeds, chopped nuts, or raisins. Add dressing just before serving. If dressing is added too early, the greens may wilt. Better still, serve the salad without dressing. Pass the dressing separately at the table so that people can add their own.

For added meal appeal and nutrition, nearly all salads can be served in edible "bowls," such as baked tortilla shells or hollowed-out fruits or vegetables. When in a rush, have your salad as a sandwich in a pita pocket.

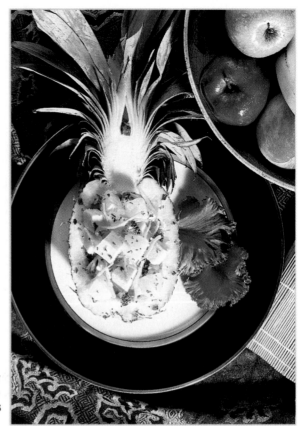

◆ Serving a mixed salad in a hollowed-out pineapple half makes a festive lunch main course. You begin by cutting the pineapple in half and carefully scooping out the fruit. Think of two other fruits or vegetables that could be used as edible "containers" for salad.

Section 20-2 Review & Activities

1. Name three kinds of salad greens. How should they be stored?

2. List three methods for assembling salads.

3. When should salad dressing be added to a green salad? Why?

4. **Analyzing.** Discuss some suggestions for cutting down on fat and calories commonly found in salad dressings.

5. **Synthesizing.** In a salad, how would you use leftover (a) chili, (b) roast beef, (c) grilled vegetables? List at least one example for each.

6. **Applying.** Describe at least two ideas for turning a small tossed salad into a main dish salad. Try one of these ideas. Write about your findings in your Wellness Journal.

RECIPE FILE

Garbanzo Salad with Honey-Mustard Dressing

Garbanzo beans, or chickpeas, provide valuable nutrients and fiber. They also combine well with other foods to create flavorful salads.

Customary	Ingredients	Metric
2 tsp.	Prepared mustard	10 mL
2 Tbsp.	Cider vinegar	30 mL
2 tsp.	Vegetable oil	10 mL
2 tsp.	Honey	10 mL
¼ tsp.	Celery seed	1 mL
8 leaves	Romaine lettuce	8 leaves
16-oz. can	Garbanzo beans, drained and rinsed	454-g can
1 large	Apple, cored and chopped	1 large
1 medium	Red or green pepper, chopped	1 medium
½ cup	Raisins	125 mL

Yield: 4 servings

Directions

1. In a small bowl, mix together mustard, vinegar, oil, honey, and celery seed. Set aside.
2. Tear lettuce into bite-size pieces.
3. In a large bowl, toss together lettuce, garbanzo beans, apple, pepper, and raisins.
4. Drizzle dressing over salad and toss.
5. Divide salad among four salad plates or bowls.
6. Serve immediately.

Nutrition Information

Per serving (approximate–salad with dressing): 233 calories, 7 g protein, 44 g carbohydrate, 5 g fat, 0 mg cholesterol, 459 mg sodium

Good source of: potassium, iron, vitamin A, vitamin E, vitamin C, B vitamins, phosphorus

Food for Thought

- Name one substitution you might make for each ingredient in the recipe.
- What could you do to keep the chopped apple from turning brown while you prepare the rest of the recipe?

Soups and Sauces

What comes to your mind when you hear the word soup? Whether you picture a soup kettle simmering away for hours, a can of your favorite flavor, or a container from a supermarket deli, soup can be a delicious, nutritious meal.

Objectives

After studying this section, you should be able to:

- Describe how to prepare clear, vegetable, and cream soups.
- Explain how to make and use white sauce and gravy.
- Explain how to make lower-fat sauce or gravy alternatives.

Look for These Terms

aromatic vegetables

stock

bouillon

white sauce

roux

au jus

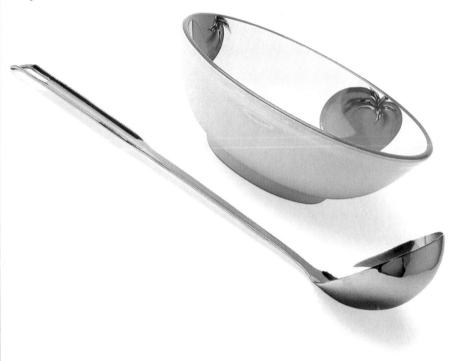

Making Soups

The first step in making most soups is to sauté **aromatic vegetables**, vegetables, such as onions, celery, and carrots, that add flavor to soups and other recipes. Sautéing vegetables before adding them helps develop the flavors. Use a stock pot and about 1 teaspoon (5 mL) of oil.

Next comes the liquid. Many soups start with **stock**, a clear, thin liquid made by simmering water flavored with the bones of meat, poultry, or fish, plus aromatic vegetables and seasonings. Many people today use canned convenience broths or bouillon cubes as a base for making

soup. You can also combine broth with a seasoned vegetable juice for additional flavor and nutrients.

Taste the soup and correct the seasonings just before serving. This will help you avoid over-seasoning the soup early in the cooking process.

Kinds of Soups

Soups are usually highly nutritious. Some B vitamins and vitamin C may be destroyed by heat, especially if the soup is cooked for a long time. Other water-soluble vitamins and minerals, however, remain in the liquid.

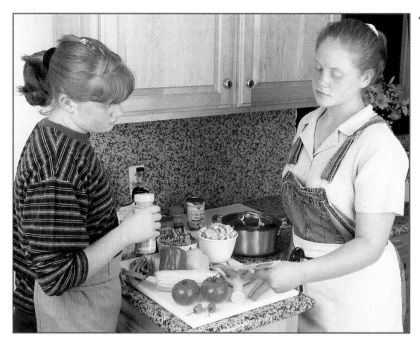

◆ Homemade soup doesn't have to take all day. Try starting with ready-made broth or vegetable juice. Add vegetables, grains, and leftover meat or poultry. What ingredients would you add to the ones shown to give your homemade soup a personal touch?

There are two main kinds of soups:

◆ **Clear soups.** These soups are usually based on unthickened, clear stock or broth. **Bouillon** (BOOL-yon) is a simple, clear soup without solid ingredients. Also called broth, the liquid is strained to remove any solids. Consommé (kahn-soh-MAY), the clearest broth, is rich and flavorful.

◆ **Thick soups.** Unlike clear soups, these soups are not transparent and they are thickened. One type, cream soup, is traditionally made with a **white sauce**—a milk-based sauce thickened with starch—plus cooked vegetables, poultry, or shellfish. Soups made this way can be high in fat.

Vegetable Soup

Vegetable soup, one of the most popular soups, is basically a clear soup with vegetables. Which vegetables are used is largely a matter of taste, although many recipes feature potatoes, tomatoes, peas, and corn, among others.

Use at least three or four different vegetables for a rich flavor and colorful appearance.

When adding the vegetables, begin with those that take the longest to cook. Then add the remaining vegetables according to the time needed for cooking. Season the soup with herbs and spices. Cover and simmer the soup only until the vegetables are tender.

For variety, flavor, and more nutrients, add cooked legumes or grain products (pasta, rice, or barley). These foods contain starch and will thicken the soup. You can also add cooked leftover meat and poultry sliced in thin strips or cut into small cubes. Making soup can be fun—and a terrific way to use leftovers.

Purées

Purées, thick, low-fat alternatives to cream soups, are unique since they are naturally thickened by mashing or grinding one or more of their ingredients. Black bean soup, made from puréed black beans, is a well-known choice.

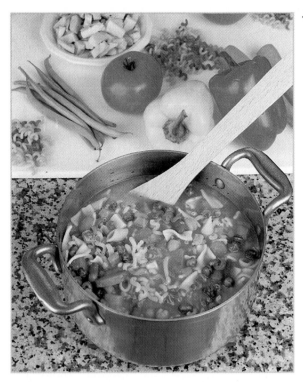

◆ A hearty soup is almost a meal in itself. Broth or cream soup might be served as a first course. What foods would you serve with the soup shown here to make a complete meal?

Vegetable soups can be prepared easily in the microwave oven. Chop the vegetables into uniform pieces, and add hot, lightly-seasoned water or broth. The hot liquid will help speed up the cooking process. Cook a larger quantity of soup in a covered, microwave-safe container to speed up cooking time. You may find, however, that larger quantities of soup take longer than on a conventional range.

Milk-based soups may foam during microwave cooking. Follow the directions in the owner's manual for the best results. Be sure to use a container that is the appropriate size.

Sauces and Gravies

Sauces and gravies are thickened liquids used to add flavor to cooked food. There are many different kinds of sauces and gravies. Most, however, are variations of a few basic types. Added ingredients and seasonings give each a distinct flavor.

Basic White Sauce

The most common sauce is white sauce. A white sauce begins with a **roux** (ROO), a blending of equal parts of flour and fat. The fat coats the starch granules to prevent them from lumping together when milk is added. Fat also adds richness to the sauce.

For a medium-thick sauce, use 2 tablespoons (30 mL) each of butter and flour for every 1 cup (250 mL) of milk. For a thinner sauce, use 1 tablespoon (15 mL) each of butter and flour.

Over medium to medium-high heat, melt the fat and whisk in the flour. Before the roux

Purées can be quick to fix, low in fat, and packed with nutrients. You can make a simple, low-fat purée using one or more puréed cooked vegetables, a starchy base, and enough stock or broth for desired consistency. Fat-free dry milk can be added, too.

You can vary the recipe by substituting different vegetables or dry legumes. Potatoes or cooked rice help thicken the soup and provide a starchy base. Purée all the cooked vegetables or legumes with the rice or potatoes for the smoothest, creamiest texture. Consider adding puréed rice or potatoes to other soups, too—for creaminess without adding cream or other high-fat products.

Cooking Soup in the Microwave Oven

Try making your own soup stock in the microwave oven. Microwaving can take less time than conventional cooking. Check a microwave cookbook for directions.

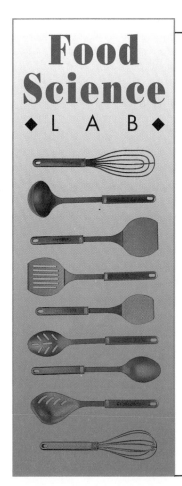

Food Science
◆ L A B ◆

What's the Best Thickener?

Cornstarch and flour are the most common thickening agents in home kitchens. Which provides the best overall thickening?

Procedure

1. In each of two pots, simmer 1 cup (250 mL) milk.

2. In separate covered jars, mix equal parts cornstarch and cold water, and flour and cold water.

3. Whisk one of the liquefied thickeners into one pot, the other thickener into the other pot. Compare the results in terms of thickness, ease of incorporation, and texture.

Conclusions

◆ How do the textures differ? Which starch would give the best results when making a clear fruit sauce?

◆ Did either starch clump up? If so, how could this affect your recipe results? How do you think the results would differ if you blended each starch with warm liquid?

◆ Which starch had more thickening ability?

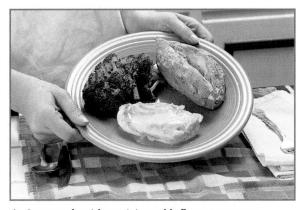

◆ **Gravy made with pan juices adds flavor to meat or poultry.** How can you reduce the fat in the gravy?

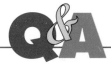

Q How can I rescue lumpy gravy or sauce?

A If a few lumps occur, put the sauce or gravy through a strainer. Reheat the mixture, stirring constantly, and serve.

browns, add the milk. Cook the mixture over low heat, stirring constantly, until it thickens. Season the sauce, as desired. The sauce should be thick enough to coat the back of a wooden spoon.

Pan Gravy

Pan gravy is made like white sauce, but with meat juices instead of milk. For traditional pan gravy, remove the meat from the pan and pour the juices that remain into a measuring cup. Skim off and reserve the fat. Measure the remaining broth. Use 2 tablespoons (30 mL) each of fat and flour for each cup (250 mL) of meat broth. Make a roux, and heat until it starts to brown. Gradually add the meat broth, and stir constantly until smooth and thickened. Scrape the bottom of the pan to loosen browned meat particles. This adds flavor to the gravy.

Lower-Fat Alternatives

White sauce and gravy are traditionally high in fat. Consider using seasoned nonfat yogurt in place of white sauce. Instead of serving roasts with gravy, try serving them **au jus**—with the pan drippings from which the fat has been skimmed. The easiest way to skim fat is to wait until the drippings have cooled. The fat, which will rise to the top, may be easily removed with a spoon.

To make lower-fat gravy, shake a mixture of 2 tablespoons (30 mL) flour or cornstarch and ¼ cup (50 mL) cold water in a covered container. Then add it to 1 cup (250 mL) of broth, and heat the mixture to boiling, stirring constantly. Cook the mixture until it thickens, about 1 minute.

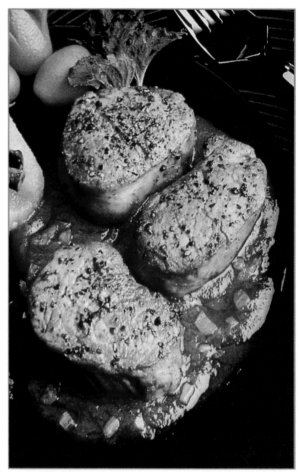

◆ Thickened, defatted pan drippings can add flavor to meat. Describe the steps involved in removing fat.

Section 20-3 Review & Activities

1. What are aromatic vegetables? Why are they sautéed?

2. Describe how to make stock.

3. What is a lower-fat alternative to serving gravy with roasted meat?

4. Comparing and Contrasting. How would a white sauce that started with a roux be different from one in which flour was added by itself to a liquid?

5. Analyzing. How might a family's food budget be stretched by serving soup as a main dish?

6. Applying. Create a recipe for a vegetable soup that you can prepare in 1 hour. What pre-preparation tasks could you do to cut down on the cooking time?

RECIPE FILE

Creamy Potato Soup

This soup is a good source of calcium with less fat than traditional cream soups.

Customary	Ingredients	Metric
1 clove	Garlic, minced	1 clove
¼ cup	Chopped onion	75 mL
¼ cup	Chopped celery	75 mL
1 Tbsp.	Vegetable oil	15 mL
3	Potatoes, peeled and cubed	3
4 cups	Reduced-sodium chicken broth	1 L
½ cup	Nonfat dry milk	125 mL

Yield: 4 servings, one cup each

Directions

1. In a Dutch oven or a stock pot, sauté garlic, onion, and celery in oil.
2. Add potatoes and chicken broth. Bring to a boil.
3. Reduce heat and simmer until potatoes are tender, about 15 minutes.
4. Carefully purée the soup in a blender or food processor.
5. Return puréed soup to pot. Stir in dry milk.
6. Simmer until thoroughly heated.
7. Season to taste and serve hot.

Note: For a chunkier soup, purée only half the soup before stirring in the dry milk.

Nutrition Information

Per serving (approximate): 192 calories, 10 g protein, 27 g carbohydrate, 5 g fat, 2 mg cholesterol, 641 mg sodium

Good source of: potassium, vitamin E, vitamin C, B vitamins, calcium, phosphorus

Food for Thought

• What is used to thicken this soup?
• What other vegetables could you add to this soup for flavor and variation?

Casseroles and Other Combinations

If you were to trace the history of food preparation to its earliest known roots, you would find a common link among the cooking habits of various primitive cultures. That link is the one-pot meal. In addition to its potential for providing servings from all five food groups, the one-pot meal—whether a stew, braised meat, stir-fry, or casserole—is a convenient solution for families with little time to cook.

Objectives

After studying this section, you should be able to:

- Plan and prepare hearty one-dish meals using a variety of ingredients.

- Explain how to prepare lower-fat one-dish meals.

- Explain several methods used to prepare one-dish meals.

Look for These Terms

extender

binder

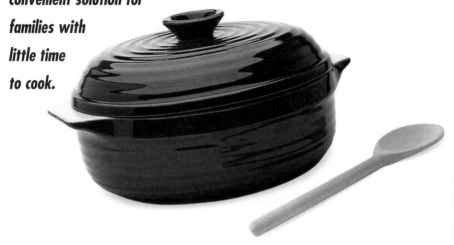

Stews

Stewing is an efficient way to cook some less tender cuts of meat or poultry. Fish and shellfish stews are delicious, too.

Stews may be made with a variety of vegetables. Potatoes or other starchy vegetables can be added for thickness. Also consider using sliced apples, dried apricots, or other fruits.

Although water is the basic liquid in stew, try substituting broth or vegetable juice for part of the water. Tomato juice, for example, contains acid, which helps tenderize meat and adds flavor.

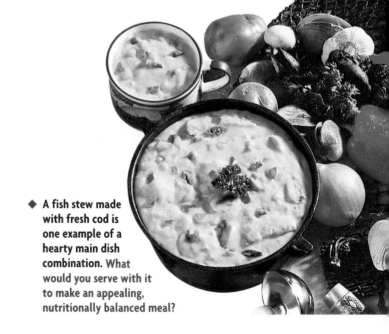

◆ A fish stew made with fresh cod is one example of a hearty main dish combination. What would you serve with it to make an appealing, nutritionally balanced meal?

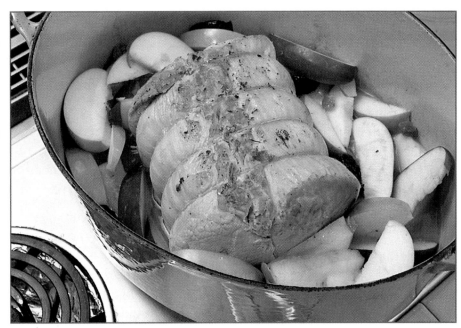

◆ **Fresh or dried fruits can be included in stewed meat dishes to perk up the flavor and add nutrients.** Consult the "Nutritive Value of Foods" table in Appendix B to determine the number of grams of food energy provided by adding a whole sliced apple to this stewed pork. How many grams of fat does the fruit add?

Cooking Time

The cooking time of a stew varies with the tenderness of the main ingredient. Fish stews, for example, take just enough time for the fish to flake and the flavors to become blended. Beef stew may need 2 or 3 hours to cook, while poultry may cook in 1 hour.

Cooking times also vary with the appliance used. A beef stew can cook in 30 minutes in a pressure cooker, 1 hour in a microwave oven, 2 to 3 hours on the range top or in a conventional oven, or about 9 hours in a slow cooker.

Vegetables and fruits may need different amounts of cooking times, depending on tenderness and the size of the pieces. Add them to the stew according to the amount of cooking time needed. Those that will take the longest to cook—chunks of fresh carrot, for instance —should be added early in the process. Items such as frozen peas or corn, which take less time to cook, can be added later. Canned vegetables or leftover cooked vegetables can be added near the end of the cooking time.

To stew meat on the range top, brown cubes of meat without added fat in a large pan. This creates a darker, more flavorful stew and helps the meat keep its shape. Remove the meat cubes to a clean plate. In the same pan, sauté aromatic vegetables in a small amount of fat; then return the browned meat to the pan. Add seasonings and enough liquid to cover the meat. Cover the pan and simmer until tender, adding the other ingredients during the cooking time, as explained above.

Before stewing poultry, cut it into parts or other large pieces. Remove the skin to reduce fat.

Braised Foods

Braising is used to cook large, less tender cuts of meat and poultry. It can also be used to give flavor to tender cuts. Fish, for example, is sometimes braised in a flavorful sauce.

Meat is often browned before braising; usually, poultry is not. Place the meat or poultry in a Dutch oven or other heavy pan. Add enough liquid to cover the bottom and create steam. Add onions, garlic, herbs, spices, and other seasonings. Cover the pan and bake at 350°F (180°C), or simmer on top of the range.

Add other vegetables as the meat braises. Large items, such as halved or quartered potatoes and carrot halves, need to be added toward the beginning. Add peas, corn, or other quick-cooking vegetables near the end of the cooking time. Consider adding fresh or canned fruit for a different flavor. Some tasty combinations are pork with peeled and quartered fresh apples (or applesauce), poultry with pineapple or orange juice, fish with lemon or grapefruit juice, beef with prunes or dried apricots, and lamb with canned plums.

Check the food at frequent intervals to be sure enough liquid remains to cover the bottom of the pan. Add water as needed. To thicken the gravy, add a diced potato an hour before serving.

The total cooking time depends on the size and cut of the meat. Cook until the ingredients are tender and the flavors are well blended.

Stir-Fries

Stir-frying is a quick and easy way to make a flavorful, nutrient-rich dish. It can be low in fat if you choose your ingredients carefully.

The secret to successful stir-fried foods is to cut up all the ingredients and assemble them in the order they are to be cooked. Because stir-frying is fast, there's no time to stop and cut up foods while you're cooking. High heat is also essential to cook food quickly and keep vegetables crisp.

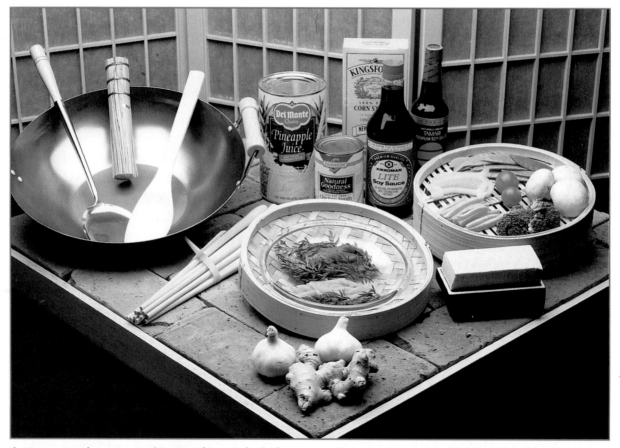

◆ You can use almost any combination of protein foods, fruits, vegetables, seasonings, and sauces in a stir-fry. Why is it important to slice each type of food uniformly?

Pre-preparation

Cut raw meat or poultry across the grain into thin, narrow strips. Meat that has been chilled in the freezer will be easier to slice. Cubes or strips of tofu or cooked meat, poultry, or fish can also be used. Vegetables should be cut into pieces of uniform size to ensure even cooking.

Stir-Frying Basics

The wok is ideal for stir-frying. It has a rounded bottom and sits on a metal ring placed on the range. Electric woks are also available. If you don't have a wok, you can use a large non-stick skillet.

The pan is ready for cooking when a few drops of water sizzle and evaporate immediately. Heat 1 to 2 tablespoons (15 to 30 mL) of oil. Add garlic, ginger, or seasonings and cook for a few seconds to flavor the oil. Next, add the meat, poultry, or fish. Keep the pieces in motion constantly so that they don't burn.

When this main ingredient has finished cooking, transfer it to a clean plate and proceed to the vegetables. Cook dense, fibrous items, such as broccoli and carrots, first. (You can also precook them in the microwave oven.) Then cook the remaining vegetables. When they are done, return the cooked main ingredient to the wok or skillet.

If you like, you can complete your stir-fry with a sauce by adding a mixture of cornstarch and stock or light, reduced-sodium soy sauce. (If you plan on stir-frying often, you may want to keep a small jar of this premixed solution handy in the refrigerator.) Stir until the sauce begins to thicken.

As you stir-fry, avoid overloading the pan. Putting too much food in the pan at one time will result in vegetables that are steamed, not stir-fried.

Stir-Fry Suggestions

In additional to being flavorful and helping you meet daily nutrient needs from several food groups, stir-fries are easy to prepare and versatile.

- **Seasonings.** ¼ to ½ teaspoon (1 to 3 mL) grated raw ginger, pressed garlic, crushed, dried thyme or marjoram.

- **Protein.** 1 cup (250 mL) cubed tofu, meat, poultry, or fish.

- **Vegetables or fruits.** 3 cups (750 mL) of at least three bite-size vegetables and fruits.

- **Sauce.** Mix 1 tablespoon (15 mL) cornstarch with 1 tablespoon (15 mL) tamari sauce, soy sauce, or prepared mustard to make a paste. Add 1 cup (250 mL) canned broth, fruit juice, or vegetable juice, and mix well. (Since cornstarch is added, this sauce will thicken when thoroughly heated.)

Pizza

Pizza is a hearty main dish served on a crust. Traditional pizza calls for a yeast bread crust topped with a tomato-based sauce, cheese (generally mozzarella), and other toppings. However, numerous variations are possible.

To bake pizza at home, use any large shallow pan. Pick your favorite flavor combinations using the following list as a guide. Be sure to add your own innovative choices to the list.

- **Base.** One ready-made or homemade crust.

- **Seasonings.** A small amount of garlic, oregano, basil, marjoram, pepper, cayenne, cinnamon, nutmeg, or chili powder.

- **Sauce.** Canned pizza, pasta, taco, or chili sauce; salsa; puréed fresh or canned fruit.

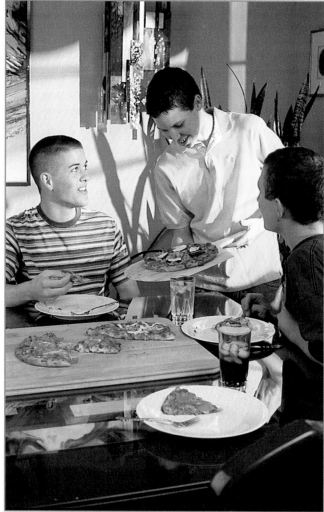

◆ Making pizza at home is easy and can be fun. These teens have come up with some combinations that feature a rice crust and vegetables as toppings. Plan a class pizza party. Have each person bring a different ingredient to include.

◆ **Toppings.** Chopped or sliced veggies; pineapple slices; cooked or canned meat, poultry, or fish.

◆ **Grated cheese.** Mozzarella, feta, gouda, cheddar, Swiss, or parmesan.

Pizza is generally baked in an oven preheated to 425°F (220°C). The cooking time may vary depending on the pizza size and the ingredients. Check a cookbook for cooking times.

Casseroles

A casserole is a tasty blend of cooked ingredients that are heated together to develop flavor.

There are three main parts to a casserole. The base of a casserole provides its main texture and flavor. It also needs an **extender**, a food ingredient that helps thicken a dish—for example, rice or pasta—and a **binder**, a liquid that holds the other ingredients together. Seasonings and aromatic vegetables give heightened flavor and added texture. Here are some suggestions for casserole combinations:

◆ **Base.** Cubed, cooked meat, poultry, or fish; browned, drained ground beef or poultry; grated or cubed cheese.

◆ **Vegetables.** Any cooked or canned vegetables.

◆ **Extenders.** Dry breadcrumbs; cooked, diced potatoes, pasta, rice, grits, or barley; cooked, mashed dry beans.

◆ **Aromatic vegetables.** Chopped celery or bell pepper; sautéed mushrooms, onions, or garlic.

◆ **Seasonings.** Dried, crushed oregano, basil, thyme, or marjoram; ground ginger, mace, cinnamon, chili powder, cayenne or black pepper. Start with ¼ teaspoon (1 mL). You can always add more to taste.

◆ **Binders.** Fat-free milk, broth, fruit juice, soup, eggs, or a thickened sauce.

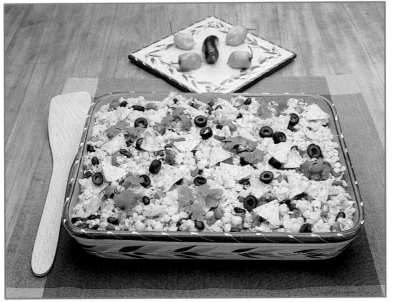

◆ Casseroles like this spicy southwestern blend of corn, rice, beans, peppers, and other ingredients make interesting and varied one-dish meals. In what ways do casseroles save time and energy when planning and preparing meals?

Cooking a Casserole

To make a casserole for four people, combine 1 cup (250 mL) of each ingredient choice (except for seasonings). Place the mixture in a 1½ quart (1.5 L) covered baking dish that has been coated with cooking oil spray. Bake the casserole about 30 minutes in an oven preheated to 350°F (180°C). Remove the cover after 20 minutes if the liquid needs to thicken.

To microwave a casserole, combine the ingredients in an ungreased baking dish with a cover. Cook the casserole at 100 percent power for 6 to 18 minutes, depending on the ingredients. Stir once or twice during cooking, and rotate the casserole halfway through the cooking time.

Casseroles can save you time and energy when planning and preparing meals. Enjoy the variety of food choices used to make casseroles —and all other combination dishes.

Section 20-4 Review & Activities

1. Stewing or braising is an ideal cooking technique for what types of meat? Give two examples.

2. Why must stir-fry ingredients be cut up and assembled before you start cooking?

3. Name three main parts of any casserole. Give an example of each.

4. Analyzing. Discuss reasons why combination foods, such as those detailed in this section, are good, economical choices for many families.

5. Synthesizing. How can stews be modified for people who need low-fat meals? How can casseroles be modified?

6. Applying. Develop a list of at least six ingredients that you could use in making three of the one-dish meals discussed in this section. What foods might you need to have on hand for "emergency" one-dish meals?

RECIPE FILE

Whitefish Stir-Fry

Stir-fried dishes can include an endless variety of ingredients. The combinations provide not only flavor, but texture and meal appeal, too.

Customary	Ingredients	Metric
1 Tbsp.	Cornstarch	15 mL
1 Tbsp.	Reduced-sodium tamari or soy sauce	15 mL
1 cup	Pineapple juice	250 mL
1 Tbsp.	Vegetable oil	15 mL
1 clove	Garlic, minced	1 clove
1 cup	Snow peas	250 mL
1 cup	Red or green pepper, chopped	250 mL
½ cup	Sliced water chestnuts	125 mL
1 cup	Pineapple chunks	250 mL
1 cup	Whitefish fillets, cooked and cubed	250 mL
	Hot cooked rice (optional)	

Yield: 4 servings, one cup each on rice

Directions

1. In a small bowl, combine cornstarch with tamari or soy sauce. Add pineapple juice and mix well. Set aside.

2. Heat oil in wok or a large, nonstick skillet. Add garlic and sauté a few seconds to flavor the oil.

3. Add snow peas, pepper, water chestnuts, and pineapple.

4. Cook, stirring constantly, until snow peas and pepper are tender-crisp.

5. Add cooked whitefish to vegetables.

6. Mix the sauce from Step 1 and pour it over the mixture.

7. Cook, stirring constantly, until mixture is thickened and fish is thoroughly heated.

8. Serve over hot cooked rice, if desired.

Nutrition Information

Per serving (approximate–stir-fry only): 169 calories, 15 g protein, 17 g carbohydrate, 4 g fat, 54 mg cholesterol, 202 mg sodium

Good source of: potassium, vitamin E, vitamin C, B vitamins, phosphorus

Food for Thought

• How could you cut the vegetables or fish to vary their appearance?
• How can you tell when the oil is hot enough for cooking?

CAREER WANTED

Individuals who communicate effectively and are willing to work long hours.

REQUIRES:

- background in purchasing or business
- problem-solving skills
- paying close attention to detail

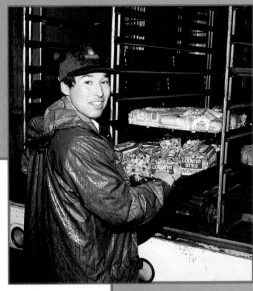

"We are changing the image of airline food,"

says Ivan Kai, Food Service Supplier

Q: Ivan, what do you do as a food service supplier?

A: My company, also known as a "provisioner," buys food from wholesalers, makes it into meals, and sells the meal packages to major airlines. There are several provisioners, all in competition for the same contracts. It means finding the best prices.

Q: What is your biggest challenge on the job?

A: It's overcoming the negative image people have of airline food. People don't understand the challenge of finding foods that can be reheated or prepared in a kitchen the size of a small closet—and that's only the tip of the iceberg!

Q: What do you mean?

A: Well, there's the need to create healthful menus that will capture people's interest. On top of that are the special needs meals, like those requested by vegetarians.

Q: What kind of credentials do you need for this line of work?

A: Most suppliers have experience in the food service industry and at least a two-year degree. Since I also supervise our kitchens, my bachelor's degree in Food Management is required.

Career Research Activity

1. Imagine that 50 years in the future there are commercial space flights between Earth and other planets. What special challenges would a food service supplier likely face? What advances in both food and nutrition and technology would be needed to face these challenges? Prepare an oral report of your view on this situation.

2. Which of the entry level jobs above would best prepare you to be a food service supplier? Why? Which of the three professional jobs would seem the most appealing to a food service supplier? Why?

Related Career Opportunities

Entry Level
- Waitperson
- Produce Worker
- Food Preparation Worker

Technical Level
- Food Service Supplier
- Passenger Service Representative

Professional Level
- Professional Chef
- Nutritionist
- Purchasing Agent

Chapter 20 Review & Activities

——— Summary ———

Section 20-1: Sandwiches, Snacks, and Packed Lunches

- Sandwiches can be as varied as the ingredients from which they are made.
- Nutritious snacks are part of a healthful eating plan.
- When packing lunches, keep hot foods hot and cold foods cold.

Section 20-3: Soups and Sauces

- There are two main types of soups: clear soups and thick soups.
- Soups often rely on aromatic vegetables for flavoring.
- You can use quick and easy methods to make low-fat soups.
- Sauces and gravies can add flavor to cooked foods. Keep sauces and gravies low in fat.

Section 20-2: Salads and Dressings

- Salads may include greens, fresh fruits or vegetables, cheese, and cooked grains, legumes, meat, poultry, fish, or eggs.
- Basic dressings include oil-based, mayonnaise, cooked, and dairy varieties. Many options for low-fat dressings exist.
- For appealing salads, find artful ways to make and serve them.

Section 20-4: Casseroles and Other Combinations

- One-dish meals can be healthful choices.
- Types of one-dish meals include stews, braised dishes, stir-fries, pizza, and casseroles.
- Combination dishes have variety and creativity in the kind and amounts of ingredients used.

Working IN THE Lab

1. **Taste Test.** Plan and prepare one or two sandwich fillings and toppings. Use a variety of breads to make up enough sandwiches so that each person can sample a piece of each sandwich. Discuss how these foods measure up to the recommendations of the Food Guide Pyramid.

2. **Foods Lab.** Plan and prepare a main dish salad that uses at least one ingredient from each of the five food groups. If possible, invite some teachers to a luncheon to share it.

Checking Your Knowledge

1. What is the difference between a fancy sandwich and a club sandwich?

2. How can you keep pocket sandwiches from absorbing moist fillings?

3. What are two ways to keep packaged lunches cold? Why is food temperature important?

4. What is the basic difference between an oil-based dressing and a mayonnaise dressing?

5. What are the base and body of a salad?

6. Name one way vegetable soups and purées are the same and one way they are different.

7. How can you keep a sauce made with flour from becoming lumpy?

8. Why is meat often browned before stewing?

9. When braising, how much liquid should you add to the pan?

10. Why is high heat essential for stir-frying?

Thinking Critically

1. Determining Accuracy. Compare the labels of several popular salad dressings, including some lower-fat varieties. Rate them in terms of fat and sodium content. How do their ratings compare with the claims or descriptions on the label?

2. Comparing and Contrasting. Examine a can of ready-made gravy, a package of gravy mix, and a can of cream soup, such as mushroom, that may be used for gravy. Using the same serving size for each, calculate the calories and fat. Which rates the highest and lowest in each category? How do your findings compare with the commonly held assumption that gravies are calorie-laden additions to meals?

Reinforcing Key Skills

1. Communication. Write a proposal to the administration of your school presenting concrete and persuasive arguments for adding a salad bar in the school lunchroom. In your proposal, point out the importance of excluding high-fat dressings and other high-fat toppings. Provide reasons for your statements.

2. Management. What specific planning and pre-preparation steps are required to prepare a soup of choice in 15 minutes or less? A stir-fry?

Making Decisions and Solving Problems

Your school sports team is leaving for an all-day tournament in the morning. The coach told each athlete to pack one meal to eat at noon and another to eat in the evening because there will be no stops along the way. What would you pack?

Making Connections

1. Social Studies. Use library references or cookbooks to find out what sandwiches are popular in other cultures. One possibility you might investigate is the *smørbrød* of Denmark. Report to the class on at least two different sandwiches. Include a description of each sandwich and a list of the ingredients in each one. If possible, prepare samples to bring to class.

2. Language Arts. Write a short essay on one of the following topics:
 a. The sandwiches I ate as a child were memorable.
 b. If I were a salad, I would be a [name a type of salad] because . . .
 c. More than just a meal, soup may help you feel better when you're not well.
 d. I recommend pizza for breakfast, lunch, dinner, and dessert.

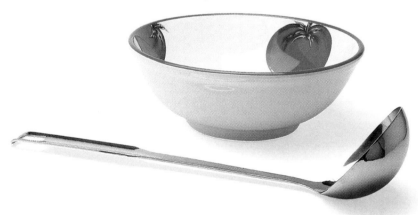

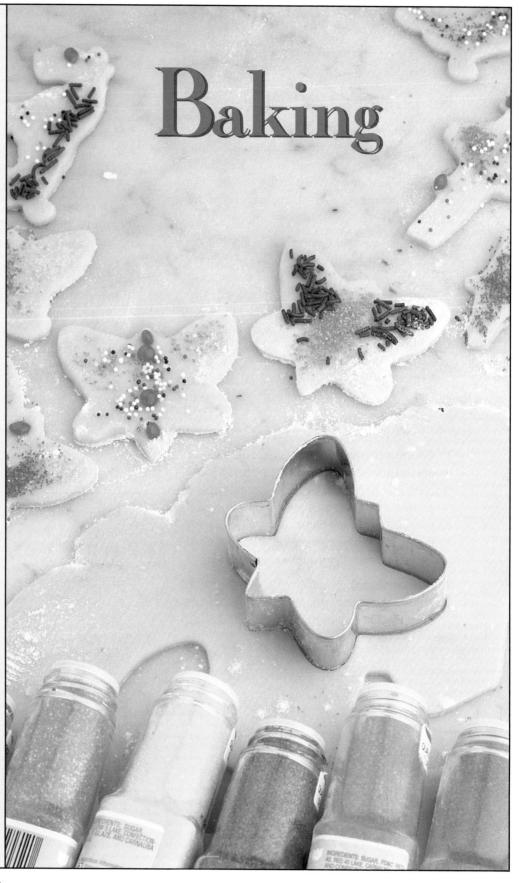

CHAPTER

21

Baking

Section 21-1
Ingredients and Techniques for Baking

Section 21-2
Quick Breads

Section 21-3
Yeast Breads and Rolls

Section 21-4
Cakes, Cookies, and Pies

How can a few ingredients make a moist, light cake or an apple pie with a flaky crust? The secret lies in the amounts of the ingredients used and how they are combined and baked. In this chapter, you will learn about ingredients and techniques used for baking.

Ingredients and Techniques for Baking

Objectives

After studying this section, you should be able to:

- Identify the basic ingredients in baking and the function of each.
- Explain how to select and prepare pans for baking.
- Compare conventional and microwave baking.

Look for These Terms

gluten

leavening agent

knead

Have you ever passed a bakery and been lured in by the aroma of cookies, cakes, and other baked goods?

Although it is hard to imagine, all these items start off with the same few basic ingredients.

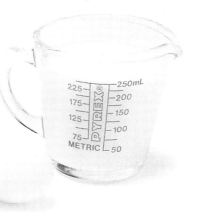

Ingredient Basics

The ingredients common to all baking are flour, liquid, leavening agents, fat, sweeteners, eggs, and flavoring. Baked goods are generally nutritious, but many are high in fat, sugar, and calories.

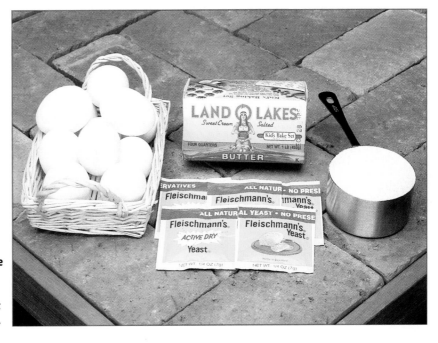

◆ **Ingredients such as these are common to many different baked goods.** Identify the specific role each ingredient shown plays in baked goods.

Flour

One ingredient you'll find in nearly every baked product is flour. The proteins and starch in flour make up most of a baked product's structure. **Gluten** (GLOO-ten), a protein that affects the texture of a baked product, helps determine how the product will rise. Starch helps absorb some of the liquid that is added in most baking recipes.

Types of Flour

There are many types of flours. All vary in gluten content.

- **All-purpose flour.** The most popular flour in American kitchens. It gives good results for most products.

- **Bread flour.** Has the highest gluten content and gives bread a strong structure.

- **Cake flour.** Contains less gluten and gives cakes a tender structure.

Whole-Grain Flour

Whole-grain flours have weaker gluten than all-purpose flour. Some whole-grain flours have no gluten at all. This explains why products made with only whole-grain flour rise less and have a heavy texture. Whole-grain flours include wheat, rye, and cornmeal.

To overcome this limitation, whole-grain flours are generally combined with all-purpose flour in equal proportions in recipes. Note that whole-grain flours need to be stirred rather than sifted—the particles are too large to go through a sifter.

Since they contain some fat, whole-grain flours should be stored in the refrigerator to keep them fresh. Store other flours in airtight containers in a cool, dry place.

Liquid

Liquids play a role in the many physical and chemical changes that occur during baking. Water and milk are the most common liquids used in baking. Milk adds flavor and nutrients, and helps baked goods brown better. To reduce fat in a recipe, use fat-free milk instead of whole milk.

Some recipes call for buttermilk, which gives a slightly tangy flavor. Buttermilk also makes the mixture more acid and affects the kind of leavening agent needed.

Leavening Agents

What is the difference between a cake that turns out flat and one that rises nicely? One answer is the use of a **leavening agent**, a substance that triggers a chemical action causing a baked product to rise. Leavening agents make most baked products less compact and give them a softer texture.

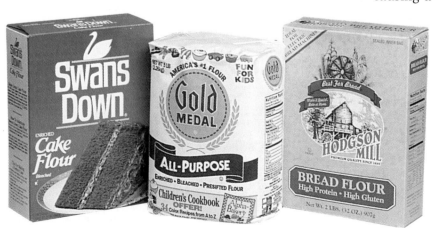

- Knowing the specific purpose of each of the many types of flour is central to becoming a versatile baker. Explain the differences among the three types of flour shown.

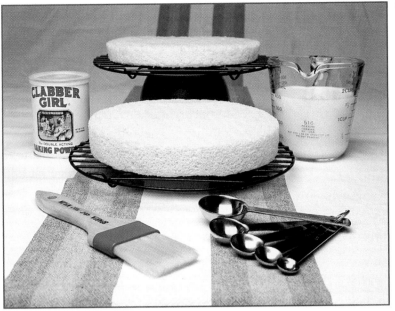

◆ Leavening agents can be the difference in whether a cake rises like the top layer or the bottom layer as seen here. Identify three different leavening agents in the school foods lab.

can be stored at room temperature. *Compressed yeast* comes in individually wrapped cakes and must be refrigerated. Use yeast before the expiration date on the package.

Types of Leavening Agents

Here is a list of leavening agents and a description of how each works:

◆ **Air.** Is trapped in mixtures as they are beaten. Creaming fat and sugar, sifting flour, and adding beaten egg whites all add air to a baked good. When the mixture is heated, the trapped air expands and the product rises. Angel food cake is leavened mainly by air in beaten egg whites.

◆ **Steam.** Leavens products that contain high amounts of water. As the product bakes, the water heats. Eventually, it turns into steam, which expands, causing the product to rise. Popovers and cream puffs use steam for leavening.

◆ **Yeast.** A microorganism that produces carbon dioxide gas as it grows. It needs food (such as flour or sugar), liquid, and a warm temperature to grow. Several forms of yeast are available. *Active dry yeast* and *quick-rising dry yeast* come as dry granules in a packet. The quick-rising type leavens the dough about twice as quickly. Both

◆ **Baking soda.** Is used whenever the recipe calls for buttermilk, yogurt, sour milk, or other acidic liquid. When combined with this type of liquid, baking soda produces carbon dioxide gas.

◆ **Baking powder.** Is made of baking soda and a powdered acid such as cream of tartar. The most common type, double-acting baking powder, releases some carbon dioxide gas when it is first mixed with a liquid. The remainder is released when it is heated.

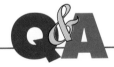

Q I baked a cake that didn't rise. What went wrong?

A One possible problem is the baking powder, which will work only if the ingredients in it are still active. You can test whether baking powder is fresh by mixing 1 teaspoon (5 mL) with ⅓ cup (75 mL) of hot water. If it bubbles quickly, it is still active.

Fat

Although it contributes calories to many baked products, fat adds richness, flavor, and tenderness. Fats can be solid or liquid.

Solid and liquid fats are not easily substituted for one another. In place of butter or shortening, you can use regular margarine, but do not use soft, whipped, or liquid margarine or spreads. They may contain air, water, or oil, which can affect the results. You can substitute solid shortening for butter or margarine. Any cooking oil may be used in baking, as long as it has a mild flavor.

Since fats play an important role in baked products, they usually can't be eliminated. However, they can often be reduced or partially substituted with other flavorful ingredients. Applesauce or puréed dried fruits are common substitutes.

Refrigerate lard, butter, and margarine. Store shortening and oils at room temperature unless the label directs otherwise.

Eggs

Eggs add flavor, nutrients, richness, and color to baked products. They also help form the structure of the baked product. When beaten, eggs add air to the mixture. To reduce fat and cholesterol, use two egg whites or ¼ cup (50 mL) liquid egg substitute in place of one whole egg.

Sweeteners

Sugar is the most commonly used sweetener. It helps make baked products tender, adds sweetness and flavor, and helps the crust brown. Granulated white sugar and brown sugar are used in many recipes. Other sweeteners include honey, corn syrup, molasses, and powdered sugar. Some sugar substitutes are suitable for baking, but others are not. Follow the manufacturers' recommendations.

Store most sweeteners in tightly covered containers in a cool place. Some sweeteners should be refrigerated after opening. Follow label directions.

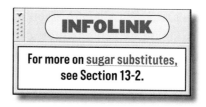

INFOLINK

For more on sugar substitutes, see Section 13-2.

◆ **Fat adds richness, flavor, and tenderness to baked goods.** List four guidelines for fat usage in baking and storage.

Flavorings

Fruits, vegetables, and nuts add flavor, texture, and nutrients to baked goods. Herbs, spices, and extracts are used in small amounts to add flavor. Some sweet spices—for instance, cinnamon and nutmeg—can actually enhance the flavor enough to allow you to cut back slightly on sugar.

Extracts are flavorings in a liquid form. Vanilla and almond are two common varieties. Store herbs, spices, and extracts in tightly closed containers in a cool, dry area.

Combining the Ingredients

The success of a baked product depends on not only the ingredients used, but also the order in which they are combined. During the mixing process, changes take place that affect the texture of the finished product.

The Role of Gluten

When flour and liquid are mixed together, the gluten in flour develops, or becomes strong and elastic. It forms a network of tiny air cells. Air, steam, or gas produced by the leavening agent is trapped by these cells. When heated, the trapped gases expand and the product rises.

The longer the mixing time, the greater the extent to which gluten is developed. For example, ingredients for cakes and quick breads are mixed only long enough to combine them. As a result, the gluten is not strong. The cells remain small and the network stretches very little. This results in a fine, tender texture.

Yeast breads, on the other hand, are mixed much longer than cakes. The dough for yeast bread is worked with the hands to develop the gluten. As a result, the gluten is very elastic and expands easily. Larger air cells are produced, giving yeast breads a coarser texture.

Batters and Doughs

The amount of liquid in relation to the amount of flour determines whether a mixture is a batter or a dough, and affects how you handle the mixture. Batters have more liquid than doughs. There are four kinds of batters and doughs:

◆ **Pour batters.** Are thin enough to pour in a steady stream. They are used to make cakes, pancakes, and waffles.

◆ **Drop batters.** Are thick and are usually spooned into pans. They are used to make some quick breads and cookies.

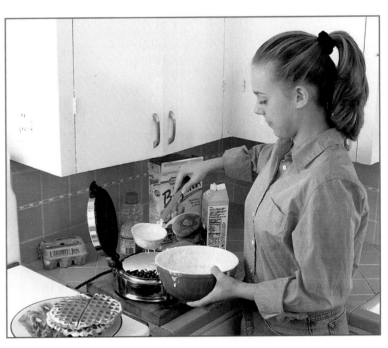

◆ Waffles are one baked product made from a batter. Identify the type of batter used to make each of the following: waffles, cookies, pancakes, quick breads.

- **Soft doughs.** Are soft and sticky but can be touched and handled. Rolled biscuits, yeast breads and rolls, and some cookies start with soft doughs.

- **Stiff doughs.** Are firm to the touch. Easy to work with and cut, they form the basis for piecrust and some cookies.

Methods of Mixing

There are several basic methods for combining ingredients. All will be explored later in this chapter. Use the method called for in the recipe you have chosen.

Unless the recipe directs otherwise, have all ingredients at room temperature before mixing. Thirty minutes is long enough to warm refrigerated items.

Kneading

After some dough is mixed, you may have to **knead** it, or work the dough with your hands to thoroughly mix ingredients and develop gluten. Kneading is a four-step process:

1. Turn the dough out on a very lightly floured surface.

2. With the heel of your hands, push down on the edge of the dough nearest you.

3. Fold the dough in half toward you and give it a quarter turn.

4. Continue pushing, folding, and turning for the time directed in the recipe.

Preparing to Bake

The baking pans you choose can affect the results of baking. Use the size and type of pan specified in the recipe. If the pan is too large or too small, the product will not bake properly.

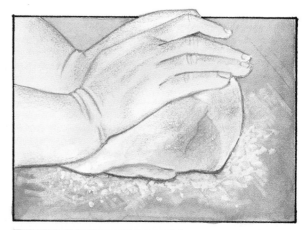

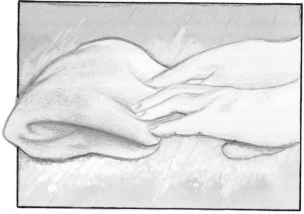

- **When making biscuits and yeast breads, knead the dough by pushing, folding, and turning it.** Describe the steps in this process.

The material the pan is made of is also important. Most recipes are developed for light-colored metal pans. If you use glass pans, lower the temperature by 25°F (14°C). Glass retains more heat than metal, and at the higher temperature, a dark, thick crust may result.

Dark pans also retain more heat than light ones and can create a thick crust. If you use dark metal pans, you may have to lower the oven temperature by about 10°F (6°C).

Glass bakeware or special microwave bakeware must always be used when baking in the microwave oven.

Pan Preparation

Baking pans must be properly prepared so that products can be easily removed from them at the end of baking. The pans should be prepared before the ingredients are mixed. Follow recipe directions carefully.

Here are several methods for preparing pans:

◆ **Grease and flour.** This means to lightly grease a pan with fat and dust it with flour. Use waxed paper to spread the fat. Sprinkle a little all-purpose flour into the pan. Tilt the pan to different angles until the flour is spread evenly. Turn the pan upside down over the sink, and tap it gently to remove any excess flour. Don't grease and flour pans for microwave baking—they become sticky.

◆ **Spray with a vegetable-oil cooking spray.** This is the easiest method, but it may not work with all products. Follow the directions on the label or in your recipe.

◆ **Line a pan with paper.** Begin by cutting a piece of cooking parchment the same shape and size as the pan bottom. Grease the pan and line the bottom with parchment paper. When the product is removed, peel the paper off the bottom. This method is used for rich cakes, such as fruitcake.

Note that some recipes required ungreased pans—otherwise the product will not rise properly. Be sure you know which method is required for your recipe.

⊕ Safety Check

The technique of lining a pan with paper requires parchment paper specially made for cooking and baking. Do not use brown paper or waxed paper. Brown paper contains chemicals that may be transferred to the food when it is heated. The wax in waxed paper may melt and possibly cause a fire.

Conventional and Microwave Baking

Most batters and doughs are baked. In a conventional oven, the dry heat creates desirable changes. The product browns, and depending on the ingredients, a crispy crust may develop. Because a microwave oven cooks with moist heat, baked products do not brown or develop a crust. They have more of a steamed texture and are very tender and moist.

Unless the recipe states otherwise, preheat the conventional oven. Before turning on the oven, be sure the oven racks are in the proper position. After you put the pans in the oven, set the timer. Begin checking the product for doneness about 5 minutes before the time is up.

Only certain kinds of cakes, quick breads, and cookies can be baked successfully in a microwave oven. Follow the directions in the owner's guide or in a microwave recipe.

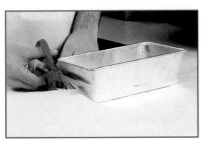 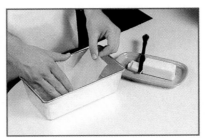 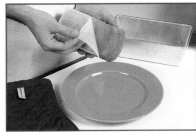

◆ In order to make the finished product easy to remove, you may need to prepare the pan for some recipes. Lining a pan with parchment paper is shown here. Why do you need to read a recipe carefully to determine whether it requires greasing the pan?

---INFOLINK---

For a review of proper <u>pan placement</u> in the oven during baking, see Section 9-3. For an update on <u>storing food</u> to prevent spoilage and nutrient loss, see Section 7-4.

Storing Baked Products

Perishable baked products, including those with cream fillings or frostings, have to be refrigerated. Studies show that other baked products get stale quickly when stored at refrigerator temperatures. Store them at room temperature if they will be eaten within three days. To store them longer, freeze them in airtight freezer containers.

Removing Baked Products from Pans

Some baked products must be removed from the pans immediately when they come out of the oven. Others need to cool for a few minutes in the pans. Still others need to remain in the pans until they are completely cool. Follow the recipe directions.

Use cooling racks so that baked goods will cool faster and stay crisp. When baked goods are allowed to cool on a solid surface, such as a cutting board, moisture collects and the product can become soggy.

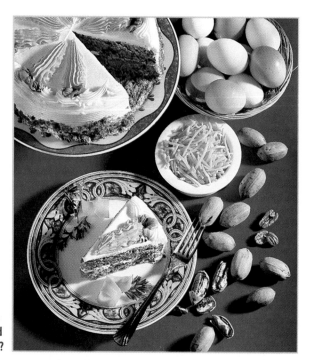

◆ This carrot cake, which has a cream cheese icing, should be refrigerated. If this cake was unfrosted, what factors would need to be considered in deciding whether to refrigerate it?

Section 21-1 Review & Activities

1. List the basic ingredients in baked products. Identify one function of each.

2. What is kneading? Briefly describe the four steps involved.

3. What are three ways of preparing pans for baking?

4. **Analyzing.** Pedro is considering cutting out half the sugar from a cake recipe to cut down on the calories. What might happen if Pedro goes through with his plan?

5. **Comparing and Contrasting.** Discuss the pros and cons of microwave baking versus conventional baking. When might you choose each?

6. **Applying.** Find a basic muffin recipe. Identify one function of each ingredient.

Quick Breads

As their name implies, quick breads are quick and easy to make. They don't require kneading, and most use baking powder as a leavening agent. Muffins, biscuits, pancakes, corn bread, and fruit breads are examples of quick breads.

Objectives

After studying this section, you should be able to:

- Suggest several additions to quick breads that increase the nutritional value.
- Discuss the differences and similarities between the muffin method and the pastry and biscuit method of mixing.
- Describe the characteristics of properly mixed and baked muffins and biscuits.

Look for These Terms

cut in

rolled biscuits

drop biscuits

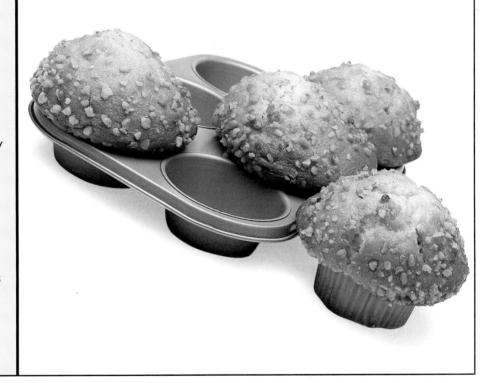

Nutrients in Quick Breads

Quick breads can be a tasty way of getting some of the nutrients your body needs. They are good sources of carbohydrates, protein, B vitamins, and iron. Using whole grains adds fiber and trace minerals. Adding fruits, vegetables, and nuts packs in even more vitamins and minerals—as well as flavor and texture. Some quick breads are high in fat. By choosing wisely, however, you can use quick breads to add variety, flavor, and nutrition to your meals and snacks.

Muffins

Muffins are prepared using the *muffin method.* The most important part of this procedure is properly mixing the liquid and dry ingredients.

Muffin Method

Muffins that are properly mixed have a rounded, pebbly top with a coarse but tender texture inside. To mix ingredients for muffins:

1. *Sift* together or mix all dry ingredients (flour, sugar, baking powder, spices) in a large bowl. Using the back of a spoon, make a well in the center of the dry ingredients.

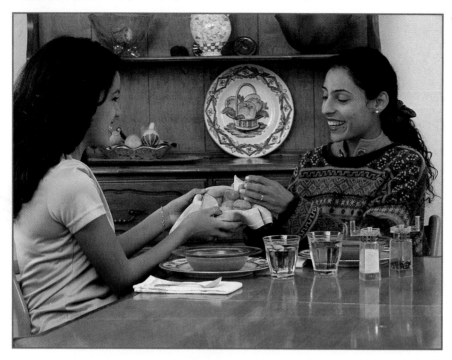

◆ Quick breads such as these muffins can add nutrients and variety to meals. Identify the common ingredients in quick breads.

2. *Beat* all liquid ingredients (eggs, milk or water, oil or melted fat, liquid flavorings) together in a small bowl until they are well blended.

3. *Pour* the liquid into the well you have made in the dry ingredients. Mix just enough to moisten the dry ingredients. A few floury spots can remain, and the batter should be lumpy.

4. *Fold* in ingredients such as chopped nuts and raisins gently.

Take care not to overmix the batter. Overmixed muffins will have peaks on top and be tough and heavy. The insides will have long, narrow tunnels.

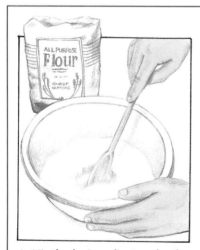

◆ Mix the dry ingredients and make a well in the center.

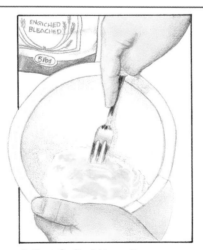

◆ Beat the liquid ingredients together.

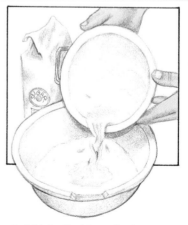

◆ Add the liquids to the dry ingredients all at once. Stir briefly—do not overmix.

Kinds of Muffins

The flavors of muffins can easily be varied with different ingredients. Fresh and dried fruits are often included. Try cranberries, blueberries, chopped dates, dried apricots, or your favorite combination. Muffin recipes may also include yogurt, tofu, shredded raw vegetables (zucchini or carrots), or cooked vegetables (such as sweet potatoes and winter squash). These ingredients add flavor as well as important nutrients. For a fiber boost, substitute ½ cup (125 mL) bran for an equal amount of flour in your muffin recipe.

Adding extra ingredients, such as fruit, to just any recipe may not work. Instead, start with a reliable recipe that already lists the ingredient you want.

Preparing and Baking Muffins

Instead of greasing muffin pans, you can line them with paper baking cups. Fill the cups only two-thirds full. If you add more than that, the batter will overflow and the muffins will have odd shapes.

When baking muffins, test them for doneness about 5 minutes before the end of the baking time. They are done when they are nicely browned. A wooden pick inserted in the center should come out clean. Muffins are best served warm.

Loaf Breads

Many quick loaf breads are mixed in the same manner as muffins. These simple cake-like breads even use many of the same basic

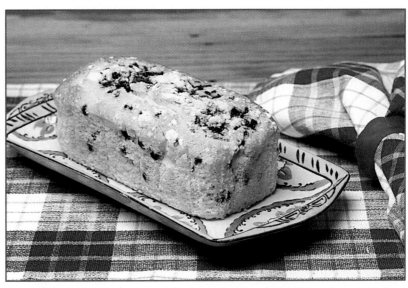

◆ **Quick loaf breads have many of the same ingredients as muffins and use the same mixing method.** Name two foods that could be served with the loaf bread shown here.

ingredients. Cranberry-orange-nut bread is a holiday favorite. Other breads, including corn bread, are less sweet. Some loaf breads are flavored with vegetables and herbs.

Quick breads are generally baked in greased loaf pans. If the bread contains dried fruits and nuts, the bottom of the pan should be lined with parchment paper so that the loaf can be removed easily.

Check for doneness as you would with muffins. Don't be surprised if the top of the loaf cracks. That is typical for quick breads.

Biscuits

Biscuits are delicate, small breads. Properly made, they have a tender but crisp crust and are an even, light brown color. The inside is slightly moist and creamy white, and peels apart in tender layers.

There are two kinds of biscuits—rolled and drop. Both are made using the *pastry and biscuit method* of mixing.

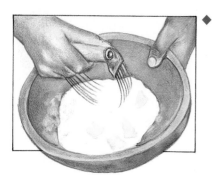

◆ **A pastry blender is a tool designed for cutting fat into flour.** Why is this tool preferable to using the hands when making baked goods?

Pastry and Biscuit Method

In the pastry and biscuit method, the fat is cut into the flour. To **cut in** means to mix solid fat and flour using a pastry blender or two knives and a cutting motion. This technique leaves the fat in fine particles in the dough. During baking, the fat melts between layers of flour, giving a flaky texture.

Handle the dough as little as possible. If the shortening and flour are overmixed, the texture will be mealy, not flaky. Mixing ingredients for biscuits is easy.

1. Sift together or mix the dry ingredients in a large bowl.

2. Cut the shortening into the flour until the particles are the size of peas or coarse bread crumbs.

3. Make a well in the center of the dry ingredients, as in the muffin method, and add the liquids. Stir just until the ingredients are blended and form a soft dough.

Rolled Biscuits

Once you have mixed the dough, you can proceed with your recipe for either rolled or drop biscuits. **Rolled biscuits** are made by rolling out dough to an even thickness and cutting it with a biscuit cutter. If you don't have a biscuit cutter, you can use the rim of a water glass.

Begin by turning the dough out on a lightly floured board and kneading about ten strokes. Knead as much as possible with the tips of your fingers, since warmth from your hands may melt the shortening, causing the biscuits to be tough. Overkneading results in tough, compact biscuits.

Next, roll the dough out to a uniform thickness of about ½ inch (1.3 cm). Cut the biscuits out with a biscuit cutter that is lightly dusted with flour. Press the cutter straight down so that the biscuits have straight sides and even shapes. Do not twist the cutter. Otherwise, the dough might tear. You can reroll any leftover dough to make more biscuits.

Place the biscuits on an ungreased baking sheet, about 1 inch (2.5 cm) apart. Bake according to recipe directions.

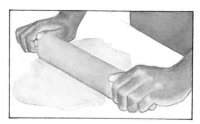

◆ **For rolled biscuits, roll the kneaded dough out to an even thickness.**

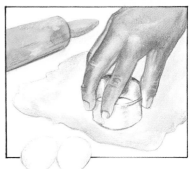

◆ **Cut the biscuits out, being careful not to pull or tear the dough.**

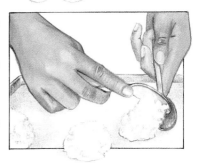

◆ **For drop biscuits, just drop the batter from a spoon in mounds onto a greased cookie sheet.** How are rolled biscuits and drop biscuits similar? How are they different?

Drop Biscuits

Drop biscuits are made by dropping dough from a spoon. Since they contain more liquid than rolled biscuits, the batter is too sticky to roll. Although these biscuits have irregular shapes, they are just as flavorful and flaky as the rolled variety.

Mix the batter for drop biscuits using the same method as for rolled biscuits. Drop the batter in mounds on a greased cookie sheet about 1 inch (2.5 cm) apart. Bake according to recipe directions. You can also spoon drop biscuits onto a casserole as a topping.

Serving Biscuits

Biscuits are delicious when they are eaten warm, right out of the oven. Serve them with meals, or use them for sandwiches. For variety, they can be topped with gravy or sweet fruit and cream. Biscuits can be made ahead of time, frozen, and then reheated in the microwave oven.

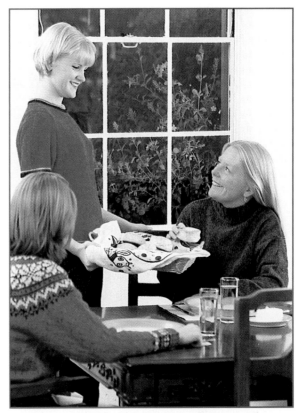

◆ Biscuits and muffins are usually served fresh from the oven or reheated. Which skill for food choices is used when planning hot biscuits as part of a meal?

Section 21-2 Review & Activities

1. List five ingredients you can add to quick breads to increase the nutritional value.

2. Name two ways that the muffin method and pastry and biscuit method of mixing are similar. In what two ways are these methods different?

3. Describe the characteristics of a well-made muffin after baking.

4. Evaluating. Josh enjoys eating a variety of sandwiches made on biscuits. He has come up with the idea of baking the sandwich ingredients right in. Tell whether you think Josh's recipe is likely to succeed, giving reasons for your answer.

5. Synthesizing. Brainstorm ways that you can use quick breads to add variety to meals.

6. Applying. Find three recipes for quick breads. Identify the mixing method used in each.

RECIPE FILE

Low-Fat Cinnamon-Oatmeal Muffins

Try serving these muffins with a fruit salad or use them as the bread in a sandwich.

Customary	Ingredients	Metric
¾ cup	Whole-wheat flour	175 mL
¾ cup	All-purpose flour	175 mL
1 cup	Uncooked rolled oats	250 mL
1 Tbsp.	Baking powder	15 mL
3 Tbsp.	Sugar	45 mL
½ tsp.	Ground cinnamon	3 mL
¼ tsp.	Salt	1 mL
1	Egg	1
1 cup	Fat-free milk	250 mL
¼ cup	Applesauce	50 mL

Yield: 12 muffins
Equipment: Muffin pan(s)
Temperature: 400°F (200°C)

Directions

1. Preheat oven.
2. Grease and flour muffin pan(s).
3. In a large bowl, combine flours, oats, baking powder, sugar, cinnamon, and salt. Mix well.
4. In a separate bowl, beat the egg.
5. Add milk and applesauce to egg. Stir well.
6. Add liquid mixture to flour mixture and stir until dry ingredients are just moistened. Do not overmix. (Batter should be lumpy.)
7. Fill muffin cups ⅔ full.
8. Bake 15 to 20 minutes or until a wooden pick inserted in the center comes out clean.

Nutrition Information

Per serving (approximate–per muffin): 107 calories, 4 g protein, 21 g carbohydrate, 1 g fat, 18 mg cholesterol, 143 mg sodium
Good source of: B vitamins, phosphorus

Food for Thought

- What would happen if the muffin batter was mixed until no lumps remained?
- Why are the muffin cups filled only two-thirds full?

SECTION
21-3

Objectives

After studying this section, you should be able to:

- Identify ways to simplify bread making.
- Describe the procedure for making yeast breads.
- Explain how to tell when yeast breads are done baking.

Look for This Term

quick-mix method

Yeast Breads and Rolls

Do you have a sandwich for lunch most days? If you do, it is probably made with a yeast bread. True to their name, yeast breads use yeast for leavening. The yeast also gives the bread a characteristic flavor and contributes to the wonderful aroma while the bread is baking.

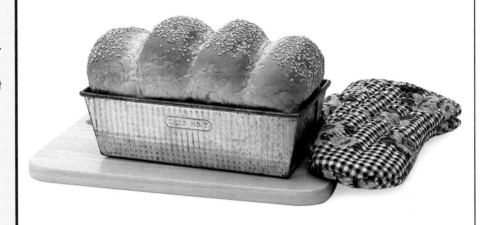

Yeast Bread

Many people believe that bread baking is too time-consuming to fit in with today's fast-paced lifestyles. With a little organization, however, bread baking can be part of regular food preparation. Making yeast dough is a flexible process. The tasks can be timed to fit into the cook's schedule.

Time-Savers

Several appliances can help speed up the bread-making process. A microwave oven can be used to heat the liquid before adding it to the yeast, to bring refrigerated ingredients to room temperature, and to let the dough rise. Check the owner's manual for specific directions, which will vary depending on the oven's power and controls.

A heavy-duty mixer with a dough hook or a powerful food processor can be used to mix yeast dough quickly. These appliances will knead it in about 6 minutes compared with the 8 or 10 minutes required to knead it by hand. Bread machines will mix, knead, and bake yeast breads. They can be set to have bread baked in time for a meal.

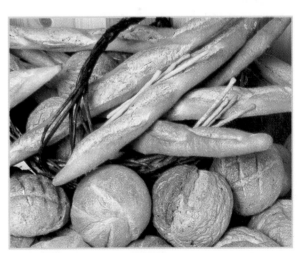

◆ **As different as these breads appear, all use yeast for leavening.** Do you know the name of the gas produced by yeast that causes breads like these to rise?

Techniques in Making Yeast Breads

There are five important techniques that should be used when making yeast breads.

Look and Learn:

For each of the techniques shown, what would happen if it was not used properly?

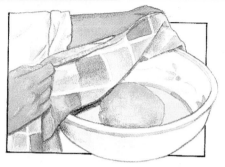

Yeast goes to work during the rising time. Cover the dough to keep it from drying out.

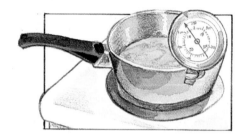

Use a thermometer to check the temperature of the liquids.

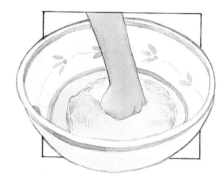

Gently "punching" the dough after the first rising eliminates excess gas bubbles.

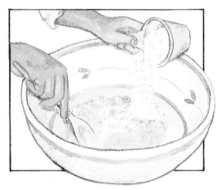

After mixing the liquid and dry ingredients, use a spoon to beat in the additional flour. The amount needed will vary. It depends on the moisture content of the flour and even the humidity in the air that day.

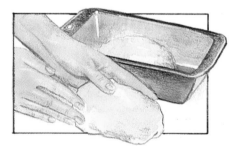

After shaping, bread dough is allowed to rise a final time in the pan.

Making Bread and Rolls

Yeast bread and rolls are both made by using the same simple five-step procedure. The steps include mixing the dough, kneading it, letting it rise, shaping it, and, finally, baking it.

Mixing the Dough

Most yeast breads are a simple mixture of flour, salt, sugar, liquid, fat, and yeast. Sugar provides food for the yeast so that it will grow. Salt controls the action of the yeast. Consult a recipe for the exact ingredients and amounts.

Although bread flour is ideal, most recipes for homemade bread call for all-purpose flour. It is more readily available than bread flour and makes a loaf with good texture. To add fiber and nutrients to recipes calling for all-purpose flour, substitute whole-grain flour for two-thirds of the total flour in the recipe. Keep amounts of other ingredients the same.

Before you begin, be sure the ingredients are at room temperature and the liquid is heated to the right temperature. Yeast will not grow if the liquid is too cold and will die if the liquid is too hot. When yeast is added to liquid at the proper temperature, the mixture becomes cloudy and begins to form a foamy layer within minutes.

Quick-Mix Method

The **quick-mix method** is a bread-making method that combines active dry yeast with the dry ingredients. A standard mixer will work for the first part of the mixing until the dough thickens and becomes too heavy for it. Beat the rest of the flour in with a wooden spoon.

1. Combine part of the flour with the undissolved active dry yeast, sugar, and salt in a large bowl.

2. Heat the liquid and fat to between 120°F and 130°F (49°C to 55°C).

3. Add the liquid to the dry ingredients, beating them with a mixer until they are well blended. At this point, the gluten is beginning to develop.

4. Beat in enough of the remaining flour to make the kind of dough specified in the recipe. You may need more or less flour than the recipe calls for. Some kinds absorb more liquid than others.

Kneading the Dough

Turn the dough out on a lightly floured surface. Knead the dough until it becomes a smooth, shiny ball, about 8 to 10 minutes. Use just enough flour to keep the dough from sticking to the work surface or to your hands. Too much flour will give a tough texture.

Don't be concerned if bubbles develop in the dough. They are a clue that gluten is developing. The cell walls are becoming elastic and expanding with carbon dioxide given off by the yeast.

Letting the Dough Rise

Shape the dough into a ball, and place it in a well-oiled bowl. Turn the ball in the bowl so that all sides are coated with oil. Place a piece of plastic wrap over the top of the dough to keep it from drying out; then cover the bowl with a clean dish towel. Set the bowl in a warm (not hot), draft-free place for about 1 to 1½ hours. The dough should rise to double its original size. Bread dough made with whole-grain flour will take longer to rise.

Once it has risen, punch the dough down by *gently* pressing your fist into the center. Gently pull the dough from the sides of the bowl toward the middle. These actions will eliminate the largest air bubbles.

When the ball has doubled in size, the dough is ready for the fourth stage—shaping. To determine whether the dough is ready, push two fingers gently into the surface. If the finger indentations remain, the dough is ready to shape. If you aren't ready to shape the dough, you can let it rise again. You can also cover it and refrigerate it overnight. It will rise in the refrigerator and be ready to shape the next day.

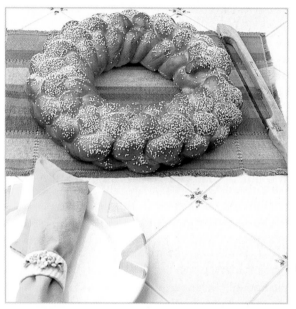

◆ Yeast dough can be shaped in many creative ways, such as this braided ring. What precautions do you think the baker took to ensure the evenly browned crust on this product?

Shaping the Dough

Shape the dough into loaves or rolls, according to recipe directions. Use kitchen scissors or a sharp knife to cut the dough into pieces. Don't pull it apart. Place it in a greased pan or on a baking sheet. Cover and let the shaped dough rise again until it doubles in size.

Baking

Since baking times vary considerably, always bake as directed in the recipe. Bread and rolls have a nicely browned crust when done baking. Check loaves for doneness by tapping them with your finger. If they sound hollow, they are done.

Remove the bread or rolls from the pans, and place them immediately on a wire cooling rack. The rack prevents moisture from forming on the bottom crust and making it soggy. Let loaves stand about 20 minutes for easier cutting.

Section 21-3 Review & Activities

1. What appliances can help speed up the bread-making process? How do they save time?

2. What happens if the liquids in yeast breads are too hot or too cool?

3. How can you tell if dough is ready to shape and bake? How can you tell if a loaf of bread is done baking?

4. **Extending.** Why do you think dough should be cut, rather than pulled apart, to be shaped into rolls?

5. **Comparing and Contrasting.** Discuss the pros and cons of making yeast breads by hand versus using an automatic bread machine or commercial frozen bread dough.

6. **Applying.** Using cookbooks or other references, describe at least five different ways of shaping yeast breads other than in a loaf.

RECIPE FILE

Honey Whole Wheat Bread

There is nothing like the aroma of freshly baked bread. The flavor is equally hard to beat, especially when the bread is served warm from the oven.

Customary	Ingredients	Metric	Customary	Ingredients	Metric
2½ to 3 cups	All-purpose flour	625 to 750 mL	1 cup	Fat-free milk	250 mL
3 cups	Whole wheat flour	750 mL	1 cup	Water	250 mL
2 tsp.	Salt	10 mL	¼ cup	Honey	50 mL
1 pkg.	Active dry yeast	1 pkg.	3 Tbsp.	Shortening	45 mL

Yield: 2 loaves
Equipment: Small saucepan; two 9 × 5 × 3 inch (23 × 3 × 8 cm) loaf pans
Oven Temperature: 400°F (200°C)

Directions

1. Mix 1 cup (250 mL) of each flour with salt and yeast in a large bowl. Set aside.
2. Combine milk, water, honey, and shortening in a small saucepan. Heat over low heat until warm, about 120°F (49°C). Shortening does not have to melt.
3. Add the heated liquid to the dry ingredients. Blend at low speed with a mixer about 2 minutes.
4. Add another ½ cup (125 mL) of each flour. Beat about 2 minutes at medium speed.
5. Stir in ¾ cup (175 mL) all-purpose flour and 1½ cups (375 mL) whole wheat flour with a wooden spoon until the mixture forms a soft dough. If necessary, add more all-purpose flour.
6. Place the dough on a lightly floured surface. Knead for 8 to 10 minutes until smooth and elastic.
7. Place the dough in a large, well-oiled bowl. Turn the dough to coat on all sides. Cover the dough with a piece of plastic wrap, and cover the bowl with a clean dish towel. Refrigerate overnight.
8. The next day, remove the dough from the refrigerator. Gently punch the dough down.
9. Turn the dough onto a lightly floured surface. Allow the dough to rest 10 to 15 minutes.
10. Divide the dough into two equal portions. Shape each portion into a loaf, and place each loaf in a well-greased loaf pan.
11. Cover the loaves with a clean dish towel, and allow them to rise in a warm place until double in size—about 1 hour, or until finger indentations remain.
12. Preheat the oven to 400°F (200°C). Bake the loaves for 25 to 30 minutes or until done.
13. Remove loaves from pans, and cool on a wire rack away from drafts.

Nutrition Information

Per serving (approximate–¹⁄₂₀ of loaf): 75 calories, 2 g protein, 14 g carbohydrate, 1 g fat, 0 mg cholesterol, 111 mg sodium
Good source of: B vitamins

Food for Thought

- Why do you suppose the flour is added a little at a time rather than all at once?
- What flavor does the honey impart to the loaf? What difference, if any, do you think would result if you used sugar instead? If you used molasses?

<table>
<tr><td>

SECTION
21-4

Objectives

After studying this section, you should be able to:

- Describe types of cakes, cookies, and pies.
- Give guidelines for preparing cakes, cookies, and pies.
- Identify ways of reducing fat in cakes, drop cookies, and piecrust.

Look for These Terms

shortened cakes

foam cakes

</td><td>

Cakes, Cookies, and Pies

Who doesn't like freshly baked cookies or a warm slice of homemade pie? Cakes, cookies, and pies are among the most popular baked goods. Unfortunately, treats like these are also traditionally high in fat, sugar, and calories. In this section, you will learn ways of eating your cake and having good nutrition, too.

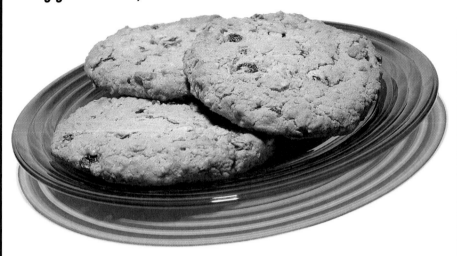

</td></tr>
</table>

Cakes

Although cakes are easy to make, accurately measuring ingredients is essential for good results.

Some cake recipes call for cake flour, which is low in gluten. If you do not have cake flour, substitute all-purpose flour, using 1 cup (250 mL) minus 2 tablespoons (30 mL) for each 1 cup of cake flour called for in the recipe.

There are two basic kinds of cakes—shortened cakes and foam cakes.

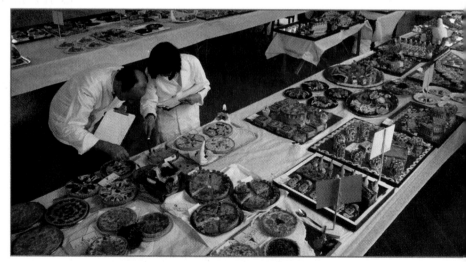

◆ Treats like this, though tempting, are high in fat, sugar, and calories. Can desserts like these be part of a healthful eating plan? Explain.

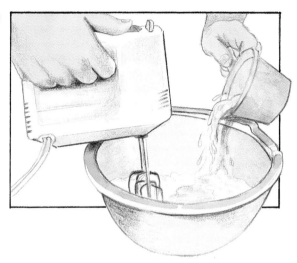

◆ The one-bowl method saves time because there are fewer steps in mixing. How else might this method save time and personal energy?

Shortened Cakes

Shortened cakes are usually made with a solid fat, though oil can also be used. The fat, which makes the cake rich and tender, is most often shortening, butter, or margarine. Shortened cakes can be made in a variety of flavors, including chocolate, lemon, and spice. Some contain chopped nuts or dried fruit.

Standard Mixing Method

Several methods can be used for mixing cakes. The most common for shortened cakes is the *standard method.* An electric mixer is helpful for creaming and beating the ingredients.

1. *Cream* the solid fat and sugar until the mixture is light and fluffy, as in whipped cream.

2. *Beat* the eggs into the mixture thoroughly, usually one at a time.

3. *Sift* the dry ingredients together.

4. *Mix* the liquids together.

5. *Add* the dry ingredients to the creamed mixture alternately with the liquid. Begin and end with the dry ingredients. This helps keep the fat from separating, which could affect the texture. Add the dry ingredients in fourths and the liquids in thirds. After each addition, beat the batter just enough to mix the ingredients.

One-Bowl Method

An alternative to the standard method for mixing shortened cakes is the *one-bowl method.* In this method, the dry ingredients are first combined by sifting and mixing. Solid fat, liquids, and flavorings are added and beaten with dry ingredients until well blended. The eggs are beaten in last.

Baking Shortened Cakes

You can bake shortened cakes in pans of many shapes and sizes, from individual cupcakes in muffin pans to large sheet cakes. Fancy molds can turn ordinary cakes into a masterpiece.

To check a shortened cake for doneness, insert a wooden pick in the center. If it comes out free of wet batter, the cake is done.

A shortened cake should have a slightly rounded top with a tender, shiny crust. When the cake is cut, it should have a fine, even grain and be moist and tender.

Foam Cakes

Foam cakes are cakes that are leavened with beaten egg whites, which give them a light, airy texture. Some foam cake recipes call for baking powder as well. Examples of foam cakes include:

◆ **Angel food cakes.** These cakes use only beaten egg whites for leavening. Because they contain neither egg yolks nor fat, they are good choices for low-fat desserts.

- **Sponge cakes.** In these cakes, beaten egg yolks are added to the batter before the batter is folded into the egg whites.

- **Chiffon cakes.** These cakes include yolks, oil, and baking powder, which are blended and then folded into beaten egg whites.

Baking Foam Cakes

Foam cakes must be baked in ungreased pans. As the batter rises during baking, it clings to the sides of a pan. If the pan were greased, the cake would not be able to rise.

A tube pan is often used for foam cakes. If the pan is in only one piece, line the bottom with parchment paper so that the cake can be easily removed.

To test a foam cake for doneness, touch the top lightly. It should spring back.

Foam cakes are generally cooled upside down in the pan to keep them from losing volume or from falling. If the tube pan does not have legs to support it upside down, use an empty glass bottle with a slender neck or a large metal funnel turned upside down. Invert the tube pan over the neck of the bottle or funnel.

When the cake is cool, gently loosen the cake from the sides with a spatula. Turn the pan upside down to remove the cake. If the pan is in two parts and has a removable bottom, use a spatula to loosen the cake from the bottom.

Decorating Cakes

Cakes are often frosted. Since frostings are usually high in fat, sugar, and calories, you may want to try one of these alternatives:

- Make a glaze with confectioners' sugar and lemon, orange, or pineapple juice. Drizzle it over the cake, letting it flow down the sides. For added eye appeal, garnish with fruit twists.

- Sift a little confectioners' sugar over the top of the cake. Try putting a cutout paper design, such as a snowflake, on top before sifting the sugar.

Another low-fat option is to skip the icing and serve the cake with fresh or frozen fruit.

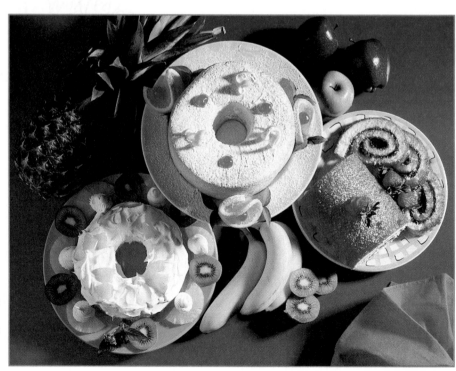

- Foam cakes like these have a light texture and airy quality. What ingredient is responsible for these properties?

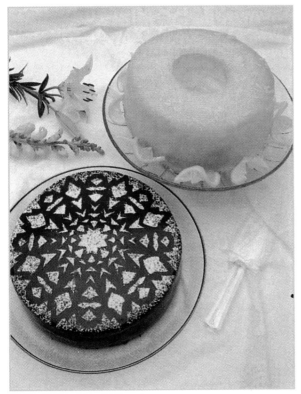

These simple cake toppings are both easy to make and easy on the eye. Identify an advantage from a nutrition standpoint of these cakes over ones with frosting.

Cookies

Cookies are easy to prepare. Many people consider homemade cookies well worth the time and effort they require. The main difference between cakes and cookies is that cookies have little, if any, liquid. This gives cookies a heavier texture than cakes.

Kinds of Cookies

Cookies vary in texture from soft to crisp. They can be made in assorted shapes and sizes, and can be decorated in many ways.

The thousands of cookie varieties can be divided into six basic kinds:

♦ **Bar cookies.** Are baked in square or rectangular pans and then cut into bars, squares, or diamonds. They can be made from a batter or a soft dough that is pressed into a pan. Textures vary from cakelike to chewy. Brownies are one popular example of bar cookies. Usually, bars are cooled in the pan and then cut.

♦ **Drop cookies.** Are made from a soft dough that is dropped from a teaspoon onto cookie sheets. During baking, the dough spreads out to make a thick cookie. Remember to allow enough space between cookies (about 2 inches [5 cm]) so that they can spread without touching. Most chocolate chip cookies are drop cookies. For reduced-fat drop cookies, replace some or all of the fat with applesauce, mashed bananas, puréed fruits, or canned pumpkin.

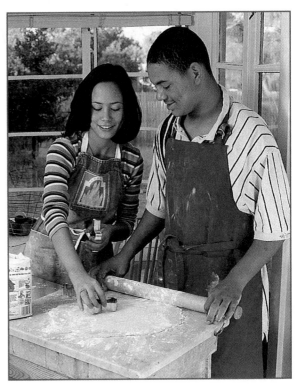

♦ There are nearly as many methods for making cookies as there are flavors. Which type of cookies are the teens in the picture making?

- **Cut-out cookies.** Also called rolled cookies. Are made from stiff dough that is rolled out and cut with cookie cutters.

- **Molded cookies.** Are formed by shaping the dough by hand into balls. These balls can be rolled in chopped nuts or other toppings before baking, or they can be flattened with a fork or the bottom of a glass. Peanut butter cookies are flattened with a fork, giving them their characteristic ridged appearance.

- **Pressed cookies.** Are made by pushing dough through a cookie press, which can create a variety of shapes. Spritz cookies are made this way.

- **Sliced cookies.** Sometimes called refrigerator or icebox cookies. Are made by forming a soft dough into a long roll and refrigerating it. When the roll is chilled and firm, the cookies are sliced and baked.

Baking Cookies

Most cookies are baked on cookie sheets—flat pans with only one edge. Let cookie sheets cool before baking more cookies. Otherwise, the warm pan will soften the dough and the cookies will lose their shape.

Bar cookies are done baking when they pull away slightly from the sides of the pan. A slight impression remains when they are tapped gently. Other cookies are done when the bottoms are lightly browned and the edges are firm.

✚ Safety Check

Although you may be tempted to do so, don't eat raw homemade cookie dough. It nearly always contains raw eggs—which can contribute to foodborne illness.

Store cooled cookies in covered containers. Waxed paper between layers will keep them from sticking together.

Pies

One dessert that has a long tradition at holiday meals is pie. A pie is a flaky crust filled with either a sweet or a savory mixture. A sweet pie may contain a fruit, custard, or cream filling, and is generally served as a dessert. A savory pie, filled with a meat or a custard and vegetable mixture, is served as a main dish. Two examples are quiche and potpie.

Pies can have one or two crusts made with flour, fat, salt, and water.

Piecrust

The key to making the piecrust is proper technique. To mix the pastry, use the pastry and biscuit method described on page 570. For a flaky pastry, handle the dough as little as possible.

Use a lightly floured surface to roll out pastry dough. Roll the dough in a large, round circle about ⅛ inch (0.3 cm) thick and 2 inches (5 cm) larger than an inverted (upside-down) pie pan. If the dough cracks or tears, patch it with another piece of dough. Moisten the area to be patched with a little water; then press a piece of dough over it. Sprinkle some flour over the patched area, and continue to roll it with a rolling pin.

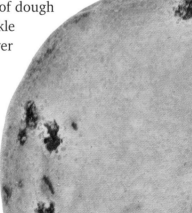

Techniques in Preparing Pie Crust

There are four techniques that are important in successfully preparing the crust for a pie.

Look and Learn:

Will the pie in the drawings be a one-crust or two-crust pie? How can you tell?

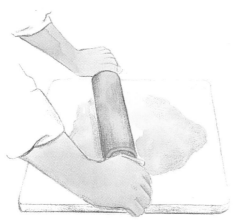

Roll pastry dough from the center outward to form a circle of even thickness.

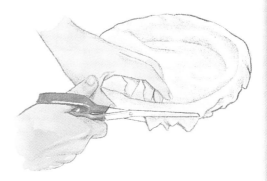

Trim the pastry with kitchen shears.

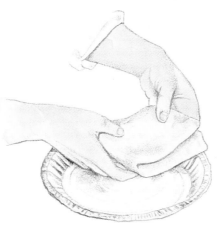

Fold the pastry so that you can transfer it to the pan without stretching or tearing it.

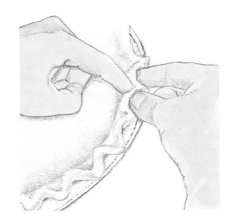

Finish the edge of the crust in some way. Making a fluted edge is shown here.

Two-Crust Pie

For a two-crust pie, fold a rolled pastry circle in half (and in half again), and gently place it in a pie pan. Unfold the circle and fit it into the pan without stretching the pastry. Trim the pastry even with the top edge of the pan. Fill it with a sweet or savory mixture. Place another circle of pastry over the filling to form the top crust. Trim it so that ½ inch (1.3 cm) extends over the edge of the pan. Moisten the bottom pastry around the edge with water. Tuck the top pastry under the edge of the bottom pastry and gently pinch the layers together. Make a decorative edge that also seals the top and bottom crusts. Make several slits in the top crust to allow steam to escape during baking.

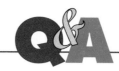

Q I have seen pies with decorative crust edges. How can I learn this technique?

A It's actually easy and can be done two ways. One is to dip the tines of a fork in flour, and then use the fork to press the pastry crust against the edge of the pan around the entire crust. The second method is to place the index finger of one hand on the inside edge of the crust and the thumb and the index finger of the other hand on the outside edge. Gently push the crust to form a curved shape, repeating this process around the entire edge.

◆ For variety, a lattice crust is sometimes used for fruit pies and savory pies. How could you make a crust have this woven appearance?

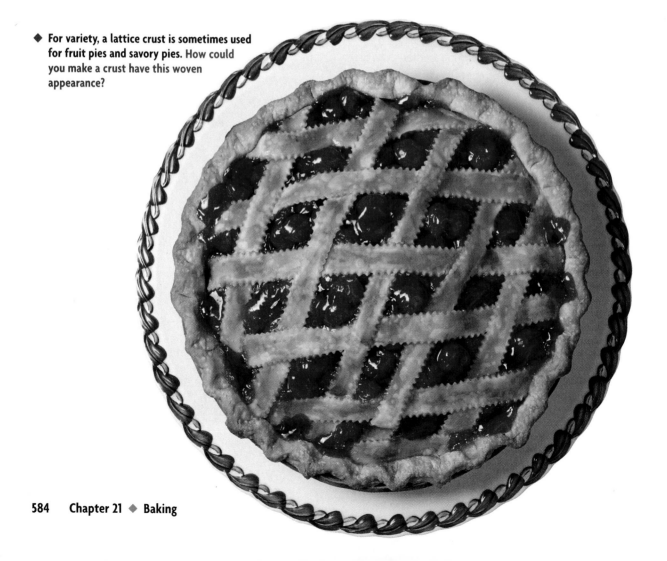

One-Crust Pie

When making a one-crust pie, roll out one pastry circle for the bottom crust. Put the pastry into the pie pan. Trim it, leaving a ½-inch (1.3-cm) overhang. Pinch the overhang under to form a double thickness along the pan rim. Flute the edge or make a forked edge.

One-crust pies can also be made with crumb crusts. Mix fine crumbs from graham crackers or gingersnaps with melted butter or margarine, and press them into the pan. These crusts, which are usually used with unbaked fillings, are popular because they're easier to make than pastry crusts. They also add flavor and texture to the pie.

Some recipes call for a baked pie shell. The filling is added later. If you bake the pie shell before filling it, pierce the bottom with a fork about every 1 inch (2.5 cm) to prevent the crust from bubbling up while baking.

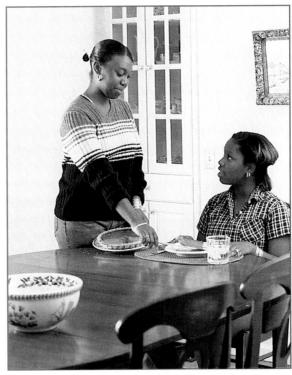

◆ Pumpkin pie is an example of a pie that is traditionally made without a top crust. Which others can you name?

Section 21-4 Review & Activities

1. What are the two basic kinds of cakes? Name two ways they are different and two ways they are alike.

2. What are the differences between cut-out cookies and drop cookies?

3. What should you do if pastry dough tears as you are rolling it?

4. **Analyzing.** Courtney has volunteered to bring cookies to a bake sale tomorrow, but she has little time for baking. What type of cookies would you suggest she bake? Give reasons for your recommendations.

5. **Evaluating.** Why do you think homemade cakes and pies were more common (and perhaps more popular) in years past?

6. **Applying.** Working in small groups, locate several pie recipes in magazines and food advertisements. Write down any shortcut ingredients or preparation methods suggested in the recipes. Make suggestions for modifying the recipes to make them lower in fat.

Apple-Bran Bars

Bar cookies are easy to prepare and are fun to eat. Try adding dried cranberries, cherries, or chopped apricots to this recipe.

Customary	Ingredients	Metric
1 cup	100 percent bran cereal	250 mL
½ cup	Fat-free milk	125 mL
1 cup	All-purpose flour	250 mL
1 tsp.	Baking powder	5 mL
½ tsp.	Ground cinnamon	3 mL
¼ tsp.	Ground nutmeg	1 mL
⅓ cup	Margarine	75 mL
½ cup	Brown sugar, packed	125 mL
2	Egg whites	2
1 cup	Pared, chopped apple	250 mL

Yield: 16 bars
Equipment: 9 × 9 inch (23 × 23 cm) baking pan
Oven Temperature: 350°F (180°C)

Directions

1. Preheat oven.
2. Grease and flour the baking pan.
3. In a large bowl, soak cereal in milk until milk is absorbed.
4. In a separate bowl, mix together flour, baking powder, cinnamon, and nutmeg.
5. In another bowl, beat margarine and sugar until creamy. Add egg whites and beat again until thoroughly combined.
6. Add the dry ingredients to the creamed mixture. Stir well.
7. Stir in apples and the cereal mixture; mix well.
8. Pour mixture into greased baking pan.
9. Bake about 30 minutes or until a wooden pick inserted in the center comes out clean.
10. Cool. Cut into 16 bars and serve.

Nutrition Information

Per serving (approximate–per bar): 92 calories, 2 g protein, 17 g carbohydrate, 2 g fat, trace cholesterol, 106 mg sodium
Good source of: Vitamin E, B vitamins, phosphorus

Food for Thought

• What are two other methods you could use to test the bars for doneness?
• How might you adapt this recipe for microwave preparation?

CAREER WANTED

Individuals with strong communication and organizational skills, lots of creativity, and a desire to solve problems

REQUIRES:

- technical degree in food science, nutrition, or related areas
- both food service and design experience

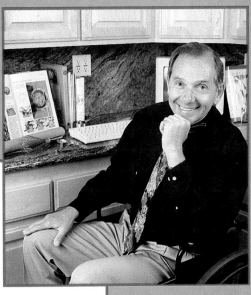

"We eat with all of our senses,"
says Food Design Consultant Thomas Biernaski

Q: Thomas, what kind of credentials does someone need to become a food design consultant?

A: A love of food and cooking is first. I create sugar-free recipes for a nutrition web site. My wife is a diabetic who loves desserts, so my job is like a paid hobby. She is my taste-tester!

Q: Have you held other jobs in your industry?

A: Yes, I've had several different kinds of jobs in the food industry. I worked in the test kitchen for a food manufacturer, and I also assisted the head chef in the kitchen of a convalescent home. Both jobs helped me understand what people expect from me in my current position.

Q: Where do you get your ideas for recipes?

A: Sometimes I modify existing recipes to fit my client's needs. Other times an idea for a new dessert will suggest itself, depending on what foods are in season and what catches my eye as I do research. Adding spices makes a recipe more appealing.

Q: What is the biggest reward that comes from the work you do?

A: It's knowing that I've helped people to enjoy food and at the same time eat healthy. It's always a joy when someone on a non-restricted eating plan praises a recipe of mine.

Career Research Activity

1. Consider a career path that begins with a position as salad worker, moves on to cookbook developer, and ends as a flavor chemist. Which high school courses would have prepared a person for this career path? Why? What are two other career options that the salad worker or cookbook developer could have pursued? How would that have changed their education or training plans?

2. Search the Internet or the library for an article on food design consulting. Do the credentials or activities described match those of Thomas Biernaski? Why might there be differences? Does this career interest you? Why or why not?

Related Career Opportunities

Entry Level
- Short-Order Cook
- Salad Worker

Technical Level
- Food Design Consultant
- Test Kitchen Worker
- Cookbook Developer

Professional Level
- Dietitian
- Geriatric Nutritionist
- Flavor Chemist

Chapter 21   Review & Activities

— Summary —

Section 21-1: Ingredients and Techniques for Baking

- Basic ingredients each play a specific role in baking.

- The strength of gluten determines what texture a baked product will have.

- Recipe directions give the mixing method, size and type of pans, and how to prepare them for baking.

- Conventional and microwave baking produce different results.

Section 21-3: Yeast Breads and Rolls

- Time-saving techniques can speed up yeast bread preparation.

- Yeast bread dough consists of flour, salt, sugar, liquid, fat, and yeast.

- After kneading and rising, the dough can be shaped and baked a number of ways.

Section 21-2: Quick Breads

- Breads, biscuits, and muffins made without yeast are called quick breads.

- They are mixed using the muffin method or the pastry and biscuit method.

- Quick breads can be nutritious, but some are high in fat and calories.

Section 21-4: Cakes, Cookies, and Pies

- Cakes, cookies, and pies are usually high in fat and calories, but can often be made with reduced-fat techniques.

- There are two basic kinds of cakes, shortened cakes and foam cakes.

- Cookies can be shaped in a variety of ways.

- Pies can have sweet or savory fillings, and can be made with one or two crusts.

Working IN THE Lab

1. **Food Science.** Demonstrate the action of leavening agents. Dissolve one package of yeast in water. Add both sugar and water to another package of yeast. Combine baking powder with water and baking soda with water. Compare the results of all the samples.

2. **Foods Lab.** Prepare yeast dough and freeze it. In the next day or two, allow the dough to thaw and rise in the refrigerator overnight. Bake it the following day. Evaluate the results.

Checking Your Knowledge

1. Name two kinds of each: batters and doughs.

2. What can air, steam, and carbon dioxide do for baked goods? How do they work?

3. What is the difference between using a dark pan for baking and using a light pan? Between using a metal pan and a glass pan?

4. Which baked goods should be refrigerated? Which should not? Why?

5. What are three kinds of quick breads?

6. Why are quick breads mixed only briefly?

7. When making whole-grain yeast dough, how much all-purpose flour should you use in the dough?

8. When and how is dough punched down?

9. What are two examples of low-fat ways to decorate a cake?

10. What are the six basic kinds of cookies?

Thinking Critically

1. Predicting Consequences. Jan is baking bread for 45 minutes in a disposable aluminum pan. Because she plans to throw the pan out after using it, she doesn't grease it, as the recipe calls for. What are two problems that using this pan might cause?

2. Determining Accuracy. Paula's friend heard that you could substitute applesauce for oil in a muffin recipe to cut down on fat. How can Paula find out whether this is true?

Reinforcing Key Skills

1. Management. Your time these days is divided among schoolwork, sports, music lessons, and several other activities. You also have finals coming up next week—just in time for your grandmother's visit. You would like to bake something that is both festive and nutritious to welcome her. What will you make?

2. Communication. Celine has just learned that her favorite uncle was diagnosed with heart disease. She is aware of his fondness for cookies. Write the dialogue of the conversation Celine has with her uncle in which she guides him in his food choices.

Making Decisions and Solving Problems

A friend invites you over to make cookies for a party. She says that she likes to bake by just "throwing a bunch of ingredients together." What would you do?

Making Connections

1. Social Studies. Use your school or public library to find out how the American colonists (or other groups) baked bread before the invention of the kitchen range.

2. Math. Make a bar graph comparing pies made in three different ways—totally from scratch, with a purchased crust and canned filling, and purchased from a bakery. Using different colors for different criteria, rate each type of pie in terms of preparation time, cost, and nutrition (fat, sugar, and calorie content). Place your graph in a location in the classroom near the foods lab.

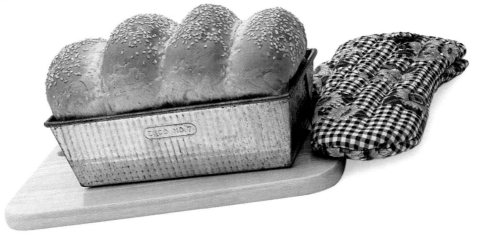

UNIT
5

Expanding

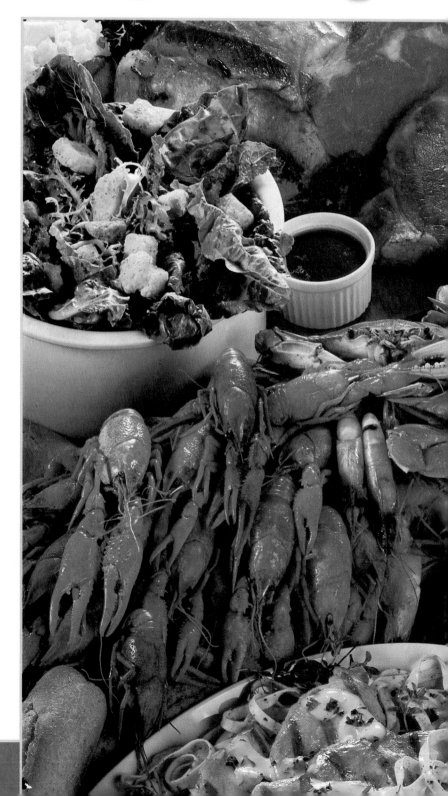

Your Horizons

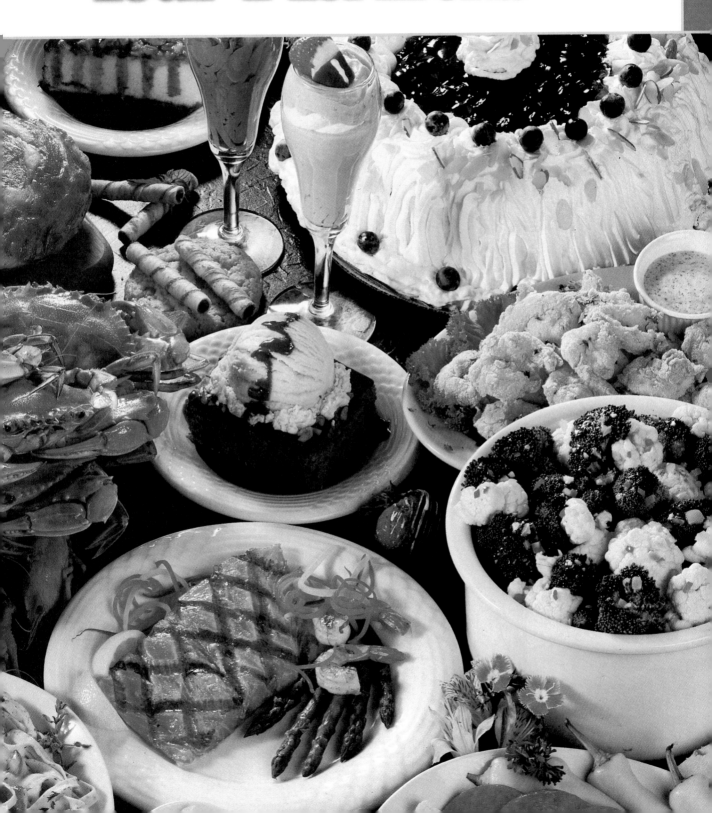

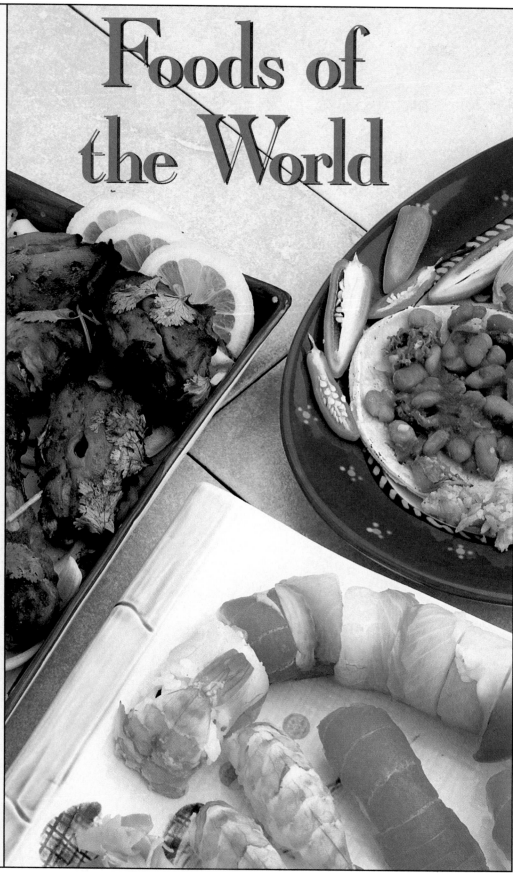

Foods of
the World

The world of food is
vast and varied. In this
chapter, you will learn
about different cultures
and the contribution
each makes to the rich
fabric of international
food customs and
preparation.

Latin America

Over twenty countries in Central and South America make up what is called Latin America. This region of over 300 million people is named because the main languages spoken there—Spanish, French, and Portuguese—are all based on Latin.

The early history of this area is dominated by three native cultures: Aztec, Inca, and Mayan. The Aztecs flourished in Mexico, the Incas in South America, and the Mayans in Central America.

Objectives

After studying this section, you should be able to:

- Describe food choices available in the various regions of Latin America.
- Identify the cultural influences on foods in Latin America.

Look for These Terms

cuisines

maize

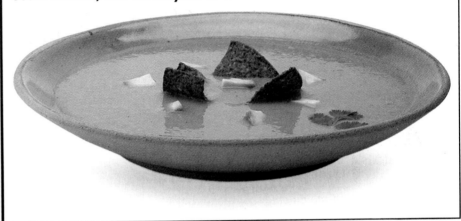

Foods of Latin America

Latin America stretches from Mexico and the islands of the Caribbean to the tip of South America. Because the area is so large, it includes climates and geographical features of all kinds—tropical rain forests, snow-capped mountains, arid deserts, and temperate zones. Foods vary according to the growing conditions. Nevertheless, many similarities exist among the **cuisines**—styles of food preparation and cooking associated with a specific group or culture.

Corn, or **maize**, is the staple grain in much of Latin America. Wheat and rice are also grown in some areas.

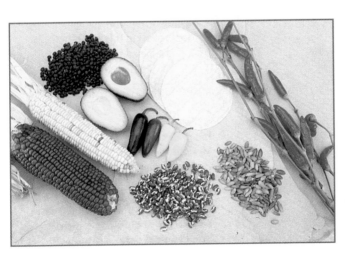

◆ Dry beans, corn products, chili peppers, and avocados are common ingredients in Latin American cooking. What is the staple grain in much of Latin America?

Mexico

Mexico's cuisine developed out of both the native foods and the influence of the Spanish conquerors. Cornmeal, rice, cooked dry beans, and chili peppers are the basics of Mexican cooking. The bland taste of corn and beans provides a contrast to the spicy taste of the various peppers.

The bread of Mexico is the tortilla. You have probably eaten tortillas in tacos, burritos, and similar foods. This flat, pounded bread is usually made from *masa*—dried corn soaked in limewater and ground while wet. In some dishes, masa is made into a dough and cooked by steaming. The best known of such dishes is *tamales*, masa formed into various shapes and often filled with finely chopped chicken and other foods. The bundles are steamed in corn husks or banana leaves.

Much of Mexican cuisine is hotly spiced. One dish that often surprises visitors to the country is *pollo con mole poblano*, chicken in a thick, dark sauce of chili peppers and chocolate.

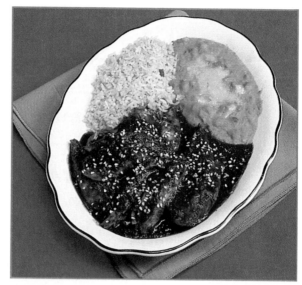

◆ *Pollo con mole poblano* is a delicious combination of braised chicken in a sauce of chili peppers, nuts, and chocolate. After reading this chapter, identify at least one other dish from another culture that contains an ingredient you would expect to find in a dessert.

Most Mexican meals include frijoles, cooked dry beans. *Frijoles refritos* are cooked dry beans that are mashed and fried in lard. Popular desserts include *flan*, a sweet baked custard topped with a sauce of caramelized sugar, and preserved guava.

INFOLINK

For more on <u>baked custard,</u> including general guidelines for preparing this and other egg-based dishes, see Section 18-4.

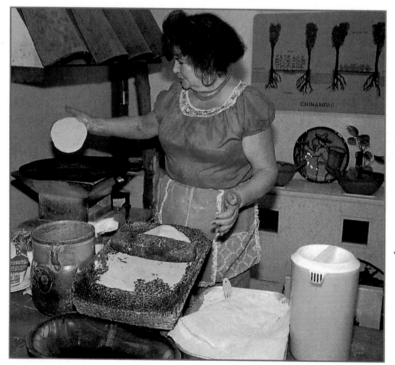

◆ Following centuries of tradition, this Mexican woman makes tortillas using the traditional tools—a *metate* to hold the dough and a *metlalpil* to roll it. Use a print or online resource to investigate the origin of the Mexican terms in the previous sentence. What does their origin reveal about Mexico's past?

Central America

A bridge of seven small countries connects Mexico to South America: Belize, Costa Rica, El Salvador, Guatemala, Honduras, Nicaragua, and Panama. This region is where the Mayan empire flourished. People who live in these countries today are of Mayan, European, African, and mixed descent. The cooking has Mayan and Aztec roots with Spanish and Caribbean influences.

Corn and beans are the staple crops. Bananas, coffee, coconuts, and cacao (the bean from which chocolate is made) are exported to other countries.

Chicken is widely eaten in Central America. It might be prepared with pineapple or in a mixture of ingredients, such as pumpkin seeds, tomatoes, and raisins.

A favorite food is *chayote*, a crisp vegetable with a delicate flavor, which is often sliced and simmered. Costa Ricans mix it with cheese and eggs, whereas cooks in the Dominican Republic fry it with eggs, tomatoes, and hot peppers.

The Caribbean

The tropical islands of the Caribbean Sea are to the south and east of Mexico, between Florida and South America. Caribbean nations include Cuba, Jamaica, Haiti, the Dominican Republic, and Puerto Rico.

Columbus landed on these islands on his voyages to find spices and a shorter route to India. The Spanish came later, as did the Dutch, Portuguese, British, and French. All these cultures left their marks on the people who live there today, in the languages they speak, their customs, and their food.

Caribbean Cuisine

The staple food is the plantain, a starchy food that looks like a banana but is cooked as a vegetable. It can be roasted, fried, boiled, baked, or combined in dishes with meat and cheese. Abundant fish and shellfish are taken from local waters. Among these are flying fish, conch, shrimp, codfish, clams, grouper, and red snapper. In the warm climate, tropical fruits—including mangoes, bananas, coconuts, papayas, and pineapples—are also plentiful. So are sweet potatoes, pumpkins, and chili peppers.

The dishes of the Caribbean vary from country to country. Some are colorfully named. For example, *Moros y Cristianos* ("Moors and Christians") is a Cuban national dish made with black beans and rice. Jamaican "Saturday Soup" consists of hot peppers (originally from Africa), carrots, turnips, and pumpkin added

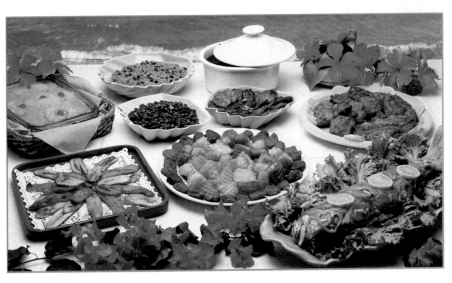

◆ This buffet from the island of Barbados includes beans, rice, plantain, fish, pineapple, and other locally available foods. Which staples of the Barbados table are common to other parts of Latin America?

◆ **Black beans are a staple in Brazil.** Can you name a popular Brazilian dish made with black beans?

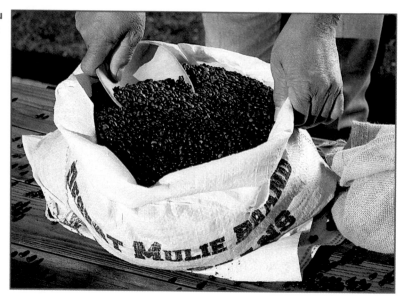

to beef stock. The cuisine of Haiti, which includes an unusual soup made of bread and pumpkin, reflects both African and French influences.

Islanders use coconut milk and fruit juice to prepare both main dishes and desserts, such as coconut custard. Ice cream made with papaya and other local fruits is also popular.

South America

Twelve nations make up South America, the southern half of the Western Hemisphere: Argentina, Bolivia, Brazil, Chili, Colombia, Ecuador, Guyana, Paraguay, Peru, Surinam, Uruguay, and Venezuela. It also includes French Guiana, a European possession.

As in the rest of Latin America, the population is of native Indian, European, and African ancestry. The climate, culture, people, and growing conditions vary greatly from country to country and from rural area to city.

Brazil

Brazil, the largest country in South America, produces great amounts of beef, coffee, and cocoa. The people trace their ethnic roots to native Indians, Portuguese, and Africans. This blend of cultures can be seen in Brazilian food. From West Africa comes *dende,* or palm oil (which gives a bright yellow-orange color to foods), *malagueta* peppers, and coconut milk. From the Portuguese come a love of sausage and the use of kale as a soup ingredient.

Sausage appears in *feijoada,* the national dish of Brazil. Links of the smoked meat are simmered—along with beef short ribs, slices of dried beef, and pork—in a pot of black beans. Side dishes of rice, collard greens, sliced oranges, and manioc flour (a toasted bread crumb-like grain) complete the rib-sticking stew. Brazil's long coastline accounts for the many fish recipes, including *mariscada,* a fish stew consisting of clams, mussels, codfish, shrimp, and crab cooked together with tomatoes and spices.

FOR YOUR HEALTH

Eating What Comes Naturally

Many of the staple foods of Latin America—such as grains, beans, and fresh fruits and vegetables—are rich in nutrients. The popularity of these foods in Latin American cultures is mainly a result of their ready availability.

Following Up

• How might the food customs that originated in the past benefit people now and in the future?

Peru

Peru is located on the Pacific coast of South America. When the Spanish conqueror Pizarro came to Peru in the sixteenth century, the local people were eating corn, potatoes, squash, beans, cassava, sweet potatoes, peanuts, tomatoes, avocados, and chili peppers. Although these foods are still popular, today Peru is also noted for its fishing industry. The potato remains its staple food. Popular meats include seafood and beef.

Peru was a Spanish colony for almost 300 years. The Spanish influence can be seen in foods such as *gazpacho,* a cold tomato-based soup of Spanish origin. *Ceviche* is a native Peruvian dish in which raw fish is marinated in lime juice. Other foods often eaten in wealthier areas include meat, poultry, vegetables, and grains, which are highly seasoned with onions, garlic, and hot peppers. Rice, potatoes, and bread accompany the main meals.

In poorer areas, meals include potatoes, corn, squash, and soups made of wheat and barley. The foods of those living in jungle areas consist of a variety of fish, small game, fruits, and nuts.

Argentina

South of Brazil, along the eastern coast of South America, lies Argentina. Today most of its inhabitants are of European descent.

Raising beef is one of Argentina's major industries, and as a result, most people eat beef. It is often grilled outdoors and served with spicy sauces. *Puchero* is a meat and vegetable stew. Another widely eaten dish is *empanadas,* turnovers of dough filled with vegetables, meat, fruit, or a combination of the three. Meats are also combined with fruits in local stews such as *carbonada criolla*—beef mixed with peaches.

Section 22-1 Review & Activities

1. What is the staple grain in most of Latin America?

2. What is the most popular type of bread in Mexican cuisine?

3. What cultures have influenced Caribbean food?

4. **Synthesizing.** Choose one of the countries or areas of Latin America covered in the section. Explain the influences of climate or geography on the cuisine of that region.

5. **Comparing and Contrasting.** Divide a sheet of paper into three columns labeled "Brazil," "Argentina," and "Both." In the columns, list unique aspects of the local cuisine for each country as well as features the two countries share.

6. **Applying.** In groups, make lists of the foods described in this section with which you are familiar. What other Latin American foods have you tasted that are not listed in the text? What ingredients appear regularly in the dishes you listed?

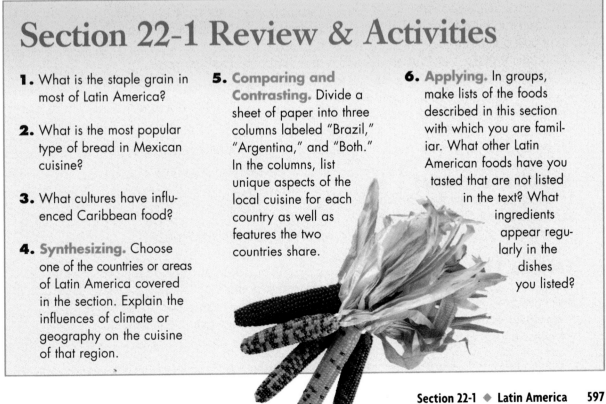

RECIPE FILE

Cuban Black Bean Soup

The variations on recipes for this Cuban signature dish are endless. This one has a creamy texture and a sharp citrus bite that makes it irresistible.

Customary	Ingredients	Metric
1	Medium onion, chopped	1
1	Rib celery, chopped	1
1	Garlic clove, minced	1
1 Tbsp.	Vegetable oil	20 mL
1 cup	Chicken or vegetable broth	250 mL
2 1-lb. cans	Black beans, drained	2 500-g cans
Dash	Cayenne pepper	Dash
1 Tbsp.	Lemon juice	20 mL
	Salt and pepper	

Yield: 4 servings
Equipment: Stock pot or Dutch oven

Directions
1. Sauté onion, celery, and garlic in oil until tender.
2. Add chicken or vegetable broth, black beans, and cayenne pepper.
3. Simmer mixture over medium heat, stirring occasionally, until heated through (about 5 minutes).
4. Carefully purée mixture in small batches in a blender or food processor. Return to stock pot.
5. Stir in lemon juice and simmer until thoroughly heated.
6. Season to taste with salt and pepper and serve hot.

Note: For a chunkier soup, purée only half the mixture before returning to stock pot.

Nutrition Information
Per serving (approximate): 286 calories, 17 g protein, 45 g carbohydrate, 5 g fat, 0 mg cholesterol, 206 mg sodium
Good source of: potassium, iron, zinc, vitamin E, B vitamins, phosphorus

Food for Thought
- Make a list of all the kitchen tools you would need to prepare and cook this soup.
- Discuss how and where in a meal you would serve this soup—for example, as an appetizer or as a main course. What would you serve along with it to make it a well-balanced, authentic Cuban meal?

Africa and the Middle East

Although Africa is an ocean away from Latin America, the two continents share some of the same foods and culinary traditions. This is the result of similarities in climate and in exploration and conquest.

Objectives

After studying this section, you should be able to:

- Describe food choices available in Africa south of the Sahara.
- Describe the cuisines of North Africa and the Middle East.
- Identify the cultural and geographical influences on the foods of Africa and the Middle East.

Look for These Terms

berbere

kibbutz

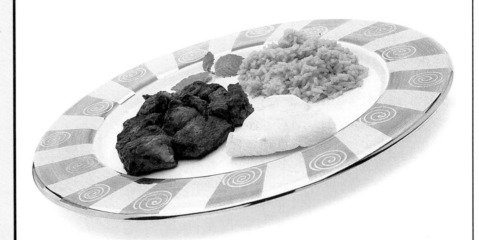

Africa

The Sahara forms a natural east-west dividing line through Africa. It separates the five nations in the north, along the Mediterranean Sea, from the rest of the continent.

The people living south of the Sahara are mainly Africans. Those living north of the Sahara are mostly Arabs, with a culture similar to that of the Middle East.

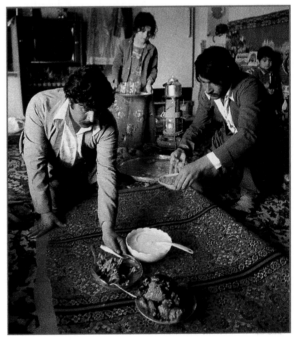

◆ **A family in Afghanistan enjoys the evening meal.** Name two differences between the dining customs in the Middle East and those common in the United States.

Sub-Saharan Africa

The area south of the Sahara is sometimes known as the sub-Saharan region. The concept of society in this region is defined by kinship groups—centuries-old networks of clans and tribes numbering sometimes in the thousands. In the past, these clans often lived together in villages and jointly owned the surrounding farmland. Food traditions are linked more with these social groups than with political boundaries past or present.

Influence of Climate

Most of sub-Saharan Africa has a tropical or subtropical climate. However, there is a wide range of geographical features, including mountains, coastlines, river valleys, tropical rain forests, and desert. Consequently, different foods are raised in these various regions.

In western and central Africa, areas that are hot and humid, the chief crops include plantains, rice, bananas, yams, and cassava. In the grasslands in the east and south, corn, millet, and sorghum are grown. Wheat is grown in many areas, along with foods such as onions, garlic, pumpkins, watermelons, cucumbers, chilies, dates, and figs.

Chickens, cattle, sheep, and goats are raised wherever possible. Small herds of animals have traditionally provided income, as well as food, for small farmers and herders. The eating of meat, however, is usually reserved for special occasions. People living along waterways, such as rivers, lakes, and seas, have an abundant supply of fish.

Influence of Settlers

Over the centuries, food crops introduced from other continents have been incorporated into African cuisines. Coconuts were introduced from Asia in the 1500s. In the same

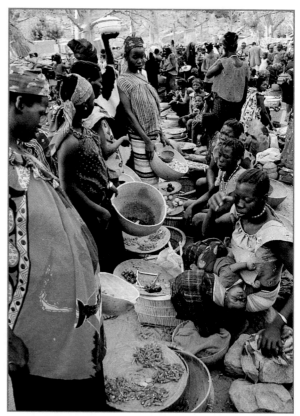

◆ At this market in the West African nation of Mali, peanuts and yams are among the foods sold. Identify two ways in which yams are prepared and eaten in Africa.

century, corn arrived from the New World. In the 1600s, cassava became an important food source. In the 1700s, peanuts were introduced, possibly from South America.

Yams have remained a staple starch throughout Africa. The traditional way to prepare them is to boil, peel, and slice or pound them until they form a paste, called *fufu*. In West Africa, cooks mash and deep-fry them, make them into croquettes, or slice and bake them. In some areas, cooks make fufu by mashing cassava and plantains.

South Africa was visited and also settled by many waves of Europeans looking for trade routes or escaping persecution. These French, Dutch, British, and German Europeans brought their own food preferences and preparation methods. African cooks modified them with local produce and techniques. *Bredie,* for example, is a stew made with meat or fish, vegetables, onions, and chili peppers.

The African Meal

Most Africans eat one large meal a day, generally in the evening. A typical meal may include a grain such as millet cooked into a porridge or a vegetable such as yams. This is served with a seasoned stew made with vegetables and flavored with meat, poultry, or fish, if available.

The evening meal is always a social occasion. The food may be served in one large bowl, which is set on the ground. People sit around the bowl, using either pieces of bread or their fingers to scoop up the food.

In many areas of Africa, spicy foods are preferred. Cooks make their own seasoning mixes, based on the many kinds of hot chili and spices available. One blend, called **berbere**, is commonly used in Ethiopia in soups and stews. It is a spicy combination of garlic, red and black peppers, salt, coriander, fenugreek, and cardamom. Other spices are added, depending on the cook's preference.

North Africa

The five main countries that make up North Africa are Libya, Egypt, Algeria, Morocco, and Tunisia. The population is clustered along the Mediterranean, in desert oases, or in irrigated parts of Egypt along the Nile. Because of its location along ancient trade routes linking Asia to Europe, this area has been well traveled. Its cuisine reflects the influence of those early travelers. The use of rice as a staple and the variety of produce are two legacies of foreign visitors. Two other staple starches grown in the region and still widely used are wheat and barley.

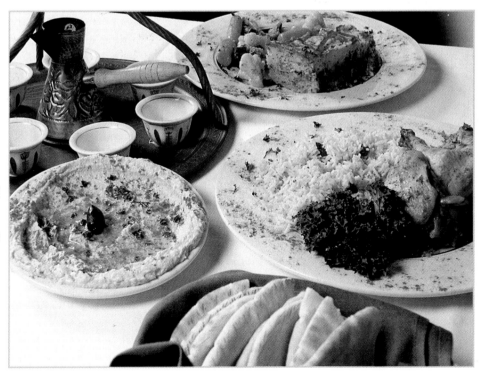

◆ The Moroccan dishes shown here are moussaka (top), made of sliced eggplant, seasoned ground beef, and potatoes topped with a special sauce and then baked; hummus (left), a dip made from blended chickpeas lightly seasoned and mixed with sesame sauce; and stuffed Cornish hen el morocco (right), a baked hen stuffed with rice, almonds, raisins, and saffron. What is the name of a sesame seed paste that is popular in this area?

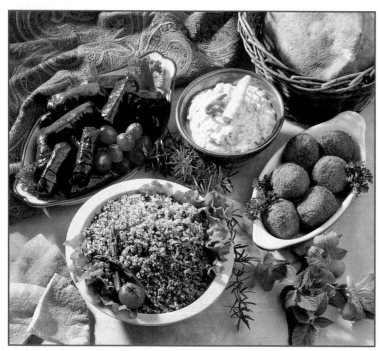

◆ Tabbouleh (in front) is a refreshing salad from the Middle East made with bulgur and accented with dill. Consult print or online resources to learn what bulgur is.

The Middle East

The Middle East is located just east of North Africa, between Southeast Europe and Southwest Asia. The main countries of the Middle East are Lebanon, Syria, Iran, Iraq, Israel, Jordan, Kuwait, Turkey, and Saudi Arabia. Most people in this area are Arabs. Israel, which is a Jewish nation, is the exception.

Middle Eastern Cuisine

There are many similarities among the foods of the various nations of the Middle East and North Africa. The names and some seasonings may vary, but the basic ingredients and cooking methods are similar.

North African Cuisine

Although there are some differences among the cuisines of North Africa, all make use of olive oil, chickpeas, fava beans, lentils, lamb, and goat. Dried fruits and nuts play a role in the cuisine, as do chili peppers and cinnamon.

One notable dish of the region is *tajine,* a Moroccan specialty. The dish is a long-cooked stew of lamb, prunes, and almonds, sometimes flavored with cinnamon. Tajine is often served with couscous, a fluffy steamed grain. *Couscous* is also the name of an entire meal featuring the grain and one of several stewed meats or poultry mixed with aromatic vegetables. Another dish that is both savory and sweet is *pastilla,* common in both Morocco and Algeria. This dish, which bears French influences, is a pigeon pie made with phyllo dough, eggs, vegetables, spices, and nuts. The finished dish is sprinkled with sugar.

Fruits include apricots, pomegranates, dates, figs, grapes, and oranges. Vegetables include eggplant, peppers, olives, cucumbers, and tomatoes. Seasonings include parsley, dill, mint, cinnamon, lemon juice, pine nuts, onion, and garlic. *Tahini,* a sesame seed paste, is popular. Lamb is commonly eaten; chicken and fish are also used when available. Chicken is sometimes an ingredient in stews made with lentils, beans, rice, and vegetables. Pork is a food forbidden by religious law throughout this region.

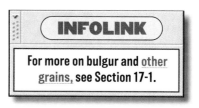

INFOLINK

For more on bulgur and other grains, see Section 17-1.

Staple Foods

Although rice and barley are eaten, the staple starch of the Middle East is wheat, especially in the form of bulgur. This grain is a featured ingredient in *tabbouleh*, a popular salad that also includes tomatoes, mint, parsley, onions, and olive oil.

Another important staple food is yogurt. Depending on where you are, you might find yogurt made from the milk of cows, goats, camels, or buffalo. In several countries, yogurt is called *leban*. Leban is often mixed with vegetables, especially cucumbers and dates, for a side dish or part of a main dish.

Here are some other dishes commonly found in this area:

♦ **Kubaybah or kibbi.** A mixture of ground lamb, bulgur, cinnamon, and all-spice.

♦ **Stuffed vine leaves.** Are filled with a rice and meat mixture and served with a sauce made of yogurt, garlic, and mint.

♦ **Herrira.** A mutton and vegetable soup. Is eaten often during Ramadan, the month when Muslims fast during daylight hours.

♦ **Chelo.** Popular especially in Iran, Iraq, and Lebanon. Steamed rice accompanied by a meat or vegetable dish.

♦ **Koresh.** A stew of meat or poultry with vegetables, fruit, nuts, seasoning, and perhaps cereal. Most Iranians will eat a *chelo koresh* for one meal a day.

Desserts of the Middle East are often fresh, seasonal fruits. The people of the Middle East also enjoy sweet desserts, such as *baklava,* phyllo dough layered with nuts and honey syrup. *Halva* is a candy made of ground sesame seeds and honey.

For a feast, such as a wedding, it is common to roast a whole sheep and serve it with couscous. A salad of tomatoes, peppers, cucumbers, mint, melon, grapes, dates, and figs might be included.

Israel

Israel includes people native to the Middle East along with others from around the world. Consequently, its food customs embrace both Middle Eastern traditions and those of many other countries. Customs also reflect Jewish food traditions and laws, including a prohibition against mixing dairy foods and meat.

Traditional condiments, which find their way into most recipes, include *shatta, zhoug,* and tahini. *Shatta* is a red chili pepper mixture. *Zhoug* is a combination of green chili peppers, parsley, coriander, cumin, garlic, olive oil, and salt and pepper.

Some Israelis live in a **kibbutz** (kee-BOOTS), a communal organization, which raises its own food. Breakfasts at a kibbutz are substantial. They may consist of fresh produce, cold meats, cheese, fish, eggs, condiments, vegetable salads, and hot coffee.

Chicken and lamb are widely used. So are chickpeas, which are enjoyed both in *falafel*— patties of the ground legume seasoned with parsley and fried—and in *hummus b'tahini,* a spread of ground chickpeas, lemon juice, and tahini. Both dishes are served with pita bread, the pocket bread popular throughout much of the Middle East.

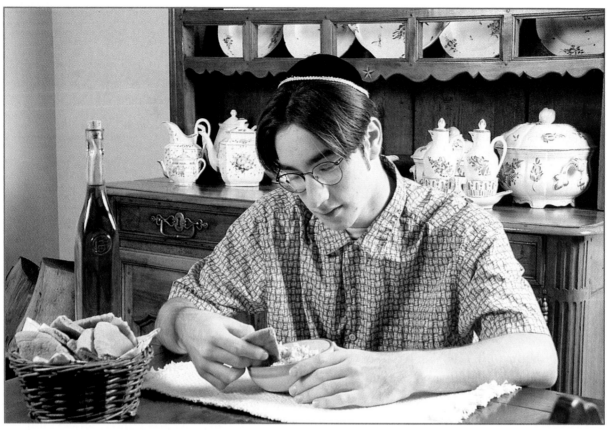

◆ **Hummus b'tahini, a mash of chickpeas, lemon juice, and tahini is a favorite in Israel and other Middle Eastern nations. What nutrients does this dish contain?**

Section 22-2 Review & Activities

1. What are two important food plants that found their way to sub-Saharan Africa from other continents?

2. Identify and describe two North African dishes.

3. Name two staple foods of the Middle East.

4. Analyzing. Give an example of how religion influences eating habits in Middle Eastern countries.

5. Synthesizing. How does global travel influence the exchange of food customs today? How does this compare with the influence of travel in the past?

6. Applying. Find a recipe for making yogurt (using milk and a small amount of cultured yogurt). Prepare a work plan for making some at home or in a foods lab.

RECIPE FILE

Couscous Tabbouleh

This refreshing salad combines a staple grain popular in North Africa and flavors of the Middle East.

Customary	Ingredients	Metric
1 cup	Reduced-sodium chicken broth	250 mL
¾ cup	Couscous	175 mL
¼ cup	Lemon juice	50 mL
1 Tbsp.	Olive oil	15 mL
¼ tsp.	Salt	1 mL
¼ tsp.	Pepper	1 mL
½ cup	Peeled, chopped cucumber	125 mL
1	Tomato, chopped	1
½ cup	Chopped green onion	125 mL
½ cup	Chopped fresh parsley	125 mL
¼ cup	Chopped fresh mint	50 mL
	Mint leaves (for garnish)	

Yield: 4 servings, ½ cup each
Equipment: Medium saucepan

Directions

1. In a medium saucepan, bring chicken broth to a boil.
2. Place couscous in a large bowl. Carefully pour hot broth over couscous. Let stand 5 minutes. (All liquid should be absorbed. Drain if necessary.) Cool to room temperature.
3. In a small bowl, whisk together lemon juice, olive oil, salt, and pepper. Set aside.
4. Add cucumber, tomato, green onion, parsley, and mint to couscous.
5. Drizzle lemon juice mixture over couscous. Toss to mix.
6. Serve, garnished with mint leaves, if desired.

Nutrition Information

Per serving (approximate):183 calories, 4 g protein, 32 g carbohydrate, 4 g fat, 0 mg cholesterol, 339 mg sodium
Good source of: iron, vitamin A, vitamin C, B vitamins

Food for Thought

- Tabbouleh is traditionally prepared with bulgur wheat. Name two other grains you could use to prepare this recipe.
- What pre-preparation tasks could be done while the couscous is cooling to room temperature?

Europe

The European countries are small, and there is considerable travel among them. They share many food customs and seasoning choices, especially neighboring countries with similar climates. On the other hand, most European countries have had distinctive histories and traditions, which give their foods unique identities.

Objectives

After studying this section, you should be able to:

- Identify foods commonly found in Western and Eastern Europe.
- Identify ways that culture, history, geography, and climate influence European foods.

Look for These Terms

scones

high tea

deglazing

haute cuisine

polenta

antipasto

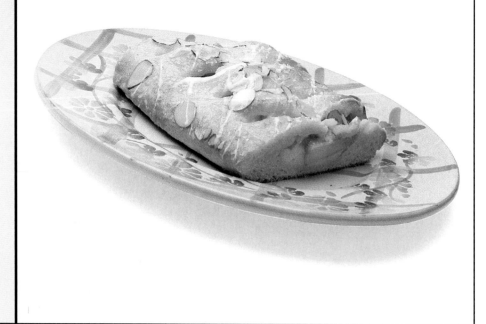

Western Europe

The cuisines of many world cultures, including our own, trace their roots to countries and regions of Western Europe, which include the British Isles, France, Spain, Portugal, Germany, Austria, Italy, Greece, and Scandinavia.

The British Isles

The British Isles are an island group just off the European continent. The two largest islands are Great Britain—which includes England, Scotland, Wales, and Northern Ireland—and Ireland. The food of this region tends to be hearty and cooked by plain, simple methods. Beef, mutton (meat from older sheep), pork, and fish are favorite foods. Many Britons eat four meals a day: breakfast, lunch, tea, and dinner (or supper).

The habit in our own country of eating hearty breakfasts is a custom inherited from Britain. Today, breakfast in the British Isles still usually includes cereal, eggs, bacon or sausage, broiled tomatoes, toast, and marmalade. Tea is more common in the morning than coffee.

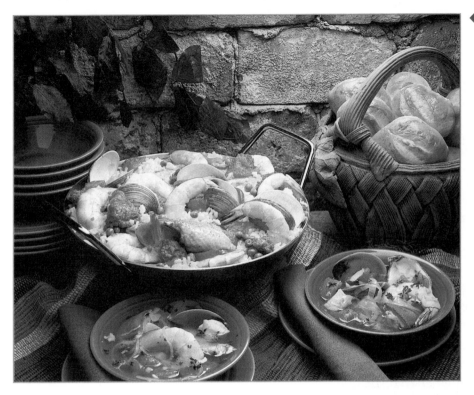

◆ Despite differences in culture and customs throughout Europe, some foods and methods of food preparation transcend national boundaries. The shellfish stew shown here is a common sight all along the Mediterranean coast. In a food encyclopedia or similar resource, look up *pizza* and *pissaladiére.* Where did the second dish originate? In what way are the two foods alike?

British Cuisine

Typical lunches and dinners in Britain revolve around meat, including:

◆ **Roast beef and Yorkshire pudding.** Beef baked in the oven, with a popover-like mixture cooked in the pan drippings. Roast beef is usually served with a horseradish sauce or mustard.

◆ **Shepherd's pie.** Leftover ground lamb or beef cooked with onions, garlic, tomatoes, and seasonings. The dish is covered with mashed potatoes and baked.

◆ **Cornish pasties** (PAS-tees). Popular in the south of England, these baked pastry turnovers—filled with steak, onions, chopped potatoes and carrots—were once carried to work by miners and eaten cold.

The British also enjoy a variety of game—pigeon, quail, pheasant, and deer. Fish is also common to British menus. *Finnan haddie,* a fish dish sometimes eaten for breakfast, is smoked haddock prepared with milk, onion, lemon juice, pepper, and parsley.

Tea

A meal that is uniquely British is four o'clock tea. Tea generally includes bread—either plain or in small finger sandwiches—and a dessert. Crumpets, which are similar to what Americans call English muffins, might also be served. So might **scones**, a tasty variation of baking-powder biscuits. Scones are often served with jam and clotted cream—a thick spread skimmed from rich, whole milk. In Scotland, tea may be served with oatcakes or oatmeal biscuits.

Sometimes, Britons have their tea served with a nonsweet dish that is somewhere between an appetizer and a main course. This meal is called **high tea**. A typical dish served at high tea is *Welsh rabbit* (or *rarebit*), seasoned, melted cheddar cheese on toast. High tea often takes the place of supper.

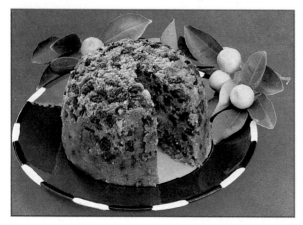

◆ Plum pudding, a Christmas tradition in England, is a dense cake made with raisins, nuts, and flavorings, steamed in cheesecloth. Despite its name, plum pudding is not made with plums. Can you name another food whose name includes an ingredient that is not present?

France

The goal of French cooking is to maximize the flavors of all ingredients in a dish so that no one flavor overpowers another. Much of French cooking is fairly simple—and frugal. The practice of **deglazing** a pan—adding stock or another liquid to a defatted sauté pan to loosen the browned-on particles—got its start in French kitchens. Deglazing is an easy and economical way of making a sauce.

Haute Cuisine

The classic dishes of France are often grouped under the heading **haute cuisine**. Literally "high cooking," this is a method of food preparation that makes use of complicated recipes and techniques, often involving costly ingredients. Originally, great chefs prepared these time-consuming dishes for aristocrats. Food preparation was considered an art. Rich sauces, elegantly decorated dishes, and exotic ingredients characterize haute cuisine. Haute cuisine exists today, usually in expensive restaurants.

Cuisine Bourgeoise

Outside of the aristocracy, a simpler form of cooking developed. *Cuisine bourgeoise* (boor-JWAHZ) is based on hearty, one-dish meals made from fresh ingredients from the local market. Cuisine bourgeoise varies from province to province. Examples include:

◆ **Ragout.** A flavorful stew made with vegetables and meat, poultry, or fish. It is often named after the region where it originated.

◆ **Pot-au-feu.** A soupy casserole of less tender cuts of beef, along with sausage and poultry, long-simmered in an earthenware pot with aromatic and root vegetables.

◆ **Cassoulet.** A hearty blend of white beans, meats, preserved duck, and garlic sausage.

◆ **Bouillabaisse.** A hearty soup that combines several types of fish and shellfish, tomatoes, and herbs.

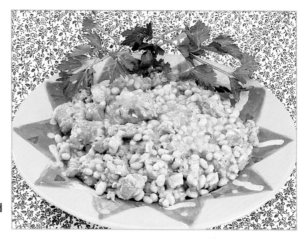

◆ Cassoulet is typical French country fare. This rib-sticking dish consists of beans, meats, poultry, and garlic sausage baked together under a breadcrumb topping. What method of cooking do you think is used to make cassoulet?

Meals in France

French people rarely eat between meals. A typical breakfast is light, consisting of coffee or hot chocolate and some kind of bread—toast, a croissant, or *brioche,* a round roll made from a rich yeast dough. Lunch or dinner might include an *hors d'oeurve* (appetizer), followed by a light fish course, followed by a main dish and vegetables. Next comes a salad of greens simply dressed with a vinaigrette. A meal concludes with either a sweet dessert or with bread and cheese. Such a menu sounds filling. Portions, however, are kept sensible, and food is eaten slowly.

Spain and Portugal

Spain and Portugal inhabit a peninsula, which provides both countries with thousands of miles of coastline. Many of the dishes of both nations are based on fish and seafood.

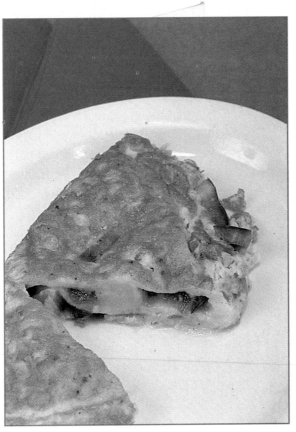

Meals in Spain

Breakfast in Spain, as in France, generally consists of coffee or hot chocolate and a bread. The bread might be *churros,* fried strips of dough.

Lunch often consists of a salad, fish, a meat course, and fruit or a light dessert. Supper at home may be a light meal, but at a restaurant, it may be another large meal. Spanish people eat out late, with dinner hour generally starting at 10:30 P.M.

A few dishes are enjoyed throughout the country. These include chicken with garlic, garlic shrimp, *gazpacho* (cold vegetable soup), and *paella*—a combination of saffron-flavored rice, poultry, and shellfish. Another dish of Spain, *tortilla española,* is an omelet made with potatoes, onions, and green peppers. The dish, served in slices at room temperature, is popular in *tapas* bars—restaurants that specialize in small servings of foods ranging from main dish to salad items.

Portuguese Cuisine

Portuguese cooking is similar to Spanish cooking, except that the Portuguese prefer foods with a spicier kick. The cuisine was greatly influenced by travelers to India, South Africa, and South America. Portuguese foods tend to be rich because they contain more cream and butter.

◆ Tortilla española is one of numerous dishes featured among the selection of tapas in Spain. It is an omelet filled with green peppers, onion, and potato, served at room temperature. Compare the above description with the recipe for frittata in Section 18-3, on page 481. What similarities can you find between the two dishes? What does this reveal about the sharing of food traditions among cultures?

Germany and Austria

Generally speaking, German food tends to be rich and heavy. Sausages abound, with different combinations and seasonings in each region. Familiar favorites include bratwurst and knockwurst.

Veal and pork are the most popular meats. Germans also eat beef and poultry, but fish is not popular.

German Cuisine

Some German dishes are characterized by a blending of fruit, vegetables, and meat to achieve sweet-sour flavors. An example is *sauerbraten,* beef marinated for several days in a sweet-sour sauce, and then simmered in the same sauce. It is served with noodles, dumplings, or boiled potatoes. *Schnitzel,* means "cutlet" in German, usually of veal. In *wienerschnitzel*—or "Viennese cutlet"—the veal is dipped in egg, breaded, and fried.

Germans are noted for their rye and pumpernickel breads as well as *stollen,* yeast bread with raisins and canned fruit. Another favorite is *streusel-kuchen,* a coffee cake topped with a mixture of flour, sugar, butter, nuts, and cinnamon.

German desserts include cakes and cookies. *Marzipan,* a rich candy made of ground almonds and sugar, has its origins in Germany. So does *nürnberger lebkuchen,* which is better known as gingerbread.

Austrian Cuisine

Austria is a nation south of Germany. The people there share not only a common language with the Germans but also many of the same food customs. Austrian cooking, in addition, bears influences of the cooking of its other Eastern European neighbors.

Austrians are famous for their rich cakes, almost always served *mitt Schlag*—with thick, sweetened whipped cream. *Linzertorte,* a cross between a pie and a cake, has a crust made in part of ground nuts and a sweet jam filling. *Sachertorte,* another famous Austrian dessert, is a rich chocolate cake spread with apricot preserves and a dark chocolate icing.

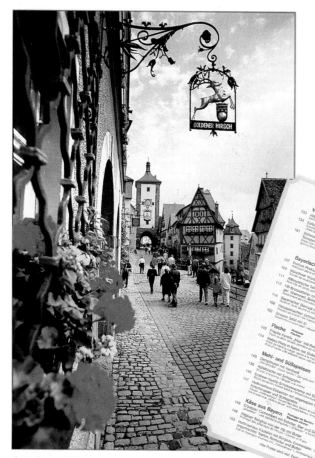

◆ Schnitzels (veal cutlets) and wursts (sausages) are staples of German cuisine. **Name a food commonly eaten with schnitzels and wursts.**

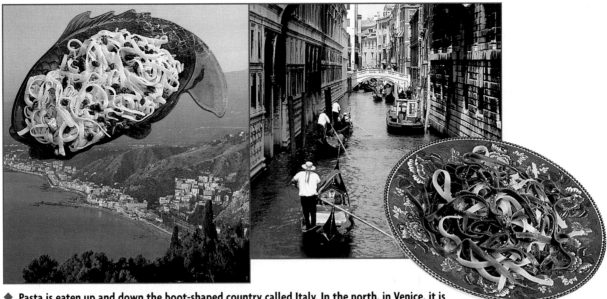

◆ Pasta is eaten up and down the boot-shaped country called Italy. In the north, in Venice, it is served as "black pasta," deriving its dark color from cuttlefish ink. In the south, in Sicily, it is served with local sardines, pine nuts, and raisins. Look at a map of Italy. Try to explain why seafood plays such a prominent role in the cuisines of this country.

Italy

Where did pasta come from? A popular explanation is that Marco Polo brought the recipe to Italy from China in the 1300s. Whatever its origins, pasta is the dish most associated with Italy. It is usually eaten, however, as a first course, not as a main course.

Italian Cuisine

In the south of Italy, pasta is often—though not always—served with tomato sauce. On the southern island of Sicily, a local favorite is *pasta con sarde,* made with sardines, raisins, and pine nuts. In some parts of northern Italy, rice is favored over pasta, in both rice balls and *risotto,* short-grained rice simmered carefully in stock. Another grain common in the north is cornmeal, served as **polenta**, cornmeal mush that is sometimes cooled, sliced, and fried.

Along Italy's northwest borders, the cooking is similar to that of France and Germany. Butter is used in place of olive oil. Italians of this region also eat *speck* (SHPEK), a local sausage with a German-sounding name.

Seafood is popular along the coastal areas. In the south, fresh bass is served mariner-style, with tomatoes, onions, and fresh basil.

No Italian meal would be complete without a *contorno* (vegetable course). Served after the main course, a large plate of eggplant, string beans, artichokes, peas, potatoes, or other vegetable is passed around the table.

Salads may begin or end a meal. They are usually served with an oil and vinegar dressing. Salads, pickled vegetables, cheeses, and other appetizers are called **antipasto**, which means "before the meal."

Italy is famous for its cheeses, from the hard parmesan and romano, which must be grated, to *ricotta* (or "recooked" cheese), which is similar to cottage cheese.

Greece

The history of Greece includes a period of nearly 400 years when it was ruled by Turkey. As a result, many Greek dishes, such as vine leaves stuffed with seasoned meat and rice, are similar to foods in the Middle East.

Greek Cuisine

Greek cooking often makes use of tomatoes, green peppers, garlic, lemon juice, and olive oil. Rice appears in many dishes. *Feta cheese,* made from sheep's or goat's milk and cured in brine, is widely eaten as an appetizer and in salads. It is also used in cooking.

Because of Greece's location on the Mediterranean, Greek cuisine makes use of fish and shellfish. Grilled octopus is eaten, and shrimp are sometimes baked with tomatoes and feta cheese. Lamb is the most popular meat, often served grilled. *Moussaka* is a layered casserole made with seasoned ground lamb and sliced eggplant. A rich white sauce is poured over the mixture before baking.

Northern Europe

Denmark, Norway, Sweden, and Finland make up the Scandinavian countries. Although these countries do not have a lavish cuisine, the people have used the foods available to them creatively and tastefully.

Foods of Scandinavia

Scandinavians rely heavily on fish for food. Dried and salted cod is a staple. Fish may also be fried, poached, or grilled, as well as used in soups and fishballs.

Dairy products are also important to Scandinavian cooks. Each country seems to have a version of thick or sour milk, which may be eaten with sugar. Milk, butter, and cream are essential ingredients in many dishes. Scandinavians also bake an array of rye and white breads.

Because the local growing season is so short, Scandinavian meals rarely include an abundance of fresh fruits and vegetables. Root vegetables such as potatoes, carrots, onions, and rutabagas are used regularly. Fresh berries (lingonberries, raspberries, and strawberries) are often used to accent desserts. *Fruksoppa,* or "fruit soup," is a mixture of dried fruit and tapioca cooked in a sweetened liquid and served cold.

Scandinavian Cuisine

The Swedish *smorgasbord* is perhaps the finest example of a bountiful buffet. Originally, the word meant "sandwich board." Now it is a collection of assorted meats and fish dishes, raw vegetables, salads, and hot dishes.

Smørrebrød are open-faced sandwiches, which the Danes eat daily. Thin slices of buttered bread are topped with pickled herring, cooked pork, raw cucumbers, onion rings, apple slices, mustard, and horseradish. The Danes are also well known for their rich, flaky, buttery pastries with touches of sugar, almonds, or jam.

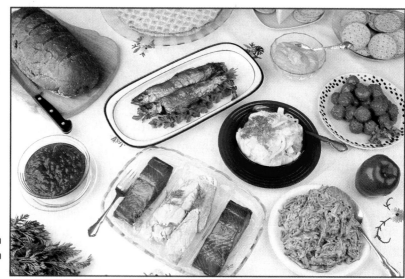

◆ Fish is a prominent part of this Swedish smorgasbord. Why is fish so common in Scandinavian cooking?

Eastern Europe

The countries of Eastern Europe underwent major changes in borders—and even names—in the late twentieth century. For ease in describing culinary history and tradition, general areas will be referred to by their traditional names. The following discussion will include the foods and culture of Russia, Czechoslovakia, Hungary, Bulgaria, Yugoslavia, and Rumania.

Russia

Russia is one of the many countries that once made up the Soviet Union. It covers a vast area, from Eastern Europe to the Pacific Coast in Asia.

Russian Cuisine

Food in Russia differs from region to region, as it does in most countries. National dishes are based mainly on available staple foods. One example is Russian black bread, a dark, heavy, moist bread of rye and wheat, flavored with chocolate, caraway, coffee, and molasses.

Hearty soups are also common. *Schchi* is a soup made from sauerkraut. Other popular soups are made with fresh cabbage and potatoes. *Borscht,* or beet soup, is one of the best-known Russian soups. If available, meat or sausage is added. Most soups either contain sour cream or are served with it.

Fish—including sardines, salted herring, and salmon—are common. Caviar is often served with *blini,* small buckwheat pancakes, and sour cream. Buckwheat is also eaten crushed and cooked as *kasha*, and is served as an accompaniment to meats.

Tea is the most popular beverage. On cold evenings, you might find a gathering of Russians drinking tea and enjoying good conversation.

Other Eastern European Nations

The food in some other nations of Eastern Europe has many similarities to that of Russia and, sometimes, to food of the Middle East. The use of wheat, kasha, and cabbage, for example, is widespread.

Poland. In Poland, the national dish, *bigos,* is a stew of game meat with mushrooms, onions, sauerkraut, sausage, apples, and tomatoes. *Krupnik* is a barley and vegetable soup to which sour cream and dill are added.

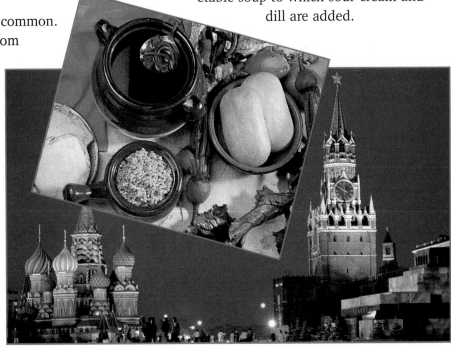

◆ This assortment from the Russian table includes borscht, piroshky, and kasha a la Gouriev. The last of these is a custard-like dessert made with farina and served warm. Which dish pictured is sometimes served cold?

Hungary. The Hungarian people enjoy grilled skewered lamb or beef in addition to the dish for which they are most famous, *gulyas* or *goulash*, in our culture. This soup-like dish is made with beef, onions, paprika, potatoes, and perhaps garlic, caraway seeds, tomatoes, and honey.

Hungarians also enjoy sauerkraut, pork-stuffed cabbage rolls, strudels, and *dobos torta,* a chocolate-filled sponge cake with many layers, glazed with caramel.

Czechoslovakia. The people of the Czechoslovakia area rely on dumplings as the cornerstone of their meals. Dumplings may be made from a variety of foods and come in many shapes and forms. Pork, beef, and game are common, as are cabbage and sauerkraut with caraway. One of the most famous Czech dishes is *kolacky,* yeast buns filled with fruit, cottage cheese, poppy seeds, or jam.

Yugoslavia. In the region of Yugoslavia, pilafs (seasoned rice dishes) are a favorite, as are cornmeal dishes, vegetables, and pasta. *Sarma,* the national dish, is rolled cabbage or sauerkraut leaves stuffed with a mixture of rice and ground pork. Also popular are thick, dark coffee; baklava; and desserts made with sweet noodles, dumplings, and fried yeast dough.

Romania. Corn is the mainstay of cooking in the area of Romania. Cornmeal mush, the national dish, is served with melted butter, sour cream, or yogurt. Romanian cooks also use peppers in their dishes and are known for their richly flavored stews.

Bulgaria. Grains, vegetables, fruit, nuts, and yogurt are mainstays of Bulgarian cuisine. Fresh vegetables are eaten widely in salads. Fruits, nuts, and herbs grow well in this region. The people prefer fish and lamb to other meats. A favorite dish is *potato musaka,* a casserole of vegetables, meat, potatoes, onions, garlic, tomato, eggs, cream, and grated cheese.

Section 22-3 Review & Activities

1. Name five foods commonly found in the countries of Western Europe.

2. What is the difference between haute cuisine and cuisine bourgeoise?

3. Identify five foods commonly found in Eastern European countries.

4. Synthesizing. Choose one of the cultures covered. What factors appear to have influenced food choices and how foods are prepared?

5. Extending. Design an international dinner. Choose an appetizer from one country, a main dish from another, a dessert from still another. Select foods that are compatible and varied, and that constitute a balanced, nutritious meal.

6. Applying. Choose a European country. Assume you are inviting two teens from that country to dinner with your family. Write a menu showing what you would serve to make these teens feel at home. Give reasons to support your selections.

RECIPE FILE

Scandinavian Marinated Cod

Cod is a staple food in Scandinavia. This recipe might be prepared for a midday meal or a light supper. The cooked cod could also be flaked and used in a salad.

Customary	Ingredients	Metric
1 lb.	Cod fillets	454 g
¼ cup	Olive oil	50 mL
2 Tbsp.	Lemon juice	30 mL
¼ cup	Finely chopped onion	50 mL
1 tsp.	Salt	5 mL
½ tsp.	Pepper	2-3 mL
2 Tbsp.	Butter or margarine, melted	30 mL
2 Tbsp.	Vegetable oil	30 mL

Yield: 4 servings
Equipment: Shallow baking dish, broiler pan

Directions

1. Wash cod fillets in cold water and pat dry. Place in shallow baking dish.
2. In a small bowl, whisk together olive oil, lemon juice, onion, salt, and pepper.
3. Pour mixture over cod fillets. Let marinade 30 minutes (15 minutes on each side). Drain marinade from fillets and discard.
4. In another small bowl, blend melted butter or margarine with vegetable oil.
5. Preheat broiler.
6. Brush cold broiler grid with 1 tablespoon of the butter and oil mixture.
7. Place cod fillets on broiler pan.
8. Broil fillets 10 minutes per inch of thickness, turning halfway through cooking time.
9. Brush fillets with remaining butter and oil mixture after turning.
10. When done, the fish should flake easily with a fork.
11. Serve immediately.

Nutrition Information

Per serving (approximate): 300 calories, 20 g protein, 1 g carbohydrate, 6 g fat, 49 mg cholesterol, 260 mg sodium
Good source of: potassium, vitamin E, B vitamins, phosphorus

Food for Thought

• What other varieties of fish might you substitute for the cod?
• What other acids, herbs, or spices could be used in the marinade for this recipe?

Asia and the Pacific

"East is East, and West is West," Rudyard Kipling *wrote over a century ago. Despite the merging of these two worlds since that time, in some ways, the East has remained separate. One way is in the food customs and traditions.*

Objectives

After studying this section, you should be able to:

- Identify foods common to the countries of Asia and the Pacific.
- Point out how culture and climate influence the foods of Asia and the Pacific.

Look for These Terms

soba

garam masala

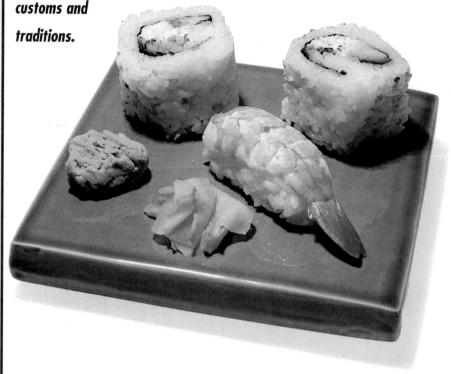

Asia

For purposes of discussion, the countries of Asia and the Pacific will be treated in four sections. The first will look at the world cultures of Japan, China, and Korea. The second will examine Southeast Asia. The third will cover the Asian subcontinent of India; the fourth, Australia and New Zealand.

Asian World Cultures

Asia is the world's largest continent in both area and population. Traditional Asian cooking emphasizes grains and legumes, and uses an abundance of fresh ingredients. The staple grain is rice, though wheat is widely used in parts of China, India, and Japan. Another staple is soybeans, which are used to make many products, such as soy sauce, tamari, and tofu. Soybean sprouts are used fresh and in cooked dishes.

The basic cooking methods include boiling, steaming, and frying. Main dishes are usually a mixture of fried or steamed vegetables, mixed with a small amount of meat, poultry, or fish. Foods are prepared and cooked in bite-size pieces, which allows them to be picked up with chopsticks. The custom of cutting foods in small pieces started centuries ago when fuel was scarce and expensive; small pieces would cook quickly.

Japan

Japanese cuisine features foods that are economical, nutritious, and attractive in appearance. Traditionally, Japanese people have eaten mainly vegetables, seaweed, and fish, as well as some fruit. Popular seafood includes squid and eel.

The Japanese dietary guidelines recommend that a person eat 30 different foods a day. Accordingly, meals usually consist of small amounts of a variety of foods. Fish is consumed both cooked and raw. It is presented the second way as sushi or sashimi, bits of very fresh raw fish combined with vinegared rice. Sushi is additionally wrapped in sheets of *nori,* or pressed seaweed.

Cooked dishes include sukiyaki—a mixture of vegetables and meat cooked quickly in a wok—and tempura—crisp batter-fried vegetables and seafood. **Soba**, buckwheat noodles, are widely eaten for lunches and snacks.

In addition to having a pleasing flavor, Japanese food must also appeal to the eye. Foods and table settings are carefully arranged.

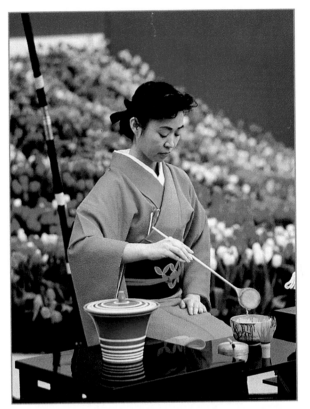

◆ The tea ceremony is a centuries-old Japanese custom. The tea is prepared and served in a ritual of grace and precision. Under what circumstances do you think this ceremony occurs?

Coastal areas enjoy an abundant variety of seafood. Seaweed is an important ingredient of Asian cooking. It is used in soups, sauces, and main dishes, and is also served as a side dish.

◆ Sushi and sashimi—assorted fish, usually served raw in combination with vinegared rice—are staples of Japan that have gained a following in the United States. What dish of Spain is similar to sushi and sashimi?

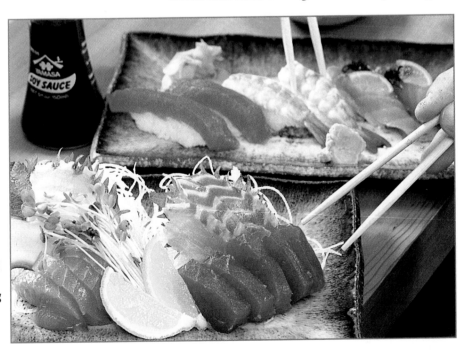

China

Chinese cuisine dates back thousands of years and goes hand in hand with Chinese philosophy. In this philosophy, the universe is seen as an interplay of opposing forces. Food preparation, therefore, balances opposites. Ingredients are carefully selected and cut into pieces to retain a sense of harmony and symmetry. Whether for a banquet or a simple family meal, the foods blend simplicity and elegance.

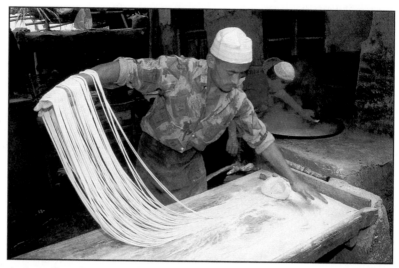

◆ **A noodle maker in Hong Kong displays the noodles he has made by swinging the dough in his hands, a traditional Chinese method.** What are some of the names by which noodles are known in the cuisines of China?

A Chinese meal does not have a main dish or a specific serving order of dishes. Instead, many dishes are arranged in the center of the table, the variety depending on the number of diners. Each person is served a bowl of rice, and then helps him- or herself to some of each food. Soup is eaten during the meal or at the end of it—sometimes, sweetened, as dessert—but never at the beginning. Hot tea is always served.

Chinese Cuisine

The foods of China, which vary from region to region, range from spicy to simple and nurturing. From the southern province of Canton comes *congee* (kahn-JEE), a "mother's-milk" dish of rice gruel flavored with meat or poultry. Congee is usually served with fried bread. *Chow fun* is broad noodles stir-fried with strips of meat, onions, and bean sprouts.

Noodle dough is known throughout China. In the northern capital of Beijing, it is made into *lo mein*—thin spaghetti-like strands—and dumplings of all shapes and sizes. The region is also home to a special-occasion dish that is one of the most complicated recipes of any

culture. That dish, *Peking duck*, requires several days of preparation, during which the duck is air-dried. The meat and crisp-roasted skin are ultimately presented ceremoniously on separate platters, along with thin pancakes.

First introduced in the United States in the 1960s and 1970s, Szechwan cooking comes from the province of the same name in central China. This area is noted for its extremely hot peppers. Other ingredients that contribute to the zesty, spicy cuisine of this region include fresh ginger and garlic.

Korea

As in much of Asia, rice is also essential in Korea. It is sometimes cooked with barley or millet, which adds nutrients, texture, and flavor to the rice.

Meals usually consist of a soup or stew plus a grilled or stir-fried dish. Fish and fish pastes appear regularly in Korean foods. Garlic, in many forms, is used in meals. In fact, some of the hottest foods in the world can be found in South Korea.

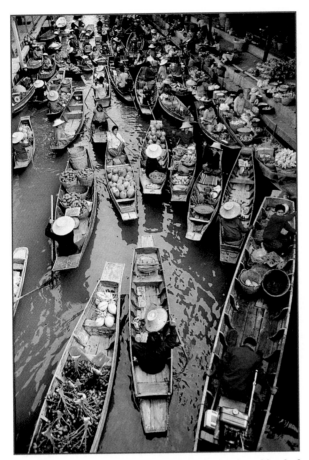

◆ Like many nations in Southeast Asia, Thailand is a blend of old and new, as this scene at the floating market shows. What can you assume about the geography of Thailand based on this picture?

Pickles add interest and flavor to Korean dishes. They might be made from almost any foods, such as pumpkins, cabbage, or ginseng. They can be rich in minerals and vitamin C.

Southeast Asia

Southeast Asia includes Myanmar (formerly Burma), Laos, Thailand, Vietnam, Cambodia, and Indonesia. These countries are in the tropics and have a variety of tropical fruits and vegetables, as well as a huge assortment of spices. The cooking reflects the influence of Chinese and European settlers.

Thailand

Coconut milk, the juice from coconuts, is frequently used as a liquid in Thai cooking, from main dishes to desserts. Noodles are a favorite and appear in casseroles and in soups. They are also mixed with sauces made of oysters, black beans, or fish. Then they are topped with chopped peanuts, coconut, and green onions.

Most food combinations in Thailand have four basic flavors—sweet, sour, salty, and spicy. They also meet four texture requirements— soft, chewy, crunchy, and crispy. Popular dishes include *pad Thai,* a mixture of rice noodles, shrimp, peanuts, egg, and bean sprouts. *Satays,* bamboo-skewered lengths of marinated and grilled chicken or beef, are served with a peanut dipping sauce.

Vietnam

Rice and fish are the staple foods in Vietnam. The Vietnamese eat rice every day, by itself and combined with other foods. Rice starch is used to make noodles and dumpling wrappers. Foods are usually seasoned with *nuoc-mam,* a pungent fish sauce.

Fish has always been the main source of protein for the Vietnamese. Fish and other foods are commonly seasoned with fresh ginger, coriander, lemon grass, and sweet basil. Many foods are rolled in lettuce or rice paper wrappers, which are easily dipped into spicy sauces.

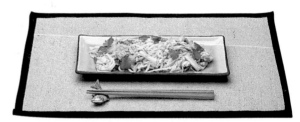

◆ Pad Thai is made with the flat noodles characteristic of Thai cooking. Name another dish common to the Thai table.

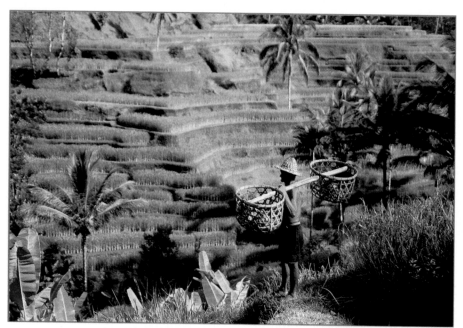

◆ Terraced rice fields like this one in Bali, Indonesia, provide the island nation with an abundant supply of its staple grain. **Explain why so much rice is grown.**

The Philippines

The inhabitants of the Philippines are a blend of Chinese, Arab, and Indian people living on 7,000 islands. The culture and food reflect the influences of those who have settled there, including the Spanish and Americans of the last few centuries.

The Chinese introduced foods such as cabbage, noodles, and soy to the Philippines. The Spaniards brought tomatoes, garlic, and peppers.

Indonesia

Indonesian foods are highly spiced. One of the most popular dishes is *nasi goreng,* a mound of fried rice surrounded by assorted meats, such as beef and shrimp, and vegetables. The diner mixes them to obtain a wide variety of flavor combinations. *Gado gado* is a salad of lettuce, hard-cooked eggs, onions, and bean sprouts, topped with a peanut butter-based dressing.

The staple foods are fish, pork, and rice, which is made into cakes, noodles, and pancakes. Fish sauces are also widely used. The national dish is *adobo,* which is pork marinated and browned in soy sauce, vinegar, garlic, bay leaves, and peppercorns.

◆ This Indian feast includes tandoori chicken, raita, dal, lamb vindaloo, and basmati rice. **Describe the role each of these dishes plays in an Indian meal.**

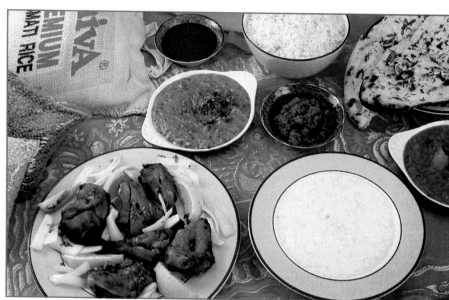

India

Cooking in India varies from region to region, according to climate and culture. In the northern and central areas, wheat is the staple grain and lamb is the most common meat. In the south, rice is the staple grain and the food is much spicier. Very little, if any, meat is eaten—especially beef, since cows are considered sacred animals. Garlic, cardamom, cumin, coriander, cloves, and other fragrant spices are widely used.

Virtually all Indian recipes begin with an exceedingly complex blend of toasted and ground spices called **garam masala**. Most cooks grind and mix their own spice blends and keep several on hand in jars. Yogurt is used widely.

India boasts a wide variety of meatless main dishes; among these is *chana baji,* sautéed chickpeas and onions liberally flavored with cumin. When poultry and fish are available, they are used sparingly in proportion to other ingredients. The dish *biryani* is a colorful plate piled high with flavorful basmati rice with almonds, raisins, and bits of either lamb, goat, or chicken.

As in Africa, breads are used as edible utensils. *Chapati,* a simple flat wheat bread, is used in some areas to scoop up rice and lentils. Breads are baked in a clay oven, or *tandoor,* which also lends its name to a famous Indian dish—*chicken tandoori.* The dish is made of chicken pieces that have been marinated in a blend of yogurt and garam masala before cooking at high heat in the tandoor.

Australia and New Zealand

The foods in Australia and New Zealand are very similar to those of the cultures who settled the coastal parts of these countries. Among these cultures are the English, the Scottish, and the French.

Menus vary according to location, from the outback of Australia, to the large cities along its coast, to the smaller cities and rural areas of New Zealand. Meals usually feature foods that are locally available. Meat and seafood are plentiful. Many people eat steaks and chops (beef or mutton) for breakfast. New Zealanders enjoy *toheroas,* which resemble clams.

One uniquely Australian dish is *Pavlova,* a rich mixture of meringue, fruit, and cream. Pies and sweet rice dishes are common desserts.

Section 22-4 Review & Activities

1. What is the staple grain throughout much of Asia and the Pacific?

2. What four food flavors are common to the foods of Thailand?

3. Name three foods eaten by the people of India.

4. **Analyzing.** Using what you read in the section, analyze this statement: "The Chinese way of eating relates to the Chinese way of thinking."

5. **Synthesizing.** Describe the role of protein in the eating plans of people in Asia and the Pacific.

6. **Applying.** Plan a meal using foods from an Asian or Pacific country. Look up the calories, grams of protein and fat, and amounts of vitamins A and C found in these foods. Are the foods in this meal a good source of these nutrients?

RECIPE FILE

Thai Chicken Satays

Satays can be eaten as an appetizer or as a main course served with rice.
Traditionally, satays are served with a peanut dipping sauce.

Customary	Ingredients	Metric
1 lb.	Boneless, skinless chicken breasts	500 g
1 Tbsp.	Lemon juice	15 mL
1 Tbsp.	Lime juice	15 mL
2 Tbsp.	Finely chopped onion	30 mL
1 Tbsp.	Garlic powder	15 mL
½ Tbsp.	Curry powder	8 mL
1 Tbsp.	Sugar	15 mL
½ cup	Coconut milk or plain, nonfat yogurt	125 mL
	Vegetable cooking spray	

Yield: About 4 servings (20 satays, about 5 satays per serving)
Equipment: Bamboo or wooden skewers; broiler pan

Directions

1. Place about 20 bamboo or wooden skewers in water to soak. Set aside.
2. Slice the chicken breast into 1- × 4-inch (2.5 × 10 cm) strips. Place in a medium bowl.
3. In a blender or food processor, blend remaining ingredients until smooth.
4. Reserve ¼ cup mixture and set aside.
5. Pour remaining mixture over chicken strips and marinate 15 minutes.
6. Preheat broiler.
7. Spray the broiler pan with the vegetable cooking spray.
8. Thread each chicken strip onto a skewer and place on cold broiler pan.
9. Broil for about 5 minutes on each side until chicken is golden brown. Brush with reserved marinade while cooking to preserve moistness.
10. Serve hot.

Nutrition Information

Per serving (approximate): 229 calories, 37 g protein, 8 g carbohydrate, 4 g fat, 98 mg cholesterol, 104 mg sodium
Good source of: potassium, magnesium, B vitamins, phosphorus

Food for Thought

• What purpose does the coconut milk or the yogurt serve in the marinade?
• What foods could you serve with this recipe to complete an Asian meal?

CAREER WANTED

Individuals who enjoy solving problems, and connecting the past with the present and the future.

REQUIRES:

- Master's degree in agricultural education or related field
- love of people, plants, and animals

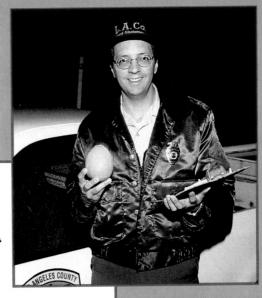

"Serving people who work the land is my mission,"

says Ed Quintero, County Extension Agent

Q: Why did you become a county extension agent?

A: I've always felt a kinship with the land. I grew up on a dairy farm, and as a youth I was an active 4-H member. Even then I knew I wanted to work with people who farmed the land.

Q: What are some of the tasks involved in your job?

A: I mainly oversee the way the environment and crop production impact each other and make sure the growing practices used in this county are as safe and efficient as they can be.

Q: What are some of the environmental factors that affect crop production?

A: Some of them relate to technology. For example, the kinds of herbicides used and whether they are carried in the groundwater. Other factors are what we call "opportunistic" and include frosts and droughts.

Q: What benefits do you receive from the work you do?

A: The most immediate benefit is seeing that the crops that come out of this soil are safe for people to eat. In the long term, our extension office strives to ensure that the soil will remain healthy enough to support the generations to come.

Career Research Activity

1. Create a star diagram that connects the careers listed on the right. Draw a star with five points and write "county extension agent" in the center. At the end of each point, write the name of another career listed. In each arm, write down at least one skill or job requirement that the two careers have in common. Consider education, training, and possible advancement.

2. Compare the careers of a county extension agent and an agronomic engineer. How are the two careers similar? How are they different? Which would you consider and why?

Related Career Opportunities

Entry Level
- Conservation Worker
- 4-H Advisor
- Recreation Assistant

Technical Level
- Forestry Technician
- USDA Lab Technician

Professional Level
- Geologist
- County Extension Agent
- Forester

Chapter 22 Review & Activities

— Summary —

Section 22-1: Latin America

- Latin American cooking combines native foods and European influences.
- Corn is the staple grain in most areas.
- Mexican meals include masa, rice, beans, and chili peppers.
- Beef is popular in the countries of South America.

Section 22-3: Europe

- The cooking of the British Isles tends to be plain but hearty.
- French cooking maximizes flavors to enhance one another.
- The foods of Spain and Portugal are based on fish and seafood.
- German cooking tends to be rich and heavy.
- Italian cuisine bears influences of its geographical neighbors.
- Eastern European cooking emphasizes root vegetables, grains, and sour cream.

Section 22-2: Africa and the Middle East

- In Africa, staples include yams, cassava, and peanuts.
- Geography, climate, native traditions, religion, and foreign influence have shaped food customs in Africa and the Middle East.
- Some food customs of the Middle East are a part of religious beliefs.

Section 22-4: Asia and the Pacific

- Rice, seafood, soybeans, and vegetables are the staples of Japanese and Chinese cooking.
- Foods in Korea and Southeast Asia are spicy and include tropical fruits and vegetables.
- Indian cuisine is known for its spicy, often meatless, recipes.
- Australian and New Zealand cuisines have European roots.

Working IN THE Lab

1. **Foods Lab.** Choose one popular food of Latin America. Find two recipes for preparing it: one traditional, the other as it is usually prepared in the United States. Prepare and sample both recipes. Tell how they differ in ingredients and flavor. Offer reasons for these differences.

2. **Demonstration.** Investigate the traditional ways of serving Japanese and Chinese meals. Then demonstrate these serving methods. Duplicate the foods, serving pieces, and serving styles as closely as possible.

Checking Your Knowledge

1. What is a plantain? How can it be prepared?

2. Name two influences on Brazilian cooking and two foods reflecting these influences.

3. Name two foods introduced to Africa in the sixteenth century and their place of origin.

4. Name and describe three dishes often eaten in the Middle East.

5. Name three traditional condiments used in Israel.

6. Name two foods usually served at British tea.

7. What is the basic philosophy behind the cooking of France?

8. What is a contorno? When in an Italian meal is it served?

9. How is the Chinese cooking of Szechwan province different from that of other regions of the country?

10. What is *nasi goreng*? How is it eaten?

Review & Activities Chapter 22

Thinking Critically

1. Predicting Consequences. Review the staple foods of the different regions of Latin America as noted in the chapter. For each food, identify one possible health advantage and one disadvantage of the typical way it is eaten in the region.

2. Comparing and Contrasting. Using recipe books, Web sites, or other information sources involving food, find examples of bean dishes served in several countries from different continents. How are they similar and different?

3. Recognizing Values. As noted in the chapter, Chinese meals reflect the Chinese people's traditional philosophy of life. What philosophies might meals in the United States reflect?

Reinforcing Key Skills

1. Communication. Ashley and her family are planning a trip to their ancestral homeland of Kenya, a country in Africa. Ashley has read that certain bacteria and other microorganisms in the foods and drinking water of some regions can cause gastric distress in visitors. What action would you advise Ashley to take to protect her and her family's well-being?

2. Leadership. You become friends with an exchange student from Eastern Europe, who tells you she is having trouble adapting to American customs. Think about particular foods and aspects of your eating habits that may be troublesome to someone from your friend's culture. Develop a strategy for helping this person overcome her difficulties.

Making Decisions and Solving Problems

Your new neighbors are a Middle Eastern family. You would like to invite them to dinner. However, you are not familiar with their food customs, their tastes, or any particular foods they may or may not eat.

Making Connections

1. Social Studies. Locate information on the controversy surrounding cattle raising in the rain forest regions of South America. What are the arguments of the opposing sides? What are the strengths and weaknesses of these arguments? Which side do you feel has the stronger case, and why? Share your findings with the class in a brief report.

2. Fine Arts. Learn more about how Japanese cuisine fits into the wider Japanese philosophy of the arts. How are the Japanese people's ideas about color, balance, and symmetry reflected in their art, music, and dance, as well as their meals? Make a presentation to the class using examples to support your conclusions.

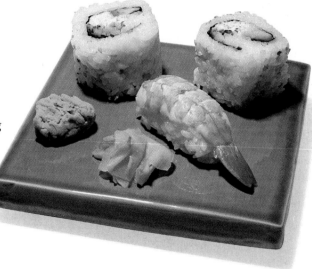

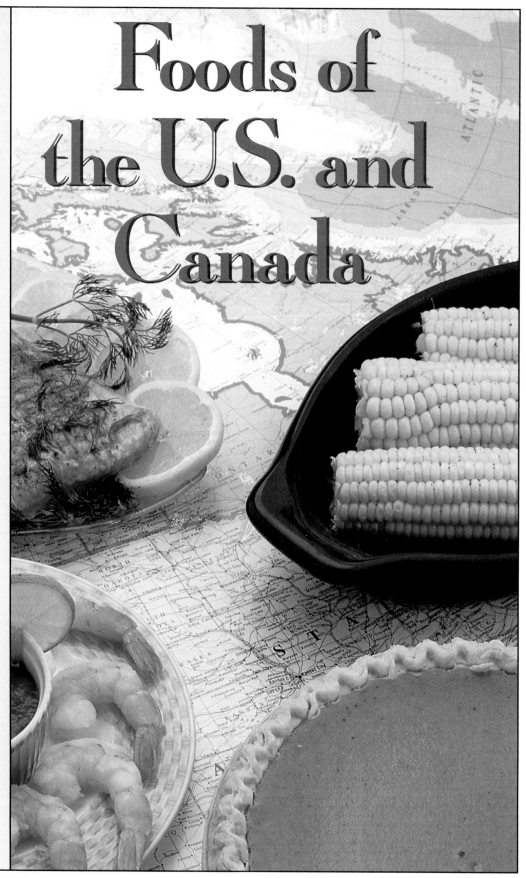

When you hear the
term *American food,*
what comes to mind?
You may picture hot
dogs and ice cream,
but hot dogs are actually
of German descent and
ice cream comes from
France and Italy.

What, then, is
American food? After
reading this chapter,
you will know the answer
to this question.

Foods of the U.S. and Canada

Regional Foods of the East, Midwest, and South

Objectives

After studying this section, you should be able to:

- List foods common to the East, Midwest, and South.
- Identify cultural and climate influences on the foods of the East, Midwest, and South.

Look for These Terms

pemmican

filé

Are there chili cook-offs where you live? Do local cooks all have their own recipes for clam chowder? Can you walk into any bakery and order a key lime pie?

These foods all have something in common. All are genuine American dishes. Today, any of these foods can be enjoyed throughout the country. However, at one time, each was known only in the region where it originated.

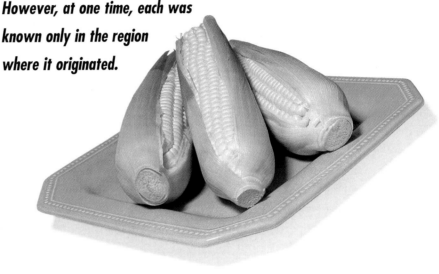

The Foundations of American Cooking

How did regional differences come about? As noted in Chapter 13, the foods common to an area depend partly on geography and climate. The way North America was settled also affected the development of food customs.

The Native Americans developed their own food customs based on locally available foods. Those foods are the foundation of much of American cooking. Later, immigrants from other parts of the world made additional contributions to the foods of America.

> **INFOLINK**
>
> For more information on the effects of geography and other factors on the staple foods of a region, see Section 13-3.

Native American Culture

Some Native Americans relied mainly on hunting, fishing, and gathering berries for meals. Others were skilled farmers and creative cooks.

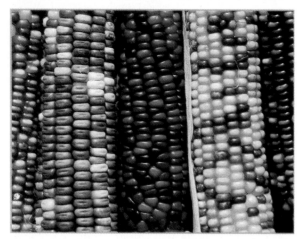

◆ Corn, or maize, was a legacy of the Native Americans to the first European settlers. How many different uses for corn can you name?

Native Americans were also early pioneers in food technology. They developed a way of cultivating wild maize (corn) so that it would yield a greater amount of food and seed. They also devised methods for storing and preserving foods. One preserved food they made was **pemmican**—dried meat, pounded into a paste with fat and preserved in cakes. Because of its nonperishable properties, pemmican could be stored for long periods of time, making meat available when hunting was scarce. The high fat content, which enabled a little of the food to go a long way, also helped sustain energy.

Native American Staples

Maize was a staple grain for many Native American groups. It was prepared in a variety of ways, some of which are still used today. Native Americans roasted and boiled the corn in the husk. Some removed the kernels and made them into a powder, which was then made into flatbread, mush, corn puddings, and beverages. Sometimes the Native Americans softened the kernels in homemade lye and made hominy, which was cooked with bits of meat.

Regional differences often determined which other foods were available. In coastal areas, seafood was a staple. Native Americans in the South concocted soups and stews from fish and small game. In the Southwest, groups grew beans to use in soups. They also roasted meats over open fires.

Colonial Cooking

In the fifteenth century, immigration from Europe began. Immigrants coming to this continent brought their food customs with them. They tended to settle as groups in areas that reminded them of their homelands. Settling in these clusters helped them preserve their traditions.

Native Americans played an important role in the survival of the first European immigrants to the New World. They introduced the immigrants to the staple foods of various regions and shared food preparation and cooking methods.

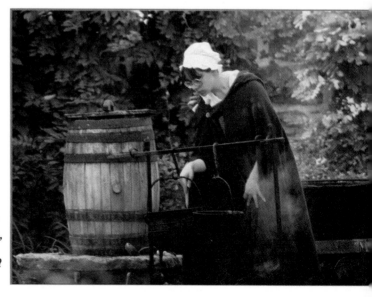

◆ A reenactment of early cooking is shown here. Cooking over an open fire outdoors preceded open hearth cooking indoors, which was the early counterpart to the kitchen stove. What foods were prepared over an open fire and in the open hearth? How are the same dishes cooked today?

Gradually, the immigrants began adapting their own recipes to available foods and the cooking and preserving methods that were used in their new homeland. Cultural exchanges also occurred between colonies and immigrant groups. Over time, this process resulted in the unique cooking styles of each region of North America.

The Northeast

Among the first European settlers in the Northeast were the English, Dutch, French, and Germans. Native Americans of the region taught the settlers to use available foods, such as deer, rabbit, wild turkey, and berries. They also taught the immigrants to plant native crops, such as corn, beans, squash, and pumpkins. Corn and dry beans provided carbohydrates and protein to help the immigrants survive in their new homeland.

New England

Because of the extremely cold winters in New England, early settlers cooked hearty foods. From the Native Americans they learned to soak dry beans and then cook them slowly for hours in a kettle over an open fire. The resulting dish, often called *Boston baked beans*, is still a favorite today.

Another New England dish inspired by the Native Americans was *chowder*, a soup made with fish or seafood, which were plentiful along the Atlantic coast. The most famous chowder—clam chowder— is made with milk, butter, onions, and clams. In some areas, cooks use tomatoes instead of milk.

Irish Influence

The Irish came to the Northeast somewhat later than other immigrants. They introduced Irish stew and corned beef with cabbage, known throughout the United States as traditional

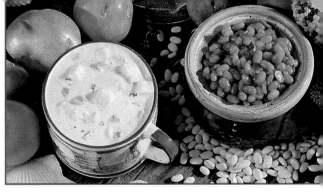

◆ **Clam chowder, Boston baked beans, and brown bread are traditional New England dishes.** What other local produce do you think appeared on the tables of settlers of the area?

Irish dishes. Such hearty and filling foods were a trademark of the Irish. These foods used a wide range of vegetables, including cabbage, carrots, and potatoes. Vegetables were combined with eggs, bread crumbs, butter, and spices to make puddings. Irish cooks also used leeks, onions, and garlic to flavor foods.

Pennsylvania Dutch

In the late 1700s, large numbers of Germans arrived in eastern Pennsylvania. They referred to themselves as *Deutsch*, the German word for "German." English-speaking settlers of the area mispronounced the word as "Dutch." The Germans in this area became known as the Pennsylvania Dutch.

These settlers were farmers, which required hard physical labor and large quantities of flavorful, filling food. They continued to prepare familiar foods from their homeland: pork, cabbage or sauerkraut, noodles, and sausage. They also were known for their hearty soups, stews, and homemade breads.

As cooks, the German immigrants were thrifty. They used everything, including the pork scraps, which were formed into a loaf that was cut into slices and fried as *scrapple*. They also enjoyed sweets. They made fruit butters and tasty baked goods. Pies, cakes, rolls, and crumb-topped cakes were shared with the neighbors over mid-morning coffee, or *kaffeeklatsch*.

The Midwest

In the eighteenth century, as the big cities in the East grew crowded, adventurous pioneers set out to explore the "wide-open spaces" farther west. Settlers followed, establishing new homes in the Midwest. During the nineteenth century, newly arrived immigrants from Europe joined this westward movement.

Soon the prairies of the heartland were supporting farms and dairies. Settlers planted familiar crops that grew well in that climate— wheat, corn, other grains, fruits, and vegetables. Farms also produced beef, pork, and poultry. Fish was available from rivers and lakes.

In general, Midwestern menus were hearty and relied on the taste of the foods themselves rather than on seasonings for flavor. The great supply of wheat made home-baked breads, cakes, and pies a way of life. Meat, potatoes, bread, vegetables, and dessert: These foods provided energy for the hard-working pioneers. It was simple fare, simply cooked, and is a part of what is now known as American cooking.

The South

In the eighteenth century, life in the South generally revolved around the plantation and other rural areas. Crops in the South were bountiful because the soil along the lakes, rivers, and deltas was rich and the temperatures were warm. These lakes and rivers, as well as the ocean, provided fish and shellfish. Corn, the staple food, was dried and ground so that it could be used in a variety of recipes, many of which originated with the Native Americans. Included were corn bread, spoon bread, corn pone, fritters, cornmeal batters, and grits. These foods are still served in the South today.

The English were the primary settlers in the area. Food customs, however, were also influenced by the Africans, French, and Spaniards.

African-American Influence

African-American cooks made their mark on Southern food. They incorporated turnip and dandelion greens, black-eyed peas, catfish, fried okra, yams, red beans, rice, and peppers into their cooking.

African Americans developed their own special recipes for foods such as pig's feet and hog jowls. Chitterlings (bits of hog intestine) were fried and dipped into a spicy sauce. Ham hocks (legs) and turnip greens became a popular dish. The backbone of the hog was simmered to make a tasty stew topped with dumplings.

The African Americans had come to appreciate chili peppers, which had been transported to Africa from Latin America. They enjoyed spicy sauces and gravies. They also depended on one-pot cooking. Dishes were cooked in an iron pot and made with a wide variety of foods, including cooking greens.

African-American cooks also combined foods to make new recipes. *Hopping John*, for instance, is a mixture of black-eyed peas and rice. *Hush puppies*, made of cornmeal batter dropped by spoonfuls into hot oil, are often served with fried catfish. According to legend, hush puppies got their name in early days when they were thrown to silence barking dogs around campfires.

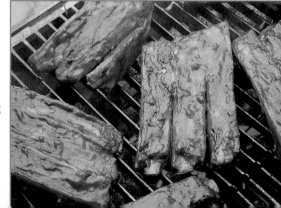

◆ In the deep South, meats and poultry are slow-roasted over open pits. These midwestern ribs, which are dry-rubbed with spices before being smoked, are being cooked on a grill. **Explain how both of these recipes reflect early American roots.**

Desserts were sweet and rich, and they included pecan pie, sweet potato pie, and peach cobbler.

Creole Cooking

Creole and Cajun are two specialized kinds of cooking that developed in southern Louisiana. Both feature ingredients such as seafood, pork, rice, peppers, celery, onions, and a variety of herbs and spices. Both are famous for their blending of flavors, which is only natural, because Creole and Cajun cooking each resulted from a blending of cultures.

Creole cooking developed in New Orleans. Many European immigrants settled there, including natives of France, Spain, and Italy. In many families, the meals were prepared by servants. To the European cuisine, these cooks added some of their own food traditions from Africa and the West Indies, as well as ingredients borrowed from Native Americans.

Creole cooking is considered by many to be a more sophisticated style than Cajun. Creole meals are likely to include a variety of separate dishes, each featuring a delicate, subtle blending of flavors. Shrimp, oysters, and crabs appear often. As in classic French cooking, sauces are often based on butter or cream. Creole cooking is sometimes described as a city-style cuisine.

Cajun Cooking

Cajun cooking, in contrast, is a country-style cuisine. The term *Cajun* is derived from *Acadian*. The Acadians were French colonists who had settled in Canada. After they were expelled from Canada by the British, some eventually found their way to the bayous and farmlands of southern Louisiana. The style of cooking that resulted combines French traditions with the locally available foods and the influences of other cultural groups.

One of the key features of Cajun cooking is improvisation. The Cajuns had to learn to

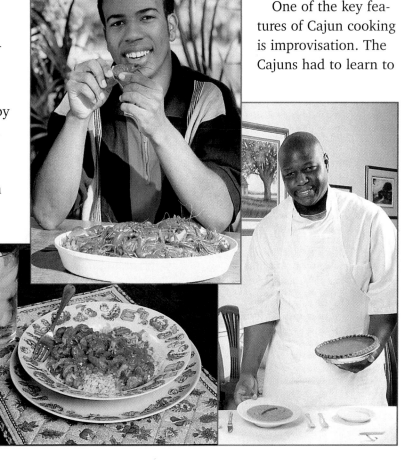

◆ Many of the dishes for which the coastal South is noted, including peanut soup and sweet potato pie, were inspired by African-American settlers to the area. The rich culinary heritage of Louisiana, influenced both by Cajun and Creole cuisines, includes étouffé, a savory stew of chicken, and shellfish such as crawfish. What other dishes are popular to these regions of the country?

live off the land, making meals from whatever they could hunt, catch, or grow on their own. Authentic Cajun cooking often includes fresh-water fish, crawfish (the Southern term for crayfish), and game such as rabbit, turtle, squirrel, and even alligator. One-dish meals made from whatever foods are on hand are common. Compared with Creole cooking, Cajun foods tend to feature stronger, hotter flavors.

Similarities

Despite these distinctions, Creole and Cajun cuisine have much in common. Many dishes owe their distinctive flavor to a brown roux. In this variation of the French thickening agent, the flour is cooked until it turns a rich, chocolate-brown color. It gives a subtle, dark, roasted flavor to sauces and dishes, such as *étouffé*, a hearty stew of chicken and shellfish. Okra is also commonly used to thicken soups and stews. The use of okra and the method of simmering foods for a long time in iron

pots are examples of the African influence on the region's cooking. Still another thickener was borrowed from the Native Americans. They used dried, crushed sassafras leaves to thicken stews and add a delicate flavor. This thickener was called **filé**, or filé powder, by the settlers.

A famous Louisiana dish is *gumbo*, a thick stew that begins with a brown roux. Many variations are possible. A Creole gumbo might include shrimp, crab, and oysters; a Cajun gumbo is more likely to feature ham and crawfish. Vegetables and seasonings are also added. Either okra or filé powder is used as a thickener. Gumbos are simmered slowly for hours, and then served over rice.

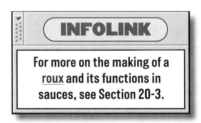

INFOLINK

For more on the making of a roux and its functions in sauces, see Section 20-3.

Section 23-1 Review & Activities

1. Name two contributions of Native Americans to the growth and development of American food.

2. Name three contributions made by the Africans to the American food culture.

3. What is a brown roux? What two cuisines of Louisiana does it link?

4. **Synthesizing.** What factors do you think encouraged the immigrants to try new foods?

5. **Comparing and Contrasting.** Make a Venn diagram, a chart with two large overlapping circles. Choose any two regional cultures identified in this section, and place their similarities in the overlapping area, their differences in the outer portions of the circles that do not overlap.

6. **Applying.** Plan a dinner meal combining different foods from the South. (You may need to check some recipe books.) Survey a supermarket and gather ingredient prices for the foods in this meal. Which items were most or least expensive? Which were the easiest and most difficult to find? What does location have to do with the price and availability of food items?

RECIPE FILE

Hopping John

Legend in the south has it that eating this dish on New Year's Day brings good luck.

Customary	Ingredients	Metric
1 cup	Chopped onion	250 mL
6 oz.	Ham, cut into 1-inch (2.5 cm) pieces	190 g
2 Tbsp.	Vegetable oil	30 mL
Dash	Ground allspice	Dash
Dash	Cayenne	Dash
1 cup	Instant rice	250 mL
2½ cups	Water	375 mL
4 cups	Canned black-eyed peas, drained and rinsed	1 L
	Salt	
	Pepper	
	Chopped green onion (optional)	

Yield: 4 servings, one cup each
Equipment: 2-quart (2-L) saucepan

Directions

1. Sauté the onion and the ham in vegetable oil until onion is golden and ham is lightly browned.
2. Stir in allspice and cayenne.
3. Add the rice, and toss until coated with the oil.
4. Add the water and bring to a boil. Reduce the heat and simmer for 15 minutes.
5. Add the black-eyed peas and simmer for another 5 minutes.
6. Remove the pan from the heat and cover. Let pan stand, covered, for 5 minutes.
7. Season to taste with salt and pepper.
8. Serve hot, garnished with chopped green onion, if desired.

Nutrition Information

Per serving (approximate): 452 calories, 21 g protein, 55 g carbohydrate, 17 g fat, 30 mg cholesterol, 854 mg sodium
Good source of: potassium, iron, zinc, vitamin E, vitamin C, B vitamins, phosphorus

Food for Thought

• What would you serve with Hopping John to meet one daily serving requirement of vegetables? Of dairy foods?
• How could you reduce the fat in this recipe? How could you reduce the sodium?

Regional Foods of the West and Canada

Early settlers in the American West brought with them the cuisine of their homelands. In adapting their traditional recipes to the climate and foods available, these early settlers developed foods that are commonly found in these regions today.

Objectives

After studying this section, you should be able to:

- Identify foods characteristic of the western United States and Canada.
- Describe the cultural influences on foods of the western United States and Canada.

Look for These Terms

sourdough starter

hibachi

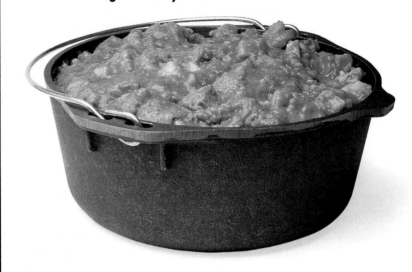

The Southwest

Most people associate the Southwest with cowboys and huge cattle ranches. Spaniards introduced cattle to this area in the sixteenth century. By the 1800s, ranches dotted the Texas plains, with large herds of longhorn cattle tended by cowboys.

Influences on Southwestern Food

Long before the Spaniards arrived, Native Americans were raising crops such as corn, beans, pumpkins, squash, and chilies. They also had an abundant supply of fish and wild game as well as berries, nuts, and seeds.

Native Americans and Spaniards influenced the cooking in the region, as did other cultures.

These included Mexicans, French, English, and other settlers from the east. Settlers moving westward found rich soil for growing abundant crops.

Cowboy Cuisine

Until the railroads came along in the later 1800s, cowboys represented the only way of getting cattle from ranch to market. These trips frequently covered 1,000 miles (1,600 km) or more.

Because cowboys couldn't go home for meals, a cook traveled with them. Food and essential equipment to cook over a campfire were carried in a chuck wagon.

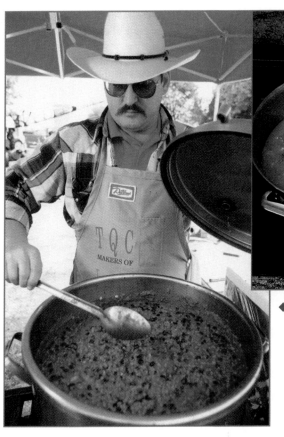

◆ Chili con carne is an all-American favorite, but nowhere is it more popular than in the Southwest, where chili "cookoffs" are periodically held. **What different ingredients can be used to vary the taste of chili?**

Cowboy cooks prepared simple meals over open fires. Meat was cooked by roasting or stewing in a pot. To save time in the morning, the cook made a biscuit mix the night before, mixing flour, salt, and baking powder in a sack. The next day, he added fat and water, and baked the biscuits over the campfire. For the cowboys, dessert was often biscuits topped with a sweet syrup or "fried" pies. Very strong coffee completed the meal.

Tex-Mex Cuisine

Because Texas had long been a territory under Mexican rule, the Mexican influence on the food remained even after the state won its independence. Beans, corn, tamales, and tacos were as popular as ever—and still are today. The cuisine of Texas, in fact, is often known as Tex-Mex.

As in Mexican cooking, corn continues to be the mainstay of Tex-Mex cooking. Corn products are usually served at every meal. In addition, beans, chili peppers, fresh vegetables, and fruit, sometimes cooked with meats, are included in Southwestern meals.

Two popular Tex-Mex dishes are *nachos*—made by smothering tortilla chips with refried beans, cheese sauce, and chilies—and *fajitas* (fah-HEE-tuhs)—tortillas wrapped around strips of marinated, grilled steak or chicken. They are usually served with grilled onions and sweet peppers, guacamole, refried beans, and salsa.

The seasoning in Tex-Mex cooking can vary from mild to fiery hot, depending on personal preference. One of the most famous Tex-Mex dishes is named for the chili pepper—*chili con carne*. There is a difference of opinion as to where this dish originated, in Texas or Mexico. There's little debate, however, over the popularity of chili, as it is now known—although there is one over whether chili should have

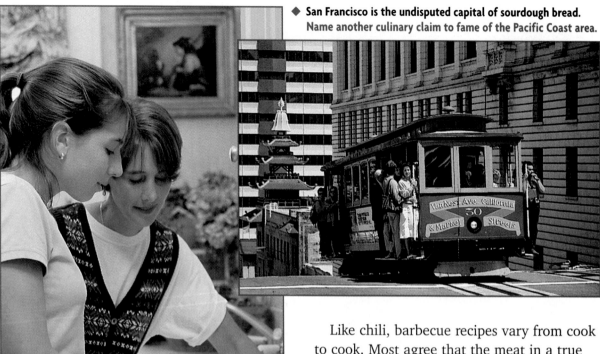

◆ **San Francisco is the undisputed capital of sourdough bread.** Name another culinary claim to fame of the Pacific Coast area.

Like chili, barbecue recipes vary from cook to cook. Most agree that the meat in a true barbecue should be seasoned only with a "dry rub" of spices. Barbecue sauce is added only at the very end of the roasting.

The Pacific Coast

Early settlers along the Pacific coast and in the Northwest found an abundant food supply. Natural resources such as seafood and game were plentiful. The settlers used simple food preparation methods to bring out the natural flavors of these foods. For example, elk and deer were grilled or roasted. Seafood was steamed, boiled, or grilled.

The coast also had a rich supply of tasty fresh fruits and vegetables. The temperate climate of southern California provided the perfect growing conditions.

Influences on Pacific Coast Food

Great shipping ports developed along the Pacific coast, including San Francisco, Seattle, and Los Angeles. When gold was discovered in California and Alaska, people from Asia

beans. Originally, chili was little more than cubed beef cooked in a spicy sauce of red chilies and marjoram. Today, cooks may use ground meat and add pinto beans, tomatoes, onions, cilantro, and spices. Local contests are held yearly from coast to coast to find out who can make the best chili.

Southwestern Barbecue

Another popular form of cooking throughout the Southwest is barbecue. Many people believe that Southerners moving to the Southwest introduced the barbecue. The word *barbecue* may be derived from the Spanish word *barbacoa*, which refers to the grid on which meat is roasted in Latin America. However, records show that meat was barbecued in Virginia as early as the seventeenth century.

flocked to the New World. These Japanese, Chinese, Russian, and Korean immigrants were joined by Mexicans, French, and Canadians.

The immigrants brought their food specialties with them and mingled them with local food customs. For example, *chow mein* is a dish created in California about 100 years ago. It is not an authentic Chinese dish, but an American dish based on Chinese cooking.

Early sailing ships brought food from China, Japan, and the Polynesian islands to America. The influence of Asian cooking is still strong in the Pacific Coast and Northwest regions.

Sourdough Bread

Sourdough bread today is considered one of the classic breads in America. Yet it had humble beginnings in the mid-nineteenth century, during the days of the gold rush. Many early settlers in California and Alaska came looking for gold. Most of the prospectors were poor and relied on bread as their staple. They had no yeast, but made bread with a **sourdough starter**, a mixture of flour, water, and salt on which wild yeast cells grew. The mixture fermented and became a leavening agent.

The prospectors never put all their starter in the bread. A small amount was always left in a crock and then replenished by adding flour and water. In this way, sourdough starter was always on hand, and the prospector was then assured of a food supply. Because they were so dependent on the starter, the prospectors came to be known as sourdoughs.

The Northwest

The northwest corner of the United States was the last part of the U.S. mainland to be settled. Settlers in Oregon and Washington came to these northwestern states by way of the Oregon Trail. Many brought seeds from fruit trees to begin orchards. Fruit orchards, which later became profitable businesses for the settlers, remain a major industry in the Northwest today. Along with raising fruits, such as pears, peaches, and apples, these settlers created delicious dishes from the abundance of fish and seafood. Dungeness crab and coho salmon were often steamed or served with creamy sauces.

Hawaii

The fiftieth state to join the Union, Hawaii has been the midway stopping point for ships traveling the long shipping lanes between Asia and North America.

Hawaiian Cuisine

The original inhabitants of Hawaii were Polynesian, but many other cultures have settled in the chain of islands, bringing their food customs with them. Today, Hawaiian cooking is a blend of Polynesian, Chinese, Japanese, Korean, Filipino, French, English, and Portuguese, as well as mainland American.

The rich soil and warm climate offer a wide variety of tropical fruits, including mango, papaya, pineapple, and bananas. The surrounding waters and inland streams provide a real bounty of flavorful fish.

Other foods were introduced by settlers. The Japanese introduced seaweed, teriyaki sauce for marinating, a new kind of noodle, and many rice and bean products. They also brought the **hibachi**, a small charcoal grill. The Chinese brought rice, soybeans, pork, and Asian vegetables such as Chinese cabbage. These, along with chicken, are the mainstays of Hawaiian cooking.

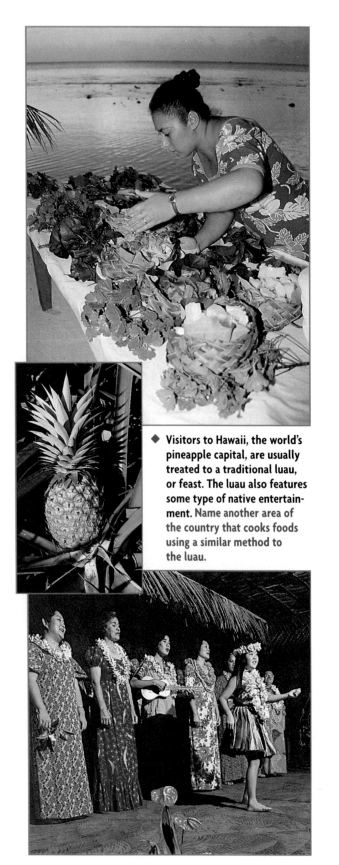

◆ Visitors to Hawaii, the world's pineapple capital, are usually treated to a traditional luau, or feast. The luau also features some type of native entertainment. Name another area of the country that cooks foods using a similar method to the luau.

The early Polynesians had no pots and pans, so they invented techniques for preparing food. One was *poi* pounding. They pounded fruits or roots into a bland, sticky paste, which was their staple. Today, poi is made from ground taro root and is often used in cooking or served as a side dish. If allowed to ferment for several days, it develops a more sour flavor. Duck may be steamed in a banana leaf with cabbage, pineapple, and poi. Taro chips, similar to potato chips, are deep-fried, thin slices of taro root.

Another cooking method was the open pit, which became famous as the *luau*, or feast. The luau is a tradition observed on special occasions, such as birthdays, marriages, and other events. Tourists visiting Hawaii are usually treated to a luau, which also features native entertainment.

The highlight of the luau is a pig roasted in an open pit. Fish and other meats are wrapped in leaves and roasted with sweet potatoes and bananas on the hot coals. Besides poi, other Hawaiian dishes that might be served include *lomi lomi salmon*—salted salmon with onions and tomatoes—and *haupia*—a sweet pudding made with arrowroot and coconut milk.

Canada

As in the United States, the foods of Canada reflect the nation's natural resources and rich cultural diversity. The natural resources include wild rice, beef, and more than 150 species of fish and shellfish. Apples and peaches lead fruit production. Just like the United States, Canada is populated by many nationalities that have retained their identities.

Atlantic Provinces

Newfoundland, New Brunswick, Nova Scotia, and Prince Edward Island make up the Atlantic provinces. The ethnic origins of the people are largely English and French, with some German, Dutch, and Irish as well. Almost half of the people speak both English and French.

Fish and seafood are the most important foods of the region. Fresh fruits and vegetables are grown locally, but the growing season is short because of the long periods of cold weather. Blueberries are an important crop.

Specialty potatoes are raised on Prince Edward Island and in New Brunswick, showing the influence of the Irish who settled the region. Potatoes were used for many things other than food by the early settlers—laundry starch, headache remedies, and bottle corks. They were an important ingredient used to help stretch soups to feed families.

A traditional Saturday night meal in the Atlantic provinces is homemade baked beans and steamed brown bread. Other popular meals include rich pea soup and a special Acadian dish called *râpée pie*, consisting of layers of cooked poultry and puréed potatoes. Another dish, *colcannon*, came from Scotland and Ireland. It is made by mashing together potatoes, turnips, and cabbage.

Quebec

As a result of its cultural and linguistic ties to France and Switzerland, Quebec shows the most European influence of any Canadian province. About one-fourth of the population of Canada resides in Quebec. These French Canadians are proud of their language and heritage. French is spoken almost exclusively in this province.

It is not surprising, then, that the food in Quebec displays a distinct French influence. Common dishes include seafood soups, special cheeses, and French breads and pastries. At the same time, there are foods that are unique to Quebec. Among these is *smoked meat*, beef

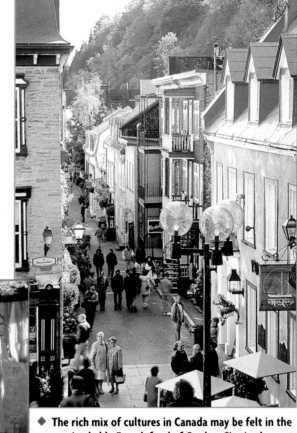

◆ **The rich mix of cultures in Canada may be felt in the unmistakably French food of Quebec City in the east and salmon smoking for use in a Native American potlatch in the west.** Read the "Connecting Food and Social Studies" feature in Section 19-4, on page 510, which describes the potlatch.

brisket smoked in a blend of spices and served thinly sliced. *Back bacon*, better known in the United States as Canadian bacon, has far less fat and a milder flavor than streaky bacon.

Quebec produces about 90 percent of Canada's maple syrup. Maple sugar was the only sweetener that early settlers had. Some Canadians still prefer blocks of maple sugar to other sweeteners. One Quebec dessert made with maple sugar is *sugar pie*. *Grand-pères* are dumplings that are served with maple syrup.

A pie made with ground pork, called *tourtière*, is another French Canadian specialty. Ground pork is also a main ingredient in *cretons*, a popular spread made with kidney and lard. The early settlers made *cipate*, a pie made with game meats. Today, however, it is made with chicken, pork, veal, and beef.

Ontario

Ontario is centrally located in Canada, lying to the north of Minnesota, Wisconsin, and Michigan. Over one-third of Canada's population lives in Ontario, making it the most heavily populated province in the country.

Beef, dairy foods, maple syrup, and wild rice are among the chief products of Ontario. Poultry, eggs, fruits, and vegetables are also plentiful. The Canadian flag's maple leaf is a clue to the abundance of maple trees. Syrup drawn from the sap of these trees is used in candy and as a popular sweetener in desserts.

Food customs in Ontario are as varied as the people who live there. Many came from Scotland, Ireland, and England. Shortbread is popular among residents with Scottish ancestors and is a common holiday gift. Swiss Mennonites, who had landed first in Pennsylvania, settled in Ontario in the late 1700s. Immigrants from most European countries, as well as India and the West Indies, came to the province. In addition, more Native Americans live in Ontario than in any other province.

The Western Provinces

To the west of Ontario are the prairie provinces of Manitoba, Saskatchewan, and Alberta. Spacious wheat fields and grazing land for cattle make the traditional foods in these provinces similar to those in the Midwestern United States. Honey and whitefish are also important products. One unique fish that is sold smoked, *Goldeye*, is known as a delicacy in many parts of the world.

In British Columbia, on the North Pacific coast, salmon is a staple. *Loganberries*, a cross between blackberries and raspberries, are also grown in British Columbia. They are a favorite in pies. Vancouver, the largest city in British Columbia, is located just north of Seattle. It has a significant Chinese population and its own Chinatown. Foods from all regions of China can be found there.

The Northwest Territories stretch across northern Canada. Native Americans and Inuit are the primary inhabitants. Until the nineteenth century, most Inuit hunted and fished for food. Seal meat, caribou, trout, and cod were staples. One fish that is unique to northern Canada is *Arctic char*, or *ilkaula*, which is a cross between salmon and trout.

As in the United States, early pioneers in northern Canada relied on sourdough starter for preparing bread. Another early bread product was *bannock*, a flat, round cake. Introduced by immigrants from Scotland and northern England, this unleavened cake was made from oatmeal, rye, or barley meal.

Cultural Diversity Today

In recent decades, the minority populations of the United States and Canada have grown significantly. Millions of immigrants have flocked to North America in search of a better life and have settled in communities across both nations. The traditions of the various cultures have merged and blended, further enriching and diversifying the area.

In addition to immigration, other factors that affect the cultural diversity in North America include:

◆ **Mobility.** People now move from one region to another more often than in the past. They carry their food traditions along with them.

◆ **Media.** Through television, magazines, and other sources, people are exposed to various cultures and their traditions.

◆ **Technology.** As a result of modern transportation and packaging methods, foods from many regions and cultures are available all across the United States and Canada.

For these and other reasons, the food in a specific region today can be as diverse as the people who live there. Many food habits and patterns now reflect the traditions of individual families more than the area in which the families live.

Section 23-2 Review & Activities

1. Briefly describe cowboy and Tex-Mex cuisines.

2. Explain two ways in which the geography of the Pacific Coast and Northwest affected the food supply.

3. Describe the contribution of the Polynesians to Hawaiian cuisine.

4. Identify one Irish influence on the foods of the Atlantic provinces of Canada. Identify two foods that are unique to Quebec.

5. Analyzing. Do you think the type of foods people were accustomed to influenced their decision about where to settle? Explain.

6. Extending. Purists are people who are resistant to change and insist on sticking with tradition. Which of the foods you learned about in this section do you think would be most likely to have a purist following? Explain your answer.

7. Applying. List ten foods that you enjoy eating. Identify the regional or ethnic source of each food.

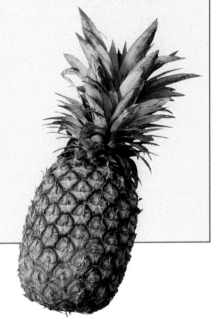

RECIPE FILE

Southwest Guacamole

Serve this recipe as a dip with tortilla chips or as a condiment with Tex-Mex foods, such as quesadillas. For added flavor, try adding sliced orange sections or hot peppers to this recipe.

Customary	Ingredients	Metric
2	Ripe avocados	2
1	Tomato, diced	1
4-oz. can	Mild green chilies, drained and chopped	112-g can
¼ cup	Minced onion	50 mL
2 Tbsp.	Lemon or lime juice	30 mL
1 Tbsp.	Cilantro, minced	15 mL
1 clove	Garlic, minced	1 clove

Yield: 8 servings, ¼ cup each

Directions
1. Peel and seed the avocados.
2. In a medium bowl, mash the avocados.
3. Stir in tomato, chilies, onion, lemon or lime juice, cilantro, and garlic.
4. Serve at room temperature or chilled.

Note: To store, cover the surface of the guacamole with plastic wrap and refrigerate.

Nutrition Information
Per serving (approximate): 87 calories, 1 g protein, 5 g carbohydrate, 8 g fat, 0 mg cholesterol, 173 mg sodium
Good source of: vitamin A, vitamin C

Food for Thought
- How could this recipe be varied to suit individual tastes?
- What purpose does the lemon or lime juice serve in this recipe?

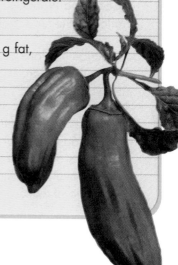

CAREER WANTED

Individuals with strong organizational skills, who are flexible and have a caring nature.

REQUIRES:

- degree in family and consumer sciences
- state teaching certification

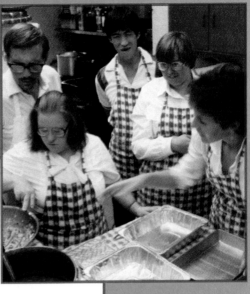

"I shape the minds of the future,"
says Family & Consumer Sciences Teacher Doreen Krebbs

Q: What do you see as your chief responsibility?

A: To help my students develop skills that they will use throughout their lives—everything from preparing nutritious meals to managing the family budget to caring for children.

Q: Describe some of the skills needed for your job.

A: As a teacher, I feel you have to know how to communicate with students. You must also be knowledgeable in your subject area. But most of all, having a genuine enthusiasm for working with young people makes the job easy.

Q: What is the biggest misconception people have about your career field?

A: Many people think teachers only work until 3 PM, Monday through Friday. The truth is that I work a 50-hour week, both in and out of the classroom. Besides actually teaching, my job involves planning lessons, grading papers, meeting with parents and school personnel, and attending in-service workshops and conferences.

Q: What is your favorite part of the job?

A: I love seeing students accomplish things. It's very rewarding to help them learn. Often, I learn from them, too!

Career Research Activity

1. Research the differences between Human Services careers and those in Family & Consumer Sciences. What do they have in common? Which career area seems to give you the most options for the future? Why? Write a synopsis of your findings.

2. What does a community health educator do? How is that career similar to a family & consumer sciences teacher? Try to interview a community health educator in person or read an article in the library or on the Internet about someone in this career field. Share your findings with the class.

Related Career Opportunities

Entry Level
- Teacher's Aide
- Clerk Typist

Technical Level
- Summer Camp Director
- Recipe Developer
- Human Services Worker

Professional Level
- Family & Consumer Sciences Teacher
- Community Health Educator
- Food Scientist

Chapter 23   Review & Activities

─────── **Summary** ───────

Section 23-1: Regional Foods of the East, Midwest, and South

- Some Native Americans were skilled farmers and cooks. They were pioneers in storing and preserving foods.

- They shared the foods and cooking methods with European immigrants, who adapted them to their own lifestyles and cooking traditions.

- British, Dutch, and German groups in the Northeast developed recipes to supply their energy needs.

- Midwestern farmers raised cattle, grains, and vegetables.

- Southern staples were incorporated into new dishes by African Americans living in the South.

- Creole and Cajun cuisines are famous for their distinctively spiced, seafood-based recipes.

Section 23-2: Regional Foods of the West and Canada

- Foods and preparation methods of the American Southwest reflect the influence of Native American and Mexican cultures.

- Along the Pacific coast and in the Northwest, shipping ports brought the influence of Asian cooking to native food supplies.

- Hawaiian cuisine combines many traditions.

- Fish, shellfish, blueberries, and potatoes are plentiful in the Atlantic provinces of Canada.

- The cuisine of Quebec reflects its historical ties to France.

- Food customs in Ontario are as varied as the residents themselves.

- Foods in Canada's Western provinces are similar to foods in the Midwestern United States.

Working IN THE Lab

1. **Foods Lab.** Find and prepare an authentic recipe for one of the regional favorites described in this chapter. Compare its basic flavor with that of the food as it is usually prepared today. Describe and give reasons for the similarities and differences you find.

2. **Foods Lab.** Combine the preferences and cooking traditions of your lab group to create your own "regional" cuisine. Prepare a meal of these favorite recipes, explaining how each one became part of the group's "heritage."

Checking Your Knowledge

1. Name three ways that Native Americans prepared corn that are still used today.

2. Describe three ways in which regional differences affected the foods and preparation methods of Native Americans.

3. Identify the three influences on the development of Midwestern cooking styles.

4. What cultures are blended in Creole cooking?

5. Name four foods that are often combined in Cajun cooking.

6. Why did cowboy cooks often make a biscuit mix before going to bed at night when on the trail? What is the origin of the barbecue?

7. *Chow mein* reflects a blending of what two cultures?

8. How is sourdough bread made? What is the advantage of this method?

9. Identify two uses of the taro root.

10. Name two foods that are unique to Quebec. Why does the Canadian flag feature a maple leaf?

Review & Activities Chapter 23

Thinking Critically

1. Recognizing Alternatives. Identify the traditional cooking methods used to prepare the regional foods described in this chapter. Suggest some modern methods that could replace the traditional methods.

2. Analyzing Behavior. What personal qualities did immigrants and settlers show by trying new foods and developing new recipes? In what other situations did those qualities help them survive? How might people today benefit from trying new foods?

3. Predicting Consequences. How do you think appreciating the food traditions of other cultures affects your attitudes and feelings toward the people of those cultures?

4. Recognizing Points of View. Do you think that being served some of their province's traditional dishes would be a problem for some health-conscious Canadians? Choose two of the Canadian specialties and think about how they might be prepared so that they would be more nutritious. Which traditional Canadian food products would be the most healthful?

Reinforcing Key Skills

1. Management. Carlita lives in a small town in New England. She has read about the nutrients in poi and would like to prepare it for her family. However, taro root is not available where Carlita lives.

2. Communication. Trying the foods of different regions and cultures of America and Canada can be an enriching experience. Imagine you have been asked to create a campaign to make people of the North American continent more aware of their rich and diverse cultural backgrounds. Write, draw, or act out your ideas for heightening awareness.

Making Decisions and Solving Problems

You are spending a few months with friends in the South. You are concerned that many of the foods they prepare—fried chicken and fish, hush puppies, meat gravy—are high in fat and calories. You would like to suggest ways of preparing foods that are more healthful, but retain the flavors and textures your friends enjoy.

Making Connections

1. Language Arts. In Willa Cather's *My Antonia*, find a passage related to food, or to the lack of food. What does the scene tell you about meals, food supplies, and preparation methods of people of that time and place? What might the scene tell you about the characters involved?

2. Social Studies. Interview people of different cultural backgrounds who live in your community. What are some traditional foods of their ethnic groups? If they originally came from another country or region, how has moving affected their cooking and eating habits? How have their cooking traditions affected the way they prepare common American dishes?

Good friends and good food—the recipe for a great time. Add some creative techniques for food preparation and presentation, and any occasion becomes special.

In this chapter, you will learn ways to give food eye appeal as well as taste appeal.

Special Topics in Food

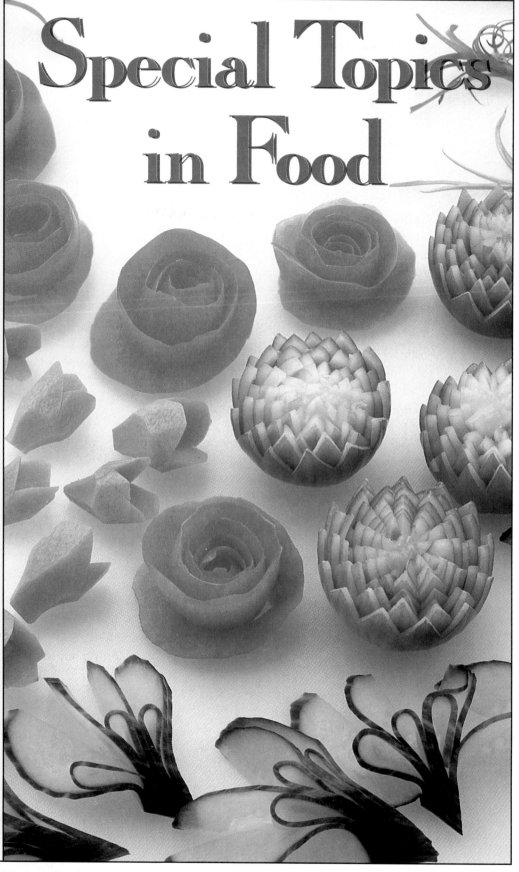

After studying this section, you should be able to:

- Describe how to use a variety of seasonings.
- Explain how to use your creativity in cooking.
- Describe ways to improve the appearance of foods with garnishes.

Look for These Terms

seasoning blends

julienne

en papillote

garnish

Creative Techniques

"This cole slaw is great, Uncle Ted!" Alonza remarked. "How did you make it so good?"

"It's a little secret I learned," her uncle said, smiling. "I added a little celery seed."

Like Alonza's uncle, many cooks know that seasonings can wake up the flavor of even basic foods.

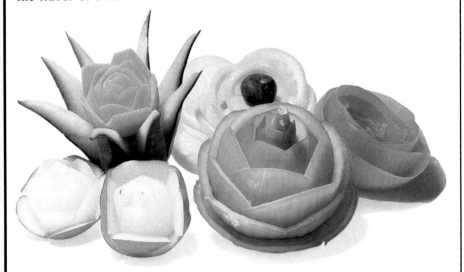

Seasoning Secrets

Seasonings are ingredients that are used in small amounts to flavor foods. They include herbs, spices, and condiments. Seasonings can be helpful for health-conscious people who are limiting their use of salt and fat by providing flavor.

When you begin to experiment with seasonings, use a small amount at first. You can always add more. If you add too much at the beginning, there's little you can do to correct the flavor.

Herbs and Spices

Herbs are the flavorful leaves and stems of soft, succulent plants that grow in the temperate zone. Some familiar examples are basil, oregano, sage, and bay leaf. Herbs are usually sold dry, but increasing numbers are available fresh in many supermarkets.

Spices are usually dried, ground buds, bark, seeds, stems, or roots of aromatic plants and trees. Most grow in tropical countries. Some—whole nutmeg, peppercorns, and cinnamon sticks, for example—are sold whole or in pieces. A few are sold fresh, such as ginger root, which is commonly used in Asian cooking.

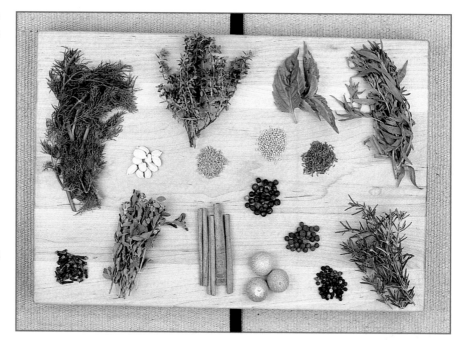

◆ Herbs and spices give many dishes an added dimension. When adding seasonings like these, remember the saying: "Less is more." Explain how the saying applies in this case.

Seasoning Blends

Seasoning blends are convenient combinations of herbs and spices. Most blends are used for specific purposes. For instance, Italian seasonings combine flavors typical in Italian cooking. You can buy blends or mix your own.

Buying and Storing Seasonings

Because herbs and spices are used in such small amounts, consider buying them in bulk. That way, you can buy only the amount you can use in a short time.

Light, air, and heat are the main enemies of herbs and spices. Store them in tightly closed, opaque containers in a cool, dark place. Do not keep them next to the range.

Dried, crushed herbs keep their flavor for about six months. To test dried herbs for freshness, rub a small amount in the palm of your hand with your thumb for about five to ten seconds. If there is little or no aroma, the herb is probably too old to use. It might give food a bitter flavor.

Ground spices keep their flavor for about a year. Whole spices may last as long as three years.

Using Herbs and Spices

Here are some guidelines for using herbs and spices:

◆ Begin with a few of the more basic herbs and spices. (The chart on pages 649 and 650 shows some of these.) Once you learn how to use these, you can add others.

◆ Herbs and spices vary in strength and are used in differing amounts. Dried herbs are more potent than fresh herbs. As a rule, you can substitute 1 tablespoon (15 mL) of fresh herbs for 1 teaspoon (5 mL) of dried, crushed herbs.

◆ When preparing hot foods, add herbs and spices at least 10 minutes before tasting or serving. This allows time for the heat to release the flavor. Do not add herbs more than 45 minutes before serving—they will lose their flavor if overcooked.

◆ When preparing cold mixtures, add herbs and spices 30 minutes to several hours before serving so that flavors can be released.

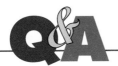

Q How can I dry my own fresh herbs?

A There are two methods—air-drying and microwaving—both of them easy. To air-dry herbs, first rinse sprigs of herbs and shake off excess water. Tie herbs into bunches, and label them. Hang them in a dry, shady, well-ventilated place. They should dry in about two weeks. To micro-wave herbs, place the rinsed herbs between several layers of paper toweling. Microwave on 100 percent power, 15 to 30 seconds at a time, until the herbs are dry and can be crumbled.

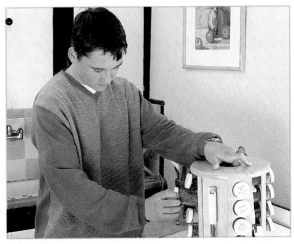

◆ **Keep in mind that dried herbs and spices go farther than fresh ones.** How many tablespoons of dried rosemary would you use in a chicken recipe that called for two tablespoons of fresh rosemary?

Basic Herbs, Spices, and Seasoning Blends

		Flavor	*Uses*
Herbs	**Basil**	Mild licorice flavor with a hint of mint	Dishes containing tomatoes, meat and poultry, carrots, peas, rice
	Bay leaf	Strong, aromatic, pungent flavor	Braised meat, stews, soups, bean dishes (Use leaf whole; remove before serving.)
	Dill weed	Sharp flavor, similar to that of caraway seeds	Cruciferous vegetables, carrots, green beans, cucumbers, fish, poultry, breads
	Marjoram	Delicate, sweet, spicy flavor with hint of mint	Soups, stews, poultry, stuffings, salads, tomato sauces
	Mint	Strong, refreshing, aromatic flavor	Yogurt dishes, tomato dishes, rice, bulgur, vegetables, lentils, fruits, tea
	Oregano	Strong, clovelike flavor	Italian and Mexican dishes, bean dishes, pork, poultry, salads, green beans

Basic Herbs, Spices, and Seasoning Blends (cont'd)

		Flavor	Uses
Herbs (cont'd)	Rosemary	Strong, piney flavor	Poultry, lamb, pork, potatoes, breads, bean dishes, pasta sauces, soups
	Sage	Strong, slightly bitter flavor	Poultry, pork, stuffings, potatoes, white beans, chowders
	Thyme	Strong, clovelike flavor	Poultry and stuffings, lamb, dry beans, stews, soups
Spices	Cinnamon	Sweet flavor	Meat dishes, desserts, legumes, sweet potatoes, squash
	Cloves	Strong, hot, pungent flavor	Meat dishes, grains, legumes, fruit desserts
	Cumin	Strong, musty flavor	Mexican and Middle Eastern foods, legumes, tomato sauces, soups, rice
	Dry mustard	Hot, sharp, spicy flavor	Meat, poultry, soups, stews, egg dishes, salad dressings
	Ground ginger	Hot, pungent, spicy flavor	Stir-fries, stews, soups, squash, sweet potatoes, grains, legumes, desserts
	Nutmeg	Mild, spicy flavor (best if purchased whole and grated fresh)	Cooked spinach, zucchini, and carrots; sweet potatoes; soups; stews; ground meat; bulgur; fruits; desserts
Seasoning Blends	Chili powder	Spicy, hot, pungent flavor	Tex-Mex cooking, chili, stews, soups, barbecue sauces, dishes made with corn
	Curry powder	Pungent, spicy flavor	East Indian cooking, poultry, meats, fish, yogurt dishes, legumes
	Italian seasoning	Blend of basil, marjoram, oregano, rosemary, sage, savory, and thyme	Italian cooking
	Poultry seasoning	Blend of lovage, marjoram, and sage	Any dishes made with poultry, including stuffing

Condiments

Condiments are liquid or semiliquid accompaniments to food. You can also use them as flavorful seasonings. Condiments vary in flavor—sweet, salty, or spicy. Mustard, salsa, and ketchup are popular condiments. Here are some others:

◆ **Soy and tamari sauces.** Are made from fermented soybeans. Soy sauce has a sharper, more pungent flavor than tamari. Low-sodium types are available.

◆ **Hot pepper sauce.** Is made from hot chili peppers. It is measured by drops because it's so strong.

◆ **Worcestershire sauce** (WOO-stuhr-shuhr). A dark, spicy sauce used in soups, stews, and meat mixtures.

Using Your Creativity

Seasonings make food taste good. What's the secret to making it *look* good? Using your creativity and your "meal appeal" skills—that's the secret. For many people, preparing food is more than just cooking. It's art. A creative cook may plan the appearance of a plate of food much as an artist plans a painting. Think about the colors and shapes of food or how the flavors blend. What would your edible work of art look like?

Creative Touches

You might want to look in a variety of cookbooks for different ways to present food. Here are a few possibilities:

◆ Swirl whipped potatoes into a fluffy mound by using a pastry bag with a decorative tip similar to those used in cake decorating.

◆ Cut foods into **julienne**—long, thin strips of food.

◆ Use a small scoop to mold fruits such as melons into balls.

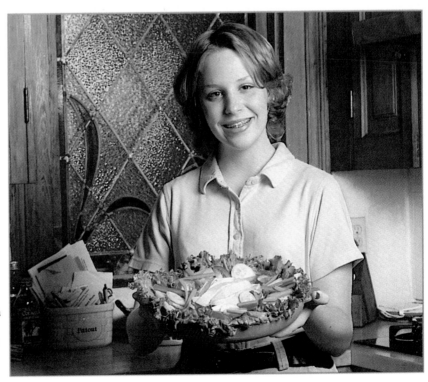

◆ Salads like this one can become a feast for the eyes as well as the palate when creative touches are used. Identify the items in this dish that have been julienned.

Cooking in parchment paper, or **en papillote** (ehn pah-pee-YOHT), is another method creative cooks use. Fish and tender cuts of meat and poultry are often cooked this way. Place one serving in the center of a square of parchment paper along with other ingredients, such as vegetables, butter, or a sauce. For each serving, fold the paper around the food to form a package. Close the ends tightly, and fold them under so that the package does not leak. Place the packages on a baking sheet and bake in the oven. As the food cooks, the flavors blend. The sealed packages retain the flavor and aroma.

To serve, place each package on a dinner plate. Cut an X in the top of the paper, and peel the paper back. As you read about garnishes, think about ways you might dress up foods served *en papillote*.

Safety Check

Do not use brown paper bags as a substitute for cooking parchment. They are not made to withstand high cooking temperatures and may burn. In addition, chemicals in the paper may be transferred to the food.

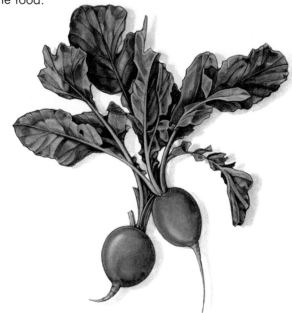

Garnishes

Have you ever been served food that had a sprig of parsley on it or next to it? Touches like that are known as garnishes. A **garnish** is any small, colorful bit of food that is used to enhance the appearance and texture of a dish. Garnishes can be used on appetizers, salads, main dishes, vegetables, desserts, and beverages. Presenting foods that are attractive, as well as tasty, helps make mealtime an enjoyable experience.

Keep size in mind when garnishing foods. If a garnish is too large, it may overpower the food. Choose colors and flavors that complement the food the garnish is added to. Here are some ideas for simple garnishes:

- **Soups.** Float a spoonful of yogurt, cucumber slices, a lemon slice, croutons, or chopped parsley or chives on soups.

- **Salads.** Top with green pepper rings, cherry tomatoes, pimiento strips, red onion rings, tomato wedges, pickle fans, radish roses, chopped nuts, or seeds.

- **Meat, poultry, and fish dishes.** Use citrus fruit slices, twists, or wedges; a small bunch of grapes; cranberry sauce; spiced crabapples; currant or mint jelly in lemon baskets; sprigs of parsley or fresh herbs; pineapple slices; or olives.

- **Sandwiches.** Use crisp vegetables—such as scored cucumber slices, carrot curls, celery fans, radish roses—and fruit slices or wedges.

- **Beverages.** Try citrus twists on a skewer, lemon or lime slices slit and slipped onto the edge of a glass, marshmallows or peppermint sticks in cocoa, or fruit slices and whole fruits frozen in an ice ring for punch.

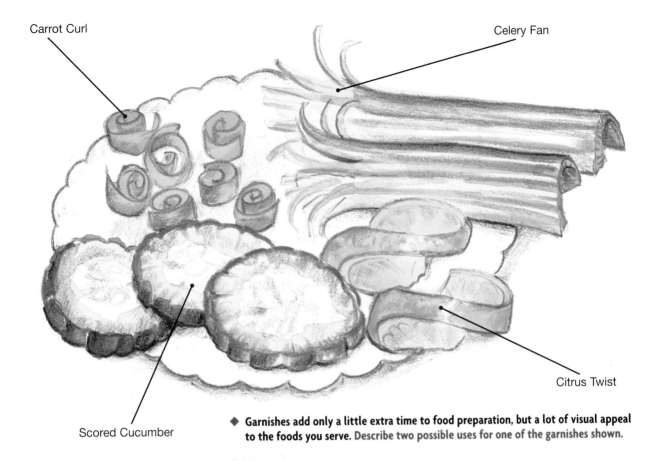

Carrot Curl

Celery Fan

Citrus Twist

Scored Cucumber

◆ **Garnishes add only a little extra time to food preparation, but a lot of visual appeal to the foods you serve.** Describe two possible uses for one of the garnishes shown.

Section 24-1 Review & Activities

1. When should herbs be added to hot foods? To cold foods?

2. In what way might cooking *en papillote* be said to be both a moist and a dry cooking method? Explain.

3. Name one way to garnish each of the following dishes: tomato soup, tossed salad, roasted whole chicken, tuna sandwich, iced tea. Explain why you would choose each garnish.

4. Analyzing. Imagine that you are teaching a food preparation class. What are some cautions you would encourage your students to be aware of when it comes to using herbs and spices?

5. Synthesizing. How can seasoning with herbs and spices replace other methods of flavoring food that are higher in fat and sodium?

6. Applying. Make a list of herbs and spices used regularly in your home. Create a recipe using some of these herbs and spices. Explain how you would use them, and describe the flavor they would give to the foods.

Beverages

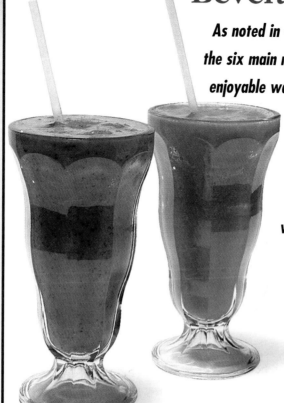

SECTION 24-2

Objectives

After studying this section, you should be able to:

- Identify various types of beverages.
- Explain how different types of beverages fit into a healthy eating plan.
- Describe procedures for preparing and serving beverages.

Look for These Terms

mulled

infuser

steep

As noted in Chapter 2, water is one of the six main nutrients. One of the most enjoyable ways of making sure your body gets the water it needs is by drinking beverages. No meal, in fact, is complete without one.

Nutrients in Beverages

In addition to being a source of water, beverages can provide other essential nutrients. Consider the following:

- Milk supplies protein, calcium, phosphorus, and vitamins D and A. Beverages that are made with milk, such as cocoa and milk shakes, also provide these same nutrients. However, they may have more sugar, fat, and calories.

- Fruit and vegetable juices provide the same vitamins and minerals found in the fruit or vegetable, and in the same amounts, except for fiber. Many types of fruit and vegetable juices are available, including fruit and vegetable juice blends. Some types

of juices are fortified with vitamin C, calcium, or other nutrients.

Juices and fruit drinks can be found on store shelves as well as in the refrigerated section. They may be in ready-to-use or concentrated form. Frozen, powdered, and liquid concentrates must be reconstituted before using. Follow the directions on the label.

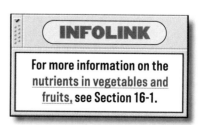

INFOLINK

For more information on the nutrients in vegetables and fruits, see Section 16-1.

FOR YOUR HEALTH

Real Juice=100%

Despite what you may hear or read in ads and commercials, not all juice products are created equal. Only products labeled "fruit juice" contain 100 percent juice. Other products, such as fruit drinks, may contain large amounts of added sugar. At the same time, some may be fortified with added nutrients. If you want to be sure you're getting the real thing, read the product label carefully.

Following Up

• Find a magazine advertisement for a juice product, or listen for a claim you might hear on TV that mentions "real juice." Find the product in your supermarket and read the label. Does it state that the product contains 100 percent juice? How will this affect you and your family's future purchases?

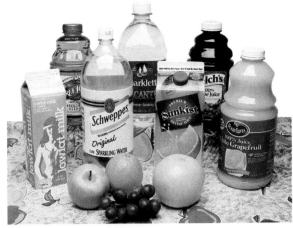

◆ **Most of the beverages shown here provide essential nutrients, as well as being a source of water.** What is missing in fruit and vegetable juices that is found in the actual fruit or vegetable?

Types of Beverages

Every beverage has water as its common denominator. Some beverages, such as punch and mulled cider, are served on festive occasions. Others, including bottled water, soft drinks, coffee and tea, are enjoyed at any time.

Punch

A punch is generally a mixture of fruit juices and carbonated beverages, such as ginger ale and seltzer, or tea. It is usually served in a punch bowl. Sherbet, ice cream, or fruit may be added. To serve the punch, ladle it from the bowl into small glasses or cups.

If the punch is to be served cold, combine all liquids except the carbonated beverages ahead of time and chill well. Chill the carbonated beverages separately; add them just

before serving the punch. If you add them ahead of time, they will go flat.

Fruit is often floated in the bowl as a garnish; the type depends on the fruit flavors in the punch. Another popular garnish is an ice ring; it also helps keep the punch cold. The ice ring is usually made with punch or water. Fruit is placed in the ring mold in a decorative design. You can also freeze fruit in ice cubes.

Punches may also be **mulled**—served hot and flavored with sweet spices, such as cinnamon, nutmeg, or cloves. This is also a popular way of preparing cider.

Bottled Water

What do you reach for when you are thirsty? Although many people reach for plain water, bottled specialty waters have become very popular in the United States. There are many different kinds, such as mineral water, spring water, seltzer water, and club soda. They vary in mineral content. Some are carbonated or have a flavoring added. Check the list of ingredients on the label.

Soft Drinks

Soft drinks represent a multibillion-dollar industry. These carbonated beverages are available with or without caffeine and sugar. These can be part of a healthful eating plan as long as you realize that they are found in the top section of the Food Guide Pyramid and should be used sparingly.

Coffee

Coffee is brewed from ground coffee beans, which are the seeds from trees grown in South and Central America, Asia, and Africa. Ground coffee can be made from just one variety of coffee beans or a blend of several varieties. Gourmet coffee is more expensive because it is made from costlier beans.

Like soda, coffee contains caffeine, a stimulant drug, which can excite the nervous system. Most forms of coffee are also available in decaffeinated (dee-KAFF-in-ay-tuhd) versions.

Instant coffee is brewed coffee that has been dried and ground. It comes as a powder or as freeze-dried crystals, regular or decaffeinated. All you do is add hot water.

Besides regular and gourmet coffee, flavored coffees are also available. Flavors include mocha, vanilla, and assorted spices.

Ground coffee comes in different grinds to suit the brewing method. Buy the grind of coffee recommended for your coffeemaker.

Unopened containers of vacuumed-packed coffee can be stored at room temperature for about a year. Once opened, refrigerate fresh coffee, whether ground or whole beans, in an airtight container. Instant coffee can be kept at room temperature.

Making and Serving Coffee

The most popular appliance for making coffee is the automatic drip coffeemaker. Most automatic drip coffeemakers have four parts—a water reservoir, a basket that holds a filter and the coffee, a carafe that catches the coffee as it brews, and a hot plate that keeps the carafe and coffee warm.

Automatic drip coffeemakers are easy to use. Just put ground coffee into a filter inside the basket, pour cold water into the reservoir, and turn on the controls.

If desired, change the amounts of water and coffee to get the strength of coffee you want. Coffeemakers usually have convenient markings on the carafe or sides of the reservoir so that you can measure the water easily.

Clean the coffee carafe and basket in hot sudsy water after every use. Coffee contains oils that cling to the inside of the carafe and basket. They can give the next carafe of coffee an unpleasant flavor.

Serve coffee piping hot, right after it is made. If coffee is held at a high temperature for too long or reheated, it loses its flavor and aroma.

Coffee can also be served iced. Make double-strength coffee, and pour it over ice cubes.

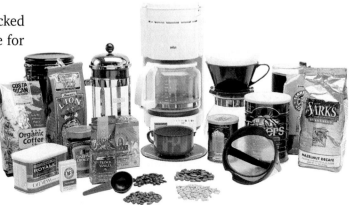

◆ The type of coffee to buy depends on the way you plan to brew it. Popular coffeemakers include the automatic drip coffeemaker and the nonautomatic drip model. Instant coffee is also an option. Name some different varieties of coffee.

Tea

Tea is a beverage made from the leaves of a shrub grown in tropical mountainous areas. Three basic kinds of tea are produced and used worldwide. *Black tea* has a dark, rich color and deep hearty flavor. *Green tea* has a delicate, light green color and a very mild flavor. *Oolong tea* is partly oxidized, so the leaves are partly brown and partly green. Its flavor and color are between those of black and green teas. Tea is sold loose or in tea bags.

Tea contains caffeine, although not as much as coffee. It is also available decaffeinated. The same processes are used to decaffeinate tea and coffee.

In addition to plain tea, you can also buy flavored and instant teas. Flavored tea includes fruit, herb, and spice flavors. Instant tea is brewed tea that has been dried and ground to a powder. It is available plain, flavored, and presweetened.

Herb teas are made from herbs and other plants. They do not contain regular tea and are caffeine-free.

Buy herb teas from reliable sources. Most supermarkets carry the major brands. Avoid teas that make health claims, such as weight-loss teas.

Brewing and Serving Tea

Tea can be brewed in a teapot or right in the cup. An automatic hot tea maker is also available. It works in much the same way as an automatic coffeemaker. It preheats the teapot, brews the tea, and keeps it at serving temperature.

To brew tea yourself, begin by heating fresh, cold water in a teakettle. Bring the water to a rolling boil.

Preheat the teapot or cup by rinsing it with hot water. Then put in the tea or tea bags. As

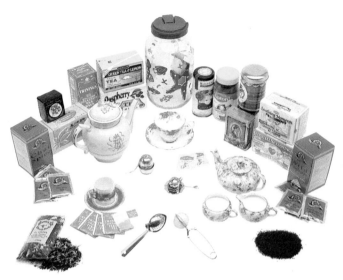

◆ **The many varieties of tea and herb tea can be purchased loose or in bags.** What tea-making utensils are shown here?

a rule, use 1 teaspoon (5 mL) of tea, or one tea bag, for each serving. To make loose tea easier to use, put it in an **infuser**—a small container with tiny holes that let water in but don't allow the tea leaves to come out. Like tea bags, the infuser is easy to remove at the end of the brewing time.

Pour boiling water over the tea. The tea will **steep**, or brew in water just below the boiling point. Follow package directions for brewing time.

Stir the tea before pouring or drinking to be sure it's uniformly strong. If the brewed tea is too strong, add a little hot water. Tea may be served with milk or lemon and sweetener.

To make iced tea, brew as for hot tea but use 50 percent more tea. That allows for melting ice when hot tea is poured into ice-filled-glasses. For six servings, use 9 teaspoons (45 mL) of tea. Steep. Remove tea and pour into ice-filled glasses.

You can use an automatic iced tea maker to prepare iced tea or iced coffee. Instant tea is another option. Just follow the directions on the label.

Sources of Caffeine

Beverages containing caffeine can fit into a healthful eating plan as long as they are used in moderation.

Beverage	Amount of Caffeine (mg)
Coffee (5-ounce serving)	
brewed	60-180
instant	30-120
decaffeinated, brewed	2-5
decaffeinated, instant	1-5
espresso (2-ounce serving)	40-170
Tea (5-ounce serving)	
brewed	25-110
instant	25-50
iced (12-ounce serving)	65-75
decaffeinated	—
Caffeinated soft drinks (12-ounce serving)	30-60
Cocoa or hot chocolate (5-ounce serving)	2-20

Section 24-2 Review & Activities

1. How do beverages meet the body's need for water?

2. Name two types of fruit or vegetable juices, and identify the nutrients they provide.

3. Why are milk and fruit and vegetable juices more healthful choices than other beverages?

4. **Extending.** Why do you think it is necessary to use double-strength coffee when serving the beverage iced?

5. **Analyzing.** What are the nutritional drawbacks of coffee, tea, and soft drinks? How do these compare with other beverage choices?

6. **Applying.** Look through cookbooks and magazines to find a punch recipe. How might you change the ingredients in this recipe to add more nutrients?

RECIPE FILE

Fruit Punch

Fruit punch can be served either chilled or hot. Try heating a cup of this punch in the microwave, adding cloves or a cinnamon stick.

Customary	Ingredients	Metric
6 oz.	Frozen lemonade concentrate, thawed	177 mL
6 oz.	Frozen orange juice concentrate, thawed	177 mL
32 oz.	Cranberry juice cocktail, chilled	1 L
2 qt.	Ginger ale or lemon-lime soda, chilled	1 L

Yield: 32 servings (approximate)
Equipment: Half-gallon (2-L) pitcher, punch bowl

Directions

1. Combine thawed juice concentrates and cranberry juice cocktail in pitcher.
2. Pour juice mixture into punch bowl.
3. Add ginger ale or lemon-lime soda and stir the mixture gently.
4. Serve chilled, garnished with citrus fruit slices or an ice ring, if desired.

Note: Do not put frozen juice concentrate directly into punch bowl—you may crack the bowl.

Nutrition Information

Per serving (approximate): 49 calories, 0 g protein, 12 g carbohydrate, 0 g fat, 0 mg cholesterol, 6 mg sodium
Good source of: vitamin C

Food for Thought

• How could you serve this punch if you didn't have a punch bowl?
• What liquids and fruits could you use to make an ice ring for the punch?

Entertaining

"Would you like to come to my house for dinner Friday?" Tamera asked. *"My dad's making his special lasagne."*

"That would be great," Leslie answered. *"Are you sure it'll be OK with your dad?"*

"He loves company!" Tamera said. *"He told us to invite a friend."*

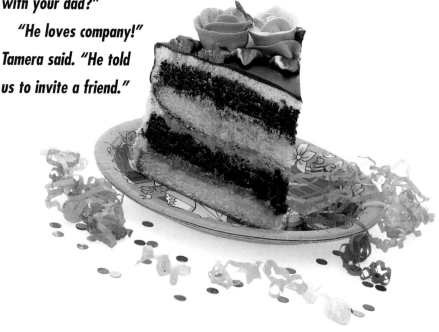

Objectives

After studying this section, you should be able to:

- Identify ways to plan for entertaining.
- Develop menus and organize food preparation and cleanup for entertaining.
- Describe different methods of serving food depending on the occasion.

Look for These Terms

modified English service

service plate

reception

Reasons for Entertaining

Like Tamera's dad, many people enjoy inviting friends into their homes. Entertaining is a way of making people feel welcome and special. Although food is generally served, entertaining involves much more than just preparing a meal.

Entertaining does not have to be elaborate. You can have a successful party with a simple soup-and-salad meal if the atmosphere is right. With planning and organization, entertaining can be as much fun for the person giving the party as it is for the guests.

Planning for Entertaining

When you think about entertaining, what comes to mind? Whether you picture a big family get-together or just having a few friends over for pizza, careful planning goes a long way when you entertain.

Informal and Formal Events

The first step in planning is to identify the type of occasion or event. The type of planning you would do for a casual party, for example, would differ from the planning necessary for a formal sit-down dinner.

◆ Parties are more memorable when both the food and decorations relate to a theme, such as a Mexican fiesta. Think of two other possible themes. List foods and decorations you would choose to go with each.

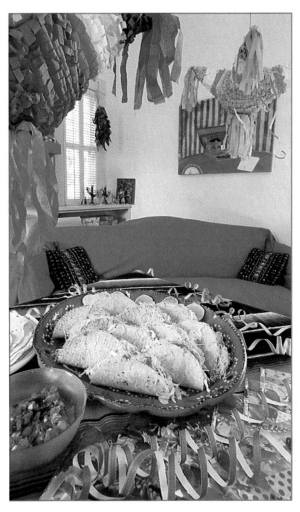

Whether the occasion is to be formal or informal also affects the menu and the way you will serve the food. Think about your skills in entertaining. If this is the first party you're giving, it's probably best to start with a simple, informal event.

Themes and Decorations

When Nikki greeted her guests at the door, she was wearing a grass skirt. She placed a *lei* around each person's neck and said, "Aloha!" Construction paper cutouts in the shape of palm trees and pineapples decorated the walls.

As Nikki knows, parties and get-togethers can be more fun when they have a theme. A theme is a specific idea on which the occasion is based. Holidays, birthdays, and graduations provide ready-made themes. For other occasions, be creative! Choose an interest you and your guests share—such as sports or old movies—or go for an ethnic theme, such as a Mexican fiesta. After you have chosen your theme, plan the menu, activities, and decorations to go with it.

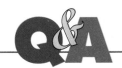

 What are some simple ways I can decorate a table?

 As with other aspects of decorating, let your imagination run free. A potted plant on a place mat, an arrangement of fresh or artificial flowers, a grouping of seashells on a wicker mat are just a few possibilities.

Invitations

As you decide on a list of guests, try to put together a combination of people who are likely to enjoy each other's company and be interesting to one another. Strive for a good blend of listeners and talkers. Whenever possible, avoid inviting people that you know don't get along.

For informal events, you will most likely invite your guests in person or by telephone about one week before the event. Of course, spur-of-the-moment gatherings are fun, too! Just be sure to check with the adults in your home first.

Invitation Specifics

Formal occasions or larger parties require sending written invitations. This will help eliminate any mix-ups about the time and date. Send your invitations ten days to two weeks before the event is to occur.

On your invitation, be sure to include the following specific information:

◆ The date, location, and time of the event.

◆ The occasion, if there is one.

◆ Your name as host.

It is customary for written invitations to include the abbreviation *R.S.V.P.* followed by the host's telephone number. These letters are short for a phrase meaning "please reply." You might also include a date by which guests are to reply so that you can buy the necessary amount of food.

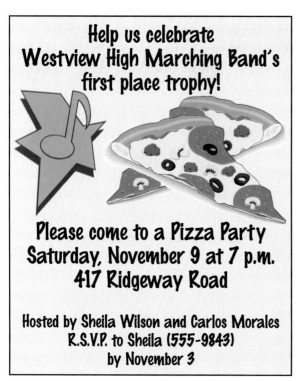

◆ Invitations need to include certain information. Refer to the list above. Find each of the pieces of information called for.

If, as an invited guest, you are asked to reply to an invitation, it is your responsibility to follow through on this request. If you can't reach a person by telephone, send a brief note in the mail.

Menus for Entertaining

When planning food for parties and other special occasions, follow the same guidelines as when planning meals. Choose a variety of nutritious foods that appeal to the eye as well as the palate. If you are planning foods for a special theme, try to choose some foods that most of your guests will like. Here are a few guidelines for selecting foods for your menu:

◆ Find out about special food needs or preferences that your guests might have.

◆ Keep food choices simple. Choose foods that can be prepared ahead of time with a minimum of last-minute preparation. For example, you might decide to prepare lasagne as the main course and do all the preparation, except for the actual baking, the day before. Add a tossed salad, bread, a beverage, and perhaps some fruit for dessert.

◆ You might want to make a simple appetizer, such as a dip and crackers or fruit, that your guests can nibble on while you make a few last-minute preparations in the kitchen.

Making a Schedule

You want to have as good a time as your guests. How can you achieve this? The one-word answer is *organization*.

After you've planned your meal or refreshments, identify the tasks you need to accomplish before the event. You might start with a list organized by categories—food shopping and preparation, decorations, setup, and cleanup.

List the tasks in order, beginning with the one you must do first. Think about ways to accomplish the items on your list efficiently. Some jobs can be done far ahead of the event. Make a special list for things to be done the day of the event. Cross each item off your list as you get it done.

Serving Food

How will you serve the meal? Will it be a sit-down meal or a buffet, informal or formal? The answer depends on the type of event, the number of people eating, the time available for serving and eating, the menu, and your personal preference.

Informal Table Service

Informal table service includes several ways to serve food. The method you choose will depend on your menu and the space that you have for serving.

One popular method of serving is family-style, bringing the food to the table in serving dishes and inviting people to help themselves. If space and tableware are limited, a good option is plate service. This means portioning out food on individual dinner plates that are then served to each person at the table. Plate service eliminates the need for serving dishes and makes cleanup easier.

Regardless of the method of service you select, you will want to set the table properly. In addition to the dinner plate, flatware, and glassware, you may want to add a bread-and-butter plate or a salad bowl above the forks on the left side of the cover.

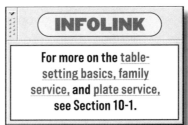

INFOLINK

For more on the table-setting basics, family service, and plate service, see Section 10-1.

Formal Service

For formal occasions, there are several ways you might handle serving food. If your guest list is limited to eight people (including yourself), you can easily handle serving the meal yourself. For larger groups, you will need help serving the meal so that all your guests are served quickly and efficiently.

For serving small groups yourself, use **modified English service**. This is a method of food service in which dinner plates and the food for the main course are brought to the table in serving dishes and placed in front of the host. If meat is to be carved, this is done by the person hosting. He or she then places the meat and vegetables on a plate and passes it to the right. The first plate is passed down to the person at the end of the table. When all the people on the right have been served, those on the left are served.

Salad is often served on individual plates from the kitchen and placed on the table before the guests are seated. Accompaniments, such as rolls and butter, are usually passed at the table.

Formal service for large groups is very rarely done at home because extra help is needed to serve the meal. This style of service is often used in fine restaurants, at hotels for banquets, and for other formal occasions.

For most formal occasions, the table is set with flatware, glassware, and a service plate for the appetizer course. A **service plate** is a large and beautifully decorated plate used for the first course only. It is removed from the table before the main course is served. Never put food directly on the service plate—serve it in a separate dish and place the dish on the service plate.

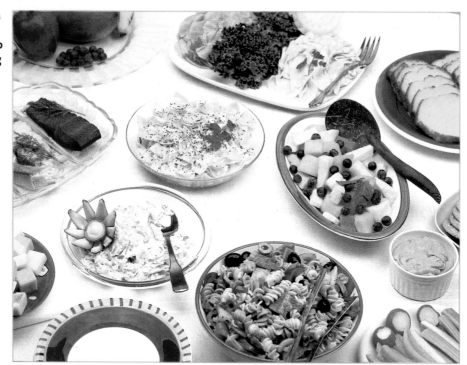

◆ When preparing foods for a buffet, arrange and garnish them attractively. Be sure to provide appropriate serving utensils where necessary. What are two important things to remember when planning a buffet meal?

As a rule, formal service includes a number of courses, each served separately on clean plates. Flatware is needed for each course. It is not uncommon to have three pieces of flatware on each side of the plate.

Buffet Service

A buffet is an easy, practical way to entertain if you don't have enough seating space at a dining table. For eating, you can set up card tables or small snack tables. People can also hold plates of food on their laps.

The prepared food is placed in the serving dishes on a large table, on the kitchen counter, or perhaps on several card tables. When setting up the buffet, stack the plates where you want guests to begin to serve themselves. After the plates, place the main dish, followed by vegetables, salad, rolls, and butter. The flatware, rolled up in a napkin, should be the last item your guests pick up.

When planning a buffet meal, choose foods that are easy to serve and that do not have to be cut with a knife. This makes the food easier to eat. Casseroles, stir-fries, sandwiches, and salads are good choices. You may want to serve beverages to your guests after they are seated.

Receptions

Receptions are social gatherings usually held to honor a person or an event, such as a wedding or a graduation. These gatherings are usually formal. Buffet service is most often used, with the food being placed on a large table. The table is covered with a floor-length tablecloth, and an eye-catching centerpiece is placed in the center.

Indicate the starting point of the reception table by where you place the plates. For large groups, divide the table in half lengthwise and offer the same food on both sides of the table. This allows people to move in two lines instead of one.

◆ **A reception table should be organized for the convenience of both servers and guests. This table is set up to handle two serving lines. What is the starting point for each line? Which direction would each line move?**

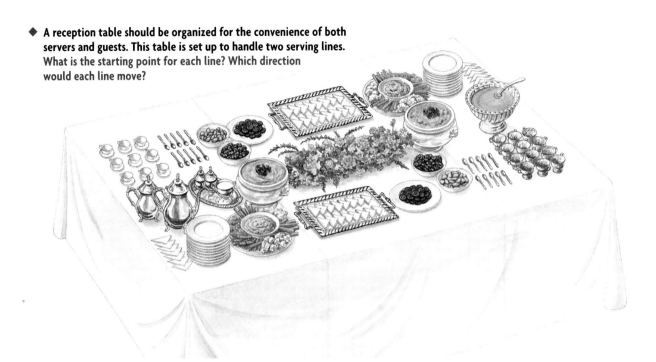

Types of Foods to Serve

Hot beverages, such as coffee or tea, are generally served at one end of the table. A cool beverage—perhaps a fruit punch—is served at the opposite end. Food choices can include finger sandwiches, cheese, crackers, fruit kabobs, or any other foods that you think your guests will enjoy.

Section 24-3 Review & Activities

1. Identify two factors that help determine whether an occasion will be formal or informal.

2. What are two reasons for finding out about the special food needs or preferences of people you're planning to invite to a party?

3. How should you set up a buffet table for serving food?

4. Extending. Suppose you want to host a sit-down dinner but have limited space. Think of a creative way of using the space available to seat your guests.

5. Synthesizing. Suppose you are hosting a buffet to celebrate an important event. After identifying the event, name three foods or dishes that you will include. Tell which factors influenced your choices.

6. Applying. In small groups, brainstorm a list of themes that might be appropriate for a party of teens. Choose one theme and describe how you would carry it out with invitations, decorations, music, and menu. How would you serve the food?

Outdoor Meals

Outdoors is a great place to share and enjoy food. Eating outdoors can take many forms, from a picnic lunch to a dinner of grilled foods. It can also occur almost anywhere—around a campfire, at the seashore, or right in your own backyard.

Objectives

After studying this section, you should be able to:

- Identify ways to cook foods safely outdoors.
- Identify foods suitable for outdoor cooking.
- Describe how to choose and pack picnic foods.

Look for This Term

micro-grill

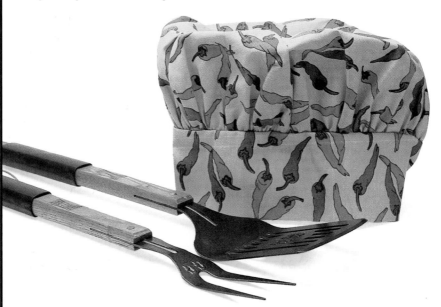

Outdoor Cooking

No matter when or where it happens, outdoor cooking uses many of the food preparation skills you have already learned. The most common form of outdoor cooking is grilling, also called barbecuing in some areas.

Grilling

Before grilling, be sure you have the proper tools and understand how to use an outdoor grill safely. The simplest grill is a round, kettle-shaped metal container that holds burning charcoal. It is topped with a wire grate for holding food above the hot coals. There are many other kinds of grills. Some cook with bottled propane gas instead of charcoal.

All grills cook by the same principle. Heat radiates upward and cooks the food held on the grate above. Grilling is a dry-heat method of cooking, similar to broiling. Cooking time depends on the kind and thickness of food and its distance from the heat.

Follow the directions in the owner's manual for using the grill. Methods vary, depending on the kind of grill you have.

Micro-Grilling

Some cooks choose to **micro-grill**. This is a cooking method that combines microwaving and grilling. The food—usually meat or poultry—is partially cooked on a rack in the microwave oven and then finished immediately afterward on the outdoor grill. Juices that collect during the microwave phase are discarded. Micro-grilling allows foods to cook faster and remain moist and juicy. An added advantage of micro-grilling is highlighted in "For Your Health" on page 668.

Accident Prevention

Home is one place where you should feel safe and secure. Yet every year, thousands of people are injured in home accidents. To lessen the risk of accidents involving grilling, follow these guidelines:

◆ Use fireproof gloves and heavy-duty grilling tools with long handles. The long handles keep your hands away from the intense heat.

◆ Set the grill on a level surface so that it won't tip over. Keep it away from buildings, shrubs, trash containers, or anything else that could catch fire.

◆ Use a clean grill. Before storing the grill after each use, remove baked-on grime from the inside and the grate with a hard-bristled brush. Baked-on food and grease can cause flames to flare up when you light the fire.

◆ Apply enough of the starter fluid (if you use it) before striking the match. Never add more fluid after the coals have been lighted—doing so could cause an explosion.

◆ Never use kerosene or gasoline as fire starters—they can explode.

◆ Fat and meat juices dripping on coals can cause flare-ups. If that happens, raise the grate, cover the grill, or use a long-handled tool to spread the coals apart. You can also remove the food from the grate and use a pump-spray bottle filled with water to spray a mist on the flare-up. Then place the food back on the grate. Don't pour water on the burning charcoal.

◆ When you have finished grilling, let the coals burn out until only ashes are left. Douse the ashes with water; then put them in a metal trash can. Don't dump hot coals or ashes on the ground. They damage the grass and can even start a fire.

Food for Grilling

Grilling is used mainly for tender cuts of meat and poultry. Cook them thoroughly, turning after half the cooking time.

Fish is also easy to grill. Place fillets skin-side down on a lightly oiled rack to keep them from sticking. Grill until the fish flakes easily. You may have to turn thick pieces.

You can grill most fruits and vegetables. Thread small pieces on metal skewers. Brush them lightly with melted butter or margarine, olive oil, or a basting sauce. Place them on the grate. Turn the skewers frequently until the foods are hot and lightly browned.

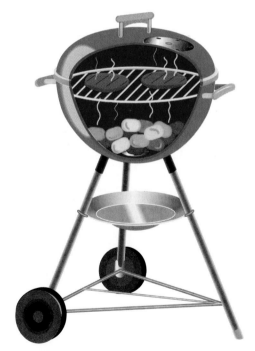

◆ **In a basic grill, hot coals provide radiant heat that cooks the food above it.** Identify three safety precautions you should take when grilling.

FOR YOUR HEALTH

"No-Deposit" Grilling

Some health experts have voiced concerns about the chemicals deposited on food as it cooks over charcoal. Studies have linked these chemicals—polycyclic aromatic hydrocarbons, or PAHs—to certain kinds of cancer. PAHs are carried in the smoke that rises after the melted fat from meat or poultry hits the heat source.

One precaution that can be taken is micro-grilling. This cooking method causes much of the fat to be lost before the meat even reaches the grill.

Another precaution is preventing fat from dripping on the heat source. Trim fat from meat before cooking. Make a drip pan from heavy-duty foil, and place it in the center of the charcoal, under the food on the grate, to catch drippings.

Following Up

• In recent years, a line of smokeless indoor grills has become available. Do research to learn whether these products produce PAHs. Is the flavor of foods cooked on them similar to that of foods prepared on an outdoor grill?

Picnic Foods

Not all food eaten outdoors is cooked there. Some food is cooked or prepared elsewhere and taken to a park, beach, or other recreational area for a picnic.

The food you choose for a picnic might depend on how far you have to travel. Avoid taking hot cooked food unless you know it will be eaten within two hours. For safety, keep hot foods in a separate insulated container.

Cooking foods on a grill at the picnic site is often safer than transporting hot food. Cook raw foods, like hamburgers, or warm up cold cooked foods. For safety, don't partially cook food at home and then finish cooking it at the picnic.

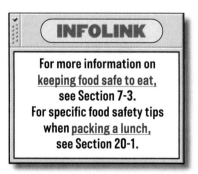

INFOLINK

For more information on keeping food safe to eat, see Section 7-3. For specific food safety tips when packing a lunch, see Section 20-1.

Packing the Picnic

If you're traveling to the picnic area, make a list of everything you'll need, including food, tableware, and cleanup equipment. Don't forget items such as premoistened cleaning wipes, can and bottle openers, a paring knife, paper towels, trash bags, and extra plastic bags for dirty utensils. As you pack for the picnic, check off each item on your list.

Be sure to follow the same food safety precautions that you would when packing a lunch. Pack nonperishable items in a basket or other container. Use an insulated cooler for perishable food. To keep the food chilled, put ice cubes or reusable frozen gel packs in the cooler. Frozen food, such as boxed frozen juices, will help keep other foods cold.

If you're taking raw meat or poultry to cook at the picnic, pack it in a separate cooler to prevent cross-contamination with ready-to-eat foods.

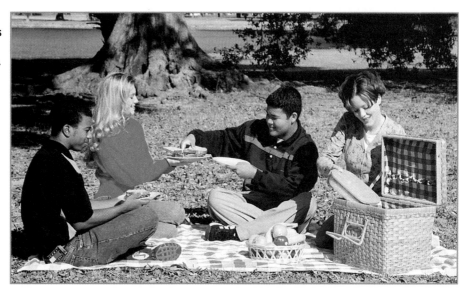

◆ A picnic can have almost any kind of food, as long as it is properly packed and kept at a safe temperature. How would you pack the foods shown here?

Packing Order

When packing the cooler and picnic basket, put the last item you will need on the bottom and the first one on the top. To pack the cooler, start with the end of the meal. Put the dessert on the bottom (if it's fragile, put it in a crush-resistant plastic container first). Packing food in this order eliminates the need to unpack the whole cooler every time you want something. Don't remove food from the cooler until you need it.

At the picnic site, keep the cooler in a cool, shady spot. Keep the cover on the cooler at all times. Don't leave the cooler in the sun, a hot car, or a car trunk. Even an insulated cooler won't stay cool under such conditions.

Section 24-4 Review & Activities

1. Give four guidelines for safe grilling.

2. Give three safety tips for choosing and preparing picnic foods.

3. After Michelle finished packing the cooler for her family's picnic, she remembered she had forgotten to pack the cookies her brother baked. Should she repack completely? Why or why not?

4. Evaluating. What are some health advantages of outdoor cooking? Some sensory advantages for the people who are eating outdoors?

5. Extending. What effect might local government regulations have on outdoor cooking in your area? Why is following posted regulations important?

6. Applying. Bring to class a favorite recipe for indoor cooking. Explain how it might be modified for preparation on a grill.

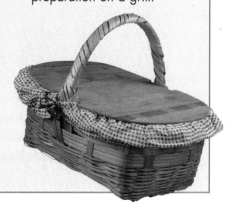

SECTION
24-5

Preserving Food at Home

Today, most foods can be purchased in either fresh, canned, frozen, or dried form. In this section, you will learn about advantages and methods of preserving fresh foods at home.

Objectives

After studying this section, you should be able to:

- Identify ways to freeze fruits and vegetables safely while retaining quality and nutrients.
- Explain how to can fruits and vegetables safely at home.
- List the benefits of drying foods at home.

Look for These Terms

dry-packing

blanching

raw-pack

hot-pack

headspace

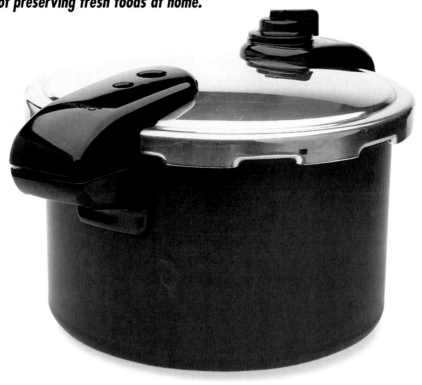

Advantages of Home Preserving

Preserving foods at home affords several real benefits to families. For many, it's a way to stretch the food budget. For others, it's a way to spend time working together and having fun. People who maintain vegetable gardens have a ready source of foods to preserve.

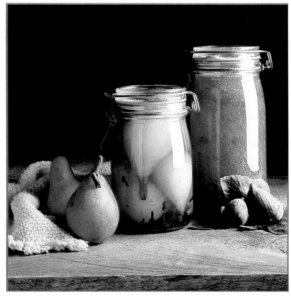

◆ **When preserving foods, choose high-quality produce for the best results.** Identify three methods for preserving foods.

Methods of Home Preserving

The preserving procedures followed today have been in use in one form or another for generations. They include freezing, canning, and drying. The method you use depends on personal preference and the equipment you have available.

If you don't grow your own food, you may be able to buy seasonal foods at low cost and save money. Farmers often have lower prices for fruits and vegetables that people pick themselves. Stores may have specials on locally grown produce.

Always use ripe, high-quality food. Freezing and canning do not improve the quality of the food. Buy only the amount you can process in the time you have available. Wash the food carefully, and prepare it according to recipe directions, keeping both cleanliness and food safety in mind.

Freezing

You may think that because freezing is so closely associated with technology, it's a modern development. However, its roots lie deep in the past. Primitive people long ago discovered that burying food under ice or snow kept it intact through the cold months.

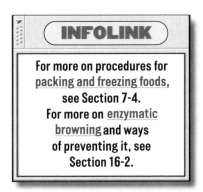

INFOLINK

For more on procedures for packing and freezing foods, see Section 7-4.
For more on enzymatic browning and ways of preventing it, see Section 16-2.

Freezing Fruits

Many fruits can be frozen. However, pears, oranges, and bananas do not freeze well. Applesauce freezes better than apples.

Before freezing any fruit, you need to know whether the fruit undergoes enzymatic browning. If it does not (which is the case with most berries, melons, pineapple, and cherries), simply dry-pack the fruit. **Dry-packing** means placing the prepared fruit on a cookie sheet, leaving space in between the pieces before placing it in the freezer. Once the food pieces are frozen solid, place them in a labeled and dated freezer package.

If you are freezing a fruit that does darken —for example, apples, figs, peaches, nectarines, or plums—use one of these two methods:

◆ Sprinkle the fruit with a ready-to-use ascorbic acid mixture according to package directions. Then dry-pack.

◆ Toss the fruits in sugar until they are well coated. Use this method—known as *sugar-packing*—whenever you want sweetened fruits or fruits in syrup to use as a sauce. When fruits defrost, their juices combine with the sugar to form a sweet syrup.

Freezing Vegetables

Before they can be frozen, vegetables require **blanching**, or partial cooking, to kill enzymes. Tomatoes do not need to be blanched. Work with 1 pound (500 g) of vegetables at a time.

To blanch vegetables, place the prepared vegetables in the strainer, and immerse them in boiling water. Allow the water to return to a rolling boil, and begin timing the vegetables. Timing depends on the type of vegetable and the size of the pieces. The larger the pieces, the longer they must blanch. (Follow the time recommended in a blanching chart.)

When the time is up, remove the strainer of vegetables and plunge them in the ice water until completely cooled. Add ice cubes as needed to keep the water ice-cold. Drain the vegetables on the clean, dry towels and pat dry. Pack them into containers and freeze.

You can also blanch vegetables in a microwave oven. Use the same method as used for microwaving vegetables. Blanching times are generally similar to those for top-of-the-range blanching.

Canning Produce

Canning methods have changed in recent years to prevent serious foodborne illness. A reliable source of information is your local cooperative extension service.

Before canning, be sure you have up-to-date recipes, instructions, and equipment. Follow the recipe directions; don't take shortcuts or change recipes.

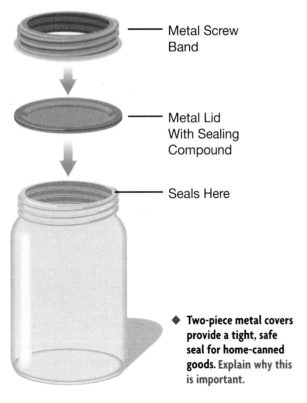

Metal Screw Band

Metal Lid With Sealing Compound

Seals Here

◆ **Two-piece metal covers provide a tight, safe seal for home-canned goods.** Explain why this is important.

Note that in many canning recipes, sugar and salt are used as preservatives. If you want low-sugar or low-sodium foods, look for those types of recipes.

Jars and Lids

Use only jars made for home canning. Be sure they are in perfect condition. Discard any that have cracks or chips that might keep the lids from sealing tightly.

Use two-piece metal covers, which combine a flat lid with a screw band. The lid is used only once. The band may be reused. Follow the manufacturer's directions for preparing the covers. Do not use one-piece covers that seal with separate rubber rings, such as glass or metal with a porcelain lining. They do not seal properly.

If filled jars are to be heated more than 10 minutes, you do not need to sterilize them before packing the food. Others should be sterilized. Follow the recipe directions.

Processing the Food

Just as in commercial food processing, food that you plan to can at home needs to be heated to stop enzyme activity and kill harmful microorganisms. There are two different heating methods. *Water-bath canning* is used for high-acid foods, such as fruits and most tomatoes. The natural acid protects the food against the growth of harmful microorganisms once the food has been canned.

Low-acid foods, such as vegetables, require *pressure canning* to be safe. A pressure canner is like a pressure cooker, only larger. It heats food under pressure to temperatures above the boiling point to kill harmful microorganisms.

Packing Methods

There are several methods you can use to pack the jars for processing. To **raw-pack** jars, place the raw foods into the jars and then pour in hot syrup, water, or juice. To **hot-pack** foods, heat the food in liquid first; then pack it into the jars.

When packing jars, leave about ½ to 1 inch (1.3 to 2.5 cm) headspace for food to expand. **Headspace** is the space between the top of the food and the rim of the jar. Run a spatula between the food and the jar to remove air bubbles. Wipe the jar top clean. Apply the covers. Screw the metal band on tightly by hand.

Processing Methods

Process the jars by using one of the recommended processing methods. Do not process canned food in conventional or microwave ovens.

♦ **Fruits.** After raw-packing or hot-packing fruits into jars, process the jars in boiling water in a water-bath canner for the time directed on the recipe. The canner is a large, covered pot with a rack to hold the jars.

♦ **Jams and fruit spreads.** Fill the jars with the prepared jam or fruit spread and apply the two-part covers. Process the jars in boiling water in a water-bath canner for the time specified in the recipe. Do not seal jars with paraffin—it does not make a tight seal.

♦ **Vegetables.** After raw-packing or hot-packing the jars with vegetables, process the jars in a pressure canner.

After processing, let the jars cool on a rack or clean dish towel away from drafts until completely cool, usually about 12 hours.

Check the covers to be sure they have sealed. Press the center of the cover, or tap it with a spoon. The cover should stay down and give a clear, ringing sound when tapped. If the jar has not sealed, reprocess or remove the food and refrigerate or freeze it.

Store home-canned foods in a clean, cool, dry place. Before tasting or using home-canned vegetables, boil them for 10 to 15 minutes to be certain that any harmful microorganisms are destroyed.

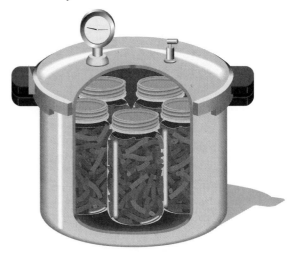

♦ **A pressure canner heats foods to temperatures higher than 212°F (100°C).** For which types of vegetables is pressure canning used?

Safety Check

A pressure canner contains a rack to hold jars, a steam-tight cover, a safety release valve, and a pressure gauge that measures accurate pressure during processing. To prevent accidents when using a pressure canner:

• *Carefully* read the manufacturer's directions.

• Process foods at the pressure indicated in the instructions for each type of food.

• Be sure the cover of the canner is fastened securely.

When the processing time is over, remove the pressure canner from the heat and allow it to cool until the pressure gauge returns to zero. Open the safety release. If no steam escapes, the pressure is down and the canner can be opened safely. *Failure to follow these instructions could result in serious injury.*

Drying Food

The easiest way to dry food at home is with a food dehydrator. Most food dehydrators have a 24-hour timer and an adjustable thermostat that allows you to dry foods between 90°F and 155°F (32°C and 69°C). Follow the manufacturer's directions for drying times and temperatures.

Foods such as fruits and vegetables, granola, and beef jerky can be dried easily at home. By taking advantage of low prices on seasonal fruits and vegetables, you can save money, too.

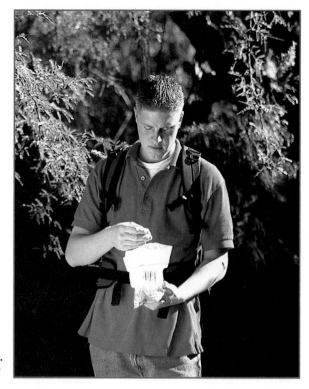

◆ Dried foods are convenient to store and make delicious snacks. They are especially popular with hikers? Can you explain why?

Section 24-5 Review & Activities

1. Anita bought a large amount of different fruits inexpensively at a food warehouse. Her plan is to freeze the fruits. How can she determine which fruits are high in natural acid?

2. Briefly explain why and how vegetables are blanched.

3. Give four guidelines for using a pressure canner safely.

4. **Analyzing.** Why do you think preserving food at home has remained popular even with today's busy lifestyles?

5. **Synthesizing.** Respond to this question: "Why bother to can food at home when you can easily buy foods in cans?"

6. **Applying.** Brainstorm a list of all the frozen, canned, and dried products your family uses regularly. Identify those that you might preserve at home. Why might it be impractical or unwise to preserve the others at home?

CAREER WANTED

Individuals who follow instructions precisely, can meet deadlines, and can work under pressure.

REQUIRES:

- degree in culinary arts or related field
- on-the-job training plus work experience

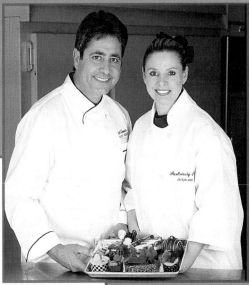

"Pastry is the crown jewel of any meal,"

says Pastry Chef Orlando Diaz

Q: Orlando, what is involved in quality baking?

A: You must start out with top-quality ingredients. Getting the most mileage out of these ingredients is key. I enjoy the creative aspect of my job. Making beautiful pastries is an art!

Q: What is your greatest challenge working in a hotel kitchen?

A: The prep time for a typical evening's dessert table can be as much as four hours. Painstaking tasks such as cake decorating also need to be figured into the equation. I'm lucky to have assistants here at this kitchen.

Q: What are working conditions like?

A: You know the saying, "If you can't stand the heat, get out of the kitchen"? Well, it's true! We have four commercial baking ovens going at all times, and I often don't notice the heat at all.

Q: How did you get into pastry work?

A: I was hired as a sauce chef to make only sauces. One day the pastry chef was sick. I was asked to make a pastry cream filling for a 6-tier wedding cake! I enjoyed that so much that I went back to culinary school and became a pastry chef.

Career Research Activity

1. Consider a career path that begins as a baker's helper, leads to a bakery manager position, and ends as a dough development director. Research the education and training necessary for each of these steps along the career path. Report your findings to the class and tell them why you would or would not pursue this career opportunity.

2. Access information from a professional group or technical school that lists the education and training requirements to be a pastry chef. What conclusions can you draw? Are the working hours desirable? Is the pay fair for the work required? Create a pamphlet promoting this career.

Related Career Opportunities

Entry Level
- Assistant Cook
- Caterer
- Baker's Helper

Technical Level
- Pastry Chef
- Bakery Manager

Professional Level
- Research & Development Specialist
- High-Volume Bakery Chef
- Dough Development Director

Summary

Section 24-1: Creative Techniques

- You can add flavors to foods with seasonings such as herbs, spices, and condiments.

- Cooking foods *en papillote,* in a sealed parchment paper package, allows the flavor of several foods to blend.

- Garnishes are colorful bits of food that complement a dish's appearance and texture.

Section 24-4: Outdoor Meals

- Safety is especially important when planning and preparing outdoor meals.

- Pack foods with care, and follow rules for safe grilling.

- Meats, fish, fruits, and vegetables can all be grilled successfully.

Section 24-2: Beverages

- Beverages help you meet your body's requirement for one of the six main nutrients—water.

- Milk and pure fruit juice are high in other nutrients, including calcium and vitamins.

- Coffee and tea come in several varieties and are easy to prepare.

Section 24-5: Preserving Food at Home

- When freezing fruits and vegetables, take steps to stop enzyme activity.

- To can safely, use up-to-date recipes and equipment, and follow recipe directions exactly.

- Some foods can be dried at home with a food dehydrator.

Section 24-3: Entertaining

- Good planning helps make any occasion, whether formal or informal, a success.

- When you plan, consider the theme, decorations, invitations, and menu.

- Options for serving the food include modified English service, formal service, and buffet service.

- Receptions are usually formal gatherings at which buffet service is used.

Checking Your Knowledge

1. What is the difference between herbs and spices?

2. Give two reasons for not using brown paper bags for cooking foods *en papillote.*

3. Identify three nutrients found in milk.

4. Identify the four main parts of an automatic drip coffeemaker.

5. Give four suggestions for making a schedule of things to do when organizing a party.

6. Describe modified English service.

7. Explain how to handle grill flare-ups.

8. Give two guidelines for packing chilled food in a cooler.

9. Describe two differences between the dry-pack plain and sugar-pack methods of freezing fruits.

10. Briefly describe how to prepare raw-packed and hot-packed jars for processing.

Working IN THE Lab

1. **Foods Lab.** Create your own herb or spice blend. Experiment with different combinations and proportions of seasonings. Prepare a recipe using your blend.

2. **Food Science.** Blanch and freeze a batch of green beans. Freeze another batch without blanching. After one week, thaw the packages and compare the appearance and texture of the beans. Cook the beans, and compare their taste. How do you explain your findings?

Thinking Critically

1. Recognizing Points of View. Aldo watched as his sister sprinkled dried oregano into the stew she was cooking. "Wouldn't that dish turn out better if you used the fresh herb?" he said. His sister replied that dried herbs have "their place in the kitchen." Based on what you learned in the chapter, explain what Aldo's sister may have meant.

2. Comparing and Contrasting. The Morabitos are shopping for a backyard grill. Charcoal grills are much less expensive than gas grills, but the store is running a clearance sale and has marked down the gas grills significantly. Make a list of the factors the Morabitos need to consider in order to make an informed decision.

Reinforcing Key Skills

1. Communication. Reggie is timid about cooking. He follows recipes to the letter, not changing a single ingredient or amount, and in general expresses the attitude that "I'm just not creative." How could you encourage Reggie to explore his creativity in cooking?

2. Management. At Luisa's dinner party, some of the guests do not seem to be enjoying themselves. They aren't eating much, they are hardly speaking, and they generally seem uncomfortable. Before you could advise Luisa on steps to take to improve the situation, what additional information would you need to have?

Making Decisions and Solving Problems

You have several items to pack in your cooler for a picnic for yourself and three family members: a large container of ham salad, a loaf of bread, a six-pack of soda, a block of cheese, a chocolate cake, and ice for the drinks. As you pack, however, you realize that there is not enough room in the cooler for everything.

Making Connections

1. Social Studies. Choose five different herbs or spices, and find out where they are commonly grown. Make a display using a world map. Identify the herb or spice, the region in which it is produced, and the geographic conditions that help it grow there.

2. Science. Find more information about one of the chemical processes involved in preserving food at home, such as oxidation, the action of enzymes, or dehydration. If possible, set up an experiment or other demonstration to illustrate the principles involved.

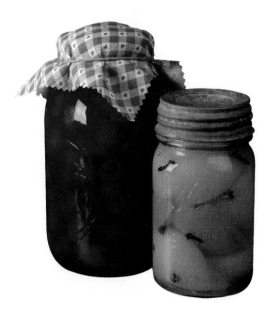

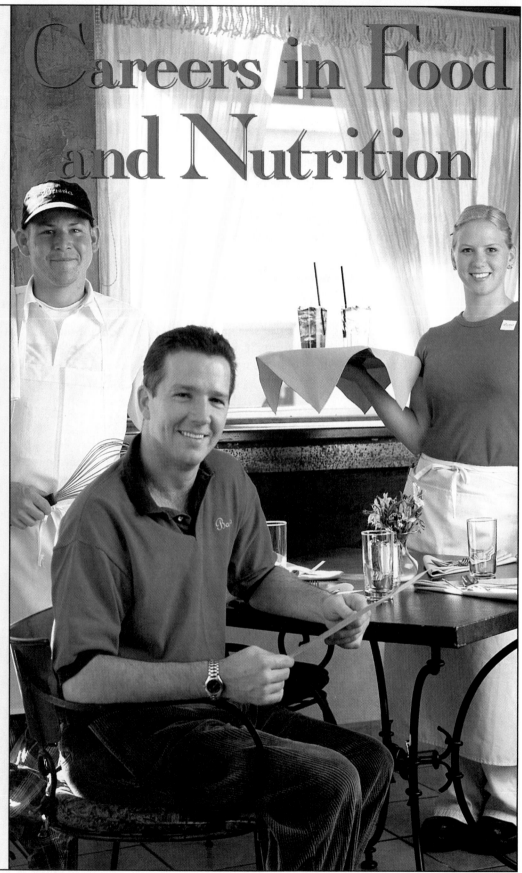

CHAPTER
25

Careers in Food and Nutrition

Section 25-1
Career Opportunities

Section 25-2
The Successful Worker

Carrie had always enjoyed preparing food for her family and friends. When she entered high school, she thought she might like to become a chef or a baker. After a few foods and nutrition courses, she discovered her opportunities in the food area were even more varied. In this chapter, you will learn, as Carrie did, about the many career possibilities in this exciting, growing field.

Career Opportunities

When you were a young child, a question you probably heard often was, "What do you want to be when you grow up?" Now that you are on the threshold of adulthood, it is the time to consider seriously the question of a career.

Objectives

After studying this section, you should be able to:

- Identify some career opportunities in food and nutrition.
- Describe the training and education needed for various careers.

Look for These Terms

career

entry-level job

entrepreneur

franchise

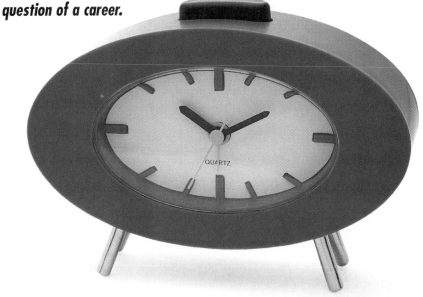

Thinking About Careers

A **career** is a profession or a life's work within a certain field. It usually begins with an **entry-level job**, a job that requires little or no experience. These jobs often lead to better-paying jobs with more responsibility.

Employees will advance in their careers by mastering the skills needed for their jobs and showing they are qualified to take on new responsibilities. Many seek additional education or training throughout their lives to further their careers.

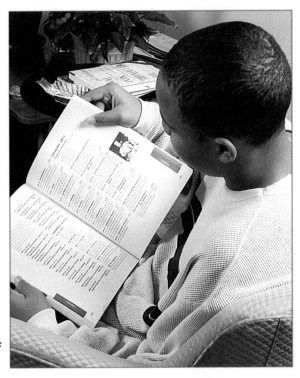

◆ An interest in food now could turn into a career someday. Identify questions you could ask yourself to determine what kind of career to pursue.

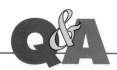

Q What's the best way to identify careers I might enjoy and do well in?

A Start by asking yourself questions. What classes and activities do you enjoy? Why do you like them? What are your skills and talents? Do any point toward a specific career you might enjoy? Working in community service or at a part-time job will also give you valuable information about yourself, your abilities, and your preferences.

Food-Related Careers

A recent study on job growth for the coming years predicted great expansion in service industries, including those pertaining to food and nutrition. The job outlook for this field is bright. Consider these trends:

◆ More people are eating out.

◆ Consumers are more interested in the relationship between food and health.

◆ The growing world population and other global factors make efficient production and use of high-quality food more important than ever.

Food Service

The food service industry includes all aspects of preparing and serving food for the public. It is expected to create more new jobs than any other retail industry in the next decade.

Jobs in food service can vary from serving food to developing recipes to merchandising food products. These jobs are usually available in every part of the country. If you like to travel, you might consider food service

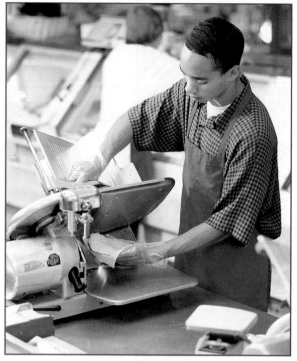

◆ **Many entry-level jobs are available in the food service industry.** List characteristics that can help a person move up the ladder to higher-paying jobs.

jobs with cruise lines or airlines, or jobs in other countries.

Educational Background

Educational requirements in food service vary, depending on the job you want. Part-time, entry-level jobs are often a good start. Food preparation classes in high school can also provide a valuable foundation. For more training, consider vocational schools, junior or community colleges, and four-year colleges and universities. Many companies offer on-the-job training to help employees advance.

Personal Qualifications

Food service jobs require certain personal traits. Employees must enjoy and be able to work successfully with people. They must be willing to do their share as part of a team. Producing quality food on a schedule can

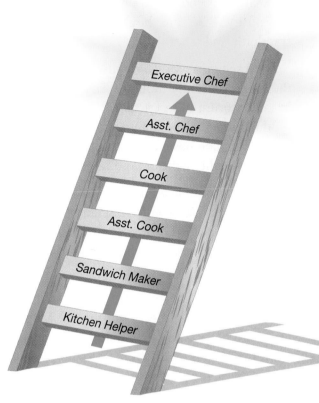

◆ Having a long-range goal, such as becoming an executive chef, can help you plan your career. An entry-level job, such as a kitchen helper, is often the first step. From there, you can work your way up the career ladder. Each promotion takes you a step closer to your long-term goal. Research another food-related career covered in this chapter or one of the careers featured at the end of each chapter. Develop a career ladder for the career chosen.

knowledge and skills to solve problems and make decisions about the home and family. Professionals with degrees in food and nutrition have many career options in addition to food service. These include teaching, communication, and research and development.

Teaching

Family and consumer sciences specialists may teach in schools, colleges, and universities. They may teach classes ranging from nutrition to ethnic foods. Nutritionists may work for county or regional extension services, teaching consumers about food preparation and related topics. They are also needed by other government agencies and health organizations to teach consumers how to make wise food choices.

Communication

This area involves communicating information to the public through television, magazines, books, and newspapers. People with strong communication skills are needed to help write speeches, articles, and advertisements about food products and services. Food stylists create attractive arrangements of foods for photographs. Employers include food producers, manufacturers, government agencies, and trade associations.

mean hard work and long hours. Good health, enthusiasm, ambition, and a sense of humor are essential. So are good work habits, such as punctuality and the ability to follow directions and accept criticism.

Job Advancement

Brent started working in a restaurant bussing tables. Through hard work and study, he moved up the career ladder to the position of assistant manager. His goal now is to become a manager.

As a rule, more education and training allow you to start on a higher rung of the career ladder. Food service offers many different career ladders.

Family and Consumer Sciences

Family and consumer sciences—called home economics, human ecology, or family studies at some universities—involves using

Research and Development

Food researchers help develop new products and appliances in test kitchens or research laboratories. They may work for universities, food producers, appliance manufacturers, or the government.

Jobs in family and consumer sciences require at least a bachelor's degree. Some, such as teaching, research, and management, may require higher degrees. Study and experience in related fields also helps. Specialists in communications, for example, might have a background in journalism or public relations.

Food Science

Food science is the study of the physical, chemical, and microbiological makeup of food. Food scientists develop food products and new ways to process and package them.

They also test foods and beverages for quality and purity to be sure they meet company standards and federal food regulations.

Food scientists are generally employed by the food processing industry. They may work in laboratories, in test kitchens, or on the production line. The many careers in food science include basic research, product development, quality control, and sales.

Food scientists need at least a bachelor's degree with a major in food science, food engineering, or food technology. Higher degrees are needed for research and managerial jobs.

Dietetics

A dietitian is a professional trained in the principles of food and nutrition. Dietitians may work for large institutions such as hospitals, health maintenance organizations, company cafeterias, and food service companies. They help develop special diets and counsel groups or individuals in making wise food choices.

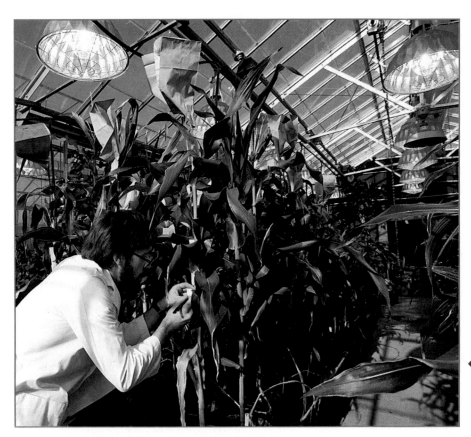

◆ A college education can lead to a rewarding career as a food scientist. What are some of the tasks a food scientist does?

Dietitians must have a bachelor's degree in food and nutrition. They must then serve a one-year internship at an approved institution. A registered dietitian (RD) must pass the Registration Examination for Dietitians. Some community colleges offer two-year programs for dietetic technicians, who work as assistants to dietitians.

Food Production, Processing, and Marketing

As noted in Chapter 13, a vast network of people is involved in producing food and getting it to the marketplace. Career opportunities vary from hydroponic farming to supermarket management.

Training and education also vary, but a combination of experience and formal education is best. Farmers, for example, need to know how to do the everyday work on the farm itself but can also benefit from studies in related topics, such as soil conservation and plant and animal genetics. A bakery owner must have experience in preparing the food as well as knowledge about business management, marketing techniques, and tax laws.

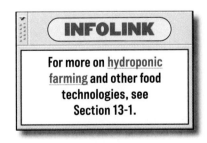

INFOLINK

For more on hydroponic farming and other food technologies, see Section 13-1.

Entrepreneurship

Many people dream of owning their own businesses. A person who runs his or her own business is called an **entrepreneur** (AHN-truh-pruh-NOOR). Successful entrepreneurs share certain personal qualities. They are willing to

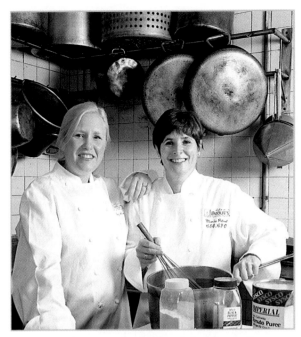

◆ Owning a business takes hard work, but the results are worthwhile. Entrepreneurs feel the special satisfaction of building their own success. Respond to the statement: "Entrepreneurs contribute to the strength and growth of their communities."

work hard and take risks. They can make sound decisions, are well organized, and understand the basic business management practices. Opportunities for entrepreneurs in food and nutrition include catering, running a snack shop, providing home delivery from restaurants or supermarkets, providing nutritional consultation, and preparing and selling food.

Franchises

Entrepreneurs sometimes invest in a **franchise**, an individually owned and operated branch of a business with an established name and guidelines. Some fast-food restaurants are franchises. Not all franchises are reliable, however, so potential owners should investigate carefully before buying. Also, the fact that the business is a franchise cannot guarantee success. It's up to the individual businessperson to provide the skills and commitment needed to succeed.

Sources of Food and Nutrition Career Information

American Association of Family
and Consumer Sciences
1555 King Street
Alexandria, VA 22314

The Institute of Food Technologists
221 N. LaSalle Street, Suite 300
Chicago, IL 60601

The American Dietetic Association
216 W. Jackson Boulevard, Suite 800
Chicago, IL 60606-6995

U.S. Department of Agriculture
14th Street and Independence Avenue, SW
Washington, DC 20250

Small Business Administration
1110 Vermont Avenue, NW, 9th floor
Washington, DC 20005

Section 25-1 Review & Activities

1. List four types of education or training for a career in food service.

2. Name three food and nutrition career options other than food service.

3. Briefly describe the educational and training requirements for registered dietitians.

4. **Synthesizing.** Identify social and cultural trends that have contributed to the increased need for workers in food and nutrition.

5. **Extending.** With a partner, brainstorm possible business opportunities for entrepreneurs. Follow up one of your hunches by speaking with a guidance counselor or with an individual in your community who is self-employed. Be prepared to share your findings in a class roundtable discussion.

6. **Applying.** Choose one food that you enjoy. List as many workers as you can that are involved in producing, processing, and distributing that food.

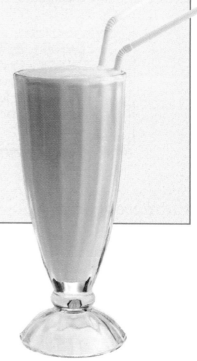

The Successful Worker

Do you have a part-time or summer job? Even if you haven't decided on a career, having a job now offers several advantages. It teaches responsibility and increases self-confidence. It sharpens your management and decision-making skills. It also lets you enjoy the benefits and pride of earning a paycheck. In addition, working can also help you decide what type of career you might enjoy.

Objectives

After studying this section, you should be able to:

- Identify qualities of successful workers.
- Describe the steps in applying for a job.
- Give guidelines for job interviews.
- Explain how to handle leaving a job.

Look for These Terms

networking

resumé

references

interview

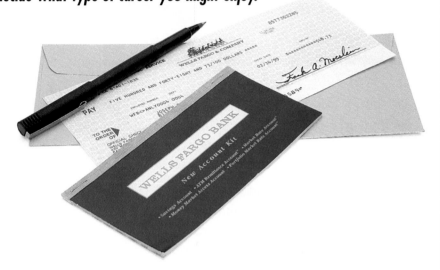

The Successful Worker

What are the qualities employers look for? Recent surveys have identified several qualities and skills, many of which you can develop while still in school:

- **Communication skills.** These include writing, reading, speaking, and listening. Employees often write reports. They must read and understand company bulletins and guidelines. They must listen carefully to instructions they receive or to customer requests.

- **Computer skills.** Most jobs involve the use of a computer in some way. In many restaurants, for instance, servers use computers to send customer food orders to the kitchen.

- **Critical thinking and problem solving skills.** Employees who can analyze situations and suggest solutions to problems are valued by their employers.

- **Positive attitude.** Employees must be enthusiastic about their work and interested in what they do.

- **Math skills.** Even though computers and calculators are widely used, employees must understand basic math. They may have to make change, keep a time schedule, or solve math-related problems.

- **Teamwork and self-responsibility.** Employees must be willing to do their share, and more, if necessary. They must work well with others to achieve common goals.

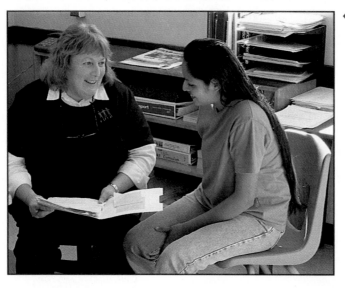

◆ **Learning to communicate effectively—for example, by speaking to adults who can help you with career decisions—is an important aspect of preparing for the future.** Name three other skills that can help you become a successful member of the workforce someday.

county extension office, and the writer of a foods column in the local newspaper. Remember, however, that other people can only help you find a job. Getting the job and keeping it are up to you.

◆ **Ability to learn.** New technology will continue to cause rapid changes in the workplace. This means learning new skills will be a lifelong process for employees.

Develop good learning and work habits while you are still in school. Volunteer work, school projects, and social activities can provide opportunities to develop essential skills.

Looking for a Job

As a student, right now you may be looking for only a part-time job. Even so, the experience of finding and keeping a job will be valuable to you personally as well as professionally.

There are many ways to find a job. Check your school employment or counseling office. Read the newspaper want ads and community bulletin boards. You can also contact employers directly and ask if they currently have any job openings.

Another idea helpful in job hunting is **networking**. This means making connections with people who can provide information about job openings. When Anton began exploring careers in food science, his network included his food science teacher, a nutritionist at a

Applying for a Job

Your next step is to apply for a specific job. This usually involves completing a job application form or letter of application and, sometimes, submitting your resumé and personal references.

A Job Application

A job application form requires basic personal information, such as your age and home address, and information about your education and experience. Remember to print your answers in ink, answering all questions as accurately as possible.

A letter of application serves the same purpose as an application form. However, you have a choice of what information to include. Include basic personal information plus any other helpful facts about yourself. As with the application form, focus on those things that will demonstrate your suitability for the job you are seeking. For example, being editor of the school yearbook shows that you can work well with other people and delegate authority. Earning good grades in food science courses indicates your knowledge of foods and any related fields.

A Resumé

For some jobs, you may need to submit a **resumé** (REH-zoo-may). This is a written summary of your experience, skills, and achievements that are related to the job you seek. A chronological resumé lists jobs and experiences in *reverse order*. That is, the list begins with the most recent experience and ends with the earliest. A functional resumé describes your skills and accomplishments as they relate to the job you are seeking.

Although a resumé is more detailed than a letter of application, it should be brief—not more than one page—and contain only relevant information. If you have no previous work experience, don't mention it. Focus instead on those activities that show your skills and abilities.

References

When applying for a job, you may be asked for **references**—people who know you well and can give information about your previous work or your character. A teacher or former work supervisor might be a good reference. Be sure to ask the people you wish to use as references for their permission for you to do so. You will need their names, addresses, and phone numbers.

Employers are prohibited by law from asking, in person or on application forms, for certain information, such as your race, gender, religion, or marital status. They may not ask questions about some aspects of your personal life or about your past.

An application form, letter of application, and resumé all demonstrate your ability to communicate in writing. All three should be carefully thought out and neatly written or typed. Be sure the grammar and punctuation are correct. Remember that this will be your potential employer's first—and possibly

---

Ginny Arnold
800 Southwest Street
Anytown, US 11111
Home Phone: (000)000-0000

OBJECTIVE: Kitchen helper, part-time.

QUALIFICATIONS:
* Received high grades in food preparation class.
* Have ability to organize work.
* Know how to use a computer.
* Would like to become a chef.

EXPERIENCE:
* Help with Friday night suppers at church.
* Organized successful pancake breakfast for parents, sponsored by the FHA/HERO Club.
* Worked at the Community Center soup kitchen, helping with meals for homeless.

EDUCATION:
* Junior at Anytown High School.
* Currently taking advanced food preparation class.

◆ A well-written resumé is brief, but provides the information that employers need in order to consider you for the job. What kind of job is the writer of this resumé seeking?

---

only—impression of you as a worker. Make it a positive one.

Working Papers

When applying for work, you may also be asked to furnish working papers. These are the documents and certificates needed for employment. Your school counselor can tell you how to obtain these important items, which include:

◆ **Social Security number.** Lifelong identification number allowing you to receive Social Security payments when you retire or if you are disabled. You may already have a number. If not, you can get one at the nearest Social Security office.

- **Work permit.** Required of students in some states.

- **Health certificates.** Necessary in some areas for working with food.

Interviewing for a Job

If the employer thinks you might be a good prospect for employment, you will be called for an **interview**. This is a meeting with an employer during which both the employer and applicant get more information and perhaps reach a conclusion regarding the job.

The impression you make at the interview should continue the one you began in your application. You want to show that you are enthusiastic, qualified, and willing to work hard. You convey this by being on time, neatly groomed, and polite.

Interview Behavior

Although interviews can be stressful, try to relax. Let the interviewer direct the conversation. Show your interest in the job and familiarity with the company. Explain how you can help the company, and be prepared to answer questions such as, "What are your strengths and weaknesses?" Remember to phrase your answers in ways that will emphasize your abilities and qualifications. Ask questions about the nature of the job, but don't focus on money or benefits yet.

At the end of the interview, thank the interviewer and repeat your interest in the job. If you are not told whether you are being offered the job, ask when you may call to find out about the decision.

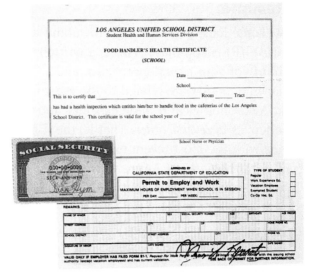

◆ These are some of the documents you may need for employment. You may already have a Social Security number. **Speak with the school counselor about where to obtain these and other necessary work documents. Record the agency names and addresses you are given in your Wellness Journal.**

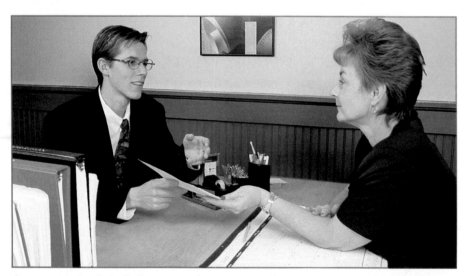

◆ It is natural to feel a little nervous when going to a job interview. Think of the interview as an opportunity to visit a workplace, learn more about an interesting job, and meet new people. **Describe how you should behave on an interview.**

After the Interview

When you get home, write the interviewer a note of thanks, again expressing your interest in the job. If you are offered the job, you have completed the first step in reaching your career goals. Now you must work to continue making progress toward those goals.

If you don't get the job, you may politely ask why. Whatever the reason, use the interview as a learning experience.

On the Job

Once you have found a job, it is up to you to keep it. These tips can help you:

◆ Get to work on time and be appropriately dressed.

◆ Follow company rules, such as those about taking breaks and eating on the job.

◆ Pay attention when receiving instruction or training.

◆ Don't be afraid to ask questions about your responsibilities.

◆ Accept criticism and suggestions without resentment.

◆ If you make a mistake, admit it and learn from it.

◆ Take pride in your work. Remember that even small jobs can make a big difference.

Leaving Your Job

There will probably come a time when you will want to leave a job. Here again, it is important to make a good impression. At least two weeks ahead of time, inform your employer with a brief but polite letter of resignation. You may mention your reasons for leaving, but do not be negative. Thank your employer for the opportunity of having worked for the company.

FOR YOUR HEALTH

TAP-ping Your Strengths

According to a popular saying, "You get only one chance to make a first impression." While this advice is useful in all social situations, it comes in especially handy in a job interview. To make a positive impression, remember the *TAP* strategy:

• **(T)horoughness.** Learn all you can about the company, including the job you are applying for. Make up an interview packet. Include your resumé (if needed), a good pen, and a small notebook.

• **(A)ppearance.** Dress neatly. Avoid jeans, excessive makeup, and excessive jewelry. Go to the interview alone. Don't bring family members or friends.

• **(P)unctuality.** Be sure to arrive on time. Write down the time and place of the interview. Be sure you know how to get there and how long the trip will take.

Following Up

• Imagine that you have a job interview at a restaurant tomorrow. Candidly assess your appearance, and decide what changes, if any, you would need to make. Specific areas include (but are not limited to) your hair length, neatness, and cleanliness; your fingernail length and cleanliness; and any facial rings or tattoos. Copy your notes into your Wellness Journal for future reference.

Continue to do your best work until your last day. Remember, you may want to use your employer as a reference in the future.

If you are fired, find out exactly why. How can you improve your job performance so that you won't have the same problem again?

When you interview for the next job, be honest about the reasons for leaving your previous job. If you were fired, explain why. Also explain how you plan to change so that you will not have the same problem again. Employers are more willing to give employees a chance if they seem eager to improve and change.

Remember, success doesn't depend on just your skills and talent. It also depends on your attitude and commitment to do the best you possibly can.

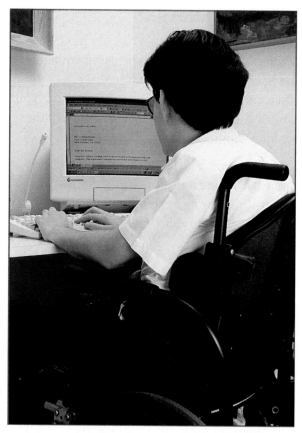

◆ When writing a letter of resignation, it is important to give careful consideration to what you say. Explain some of the negative future fallout that might come of writing a letter of resignation that was critical or angry toward an employer.

Section 25-2 Review & Activities

1. Name six qualifications of a successful worker.

2. How are a job application form and a letter of application similar? How do they differ?

3. Give five suggestions for interviewing successfully.

4. How much notice should you give an employer before leaving a job?

5. Evaluating. What do you think is the most serious mistake people make when they interview for a job?

6. Analyzing. When Gil learned he had made the varsity basketball team, he left his job at the hardware store without a word. When his mother urged him to at least place a call to the store owner, Gil replied, "Why should I? I'll never need him for anything." How would you respond as Gil's mother?

7. Applying. Review the qualities of successful workers described in this section. Using job listings from the newspaper want ads, give specific examples of how each skill might be needed in a particular job.

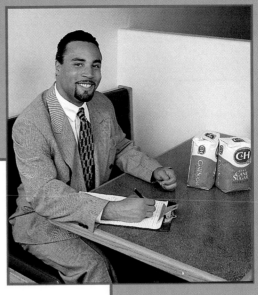

CAREER WANTED

Individuals who are self-motivated, energetic, and ambitious.

REQUIRES:
- computer knowledge
- sales experience

"Know your client,"

says Restaurant Sales Representative Charles Maysch

Q: Charles, what kinds of products do you sell to restaurants?

A: My company is a full-service supply organization with over 15,000 products, from meat to produce to seasonings. We also feature ready-made entrées, tablecloths, and ovens. I need to sell a combination of products to make my quota each month.

Q: You mentioned ready-made entrées. Where do these come from?

A: We create them in our own test kitchen. This enables sales reps like me to help restaurants capitalize on current market trends: what is "hot" with children and what is required by senior citizens or vegetarians.

Q: What is the most important trait of a restaurant sales rep?

A: I'd say flexibility. We deal with all different-sized clients. I have to be prepared to service every client with the same consideration, regardless of that account's income potential.

Q: What is the most significant change you have seen in the restaurant business in the past 20 years?

A: "Healthful eating" seems to be lasting longer than other trends. We serve more fruits and vegetables and smaller servings of meat, fish, and poultry. We also sell a lot of pasta every day.

Career Research Activity

1. Write a short paragraph describing what you think a menu creator does for a living. Then access information about that career. How does it compare with restaurant sales? In what way do both careers require creativity? Write another short paragraph contrasting the two careers.

2. Create a sales portfolio that you would carry as the restaurant sales representative for a restaurant. Be sure the portfolio contains a list of the products you offer. After presenting your portfolio, ask the class members whether they would buy your products and why or why not.

Related Career Opportunities

Entry Level
- Food Broker
- Wholesaler
- Menu Creator

Technical Level
- Restaurant Sales Representative
- Assistant Buyer

Professional Level
- Restaurant Purchasing Executive
- Sanitation Officer
- Hotel Concierge

Chapter 25   Review & Activities

──── Summary ────

Section 25-1: Career Opportunities

- Career opportunities in food and nutrition are growing and varied.

- Food service jobs include all those needed to prepare and serve food for the public. Food and consumer science specialists are needed to inform consumers about food, food choices, and related topics. Food scientists develop new foods and test foods for safety and quality. Dietitians help develop special diets for individuals or large groups. Many opportunities exist in food production, processing, and marketing.

- The food industry offers many options for entrepreneurs.

- The training and education needed for these careers varies.

Section 25-2: The Successful Worker

- Successful workers share certain qualities. They can communicate well, solve problems, and learn new things. They have a positive attitude and work well with others.

- Applying for a job may involve filling out an application form, writing a letter of application, and/or submitting a resumé.

- Interviews can be successful if you are relaxed, display a positive attitude, and show an interest in the job and a willingness to learn.

- Even deciding to leave a job or being fired can be a learning experience.

Working IN THE Lab

1. **Computer Lab.** Design and print a form that might be used by an entrepreneur in the food industry, such as an inventory report or an employee schedule.

2. **Foods Lab.** Suppose you are a dietitian working in an institution. Think of the special diets that might be needed by people in that setting. Create one such diet, and prepare one of your recipes.

3. **Demonstration.** Working in pairs, demonstrate how to successfully interview for a job. Have the rest of the class identify the positive points of the interview.

Checking Your Knowledge

1. Give three reasons for the expected job growth in food and nutrition.

2. Name six personal traits needed to succeed in food service.

3. Identify two career options for family and consumer scientists in teaching and two in communications.

4. What degrees and majors are needed to become a food scientist?

5. Identify two risks of investing in a franchise.

6. Name three benefits of having a job.

7. Identify three instances when employees need good communication skills.

8. What is networking?

9. Give three tips for preparing for an interview.

10. Give four tips for being a valuable employee.

Thinking Critically

1. Recognizing Stereotypes. You have accepted a summer job bussing tables in a local restaurant. You share your news with a friend, who comments that he thinks it's an unimportant, dead-end job. How do you respond?

2. Comparing and Contrasting. How might the training and communication skills needed by a family and consumer sciences teacher be similar to those needed by a family and consumer sciences professional in research and development? How might they differ?

3. Predicting Consequences. Paul and José work for the same catering firm. Lately, Paul has begun to grumble a lot about his responsibilities and often shows up late for work, asking José to cover for him. Paul's poor work habits are affecting his working relationship with José. What are some possible negative long-term consequences to the business if Paul's slacking off continues?

Reinforcing Key Skills

1. Directed Thinking. Jared has worked as a counselor at the same summer camp for three years in a row and has worked in a fast-food restaurant part-time. He has maintained a low B average through his school years. He has always been weak in math but strong in language arts. When applying for a job as a waiter in an exclusive French restaurant, what personal resources can Jared mention that will make him a candidate worth considering for the position?

2. Communication. Amanda, a high school student, is checking the help wanted ads for summer jobs. She has always enjoyed baking and would like to learn more about it, with an eye toward a possible career in this field one day. Most of the ads state that applicants must have prior job experience. Do you think Amanda should abandon her goal? If not, what would you advise her to do?

Making Decisions and Solving Problems

You have been working for almost a year as a cook in a fast-food restaurant, hoping to work your way up the career ladder. However, others who have been working at the restaurant less time than you have are being promoted ahead of you.

Making Connections

1. Economics. Interview at least two local entrepreneurs about the economic aspects of their businesses. What economic factors encouraged them to start their businesses? What social and economic trends affect their business decisions? What role do their businesses play in the local or national economy? Do they feel the economy is a good one now for starting a business? If so, what kind? Write a transcript or a summary of your interview, including an explanation of what you learned from it.

2. Social Studies. Trace the history of child labor and child labor laws in this country. At what jobs and under what conditions have children worked in the past? How have attitudes toward child labor changed over time? What circumstances led to the enactment of child labor laws? How do these laws protect children in the workplace? Are there any disadvantages to these laws? Share your findings in a short report to the class.

Glossary

A

aerobic (uh-ROH-buhk) exercise. Vigorous activity in which oxygen is continuously taken in for a period of at least 20 minutes. Activities including walking, jogging, bicycling, etc. (Section 5-3)

AIs. Stands for "Adequate Intake." Approximate nutrient measures set when an RDA cannot be established. (Section 2-1)

albumen (al-BYOO-muhn). A thick, clear fluid inside an egg; also known as egg white. (Section 18-3)

al dente (ahl DEN-tay). Term meaning firm to the bite, often referring to cooked pasta. (Section 17-2)

amino (uh-MEE-noh) acids. Chains of chemical building blocks from which proteins are made. (Section 2-2)

anabolic steroids (AN-uh-bahl-ik STEHR-oydz). Prescription medicines used to help build muscle strength in patients with chronic diseases. When used illegally, dangerous side effects can occur. (Section 5-4)

anaerobic (AN-uh-ROH-buhk) exercise. Exercise, which builds flexibility and endurance, involving intense bursts of activity in which the muscles work so hard that they produce energy without using oxygen. (Section 5-3)

analogues (AN-uh-logs). Foods made from a vegetable protein and processed to resemble animal foods. (Section 15-1)

annual percentage rate (APR). The yearly cost of a loan. (Section 14-1)

anorexia nervosa (an-uh-REK-see-yuh ner-VOH-suh). A type of eating disorder that involves an irresistible urge to lose weight through self-starvation. (Section 6-3)

antioxidants. Substances that protect body cells and the immune system from harmful chemicals in the air, certain foods, and tobacco smoke. (Section 2-4)

antipasto. Italian for "before the meal"; referring to appetizers. (Section 22-3)

appetite. A desire to eat. (Section 4-2)

aquaculture. A method of growing fish or seafood in enclosed areas of water. (Section 13-1)

arcing. Electrical sparks produced when metal is used in a microwave oven; can damage the oven or start a fire. (Section 9-4)

aromatic vegetables. Vegetables that add flavor to soups and other recipes; includes onions, garlic, celery, and green peppers. (Section 20-3)

assembly directions. The step-by-step procedure that explains how to put the ingredients in a recipe together. (Section 8-1)

au jus. Serving food with the pan drippings from which the fat has been skimmed. (Section 20-3)

B

bakeware. Equipment for cooking food in an oven. (Section 9-1)

basal metabolism (BAY-suhl muh-TAB-uh-lih-zuhm). Minimum amount of energy required to maintain the life processes in a living organism. (Section 2-5)

base. A foundation of greens for a salad. (Section 20-2)

behavior modification. Making gradual, permanent changes in your eating and activity habits. (Section 5-2)

berbere. A spicy combination of garlic, red and black peppers, salt, coriander, fenugreek, and cardamom. (Section 22-2)

bias. A tendency to be swayed toward a particular conclusion. (Section 3-3)

binder. A liquid that holds the other ingredients of a casserole together. (Section 20-4)

binge eating disorder. A type of eating disorder involving a lack of control while eating huge quantities of food at one time. (Section 6-3)

blanching. Partial cooking of food, usually vegetables, to kill enzymes. (Section 24-5)

body. Main part of the salad. (Section 20-2)

body mass index (BMI). Uses a ratio of weight and height. (Section 5-1)

bouillon (BOOL-yon). A simple, clear soup without solid ingredients. (Section 20-3)

bran. The edible, outer protective layers of a seed. (Section 17-1)

budget. Plan for managing money in order to cover the costs of life's necessities. (Section 11-3)

bulimia nervosa (byoo-LIM-ee-yuh ner-VOH-suh). A type of eating disorder that involves episodes of binge eating followed by purging. (Section 6-3)

bulk foods. Shelf-stable foods that are sold loose in covered bins or barrels. (Section 12-3)

C

calorie. The amount of energy needed to raise the temperature of 1 kilogram of water 1 degree Celsius. (Section 2-1)

carbohydrates (kar-boh-HY-drayts). Nutrients that are the body's main source of energy. (Section 2-1)

career. A profession or a life's work within a certain field. (Section 25-1)

certified nurse midwife. An advanced practice nurse who, in addition to providing prenatal care, specializes in the delivery of healthy babies. (Section 6-1)

chalazae (kuh-LAH-zuh). Twisted, cordlike strands of albumen which anchor the yolk in the center of the egg. (Section 18-3)

chlorophyll (KLOR-uh-fil). The chemical compound that plants use to turn the sun's energy into food. (Section 16-3)

cholesterol (kuh-LES-tuhr-ol). A fatlike substance present in all body cells that is needed for many essential body processes. (Section 2-3)

club sandwich. A sandwich made with three slices of toasted bread and filled with chicken or turkey breast, bacon, tomato, lettuce, and mayonnaise. (Section 20-1)

coagulate. To become firm. (Section 18-3)

code dating. A series of numbers or letters that indicate where and when the product was packaged. (Section 12-2)

colostrum (kuh-LAH-strum). A special form of thick, yellowish milk that is produced three days after birth and is rich in nutrients and antibodies. (Section 6-1)

comparison shop. Compare prices and characteristics of similar or like items to determine which offers the best value. (Section 12-3)

complete proteins. Proteins that supply all nine essential amino acids. (Section 2-2)

conduction. Heat transfer by direct contact. (Section 9-2)

conservation. Concern about and action taken to ensure the preservation of the environment. (Section 7-5)

contaminants. Harmful substances that accidentally get into food as it moves from the farm to the table. (Section 13-2)

continuous cleaning. An oven that has special rough interior walls that absorb spills and splatters. (Section 14-2)

convection. Transfer of heat by the movement of air or liquid. (Section 9-2)

convection current. A circular flow of air or liquid resulting from uneven heating. (Section 9-2)

cookware. Equipment for cooking food on top of the range. (Section 9-1)

cover. The arrangement of a place setting for one person. (Section 10-1)

CPR. Stands for cardiopulmonary resuscitation (KARD-ee-oh-PUL-muh-nayr-ee ree-SUS-uh-TAY-shun), a technique used to revive a person whose breathing and heartbeat have stopped. (Section 7-2)

credit. Money you borrow from a lender. (Section 14-1)

critical thinking. Examination of printed and spoken language in order to gain insights into meanings and interpretations. (Section 1-5).

cross-contamination. Letting microorganisms from one food get into another. (Section 7-3)

cruciferous (kroo-SIH-fur-uhs) **vegetables.** Vegetables in the cabbage family. (Section 16-1)

crustaceans. Shellfish that have long bodies with jointed limbs, covered with a shell; includes crabs, crayfish, lobsters, and shrimp. (Section 19-4)

cuisine. Styles of food preparation and cooking associated with a specific group or culture. (Section 22-1)

culture. The shared customs, traditions, and beliefs of a large group of people which defines a group's unique identity. (Section 1-2)

cultured. Fermented by a harmless bacteria added after pasteurization. (Section 18-1)

cut. A particular edible part of meat, poultry, or fish. (Section 19-1)

cut in. To mix solid fat and flour using a pastry blender or two knives and a cutting motion. (Section 21-2)

D

Daily Value (DV). A specific nutrition reference amount recommended by health experts. (Section 12-2)

deglazing. Adding stock or another liquid to a defatted sauté pan to loosen the browned-on particles. (Section 22-3)

dehydration (dee-hy-DRAY-shun). Lack of adequate fluids in the body. (Section 5-4)

desired yield. Number of servings you need. (Section 8-3)

developing nations. Countries that are not yet industrialized or are just beginning to become so. (Section 13-3)

diabetes. A condition in which the body cannot control blood sugar levels. (Section 6-2)

dietary fiber. A mixture of plant materials that is not broken down in the digestive system; necessary for good health. (Section 2-1)

dietary supplements. Nutrients taken in addition to foods eaten. (Section 6-2)

digestion. Process of breaking down food into usable nutrients. (Section 2-5)

doneness. Having cooked food long enough for the necessary changes to take place so that a cut tastes good and is safe to eat. (Section 19-5)

dovetail. To fit different tasks together smoothly. (Section 8-5)

DRIs. Stands for "Dietary Reference Intakes"; A series of standards for assessing nutrient needs among people of different age and gender groups. (Section 2-1)

drop biscuits. Biscuits made by dropping dough from a spoon. (Section 21-2)

dry heat cooking. Cooking food uncovered without added liquid or fat. (Section 9-3)

dry-packing. Leaving spaces between the pieces of food before placing it in the freezer. (Section 24-5)

E

eating disorder. An extreme, unhealthful behavior related to food, eating, and weight. (Section 6-3)

eating patterns. Food customs and habits, including when, what, and how much people eat. (Section 4-1)

electrolytes (ee-LEK-troh-lyts). Specific major minerals that work together to maintain the body's fluid balance; includes sodium, potassium, and chloride. (Section 2-4)

emulsion. An evenly blended mixture of two liquids that do not normally stay mixed. (Section 20-2)

endosperm. Food supply, made of protein, for a seed's embryo. (Section 17-1)

EnergyGuide label. Label on a large appliance that gives consumers information about estimated yearly energy costs. (Section 14-1)

en papillote (ehn pah-pee-YOHT). Cooking foods in parchment paper. (Section 24-1)

enrichment. A process in which some nutrients lost as a result of processing are added back to the product. (Section 17-1)

entrée (AHN-tray). The term used for main dishes on many restaurant menus. (Section 4-3)

entrepreneur (AHN-truh-pruh-NOOR). A person who runs his or her own business. (Section 25-1)

entry-level job. A job that requires little or no experience. (Section 25-1)

enzymatic (EN-zih-mat-ik) **browning.** Discoloration of fruits which results when the fruit is exposed to air. (Section 16-2)

equivalent. The same amount expressed in different ways by using different units of measure. (Section 8-2)

ergonomics. The study of ways to make tools and equipment easier and more comfortable to use. (Section 1-4)

esophagus (ih-SOFF-uh-gus). A long tube connecting the mouth to the stomach. (Section 2-5)

ethnic group. A cultural group based on common heritage. (Section 1-3)

extender. A food ingredient that helps thicken a dish. (Section 20-4)

F

fad diets. Popular weight-loss methods that ignore sound nutrition principles. (Section 5-2)

famine. Food shortages that continue for months or years, frequently resulting in starvation. (Section 13-3)

fats. A nutrient that provides a concentrated source of energy. (Section 2-1)

fat-soluble vitamins. Vitamins that are absorbed and transported by fat; includes vitamins A, D, E, and K. (Section 2-4)

fetus (FEE-tus). An unborn baby. (Section 6-1)

filé. Dried, crushed sassafras leaves used to thicken stews and add a delicate flavor. (Section 23-1)

finance charge. The total amount a person is charged for borrowing money; includes interest plus any service charges or insurance premiums. (Section 14-1)

foam cakes. Cakes that are leavened with beaten egg whites, which give them a light texture. (Section 21-4)

folding. A technique used to gently mix delicate ingredients. (Section 8-4)

food additives. Chemicals added to food to preserve freshness or enhance color and flavor. (Section 13-2)

food allergy. An abnormal, physical response to certain foods by the body's immune system. (Section 6-2)

food cooperatives. Food distribution organizations mutually owned and operated by a group of people. (Section 12-1)

Food Guide Pyramid. A pyramid-shaped food grouping system that is designed to help you choose a variety of foods in moderate amounts. (Section 3-2)

food safety. Following practices that help prevent foodborne illness and keep food safe to eat. (Section 7-3)

food science. The scientific study of food and its preparation. (Section 1-4)

food tolerance. A physical reaction to food not involving the immune system. (Section 6-2)

formed product. A food made from an inexpensive food source processed to resemble a more expensive one. (Section 15-1)

fortification. A process of adding 10 percent or more of the Daily Value for a specific nutrient to a product by the manufacturer. (Section 17-1)

franchise. An individually owned and operated branch of a business with an established name and guidelines. (Section 25-1)

freezer burn. A condition that results when food is improperly packaged or stored in the freezer too long; food dries out and loses flavor and texture. (Section 7-4)

frying. Cooking food in oil or melted fat. (Section 9-3)

G

garam masala. A complex blend of toasted and ground spices that most Indian recipes begin with. (Section 22-4)

garnish. Any small, colorful bit of food that is used to enhance the appearance and texture of a dish. (Section 24-1)

generic. Items produced without a commercial or store brand name which are less expensive and have a plain label. (Section 12-3)

genetic engineering. A method of enhancing specific natural tendencies of plants and animals. (Section 13-2)

germ. A tiny embryo in a seed that will grow into a new plant. (Section 17-1)

giblets (JIB-luhts). Edible poultry organs such as the liver, gizzard, and heart. (Section 19-3)

glucose (GLOO-kohs). The body's basic fuel supply. (Section 2-5)

gluten (GLOO-ten). A protein that affects the texture of a baking product. (Section 21-1)

glycogen (GLY-kuh-juhn). A storage form of glucose that is stored in the liver and the muscles. (Section 2-5)

gratuity (grah-TOO-uh-tee). Extra money given to a server in appreciation of good service; also known as a tip. (Section 10-2)

grazing. An eating pattern in which people eat five or more small meals throughout the day. (Section 4-1)

grounding. A method of minimizing the risk of electrical shock by providing a path for current to travel back through the electrical system. (Section 14-3)

H

haute cuisine. Literally means "high cooking"; a method of food preparation that makes use of complicated recipes and techniques. (Section 22-3)

HDL. Stands for "high-density lipoprotein"; a chemical that picks up excess cholesterol and takes it back to the liver, keeping it from causing harm. (Section 2-3)

headspace. In canning, the space between the top of the food and the rim of the jar. (Section 24-5)

heating units. Energy sources in ranges used to heat foods. (Section 9-1)

Heimlich maneuver. Technique used to rescue victims of choking. (Section 7-2)

herbal remedies. Nonstandardized products containing herbs known to have medicinal-like qualities. (Section 6-2)

hibachi. A small charcoal grill. (Section 23-2)

high tea. A meal when tea is served with a nonsweet dish that is somewhere between an appetizer and a main course; originated in England. (Section 22-3)

HIV/AIDS. A disorder that interferes with the immune system's ability to combat disease-causing pathogens. (Section 6-2)

home-meal replacement. A term used by the food service industry that refers to take-out or carry-out meals. (Section 4-3)

homogenization. The process whereby fat is broken down and evenly distributed in milk. (Section 18-1)

hot-pack. A method of filling jars for canning. The food is first heated in liquids and then packed into jars. (Section 24-5)

hot spot. An area of concentrated heat. (Section 9-4)

hydrogenation (hy-DRAH-juh-NAY-shun). A process in which missing hydrogen atoms are added to an unsaturated fat to make it firmer in texture. (Section 2-3)

hydroponic (high-druh-PAH-nik) farming. Using nutrient-enriched water to grow plants without soil. (Section 13-1)

I

impulse buying. Buying items you didn't plan to purchase and don't really need because it seems appealing at the time. (Section 12-1)

incomplete proteins. Proteins lacking one or more essential amino acids; foods from plant sources provide incomplete proteins. (Section 2-2)

industrialized nations. Countries that rely on a sophisticated, organized food industry to supply their citizens with food. Also called "developed countries." (Section 13-3)

infuser. A small container with tiny holes that let water in but don't allow tea leaves to come out. (Section 24-2)

insoluble fiber. A type of fiber that will not dissolve in water but will absorb water; helps move waste through the digestive system. (Section 2-2)

interest. The amount of money a lender charges as a fee for the loan; equals a specific percentage of the amount borrowed. (Section 14-1)

interview. A meeting with a potential employer in which both the employer and applicant get more information and perhaps reach a conclusion regarding the job. (Section 25-2)

inventory. Ongoing record of the food stored in the freezer. (Section 7-4)

irradiation. Process of exposing food to gamma rays to increase its shell life and kill harmful microorganisms. (Section 13-2)

island. A freestanding unit, often in the center of a kitchen. (Section 14-3)

J K L

julienne. Long, thin strips of food. (Section 24-1)

kibbutz (kee-BOOTS). An Israeli communal organization that raises its own food. (Section 22-2)

knead. To work dough with your hands to thoroughly mix ingredients and develop gluten. (Section 21-1)

lacto-ovo vegetarians. People who eat foods from plant sources, dairy products, and eggs. (Section 4-4)

lacto vegetarians. People who eat dairy products in addition to foods from plant sources. (Section 4-4)

LDL. Stands for "low-density lipoprotein"; a chemical that takes cholesterol from the liver to wherever it is needed in the body. (Section 2-3)

leavening agent. A substance that triggers a chemical action causing a baked product to rise. (Section 21-1)

legumes. Plants whose seeds grow in pods that split along both sides when ripe; includes dry beans and peas, lentils, and peanuts. (Section 17-3)

life span. Constant progression from one stage of development to the next. Stages include prenatal period, infancy, childhood, adolescence, and adulthood. (Section 6-1)

life-span design. A design approach in which living space is adapted to the needs of people of various ages and degrees of physical ability. (Section 14-3)

lifestyle. A person's typical way of life, which includes how you spend your time and what is important to you. (Section 1-2)

lifestyle activities. Forms of physical activity that are a normal part of your daily routine or recreation that promote good health throughout a lifetime. (Section 5-3)

lifestyle diseases. Illnesses that relate to how a person lives and the choices he or she makes. Examples include high blood pressure, heart disease, stroke, diabetes, and certain kinds of cancer. (Section 3-1)

M

maize. Corn; a staple crop in many countries. (Section 22-1)

major appliance. A large device that gets its energy from electricity or gas. (Section 7-1)

major minerals. Minerals needed in relatively large amounts. (Section 2-4)

malnutrition. Serious health problems caused by poor nutrition over a prolonged period of time. (Section 2-1)

management. Specific techniques that help you use resources wisely. (Section 1-5)

manufactured food. A product developed to serve as a substitute for another food. (Section 15-1)

marbling. Small white flecks of internal fat that may appear within the muscle tissue of meat. (Section 19-1)

marinades (MAR-uh-nayds). Flavorful liquids in which food is steeped. (Section 19-5)

marinating. A method of tenderizing and adding flavor to foods before you cook them by steeping the foods in a liquid. (Section 19-5)

mature fruits. Fruits that have reached their full size and color. (Section 16-1)

meal appeal. Characteristics that make a meal appetizing and enjoyable. (Section 11-1)

media. A multitude of communication sources, including television, radio, movies, newspapers, magazines, advertisements, and the Internet. (Section 2-1)

medical nutrition therapy. An assessment of the nutritional status of a patient with a condition. (Section 6-2)

megadose (MEH-guh-dohs). An extra-large amount of a supplement thought to prevent or cure diseases. (Section 6-2)

meringue (muhr-ANG). A foam made of beaten egg whites and sugar. (Section 18-4).

micro-grill. A cooking method that combines microwaving and grilling. (Section 24-4)

microorganisms. Tiny living creatures, such as bacteria, visible only through a microscope. (Section 7-3)

minerals. Nonliving substances that help the body work properly and may become part of body tissues. (Section 2-1)

moderation. Avoiding extremes, such as eating adequate amounts of a variety of foods. (Section 3-1)

modified English service. A method of food service in which dinner plates and the food for the main course are brought to the table in serving dishes and placed in front of the host. (Section 24-3)

moist heat cooking. Method in which food is cooked in hot liquid, steam, or a combination of both. (Section 9-3)

mollusks. Shellfish with soft bodies that are covered by at least one shell such as clams, mussels, oysters, scallops, and squid. (Section 19-4)

monounsaturated (MAH-no-un-SAT-chur-ay-ted) **fatty acids.** Fats that appear to lower LDL cholesterol levels and may help raise levels of HDL. (Section 2-3)

mulled. Beverages that are served hot and flavored with sweet spices. (Section 24-2)

N

net weight. The weight of the food itself, not including the packaging. (Section 12-2)

networking. Making connections with people who can provide information about job openings. (Section 25-2)

nutrient deficiency. A severe nutrient shortage. (Section 2-1)

nutrient-dense. Describes foods that are low or moderate in calories yet rich in important nutrients. (Section 3-2)

nutrients. Chemicals from food that your body uses to carry out its functions. (Section 1-1)

nutrition. The study of nutrients and how they are used by the body. (Section 1-1)

O

obese (oh-BEESE). A term that means having excess body fat. (Section 5-1)

obstetrician (ob-stuh-TRISH-un). A physician who specializes in pregnancy. (Section 6-1)

open dating. A practice in which a date is stamped directly on the product for the benefit of the consumer, such as a "sell by" or expiration date. (Section 12-2)

osteoporosis (AH-stee-oh-puh-ROH-sis). A condition in which bones lose their minerals and become porous, making them weak and fragile. (Section 2-4)

over-the-counter drugs. Drugs that can be obtained without a prescription. (Section 5-2)

overweight. Weighing more than 10 percent over the standard weight for one's height. (Section 5-2)

ovo vegetarians. People who eat eggs in addition to foods from plant sources. (Section 4-4)

oxidation (AHKS-ih-day-shuhn). A process in which fuel is combined with oxygen to produce energy. (Section 2-5)

P

pare. To cut a very thin layer of peel or outer coating of a food. (Section 8-4)

pasteurized. A heat treatment that kills enzymes and harmful bacteria. (Section 18-1)

pediatrician. A physician who cares for infants and children. (Section 6-1)

pemmican. Dried meat, pounded into a paste with fat and preserved in cakes. (Section 23-1)

peninsula. An extension of a countertop. (Section 14-3)

peristalsis (PEHR-uh-STAHL-suhs). A series of wavelike movements that force food into the stomach. (Section 2-5)

place setting. Pieces of tableware used by one person to eat a meal. (Section 10-1)

phytochemical. A disease-fighting nutrient found in plant foods. (Section 2-4)

poaching. Simmering whole foods in a small amount of liquid until done. (Section 9-3)

polarized plugs. Electrical plugs made with one plug wider than the other and designed to fit in the outlet in only one way as a safety measure. (Section 7-2)

polenta. A cornmeal mush that is sometimes cooled, sliced, and fried. (Section 22-3)

polyunsaturated (Pah-lee-un-SAT-chur-ay-ted) **fatty acids.** Fats that seem to help lower cholesterol levels. (Section 2-3)

preheating. Turning the oven on about 10 minutes before using it so that it will be at the desired temperature when the food is placed inside. (Section 9-3)

pre-preparation. Refers to tasks done before assembling the actual recipe. (Section 8-5)

principal. The amount of money that is borrowed from a lender. (Section 14-1)

proteins. Nutrients that help build, repair, and maintain body tissues; also a source of energy. (Section 2-1)

psychological (sye-kuh-LODGE-ih-kuhl). Having to do with the mind and emotions. (Section 1-1)

purée. To make food smooth and thick by putting it through a strainer, blender, or food processor. (Section 8-4)

Q

quiche (KEESH). A pie with a custard filling that contains foods such as chopped vegetables, cheese, and chopped cooked meat. (Section 18-4)

quick-mix method. A bread-making method that combines active dry yeast with the dry ingredients. (Section 21-3)

R

radiation. A heat transfer method that uses infrared rays to strike and warm an object. (Section 9-2)

raw-pack. In canning, placing the raw foods into jars and then pouring in hot syrup, liquid, or juice. (Section 24-5)

RDAs. Stands for "Recommended Daily Allowances"; the amount of a nutrient needed by 98 percent of the people in a given age and gender group. (Section 2-1).

rebate. A partial refund from the manufacturer of a purchased good. (Section 12-1)

recall. The immediate removal of a product from store shelves and the notification of the public through the media by the government or the manufacturer. (Section 13-2)

receptions. Social gatherings usually held to honor a person or an event. (Section 24-3)

recipe. A set of directions for preparing a food or beverage. (Section 8-1)

reconstitute. To add back the liquid in a food that was removed in processing. (Section 15-2)

recycling. The treating of waste so that it can be reused; an awareness of such practices. (Section 7-5)

references. People who know you well and can give you information about your previous work or your character. (Section 25-2)

refined sugars. Sugars that are extracted from plants and used as a sweetener. (Section 2-2)

reservation. An arrangement made ahead of time for a table at a restaurant. (Section 10-2)

resource. An object and quality that can help you reach a goal; includes time, money, skills, knowledge, and equipment. (Section 1-2)

resumé (REH-zoo-may). A written summary of your experience, skills, and achievements that are related to the job you seek. (Section 25-2)

retail cuts. The smaller cuts of meat from wholesale cuts found in the supermarket. (Section 19-2)

ripe fruits. Fruits that are tender and have a pleasant aroma and fully developed flavor. (Section 16-1)

ripened cheese. Aged cheese that is made from curds to which ripening agents—bacteria, mold, yeast, or a combination of these—have been added. (Section 18-1)

rolled biscuits. Biscuits made by rolling out dough to an even thickness and cutting it. (Section 21-2)

roux (ROO). A blending of equal parts of flour and fat. (Section 20-3)

S

saturated (SAT-chur-ay-ted) **fatty acids.** Fats that appear to raise the LDL cholesterol in the blood stream. (Section 2-3)

sauté (saw-TAY). To brown or cook foods in a skillet with a small amount of fat. (Section 9-3)

scalded milk. Milk that is heated to just below the boiling point. (Section 18-2)

scones. A variation of baking-powder biscuits; popular in parts of Britain. (Section 22-3)

score. To make shallow, straight cuts in the surface of a food. (Section 8-4)

seasoning blends. Convenient combinations of herbs and spices; examples are chili powder and Italian seasoning. (Section 24-1)

self-cleaning. An oven with a special cleaning cycle using high heat to burn off food stains. (Section 14-2)

serrated. Refers to a knife with sawtooth notches along the edge of its blade. (Section 8-4)

service contract. Repair and maintenance insurance purchased to cover a product for a specific length of time. (Section 14-1)

service plate. A large, decorative plate used for the first course of a formal meal. (Section 24-3)

serving pieces. Platters, large bowls, and other tableware used for serving food. (Section 10-1)

sharpening steel. A long, steel rod on a handle used to help keep knives sharp. (Section 8-4)

shelf life. The length of time food can be stored and still retain its quality. (Section 7-4)

shelf-stable. Foods that will last for weeks or even months at room temperatures below 85°F (29°C). (Section 7-4)

shirred eggs. Baked eggs. (Section 18-3)

skinfold calipers. A device that pinches the skin to measure body fat. (Section 5-1)

shortened cakes. Cakes usually made with a solid fat. (Section 21-4)

small appliance. A small electrical household device used to perform simple tasks such as mixing, chopping, and cooking. (Section 7-1)

smoking point. A temperature at which fat begins to smoke and break down chemically. (Section 9-3)

soba. Buckwheat noodles. (Section 22-4)

soluble fiber. Dietary fiber that dissolves in water; may help lower blood cholesterol levels. (Section 2-2)

soufflé (soo-FLAY). A dish made by folding stiffly beaten egg whites into a sauce or batter, and then baking the mixture in a deep casserole until it puffs up. (Section 18-4)

sourdough starter. A mixture of flour, water, and salt on which wild yeast cells grow. (Section 23-2)

spores. Cells that will develop into bacteria if conditions are right. (Section 7-3)

standing time. Period during which heat build-up in a microwaved food completes its cooking. (Section 9-4)

staple foods. Foods that make up a region's basic food supply. (Section 13-3)

staples. Items used on a regular basis such as flour and honey. (Section 12-1)

steep. To brew in water just before the boiling point. (Section 24-2)

stewing. To cover small pieces of food with liquid, then simmer until done. (Section 9-3)

stock. A clear, thin liquid made by simmering water flavored with the bones of meat, poultry, or fish, plus aromatic vegetables and seasonings. (Section 20-3)

store brands. Brands specially produced for the store; also called "private labels." (Section 12-3)

stress. Physical or mental tension triggered by an event or situation in your life. (Section 6-2)

study design. The approach used by researchers to investigate a claim. (Section 3-3)

subsistence farming. Practice of maintaining a small plot of land on which a family grows its own food. (Section 13-3)

sustainable farming. The cutting back on, or elimination of, chemicals in farming. (Section 13-1)

T

table etiquette. Courtesy shown by good manners at a meal. (Section 10-2)

tableware. Includes any items used for serving and eating foods. (Section 10-1)

task lighting. Bright, shadow-free light over specific work areas. (Section 14-3)

technology. The practical application of scientific knowledge. (Section 1-2)

texture. Way food feels when you chew it. (Section 11-1)

tolerance levels. Maximum safe levels for certain chemicals in the human body. (Section 13-2)

toxins. Poisons produced by bacteria. (Section 7-3)

trace minerals. Minerals needed in very small amounts. (Section 2-4)

tuber. A large underground stem that stores nutrients. (Section 16-1)

U

underweight. Weighing 10 percent or more below the standard weight for one's height. (Section 5-2)

unit price. An item's price per ounce, quart, pound, or other unit of measurement. (Section 12-3)

unripened cheese. Cheese made from curds that have not been aged. (Section 18-1)

UPC. Universal Product Code. A bar code on food labels and other products; it carries coded information that can be read by a scanner. (Section 12-2)

utensils. Tools or containers used for specific tasks in food preparation. Examples include measuring cups, peelers, and cookware. (Section 7-1)

V

vacuum bottle. A glass or metal bottle with a vacuum space between the outer container and the inner liner; used to keep food hot. (Section 20-1)

variety meats. Edible animal organs. (Section 19-2)

vegans (VEE-guns or VEH-juns). Also known as pure vegetarians. People who eat only food from plant sources, such as grain products, dry beans and peas, fruits, vegetables, nuts, and seeds. (Section 4-4)

vegetarians. People who do not eat meat, poultry, or fish; some do not eat dairy foods or eggs. (Section 4-4)

versatility. Capability of being adapted to many uses. (Section 11-2)

vitamins. Chemicals in food that help regulate many vital body processes and aid other nutrients in doing their jobs. (Section 2-1)

volume. The amount of three-dimensional space something takes up. (Section 8-2)

W

waist-to-hip ratio. A measure of how fat is distributed in the body. (Section 5-1)

warranty. Manufacturer's written guarantee that a product will perform as advertised; it will repair or replace the product that does not perform properly. (Section 14-1)

water-soluble vitamins. Vitamins that dissolve in water and pass easily into the bloodstream in the process of digestion; include B vitamins and vitamin C. (Section 2-4)

watts. Units by which electrical power is measured. (Section 9-4)

wellness. A philosophy that encourages people to take responsibility for their own physical, emotional, and mental health. (Section 1-1)

whisk. A balloon-shaped device made of wire loops held together by a handle which is used for mixing, stirring, beating, and whipping. (Section 8-4)

white sauce. A milk-based sauce thickened with a starch. (Section 20-3)

whole grain. The entire grain kernel. (Section 17-1)

wholesale cuts. Large cuts of meat for marketing; also called primal cuts. (Section 19-2)

WIC program. Stands for "Women, Infants, and Children"; a government-sponsored program designed to improve the health of low-income pregnant and breast-feeding women, infants, and children up to five years of age. (Section 11-3)

wok. A special bowl-shaped pan used for stir-frying. (Section 9-3)

work center. An area in the kitchen designed for specific tasks; includes equipment needed for the task and adequate storage and work space. (Section 7-1)

work flow. Recurring patterns of activities and repetitive tasks associated with any type of job routine. (Section 14-3)

work plan. A list of all the tasks required to complete a recipe and an estimate of how long each task will take. (Section 8-5)

X Y Z

yield. Number of servings or the amount a recipe makes. (Section 8-1)

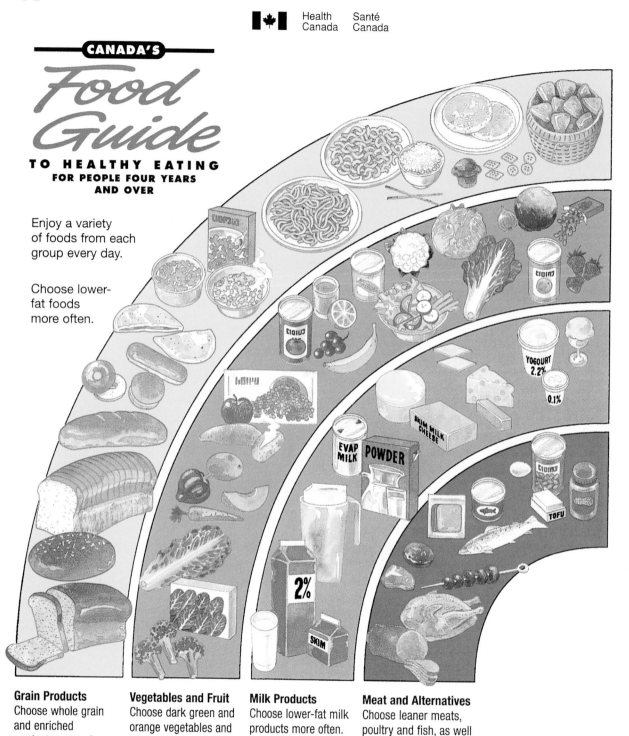

Health Canada Santé Canada

CANADA'S Food Guide

**TO HEALTHY EATING
FOR PEOPLE FOUR YEARS
AND OVER**

Enjoy a variety
of foods from each
group every day.

Choose lower-
fat foods
more often.

Grain Products
Choose whole grain
and enriched
products more often.

Vegetables and Fruit
Choose dark green and
orange vegetables and
orange fruit more often.

Milk Products
Choose lower-fat milk
products more often.

Meat and Alternatives
Choose leaner meats,
poultry and fish, as well
as dried peas, beans
and lentils more often.

Canadä

Grain Products

5–12 SERVINGS PER DAY

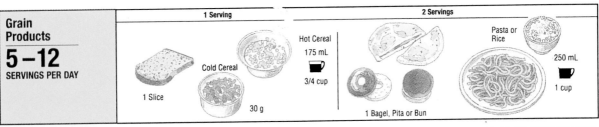

1 Serving

1 Slice

Cold Cereal
30 g

Hot Cereal
175 mL
3/4 cup

2 Servings

1 Bagel, Pita or Bun

Pasta or Rice
250 mL
1 cup

Vegetables and Fruit

5–10 SERVINGS PER DAY

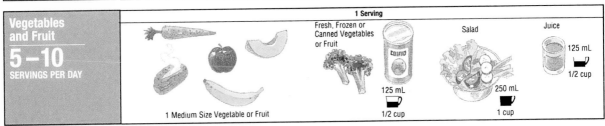

1 Serving

1 Medium Size Vegetable or Fruit

Fresh, Frozen or Canned Vegetables or Fruit
125 mL
1/2 cup

Salad
250 mL
1 cup

Juice
125 mL
1/2 cup

Milk Products

SERVINGS PER DAY
Children 4–9 years: 2–3
Youth 10–16 years: 3–4
Adults: 2–4
Pregnant and Breast-feeding Women 3–4

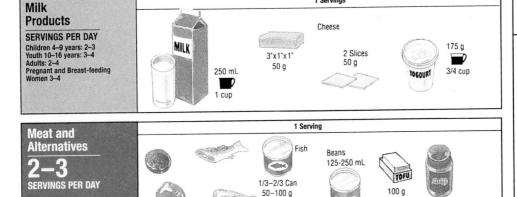

1 Servings

MILK
250 mL
1 cup

Cheese
3"x1"x1"
50 g

2 Slices
50 g

YOGOURT
175 g
3/4 cup

Meat and Alternatives

2–3 SERVINGS PER DAY

1 Serving

Meat, Poultry or Fish
50–100 g

Fish
1/3–2/3 Can
50–100 g

1–2 Eggs

Beans
125–250 mL
1/3 cup

TOFU
100 g

Peanut Butter
30 mL 2 tbsp

Other Foods

Taste and enjoyment can also come from other foods and beverages that are not part of the 4 food groups. Some of these foods are higher in fat or Calories, so use these foods in moderation.

Different People Need Different Amounts of Food

The amount of food you need every day from the 4 food groups and other foods depends on your age, body size, activity level, whether you are male or female and if you are pregnant or breast-feeding. That's why the Food Guide gives a lower and higher number of servings for each food group. For example, young children can choose the lower number of servings, while male teenagers can go to the higher number. Most other people can choose servings somewhere in between.

Enjoy eating well, being active and feeling good about yourself. That's VITALIT

© Minister of Public Works and Government Services Canada, 1997
Cat. No. H39-252/1992E   ISBN 0-662-19648-1
No changes permitted. Reprint permission not required.

Appendix B: Nutritive Value of Foods

							Nutrients in Indicated Quantity					
Item No.	Food Description	Approximate Measure	Weight	Food energy	Protein	Fat	Cho-les-terol	Calcium	Iron	Sodium	Vita-min A value*	Vita-min C
			Grams	Calories	Grams	Grams	Milli-grams	Milli-grams	Milli-grams	Milli-grams	Retinol equiva-lents	Milli-grams
Beverages												
9	Club soda	12 fl oz	355	0	0	0	0	18	Tr	78	0	0
10	Regular cola	12 fl oz	369	160	0	0	0	11	0.2	18	0	0
11	Diet, artificially sweetened cola	12 fl oz	355	Tr	0	0	0	14	0.2	32	0	0
20	Fruit punch drink	6 fl oz	190	85	Tr	0	0	15	0.4	15	2	61
Dairy Products												
	Natural Cheese:											
32	Cheddar, cut pieces	1 oz	28	115	7	9	30	204	0.2	176	86	0
38	Cottage cheese, lowfat (2%)	1 cup	226	205	31	4	19	155	0.4	918	45	Tr
43	Mozzarella, part skim milk	1 oz	28	80	8	5	15	207	0.1	150	54	0
46	Parmesan, grated	1 tbsp	5	25	2	2	4	69	Tr	93	9	0
52	Pasteurized process American cheese	1 oz	28	105	6	9	27	174	0.1	406	82	0
	Milk, fluid:											
78	Whole (3.3% fat)	1 cup	244	150	8	8	33	291	0.1	120	76	2
79	Lowfat (2%)	1 cup	244	120	8	5	18	297	0.1	122	139	2
83	Nonfat (skim)	1 cup	245	85	8	Tr	4	302	0.1	126	149	2
85	Buttermilk	1 cup	245	100	8	2	9	285	0.1	257	20	2
88	Evaporated skim milk	1 cup	255	200	19	1	9	738	0.7	293	298	3
91	Dried, nonfat, instantized	1 cup	68	245	24	Tr	12	837	0.2	373	483	4
	Milk beverages:											
94	Chocolate milk, lowfat (1%)	1 cup	250	160	8	3	7	287	0.6	152	148	2
105	Shakes, thick: Vanilla	10 oz	283	315	11	9	33	413	0.3	270	79	0
	Milk desserts, frozen:											
	Ice cream, vanilla, regular (about 11% fat):											
107	Hardened	1 cup	133	270	5	14	59	176	0.1	116	133	1
109	Soft serve (frozen custard)	1 cup	173	375	7	23	153	236	0.4	153	199	1
	Ice cream, vanilla, low-fat:											
113	Hardened (about 4% fat)	1 cup	131	185	5	6	18	176	0.2	105	52	1
116	Sherbet (about 2% fat)	1 cup	193	270	2	4	14	103	0.3	88	39	4
	Yogurt, made with lowfat milk:											
117	Fruit-flavored	8 oz	227	230	10	2	10	345	0.2	133	25	1
118	Plain	8 oz	227	145	12	4	14	415	0.2	159	36	2

Eggs

#	Food	Measure	Grams								
	Eggs, large (24 oz. per dozen):										
	Cooked:										
124	Fried in margarine	1 egg	46	90	6	7	211	25	0.7	162	114	0
125	Hard-cooked, shell removed	1 egg	50	75	6	5	213	25	0.6	62	84	0

Fats and Oils

#	Food	Measure	Grams								
129	Butter (4 sticks per lb) (⅛ stick)	1 tbsp	14	100	Tr	11	31	3	Tr	116	106	0
138	Margarine (⅛ stick)	1 tbsp	14	100	Tr	11	0	4	Tr	132	139	Tr
147	Corn oil	1 cup	218	1,925	0	218	0	0	0.0	0	0	0
	Salad dressings, commercial:										
162	French, Regular	1 tbsp	16	85	Tr	9	0	2	Tr	188	Tr	Tr
163	French, Low calorie	1 tbsp	16	25	Tr	2	0	6	Tr	306	Tr	Tr

Fish and Shellfish

#	Food	Measure	Grams								
177	Fish sticks, frozen, reheated, (stock, 4 by 1 by ½ in.)	1 fish stick	28	70	6	3	26	11	0.3	53	5	0
181	Haddock, breaded, fried	3 oz	85	175	17	9	75	34	1.0	123	20	0
182	Halibut, broiled, with butter and lemon juice	3 oz	85	140	20	6	62	14	0.7	103	174	1
195	Tuna, canned, oil pack, chunk light	3 oz	85	165	24	7	55	7	1.6	303	20	0
196	Tuna, canned, water pack, solid white	3 oz	85	135	30	1	48	17	0.6	468	32	0

Fruits and Fruit Juices

#	Food	Measure	Grams								
198	Apples, raw, unpeeled, 2¾-in. diam.	1 apple	138	80	Tr	Tr	0	10	0.2	Tr	7	8
202	Apple juice, bottled or canned	1 cup	248	115	Tr	Tr	0	17	0.9	7	Tr	2
204	Applesauce, canned, unsweetened	1 cup	244	105	Tr	Tr	0	7	0.3	5	7	3
215	Bananas, raw, without peel, whole	1 banana	114	105	1	1	0	7	0.4	1	9	10
229	Fruit cocktail, canned, juice pack	1 cup	248	115	1	Tr	0	20	0.5	10	76	7
230	Grapefruit, raw, without peel, 3¾-in. diam.	½ grapefruit	120	40	1	Tr	0	14	0.1	Tr	1	41
233	Grapefruit juice, canned, unsweetened	1 cup	247	95	1	Tr	0	17	0.5	2	2	72
237	Grapes, Thompson Seedless	10 grapes	50	35	Tr	Tr	0	6	0.1	1	4	5
239	Grape juice, canned or bottled	1 cup	253	155	1	Tr	0	23	0.6	8	2	Tr
242	Kiwifruit, raw, without skin	1 kiwifruit	76	45	1	Tr	0	20	0.3	4	13	74
250	Mangos, raw, without skin and seed	1 mango	207	135	1	1	0	21	0.3	4	806	57
251	Cantaloupe, orange-fleshed, 5-in. diam.	½ melon	267	95	2	1	0	29	0.6	24	861	113
253	Nectarines, raw, without pits	1 nectarine	136	65	1	1	0	7	0.2	Tr	100	7
254	Oranges, raw, whole	1 orange	131	60	1	Tr	0	52	0.1	Tr	27	70
260	Orange juice, frozen concentrate, diluted	1 cup	249	110	2	Tr	0	22	0.2	2	19	97
262	Papayas, raw, ½-in. cubes	1 cup	140	65	1	Tr	0	35	0.3	9	40	92
263	Peaches, raw, whole, 2½-in. diam.	1 peach	87	35	1	Tr	0	4	0.1	Tr	47	6
273	Pears, raw, with skin, cored, Bartlett, 2½-in. diam.	1 pear	166	100	1	1	0	18	0.4	Tr	3	7
283	Pineapple, chunks or tidbits, juice pack	1 cup	250	150	1	Tr	0	35	0.7	3	10	24
287	Plantains, without peel, cooked, boiled, sliced	1 cup	154	180	1	Tr	0	3	0.9	8	140	17
288	Plums, raw, 2⅛-in. diam.	1 plum	66	35	Tr	Tr	0	3	0.1	Tr	21	6
297	Raisins, seedless, cup, not pressed down	1 cup	145	435	5	1	0	71	3.0	17	1	5

Nutrients in Indicated Quantity

Item No.	Food Description	Approximate Measure	Weight (Grams)	Food energy (Calories)	Protein (Grams)	Fat (Grams)	Cholesterol (Milligrams)	Calcium (Milligrams)	Iron (Milligrams)	Sodium (Milligrams)	Vitamin A value* (Retinol equivalents)	Vitamin C (Milligrams)
303	Strawberries, raw, capped, whole	1 cup	149	45	1	1	0	21	0.6	1	4	84
309	Watermelon, 4 by 8 in. wedge	1 piece	482	155	3	2	0	39	0.8	10	176	46
	Grain Products											
311	Bagels, plain or water, enriched	1 bagel	68	200	7	2	0	29	1.8	245	0	0
314	Biscuits, from mix, 2-in. diam.	1 biscuit	28	95	2	3	Tr	58	0.7	262	4	Tr
	Breads:											
319	Cracked-wheat bread (18 per loaf)	1 slice	25	65	2	1	0	16	0.7	106	Tr	Tr
332	Pita bread, enriched, white, 6½-in. diam.	1 pita	60	165	6	1	0	49	1.4	339	0	0
346	White bread, enriched (18 per loaf)	1 slice	25	65	2	1	0	32	0.7	129	Tr	Tr
353	Whole-wheat bread (16 per loaf)	1 slice	28	70	3	1	0	20	1.0	180	Tr	Tr
355	Bread stuffing, dry type, from mix	1 cup	140	500	9	31	0	92	2.2	1,254	273	0
	Breakfast cereals:											
359	Cream of Wheat®, cooked	1 cup	244	140	4	Tr	0	54	10.9	5	0	0
367	Cheerios®	1 oz	28	110	4	2	0	48	4.5	307	375	15
368	Kellogg's® Corn Flakes	1 oz	28	100	2	Tr	0	1	1.8	351	375	15
383	Shredded Wheat	1 oz	28	100	3	1	0	11	1.2	3	0	0
386	Sugar Frosted Flakes, Kellogg's®	1 oz	28	110	1	Tr	0	1	1.8	230	375	15
390	Wheaties®	1 oz	28	100	3	Tr	0	43	4.5	354	375	15
	Cakes prepared from cake mixes:											
394	Angelfood, 1/12 of cake	1 piece	53	125	3	Tr	0	44	0.2	269	0	0
396	Coffeecake, crumb, 1/6 of cake	1 piece	72	230	5	7	47	44	1.2	310	32	Tr
398	Devil's food with chocolate frosting, 1/16 of cake	1 piece	69	235	3	8	37	41	1.4	181	31	Tr
	Cookies, commercial:											
424	Brownies with nuts and frosting	1 brownie	25	100	1	4	14	13	0.6	59	18	Tr
426	Chocolate chip, 2¼-in. diam.	4 cookies	42	180	2	9	5	13	0.8	140	15	Tr
429	Fig bars, square, 1⅝ in. square	4 cookies	56	210	2	4	27	40	1.4	180	6	Tr
430	Oatmeal with raisins, 2⅝-in. diam.	4 cookies	52	245	3	10	2	18	1.1	148	12	0
437	Corn chips	1-oz pkg.	28	155	2	9	0	35	0.5	233	11	1
	Crackers:											
444	Graham, plain, 2½ in. square	2 crackers	14	60	1	1	0	6	0.4	86	0	0
448	Snack-type, standard	1 cracker	3	15	Tr	1	0	3	0.1	30	Tr	0
449	Wheat, thin	4 crackers	8	35	1	1	0	3	0.3	69	Tr	0
	Doughnuts, made with enriched flour:											
456	Cake type, plain, 3¼-in. diam.	1 doughnut	50	210	3	12	20	22	1.0	192	5	Tr
457	Yeast-leavened, glazed, 3¾-in. diam.	1 doughnut	60	235	4	13	21	17	1.4	222	Tr	0

No.	Food	Amount										
458	English muffins, plain, enriched	1 muffin	57	140	5	1	0	96	1.7	378	0	0
461	Macaroni, enriched, cooked	1 cup	130	190	7	1	0	14	2.1	1	0	0
	Muffins, 2½-in. diam., commercial mix:											
467	Blueberry	1 muffin	45	140	3	5	45	15	0.9	225	11	Tr
468	Bran	1 muffin	45	140	3	4	28	27	1.7	385	14	0
470	Noodles (egg noodles), enriched, cooked	1 cup	160	200	7	2	50	16	2.6	3	34	0
	Pancakes, 4-in. diam.:											
474	Plain, from mix (with enriched flour), egg, milk, and oil added	1 pancake	27	60	2	2	16	36	0.7	160	7	Tr
	Pies, 9-in. diam.:											
478	Apple, ⅙ of pie	1 piece	158	405	3	18	0	13	1.6	476	5	2
488	Lemon meringue, ⅙ of pie	1 piece	140	355	5	14	143	20	1.4	395	66	4
494	Pumpkin, ⅙ of pie	1 piece	152	320	6	17	109	78	1.4	325	416	0
	Popcorn, popped:											
497	Air-popped, unsalted	1 cup	8	30	1	Tr	0	1	0.2	Tr	1	0
498	Popped in vegetable oil, salted	1 cup	11	55	1	3	0	3	0.3	86	2	0
499	Sugar syrup coated	1 cup	35	135	2	1	0	2	0.5	Tr	3	0
500	Pretzels, stick, 2¼ in. long	10 pretzels	3	10	Tr	Tr	0	1	0.1	48	0	0
	Rice:											
503	Brown, cooked, served hot	1 cup	195	230	5	1	0	23	1.0	0	0	0
505	White, enriched, cooked, served hot	1 cup	205	225	4	Tr	0	21	1.8	0	0	0
	Rolls, enriched, commercial:											
509	Dinner, 2½-in. diam.	1 roll	28	85	2	2	Tr	33	0.8	155	Tr	Tr
510	Frankfurter and hamburger	1 roll	40	115	3	2	Tr	54	1.2	241	Tr	Tr
514	Spaghetti, enriched, cooked	1 cup	130	190	7	1	0	14	2.0	1	0	0

Legumes, Nuts, and Seeds

No.	Food	Amount										
526	Almonds, shelled, whole	1 oz	28	165	6	15	0	75	1.0	3	0	Tr
	Beans, dry, cooked, drained:											
527	Black	1 cup	171	225	15	1	0	47	2.9	1	Tr	0
528	Great Northern	1 cup	180	210	14	1	0	90	4.9	13	0	0
531	Pinto	1 cup	180	265	15	1	0	86	5.4	3	Tr	0
536	Black-eyed peas, dry, cooked (with cooking liquid)	1 cup	250	190	13	1	0	43	3.3	20	3	0
544	Chickpeas, cooked, drained	1 cup	163	270	15	4	0	80	4.9	11	Tr	0
550	Lentils, dry, cooked	1 cup	200	215	16	1	0	50	4.2	26	4	0
553	Mixed nuts, dry roasted, with peanuts, salted	1 oz	28	170	5	15	0	20	1.0	190	Tr	0
555	Peanuts, roasted in oil, salted	1 cup	145	840	39	71	0	125	2.8	626	0	0
557	Peanut butter	1 tbsp	16	95	5	8	0	5	0.3	75	0	0
564	Refried beans, canned	1 cup	290	295	18	3	0	141	5.1	1,228	0	17
	Soy products:											
567	Miso	1 cup	276	470	29	13	0	188	4.7	8,142	11	0
568	Tofu, piece 2½ by 2¾ by 1 in.	1 piece	120	85	9	5	0	108	2.3	8	0	0
569	Sunflower seeds, dry, hulled	1 oz	28	160	6	14	0	33	1.9	1	1	Tr
570	Tahini	1 tbsp	15	90	3	8	0	21	0.7	5	1	1

Nutrients in Indicated Quantity

Item No.	Food Description	Approximate Measure	Weight	Food energy	Protein	Fat	Cholesterol	Calcium	Iron	Sodium	Vitamin A value* (Retinol equivalents)	Vitamin C
			Grams	Calories	Grams	Grams	Milligrams	Milligrams	Milligrams	Milligrams		Milligrams
Meat and Meat Products												
	Beef, cooked, braised, or pot roasted:											
575	Chuck blade, lean and fat, piece	3 oz	85	325	22	26	87	11	2.5	53	Tr	0
577	Round, bottom, lean and fat, piece	3 oz	85	220	25	13	81	5	2.8	43	Tr	0
578	Lean only from item 577	2.8 oz	78	175	25	8	75	4	2.7	40	Tr	0
580	Ground beef, regular, broiled, patty	3 oz	85	245	20	18	76	9	2.1	70	Tr	0
585	Round, eye of, lean and fat, roasted	3 oz	85	205	23	12	62	5	1.6	50	Tr	0
587	Sirloin, steak, broiled, lean and fat	3 oz	85	240	23	15	77	9	2.6	53	Tr	0
590	Beef, dried, chipped	2.5 oz	72	145	24	4	46	14	2.3	3,053	Tr	0
	Lamb:											
593	Chops, loin, broiled, lean and fat	2.8 oz	80	235	22	16	78	16	1.4	62	Tr	0
	Pork, cured, cooked:											
599	Bacon, regular	3 slices	19	110	6	9	16	2	0.3	303	0	6
601	Ham, light cure, roasted, lean and fat	3 oz	85	205	18	14	53	6	0.7	1,009	0	0
	Luncheon meat:											
605	Chopped ham (8 slices per 6 oz pkg)	2 slices	42	95	7	7	2`	3	0.3	576	0	8
	Pork, fresh, cooked:											
610	Chop, loin, pan fried, lean and fat	3.1 oz	89	335	21	27	92	4	0.7	64	3	Tr
614	Rib, roasted, lean and fat	3 oz	85	270	21	20	69	9	0.8	37	3	Tr
	Sausages											
618	Bologna, slice (8 per 8-oz pkg)	2 slices	57	180	7	16	31	7	0.9	581	0	12
620	Brown and serve, browned	1 link	13	50	2	5	9	1	0.1	105	0	0
621	Frankfurter cooked (reheated)	1	45	145	5	13	23	5	0.5	504	0	12
Mixed Dishes and Fast Foods												
	Mixed dishes:											
629	Beef and vegetable stew, home recipe	1 cup	245	220	16	11	71	29	2.9	292	568	17
631	Chicken a la king, home recipe	1 cup	245	470	27	34	221	127	2.5	760	272	12
642	Spaghetti in tomato sauce with cheese, home recipe	1 cup	250	260	9	9	8	80	2.3	955	140	13
	Fast food entrees:											
645	Cheeseburger, regular	1 sandwich	112	300	15	15	44	135	2.3	672	65	1
648	English muffin, egg, cheese, bacon	1 sandwich	138	360	18	18	213	197	3.1	832	160	1
649	Fish sandwich, regular, with cheese	1 sandwich	140	420	16	23	56	132	1.8	667	25	2
651	Hamburger, regular	1 sandwich	98	245	12	11	32	56	2.2	463	14	1
653	Pizza, cheese, ⅛ of 15-in. diam.	1 slice	120	290	15	9	56	220	1.6	699	106	2
654	Roast beef sandwich	1 sandwich	150	345	22	13	55	60	4.0	757	32	2
655	Taco	1 taco	81	195	9	11	21	109	1.2	456	57	1

Poultry and Poultry Products

No.	Food	Measure										
	Chicken:											
	Fried, flesh, with skin and bones:											
656	Breast, ½ breast, batter dipped	4.9 oz	140	365	35	18	119	28	1.8	385	28	0
657	Drumstick, batter dipped	2.5 oz	72	195	16	11	62	12	1.0	194	19	0
	Roasted, flesh only:											
660	Breast, ½ breast	3.0 oz	86	140	27	3	73	13	0.9	64	5	0
662	Stewed, flesh only, light and dark meat	1 cup	140	250	38	9	116	20	1.6	98	21	0
	Turkey, roasted, flesh only:											
665	Dark meat, piece, 2½ by 1⅝ by ¼ in.	4 pieces	85	160	24	6	72	27	2.0	67	0	0
666	Light meat, piece, 4 by 2 by ¼ in.	2 pieces	85	135	25	3	59	16	1.1	54	0	0
667	Chopped or diced	1 cup	140	240	41	7	106	35	2.5	98	0	0

Soups, Sauces, and Gravies

No.	Food	Measure										
	Soups, condensed:											
	Canned, prepared with milk:											
679	Cream of mushroom	1 cup	248	205	6	14	20	179	0.6	1,076	37	2
680	Tomato	1 cup	248	160	6	6	17	159	1.8	932	109	68
	Canned, prepared with water:											
681	Bean with bacon	1 cup	253	170	8	6	3	81	2.0	951	89	2
682	Beef broth, bouillon, consomme	1 cup	240	15	3	1	Tr	14	0.4	782	0	0
684	Chicken noodle	1 cup	241	75	4	2	7	17	0.8	1,106	71	Tr
693	Vegetarian	1 cup	241	70	2	2	0	22	1.1	822	301	1
	Dehydrated, prepared with water:											
697	Onion	1 pkt (6-fl-oz)	184	20	1	Tr	0	9	0.1	635	Tr	Tr
	Sauces, ready to serve:											
703	Barbecue	1 tbsp	16	10	Tr	Tr	0	3	0.1	130	14	1
704	Soy	1 tbsp	18	10	2	0	0	3	0.5	1,029	0	0
	Gravies:											
708	Brown, from dry mix	1 cup	261	80	3	2	2	66	0.2	1,147	0	0
709	Chicken, from dry mix	1 cup	260	85	3	2	3	39	0.3	1,134	0	3

Sugars and Sweets

No.	Food	Measure										
	Candy:											
711	Chocolate, milk, plain	1 oz	28	145	2	9	6	50	0.4	23	10	Tr
712	Chocolate, milk, with almonds	1 oz	28	150	3	10	5	65	0.5	23	8	Tr
717	Fondant, uncoated (mints, other)	1 oz	28	105	Tr	0	0	2	0.1	57	0	0
720	Hard candy	1 oz	28	110	0	0	0	Tr	0.1	7	0	0
723	Custard, baked	1 cup	265	305	14	15	278	297	1.1	209	146	1
724	Gelatin dessert	½ cup	120	70	2	0	0	2	Tr	55	0	0
726	Honey, strained or extracted	1 tbsp	21	65	Tr	0	0	1	0.1	1	0	Tr
727	Jams and preserves	1 tbsp	20	55	Tr	Tr	0	4	0.2	2	Tr	Tr
739	Pudding, vanilla, instant	½ cup	130	150	4	4	15	129	0.1	375	33	1

Nutrients in Indicated Quantity

Item No.	Food Description	Approximate Measure	Weight Grams	Food energy Calories	Protein Grams	Fat Grams	Cholesterol Milligrams	Calcium Milligrams	Iron Milligrams	Sodium Milligrams	Vitamin A value* Retinol equivalents	Vitamin C Milligrams
	Sugars:											
741	Brown, pressed down	1 cup	220	820	0	0	0	187	4.8	97	0	0
742	White, granulated	1 tbsp	12	45	0	0	0	Tr	Tr	Tr	0	0
745	White, powdered, sifted	1 cup	100	385	0	0	0	1	Tr	2	0	0
	Syrups:											
748	Molasses, cane, blackstrap	2 tbsp	40	85	0	0	0	274	10.1	38	0	0
749	Table syrup (corn and maple)	2 tbsp	42	122	0	0	0	1	Tr	19	0	0
	Vegetables and Vegetable Products											
750	Alfalfa seeds, sprouted, raw	1 cup	33	10	1	Tr	0	11	0.3	2	5	3
	Beans, snap, cooked, drained:											
761	From frozen (cut)	1 cup	135	35	2	Tr	0	61	1.1	18	71	11
	Broccoli:											
771	Raw	1 spear	151	40	4	1	0	72	1.3	41	233	141
772	Cooked	1 spear	180	50	5	1	0	82	2.1	20	254	113
	Cabbage, common varieties:											
778	Raw, coarsely shredded or sliced	1 cup	70	15	1	Tr	0	33	0.4	13	9	33
	Cabbage, Chinese:											
780	Pak-choi, cooked, drained	1 cup	170	20	3	Tr	0	158	1.8	58	437	44
	Carrots:											
784	Whole, 7½ by 1⅛ in.	1 carrot	72	30	1	Tr	0	19	0.4	25	2,025	7
786	Cooked, sliced, drained, from raw	1 cup	156	70	2	Tr	0	48	1.0	103	3,830	4
	Celery, pascal type, raw:											
792	Stalk, large outer, 8 by 1½ in.	1 stalk	40	5	Tr	Tr	0	14	0.2	35	5	3
	Collards, cooked, drained:											
795	From frozen (chopped)	1 cup	170	60	5	1	0	357	1.9	85	1,017	45
	Corn, sweet:											
	Cooked, drained:											
796	From raw, ear 5 by 1¾ in.	1 ear	77	85	3	1	0	2	0.5	13	17	5
798	From frozen kernels	1 cup	165	135	5	Tr	0	3	0.5	8	41	4
	Canned:											
799	Cream style	1 cup	256	185	4	1	0	8	1.0	730	25	12
800	Whole kernel, vacuum pack	1 cup	210	165	5	1	0	11	0.9	571	51	17
801	Cucumber, with peel, slices ⅛ in. thick, 2⅛-in. diam.	6 slices	28	5	Tr	Tr	0	4	0.1	1	1	1
806	Kale, cooked, drained, from raw	1 cup	130	40	2	1	0	94	1.2	30	962	53

No.	Food	Measure										
	Lettuce, raw:											
813	Crisp head, as iceberg, chopped	1 cup	55	5	1	Tr	0	10	0.3	5	18	2
814	Loose leaf, chopped or shredded	1 cup	56	10	1	Tr	0	38	0.8	5	106	10
830	Peas, green, frozen, cooked, drained	1 cup	160	125	8	Tr	0	38	2.5	139	107	16
832	Peppers, sweet, raw	1 pepper	74	20	1	Tr	0	4	0.9	2	39	95
	Potatoes, cooked:											
834	Baked, with skin	1 potato	202	220	5	Tr	0	20	2.7	16	0	26
	French fried, strip, frozen:											
838	Oven heated	10 strips	50	110	2	4	0	5	0.7	16	0	5
839	Fried in vegetable oil	10 strips	50	160	2	8	0	10	0.4	108	0	5
849	Potato chips	10 chips	20	105	1	7	0	5	0.2	94	0	8
852	Radishes, raw	4 radishes	18	5	Tr	Tr	0	4	0.1	4	Tr	4
	Spinach:											
856	Raw, chopped	1 cup	55	10	2	Tr	0	54	1.5	43	369	15
858	Cooked, drained, from frozen (leaf)	1 cup	190	55	6	Tr	0	277	2.9	163	1,479	23
	Squash, cooked:											
861	Summer, sliced, drained	1 cup	180	35	2	1	0	49	0.6	2	52	10
862	Winter, baked, cubes	1 cup	205	80	2	1	0	29	0.7	2	729	20
863	Sweet potatoes, baked in skin, peeled	1 potato	114	115	2	Tr	0	32	0.5	11	2,488	28
	Tomatoes:											
868	Raw, 2⅗-in. diam.	1 tomato	123	25	1	Tr	0	9	0.6	10	139	22
869	Canned, solids and liquid	1 cup	240	50	2	1	0	62	1.5	391	145	36
870	Tomato juice, canned	1 cup	244	40	2	Tr	0	22	1.4	881	136	45
877	Vegetable juice cocktail, canned	1 cup	242	45	2	Tr	0	27	1.0	883	283	67

Miscellaneous Items

No.	Food	Measure										
885	Catsup	1 cup	273	290	5	1	0	60	2.2	2,845	382	41
894	Mustard, prepared, yellow	1 tsp	5	5	Tr	Tr	0	4	0.1	63	0	Tr
895	Olives, canned, green, medium	4	13	15	Tr	2	0	8	0.2	312	4	0
	Pickles, cucumber:											
901	Dill, medium, whole, 3¾ in.	1 pickle	65	5	Tr	Tr	0	17	0.7	928	7	4
903	Sweet, small, whole, 2½ in. long	1 pickle	15	20	Tr	Tr	0	2	0.2	107	1	1

*1 RE = 3.33 IU from animal foods or 1 mcg retinol.
1 RE = 10 IU from plant foods or 6 mcg beta carotene.
Tr = Trace amount.
Source: USDA Home and Garden Bulletin No. 72, "Nutritive Value of Foods"

NOTE: Nutritive values of most packaged foods may be obtained from the "Nutrition Facts" label on the container.

Index

A

Absorption, 83
Accident prevention. *See* Safety
Accompaniment salad, 537
Acesulfame-K, 364
Activity
    benefits of, 148
    getting in habit of, 150
    types of, 148–49
Adequate Intake (AI), 56, 694
Adolescence, 166
Adulthood, 166
Advertisements
    evaluating, 103–4
    for food, 29
Aerobic exercise, 149, 694
Aflatoxins, 366
African American cuisine, 630–31
African cuisine, 599–603
Aging adults
    accident prevention in, 196
    nutritional problems for, 167
Agriculture, U.S. Department of, 684
Air
    as leavening agent, 561
    and spoilage, 206
Albumen, 475, 694
Al dente, 449, 694
Allyl sulfides, 78
American Association of Family and
    Consumer Sciences, 684
American cuisine, 627
    African-American influence on,
      630–31
    colonial, 628–29
    cultural diversity in, 641
    Hawaiian, 637–38
    Irish influence on, 629
    in Midwest, 630
    Native American influence on,
      627–28
    in New England, 629
    in Northeast, 629
    in Northwest, 637
    in Pacific coast, 636–37
    Pennsylvania Dutch influence on, 629
    in South, 630
    in Southwest, 634–36
    Tex-Mex, 635–36
American Dietetic Association, 60, 684
American Gas Association seal, 379
Amino acids, 62, 83, 451, 694
    essential, 62
Anabolic steroids, 155–56, 694
Anaerobic exercise, 150, 694
Analogues, 402, 694
Anemia, iron-deficiency, 75
Annual percentage rate (APR), 378, 694
Anorexia nervosa, 176–77, 179, 694
Antioxidants, 69, 77, 417, 694
Antipasto, 611, 694
Appetite, 116, 694
Appliances
    buying, 383–85

cleanup, 201
    major, 187, 261–64, 698
    plugged-in, 192
    small, 187, 264, 385, 700
Aquaculture, 358, 694
Arcing, 287, 694
Argentinean cuisine, 597
Aroma
    effect of heat on, 273
    in meal appeal, 315
Aromatic vegetables, 542, 694
Ascorbic acid, 70, 72, 90, 129, 417
Aseptic packages, 359
Asian cuisine, 616–619
Aspartame, 364
Assembly directions, 226, 694
Athletes
    myths for, in eating, 154–55
    nutrient needs of, 152–55
    timing of meals for, 155
Au jus, 546, 694
Australian cuisine, 621
Austrian cuisine, 610

B

Baked products
    removing, from pans, 566
    storing, 566
Bakeware, 264, 268, 694
    buying, 385
Baking, 279–80, 518
    combining ingredients in, 563–64
    conventional, 565
    fruits in, 433
    ingredients for, 559–63
    microwave, 565
    pan preparation in, 565
    preparing to, 564
    vegetables in, 430–31
Baking powder, 561
Baking soda, 561
Barley, 442, 448
Barrier-free kitchens, 393–94
Basal metabolic rate (BMR), 84
Basal metabolism, 84, 694
Base
    of casseroles, 552
    of salad, 538–39, 694
Basic white sauce, 544–45
Batters, 563
Beans
    simmering, 455
    soaking, 454
Beef, 497
Behavior modification, 144, 694
Belonging, sense of, 25–26
Berbere, 601, 694
Beta carotene, 77, 78, 417
Beverages, 652
    nutrients in, 654
    types of, 655–57
Bias, 103, 694
Bile, 82
Binders in casseroles, 552, 694
Binge eating, 177, 179, 694
Biotin, 72
Biscuits, 569
    drop, 571

rolled, 570
    serving, 571
Blanching, 671, 694
Body
    myth of ideal, 137
    of salad, 539, 694
Body fat percentage, 139
Body mass index (BMI), 138, 694
Boiling, 277
Bottle-feeding, 163–64, 164
Bouillabaisse, 608
Bouillon, 543, 694
Braising, 282, 522, 549–50
Brans, 439, 442, 694
Brazilian cuisine, 596
Breads, 445. *See also* Biscuits
    quick, 567–71
    yeast, 563, 573–76
Breast-feeding, 163–64
British Isles cuisine, 606–7
Broiler, 264
Broiling, 281, 519
Budget, 694
    food, 326–29
Buffet service, 664
Bulbs, 419
Bulgarian cuisine, 614
Bulgur, 442, 448
Bulimia nervosa, 177–78, 179, 694
Bulk foods, 347, 694
Butter, 469
Buttermilk, 465

C

Caffeine, sources of, 658
Cajun cooking, 631–32
Cakes, 578
    decorating, 580
    foam, 579–80
    shortened, 579
Calcium, 72, 74, 75, 129
Calories, 56, 342, 694
    burning of, in activities, 144
    recommended sources of, 57
Campylobacter jejuni, 199
Canada's Food Guide, 702–3
Canadian foods, 638
    in Atlantic Provinces, 639
    cultural diversity in, 641
    in Ontario, 640
    in Quebec, 639–40
    in Western Provinces, 640
Canned foods, 406
Canning, 358
    produce, 672–73
Carbohydrate loading, 152–53
Carbohydrates, 59, 82, 694
    complex, 59–60, 152
    as nutrient, 53
    simple, 59, 61
Cardiopulmonary resuscitation (CPR),
    197, 695
Careers, 679, 694
    agronomic engineer, 487
    athletic trainer, 157
    caterer, 293
    consumer advocate, 353
    county extension agent, 623

and food choices, 48
  steps in, 47
Deep-fat frying, 282
Deglazing, 608, 695
Dehydration, 153, 695
Desired yield, 695
Developing nations, 368, 695
Diabetes, 173, 695
Dietary fiber, 53, 59, 60, 91, 695
Dietary Guidelines for Americans,
  89–94, 129
Dietary laws, 33
Dietary Reference Intakes (DRIs), 55–56,
  695
Dietary supplements, 171–72, 695
Dietetics, 682–83
Diet pills, 142
Diets
  fad, 142, 696
  weight-management, 141
Digestion, 81–83, 695
Diseases
  lifestyle, 90
  prevention and nutrients, 171–72
Dishes, washing, by hand, 201–2
Doneness, 515–18, 695
Double boiler, 265
Dough, 564
Dovetail, 254, 695
Dried foods, 406
Drop biscuits, 571, 695
Dry-heat cooking, 279, 695
  baking as, 279–80
  broiling as, 281
  frying as, 282
  pan-broiling as, 282
  roasting as, 279–80
Drying, 359
  food, 674
Dry ingredients, measuring, 233–34
Dry measuring cup method, 234
Dry mixes, 407
Dry-packing, 671, 696

E

Eastern European cuisine, 613–14
Eating areas, cleaning, 202
Eating at school, 125
Eating disorders, 696
  anorexia nervosa, 176–77
  binge, 177
  bulimia nervosa, 177–78
  effects of, 178
  getting help, 179–80
  recognizing, 179
  treatment options, 180
Eating habits
  changing, 146
  improving your, 118
  promoting, 165–66
Eating patterns, 111, 696
  breakfast in, 112–13
  dinner in, 114
  evening meals in, 113
  grazing in, 115
  midday meals in, 113
  snacks in, 114–15

Eating plans
  adjusting to special, 174–75
  special, 172–74
Economics, 369
Efficiently, working, 254
Eggs, 562
  buying, 476
  cholesterol in, 66
  cooked in shell, 478
  and food safety, 77, 476, 477, 484
  freezing, 477
  nutrients in, 476
  preparing, 477–80
  in recipes, 482–86
  separating, 483
  storing, 476–77
  structure of, 475
Egg substitutes, 402
Egg whites
  beating, 484
  effect of temperature on, 40
Elastin, 494
Elderly Nutrition Program (ENP), 330
Electrical resistance, 263
Electrical system, 392
Electricity, safe use of, 192
Electrolytes, 72, 76, 696
Electronic Benefits Transfer (EBT) card,
  329
Elements, 262
Emotions, 31
Employees, skills desired in, 685–90
Emulsification, 537
Emulsion, 536, 696
Endosperm, 439, 696
Energy
  getting, from nutrients, 56–58
  needs of athletes, 152–53
EnergyGuide labels, 380, 696
En papillote, 652, 696
Enrichment, 440, 696
Entertaining
  decorations in, 661
  invitations for, 661–62
  making schedule for, 662–63
  menus for, 662
  planning for, 660–66
  reasons for, 660
  serving food in, 663–65
  themes in, 661
Entrée, 124, 696
Entrepreneurship, 683, 696
Entry-level job, 679, 696
Environmental Protection Agency (EPA),
  363
Enzymatic browning, 426, 696
Enzymes in food, 207
Equipment. *See* Kitchen equipment
  proper use of, 254
Equivalents, 229–30, 696
Ergonomics, 38, 40, 696
Escherichia coli, 199
Esophagus, 82, 696
Essential amino acids, 62
Essential fatty acids, 64
Ethnic cuisine, 131
Ethnic group, 32, 696
Etiquette, cultural, 34

Exercise
  and safety, 149
  types of, 149–50
Extenders in casseroles, 552, 696

F

Fad diets, 142, 696
Falls, preventing, 191
Families, food customs in, 28
Family and consumer sciences, jobs in,
  681–82
Family meals
  general guidelines for, 300
  mealtime atmosphere in, 297–98
  plate service in, 300
  service, 299
  settings for, 299
  setting table for, 298
  table-setting basics, 298–99
Famine, 369, 696
Farmer's markets, 336
Farming, 357–58
  inefficient methods of, 370
  subsistence, 369
Fats, 129, 696
  in baked products, 562
  functions and sources of, 64–65
  invisible, 92, 93
  limiting, 92
  lowering, 92, 93
  measuring, 234–35
  in milk, 464, 465
  as nutrient, 53
  reducing saturated, 68
  saturated, 92
  tips for reducing, 239
  types of, in meats, 492
  visible, 92
Fat-soluble vitamins, 70, 73, 83, 696
Fat substitutes, 238, 364–65
Fatty acids
  monounsaturated, 66
  polyunsaturated, 66
  saturated, 66
  trans, 67
Federal Trade Commission (FTC), 381
Fetus, 161, 696
Fiber
  amount consumed, 60
  dietary, 53, 60, 91
  insoluble, 60
  soluble, 60
Filé, 632, 696
Finance charge, 378, 696
First aid techniques, 197
Fish and shellfish
  buying, 511
  in Caribbean cuisine, 595
  comparing costs of, 495–96
  composition of, 495
  cooking, 512–22
  cuts in, 491
  fat and cholesterol in, 492
  and food safety, 496
  garnishes for, 652
  inspection and grading, 510–11
  market forms of, 508
  microwaving, 521